PROVE IT!
EVIDENCE-BASED ANALYSIS OF COMMON SPINE PRACTICE

PROVE IT!
EVIDENCE-BASED ANALYSIS OF COMMON SPINE PRACTICE

CHRISTOPHER M. BONO, MD

Chief of the Orthopaedic Spine Service
Brigham and Women's Hospital
Boston, Massachusetts

CHARLES G. FISHER, MD, MHSc(Epi), FRCSC

Director Spine Fellowship Program (CNOSP)
Vancouver General Hospital
Vancouver, British Columbia

Wolters Kluwer | Lippincott Williams & Wilkins
Health

Philadelphia • Baltimore • New York • London
Buenos Aires • Hong Kong • Sydney • Tokyo

Acquisitions Editor: Robert Hurley
Product Manager: Elise M. Paxson
Production Manager: Bridget Dougherty
Senior Manufacturing Manager: Benjamin Rivera
Marketing Manager: Lisa Lawrence
Design Coordinator: Doug Smock
Production Service: SPi Technologies

© 2010 by LIPPINCOTT WILLIAMS & WILKINS, a WOLTERS KLUWER business

Two Commerce Square
2001 Market Street
Philadelphia, PA 19103 USA
LWW.com

Printed in China

Library of Congress Cataloging-in-Publication Data
Prove it! : evidence-based analysis of common spine practice / [edited by] Christopher M. Bono, Charles G. Fisher.
p. ; cm.
Other title: Evidence-based analysis of common spine practice
Includes bibliographical references.
ISBN 978-1-60547-027-6
1. Spine—Surgery—Case studies. 2. Evidence-based medicine. I. Bono, Christopher M. II. Fisher, Charles G. III. Title: Evidence-based analysis of common spine practice.
[DNLM: 1. Spinal Diseases—diagnosis—Case Reports. 2. Evidence-Based Medicine—methods—Case Reports. 3. Spinal Diseases—therapy—Case Reports. WE 725]

RD768.P76   2010
616.7'3—dc22

2010029497

To purchase additional copies of this book, call our customer service department at (800) 638-3030 or fax orders to (301) 223-2320. International customers should call (301) 223-2300.

Visit Lippincott Williams & Wilkins on the Internet: at LWW.com. Lippincott Williams & Wilkins customer service representatives are available from 8:30 am to 6 pm, EST.

10 9 8 7 6 5 4 3 2 1

To my understanding and supportive wife, Terri, and our beautiful children, Alissa, Annabella, and Christopher, whose love gave me the inner peace and confidence to complete such a project; to my father, who without question embodies the definition of perseverance and the will to live, and to my mother who is an enduring example of strength and the work ethic—**C.M.B.**

To my lovely wife Carolyn and our wonderful family Zach, Charlotte, Anabelle and Olivia for their love and unwavering support in putting together this book. To Eloise and John Fisher for providing the work ethic and values necessary for such a venture and to my colleague and friend Marcel Dvorak whose mentorship helped provide me with the tools and knowledge necessary to undertake such a rewarding and worthwhile endeavor—**C.G.F.**

CONTRIBUTORS

Paul A. Anderson, MD
Professor
Department of Orthopedics & Rehabilitation
University of Wisconsin
Madison, Wisconsin

Paul M. Arnold, MD, FACS
Professor of Neurosurgery
Department of Neurosurgery
University of Kansas Medical Center
Director
Spinal Cord Injury Center
Department of Neurosurgery
University of Kansas Hospital
Kansas City, Missouri

Harel Arzi, MD
Fellow
Department of Neurosurgery
University of Kansas Medical Centre
Fellow
Department of Neurosurgery
University of Kansas Hospital
Kansas City, Missouri

Christopher S. Bailey, MD, FRCSC, MSc
Assistant Professor
Department of Surgery
University of Western Ontario
Department of Surgery
London Health Science Center
London, Ontario, Canada

Mark H. Bilsky, MD
Attending
Department of Neurosurgery
Memorial Sloan-Kettering Cancer
Professor
Department of Neurosurgery
Weill Cornell Medical College
New York, New York

Eugene Carragee, MD
Professor
Department of Orthopaedic Surgery
Stanford University
Stanford, California

Leah Y. Carreon, MD, MSc
Norton Leatherman Spine Center
Louisville, Kentucky

John Chi, MD, MPH
Assistant Professor
Department of Neurosurgery
Harvard Medical Surgery
Associate Surgeon
Department of Neurosurgery
Brigham Women's Hospital
Boston, Massachusetts

Sean Comstock, MD, FRCSC
Orthopaedic Spine Surgeon
Department of Orthopaedics
Moncton Hospital
Moncton, New Brunswick

Terrence T. Crowder, MD
Sonoran Spine Center
Phoenix, Arizona

Vincent J. Devlin, MD
Orthopaedic Spine Surgeon
Department of Oklahoma Sports, Science and
    Orthopaedics (OSSO) Spine Center
Oklahoma City, Oklahoma

John R. Dimar II, MD
Professor
Department of Orthopaedic Surgery
University of Louisville School of Medicine
Norton Leatherman Spine Center
Louisville, Kentucky

Marcel F. Dvorak, MD, FRCSC
Professor and Head, Division of Spine
Department of Orthopaedics
University of British Columbia
Head Division of Spine
Combined Neurosurgical and Orthopaedic Spine
    Program
Vancouver General Hospital
Vancouver, British Columbia

Daniel R. Fassett, MO, MBA
Associate Professor
Department of Neurosurgery
UICOMP
Director of Spinal Surgery
Department of Neurosurgery
Illinois Neurological Institute
Peoria, Illinois

Charles G. Fisher, MD, MHSc(Epi), FRCSC
Director Spine Fellowship
    Program (CNOSP)
Vancouver General Hospital
Vancouver, British Columbia

Daryl R. Fourney, MD, FRCSC, FACS
Associate Professor
Division of Neurosurgery
University of Saskatchewan
Royal University Hospital
Saskatoon, Saskatchewan

John C. France, MD
Professor of Orthopaedic Surgery
West Virginia University
Morgantown, West Virginia

Steven R. Garfin, MD
Professor and Chair
Department of Orthopaedics
University of California, San Diego
San Diego, California

Hossein Ghofrani, MD
Assistant Professor
Department of Internal Medicine
University of Giessen Lung Center
Giessen, Germany

Steven D. Glassman, MD
Professor
Department of Orthopaedic Surgery
University of Louisville School of Medicine
Norton Leatherman Spine Center
Louisville, Kentucky

Collin B. Harris, MD
Resident
Department of Orthopaedics
University of Medicine and Dentistry
New Jersey Medical School
Newark, New Jersey

Mitchel B. Harris, MD
Department of Orthopaedic Surgery
Brigham and Women's Hospital
Boston, Massachusetts

Christopher C. Harrod, MD
Chief Resident
Department of Orthopaedic Surgery
Harvard Combined Orthopaedic Residency Program
Harvard Medical School
Boston, Massachusetts

James S. Harrop, MD
Associate Professor
Department of Neurological and Orthopedic Surgery
Jefferson Medical College
Chief
Division of Spine and Peripheral Nerve Surgery
Department of Neurological and Orthopedic Surgery
Jefferson Hospital
Philadelphia, Pennsylvania

Harry N. Herkowitz, MD
Chairman, Department of Orthopaedic Surgery
Fellowship Coordinator for Spine and Sports
    Medicine
William Beaumont Hospital
Royal Oak, Michigan

Christopher Hume, DO
Spine fellow
Department of Orthopaedic Spine Surgery
Texas Back Institute
Plano, Texas

Shiveindra Jeyamohan, MD
Resident
Department of Neurological Surgery
Albany Medical College
Albany Hospital
Albany, New York

David Kaye I., BS
MSIV
Albert Einstein College of Medicine
Bronx, New York

David H. Kim, MD
Department of Orthopaedic Surgery
New England Baptist Hospital
Boston, Massachusetts

Stephen P. Kingwell, MD, FRCSC
Assistant Professor
Department of Surgery
University of Ottawa
Orthopaedic Surgeon
Department of Surgery
Ottawa Hospital
Ottawa, Ontario

Ilya Laufer, MD
Clinical Instructor
Neurological Surgery
Johns Hopkins
Baltimore, Maryland

Yu-Po Lee, MD
Department of Orthopaedic Surgery
University of California at San Diego
La Jolla, California

Brian Lenehan, MB, MCh, FRCS
Consultant Orthopaedic/Spine Surgeon
Department of Orthopaedics
Mid-Western Regional Hospitals
Limerick, Ireland

Gang Li, MD
Honorary Consultant Surgeon
Queen's University Belfast
Belfast, Ireland

Ning Lin, MD
Resident
Department of Neurosurgery
Brigham Women's Hospital
Boston, Massachusetts

Eric Lis, MD
Associate Professor
Department of Radiology
Weill-Cornell Medical College
Associate Attending
Department of Radiology
Memorial Sloan-Kettering Cancer Center
New York, New York

Amy Marcini, MD
Department of Orthopaedic Surgery
Grant Medical Center
Columbus, Ohio

Todd D. McCall, MD
Assistant Professor
Department of Neurosurgery
University of Illinois
Neurosurgeon
Department of Neurosurgery
Illinois Neurological Institute
Peoria, Illinois

Kevin J. McGuire, MD, MS
Instructor
Department of Orthopedic Surgery
Harvard Medical School
Chief Orthopedic Spine Service
Department of Orthopedic Surgery
Beth Israel Medical Center
Boston, Massachusetts

Gregory S. McLoughlin, MD
Division of Neurosurgery
University of Saskatchewan
Saskatoon, Saskatchewan

Harsh Parikh, BA
University of Illinois
College of Medicine at Peoria
Peoria, Illinois

Don Young Park, MD
Clinical Instructor
Orthopaedic Surgery
Stanford University
Stanford, California

Peter G. Passias, MD
Clinical Assistant Professor
Department of Orthopaedic Surgery
New York University
Langone Medical Center
New York, New York

Oma Persaud, MSc
Research Coordinator
Department of Orthopaedics
Toronto Western Hospital
University Health Network
Toronto, Ontario

Raja Rampersand, MD, FRCSC
Associate Professor
Department of Surgery
University of Toronto
Spine Surgeon
Department of Orthopaedics
Toronto Western Hospital
University Health Network
Toronto, Ontario

Ciro G. Randazzo, MD, MPH
Instructor
Department of Neurological Surgery
Jefferson Medical College
Division of Cerebrovascular Surgery
Department of Neurological Surgery
Jefferson Hospital
Philadelphia, Pennsylvania

Daniel K. Resnick, MD, MS
Associate Professor and Vice Chairman
Department of Neurosurgery
University of Wisconsin School of Medicine and
    Public health
Attending Physician
Department of Neurosurgery
University of Wisconsin Hospital and Clinics
Madison, Wisconsin

John M. Rhee, MD
Associate Professor
Orthopedic Surgery
Emory University School of Medicine
Emory Spine Center
Atlanta, Georgia

Chintan Sampat, MD
Spine Surgeon
Department of Orthopaedic Surgery
Parkview Musculoskeletal Institute
Joliet, Illinois

Andrew J. Schoenfeld, MD
Assistant Professor
Department of Orthopaedic Surgery
Texas Tech University Health Sciences Center
Department of Orthopaedic Surgery
William Beaumont Army Medical Center
El Paso, Texas

Joseph H. Schwab, MD
Department of Orthopaedic Surgery
Massachusetts General Hospital
Boston, Massachusetts

Manish K. Sethi, MD
Fellow
Division of Orthopaedic Trauma Surgery
Orthopaedic Surgery
Vanderbilt University Medical Center
Nashville, Tennessee

Alok D. Sharan, MD
Assistant Professor
Department of Orthopedic Surgery
Albert Einstein College of Medicine
Chief
Orthopedic Spine Service
Department of Orthopedic Surgery
Montefiore Medical Center
Bronx, New York

John Street, MD, PhD
Associate Professor
Department of Orthopedics
University of British Columbia
Spine Surgeon
Combined Neurosurgical and Orthopedic Spine
    Program
Vancouver, British Columbia

Eeric Truumees, MD
Attending Spine Surgeon
Director of Research
Seton Spine and Scoliosis Center
Brackenridge University Hospital
Austin, Texas

Alexander Vaccaro, MD
Department of Orthopaedic Surgery
Thomas Jefferson University
Philadelphia, Pennsylvania

Michael J. Vives, MD
Associate Professor
Department of Orthopedics
University of Medicine & Dentistry
New Jersy Medical School
Newark, New Jersy

William C. Watters III, MS, MMS, MD
Clinical Assistant Professor
Department of Orthopedic Surgery
Baylor College of Medicine
Senior Attending
Department of Orthopedic Surgery
Saint Luke's Episcopal Hospital
Houston, Texas

Andrew P. White, MD
Instructor Harvard Medical School
Department of Orthopaedic Surgery
Beth Israel Deaconess Medical Center
Boston, Massachusetts

Kirkham B. Wood, MD
Associate Professor
Department of Orthopaedic Surgery
Massachusetts General Hospital
Harvard Medical School
Boston, Massachusetts

PREFACE

Evidence-based medicine (EBM) was initially defined and is currently perceived as "the explicit, judicious, and conscientious use of current best evidence from health care research in decisions about the care of individuals and populations". The current definition of EBM, however, integrates *best available evidence* with *clinical expertise* and *patient preference in making the best decisions about patient care*. EBM occurs at both an organizational (e.g. professional societies that develop clinical practice guidelines) and individual practitioner level. It is the latter that is perhaps most demanding in this era of unprecedented technology advancement, strong consumer demand, cost restraint, and limited scientific evidence. Because of this there has never been a greater need to provide the spine surgeon with guidance and support in the practice of EBM; thus EBM spine surgery is the focus of this textbook.

The concept of EBM has become commonplace and represents the hallmark of excellence in clinical practice. Firmly established in the medical realm, EBM's integration into the spine surgery domain has been sometimes awkward and misguided due to a poor understanding or misinterpretation of the concept. Although EBM must be fully integrated into the practice of spine surgery, it is essential that the term is properly understood and applied by all stakeholders including surgeons, researchers, governmental agencies, insurance companies, and professional societies. This will lead to necessary, appropriate questioning and scrutiny of indications for and results of common spine surgical procedures. Furthermore, it will help standardize and optimize clinical research and education at all levels.

Though often considered the antithesis of EBM, textbooks continue to be a highly utilized and succinct educational resource for practicing spine surgeons, fellows, and residents. Considering this, it was our intention to bridge the gap between conventional textbooks and EBM practice, in a distinctive manner. Unlike traditional textbooks in which an author diligently prepares a narrative review about a particular topic, the authors of *Prove It!* were asked to do something uniquely different. For each chapter, the authors were supplied with a clinical vignette of an actual patient seen by one of us in our practice that included a history, physical examination findings, and imaging studies. Next, they were asked to describe their interpretation of the findings, declare a diagnosis, and perform a systematic literature review based on the specific management question. The results of the systematic review were then integrated with their clinical expertise to determine a precise treatment plan or recommendation for the specific patient. In this way, the reader gains EBM recommendations for treatment of common spinal disorders and appreciates and gains understanding into the merits and limitations of practicing EBM at an *individual* level.

There is a necessary and growing demand from all the stakeholders involved in spine care for clinicians to practice EBM when managing their patients. This is a daunting requirement for the busy clinician given the time and effort needed to properly understand the essential concepts of EBM, the level of sophistication needed to interpret the expanding breadth of spine literature, and the invaluable impact of shared or consensus expert opinion in determining the appropriate treatment. Organizational EBM helps this process from a guideline perspective. However, if we are to ensure and optimize personalized medicine for our patients then clinicians need further support to practice EBM at an individual level. *Prove It!* fulfills this role for the practicing spinal surgeon by providing relevant, unbiased, and rigorous analyses of the current literature based on questions concerning treatments of common clinical disorders framed by clinical expertise, experience, and, when possible, patient preference. Furthermore, the reader will learn the process by which evidence-based treatment decisions are formulated, and will hopefully incorporate this process into his or her own clinical practice and disseminate it to others. Finally we have tried to ensure that the reader is left with a practical treatment recommendation rather than the frequent (and not too helpful) take home message of "more research is needed". Clearly more research is needed, but we must provide the best possible care for our patients now. ***We feel Prove It! does this and provides a new standard in facilitating evidence-based care for our patients.***

CONTENTS

SECTION

I

DEGENERATIVE CERVICAL SPINE

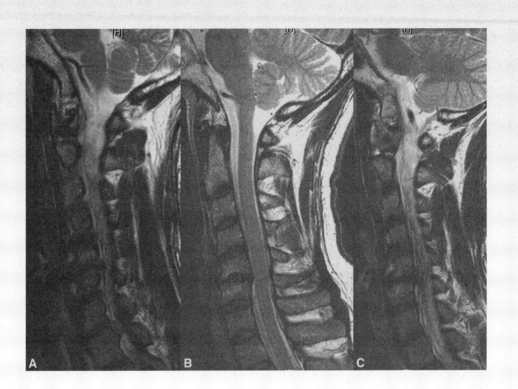

Cervical Stenosis with Multiple Subluxations

TERRENCE T. CROWDER, MD
AND HARRY N. HERKOWITZ, MD

An 81-year-old man presents with a primary complaint of right shoulder pain along with low back and right buttock pain. He indicates that he has had progressive imbalance with walking and has had a couple of recent falls. In addition, he has a complaint of substantial weakness in the upper extremities, difficulty with manual dexterity, and dropping objects from his hand due to numbness and tingling. He has no bowel or bladder complaints.

Upon exam, he is only slightly overweight. He displays profound imbalance upon walking and uses a wide-based gait. He stumbles with turning. He has weakness and pain in his right upper extremity to a level that it is difficult to hold his arm out for a handshake. Motor testing demonstrates 3/5 right grip strength, 4/5 right biceps, and 3/5 right deltoid. Finger dexterity is diminished. The man has a negative Lhermitte sign but a positive Spurling test with rotation to the right side. He has positive Hoffmann reflexes, more on the right than the left, and hyperreflexia in the upper and lower extremities of 3+. Though flexion is full and reasonably painless, he has pain at the extreme of extension, which also exacerbates his shoulder pain.

Radiographic imaging studies are shown in Figure 1.1A–G.

INTERPRETATION OF CLINICAL PRESENTATION

The patient in this case presents with a chief complaint of pain in the right upper and lower extremities with no history of trauma. The more important parts of his history

are his progressive difficulty walking and imbalance, the weakness in his upper extremities, his decreased hand dexterity, and his paresthesias. These historical findings are suggestive of a spinal cord lesion.

The patient's difficulty with walking and waddling gait suggest cervical lesion versus lumbar. A lumbar lesion would be less likely to cause change in gait and more likely to cause lower extremity weakness and radiculopathy. Changes in gait are indicative of spinal cord long tract dysfunction. He has a positive Spurling test which suggests a cervical root compression. The patient's weakness in his right upper extremity could also be the result of cervical root compression. However, the patient demonstrates weakness in several muscle groups which are innervated by varying roots. This would suggest multilevel disease.[1] A positive Hoffman's and hyperreflexia point to decreased spinal cord inhibition and strengthened the diagnosis of myelopathy.[2] Painless flexion and pain with hyperextension which decreases the functional diameter of the spinal canal suggest compression pathology.[1]

The radiographic images are T2 weighted sagittal and axial magnetic resonance imaging (MRI) scans of the cervical spine. Figure 1.1A and B demonstrate severe cervical stenosis at C3-4 and moderate stenosis at C4-5. At C3-4, the cord is being compressed anteriorly by a bulging disc and posteriorly by the ligamentum flavum. Subluxations are also noted at C3-4 and C4-5. These images also demonstrate a loss of normal lordosis resulting in a straight spine. T2 increased signal intensity is seen in the spinal cord at C3-4. At C5-6, a disc herniation and posterior osteophytes can be seen causing moderate canal stenosis. Figure 1.1C–G demonstrate T2 axial images of each disc space from C2-7. At C2-3, Figure 1.1C, there is mild canal stenosis and posterior spinal cord compression. Figure 1.1D, C3-4, demonstrates severe canal stenosis. There is significant cord compression anteriorly and posteriorly resulting in cord deformation. No cerebrospinal fluid (CSF) can be visualized in this image. At C4-5, Figure 1.1E, the spinal cord is being compressed on the

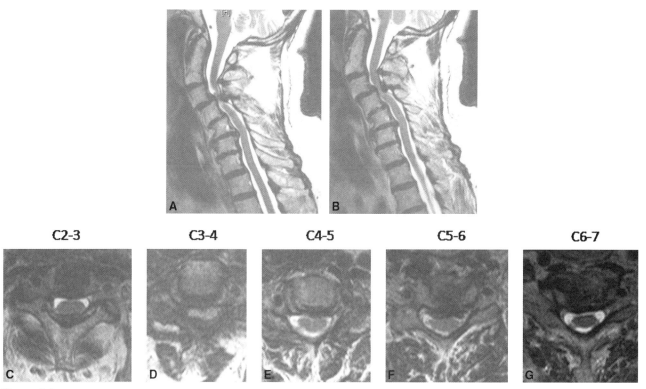

Figure 1.1.

left side anteriorly by a disc herniation but CSF is seen posteriorly. Figure 1.1F, C5-6, shows significant canal stenosis and cord compression bilaterally by an anterior disc complex. The left C6 root appears more compressed than the right. C6-7, Figure 1.1G, shows mild canal stenosis with CSF visible around the entire cord. Interestingly, the patient has more right sided symptoms. Figure 1.1E and F suggest more left sided foraminal stenosis than right. These images represent multilevel cervical spinal stenosis with subluxations and myelomalacia.

DECLARATION OF SPECIFIC DIAGNOSIS

The patient has symptomatic multilevel cervical stenosis with subluxations. Degenerative disc disease has resulted in compression anteriorly and posteriorly from the ligamentum flavum hypertrophy and infolding.

BRAINSTORMING: WHAT ARE THE TREATMENT GOALS AND SURGICAL OPTIONS?

The treatment goals are

1. To alleviate or decrease the pain
2. Stabilize the cervical spine
3. Halt the progression of myelopathic changes
4. Rehabilitation and recovery
5. Improve neurologic function

The treatment options are

1. Bracing, therapy, and cervical injections
2. Multilevel anterior cervical discectomy and fusion (ACDF)
3. Multilevel anterior corpectomy and fusion (ACCF)
4. Hybrid construct of ACDF and ACCF
5. Laminoplasty
6. Multilevel laminectomy with or without fusion
7. Anterior/posterior combined
8. Cervical disc arthroplasty

EVALUATION OF THE LITERATURE

A search of Ovid Web was performed to find and evaluate the literature on cervical spondylotic myelopathy with multiple subluxations. Using a reference period from 1950 to 2009, a Medline search was performed using the keyword "cervical." This was then combined with cervical. The search was further narrowed by combining "myelopathy." The results revealed 2,743 potential articles. When "subluxation" was combined with the previous key words, 103 articles were found. The articles were searched and reviewed electronically. The Cochrane Library of evidence based medicine was then searched. A total of 25 articles were identified. One-hundred ten abstracts were reviewed and 38 full text articles were read.

DETAILED REVIEW OF PERTINENT ARTICLES

Operative or Nonoperative Treatment

A large volume of literature on cervical myelopathy has been published; however, there are few prospective, randomized studies regarding treatment. After a thorough literature search, only a few articles were found regarding degenerative spondylolisthesis and cervical myelopathy.[3,4] These articles were reviewed in order to present the best possible data to make a decision concerning treatment.

When deciding between operative and nonoperative treatment for cervical spondylitic myelopathy with multiple subluxations, the natural history must be considered. In general, most patients experience a slowly progressive decline in function with prolonged periods of stable neurologic function. A majority of patients experience stepwise decline between these periods of quiescent disease.[5] Currently, no methods of predicting neurologic decline exist. Therefore, it is imperative to arrest disease in those patients already experiencing significant neurologic symptoms. Considering this unfavourable and unpredictable natural history, many authors recommend surgical treatment. Surgically treated patients appear to have better outcomes than those treated nonoperatively.[6]

Without prospective, controlled, randomized studies, it is difficult to predict outcomes after treatment for cervical myelopathy. A nonrandomized, multicenter, prospective investigation by the Cervical Spine Research Society provides the best data to date on outcomes of cervical myelopathy.[6] Sampath et al. compare the outcomes of patients treated surgically and those treated conservatively and suggest that surgical treatment improves outcome. Surgically patients demonstrated significant improvements in functional status (social and work activities) and pain but not in neurologic outcome. Conversely, medical treatment significantly decreased ADL performance but had no effect on pain, functional status, or neurologic outcome.[6] When combined with previously cited studies, surgically treated patients can expect arrest of myelopathic symptoms and some neurologic improvement, whether anterior or posterior surgery is performed.[9,7] These outcomes are maintained at up to 10 years after treatment.[8]

After the decision has been made to proceed with operative management, the next step involves deciding on the appropriate approach and procedure. Patient factors, neurologic status, and clinical expertise will be considered in this process.

Patient Factors

The patient has cervical myelopathy from spondylotic stenosis with degenerative spondylolisthesis. The patient's symptoms are progressive.

Neurologic Status

The patient already demonstrates significant myelopathy symptoms. He has an unsteady gait, loss of hand dexterity, weakness, a positive Hoffman's. His shoulder pain and positive Spurling's suggest radiculopathy as well. Considering he is already experiencing significant neurologic dysfunction, it is unlikely he will improve without intervention.[5]

Anterior Decompression and Fusion

Anterior decompression and fusion for cervical myelopathy has been shown to be a highly effective treatment.[7] Emery el al.[9] reviewed 108 patients with cervical myelopathy that were treated with anterior decompression and fusion. Average follow-up was 5 years. Both ACDF and ACCF were able to significantly improve Nurick grade. More than 80% had an improvement in their gait. Ninety percent had improvement in their neurologic deficits. Development of a pseudoarthrosis predicted a poor outcome. Older patients tended to have more severe myelopathy at presentation. Those patients with less severe myelopathy preoperatively had better postoperative neurologic outcomes. Interestingly, men had better improvement in neurologic grade than women.[9] This study suggests that anterior decompression with fusion is safe and is associated with a high rate of pain relief and neurologic improvement.

The patent has a kyphotic deformity. When loss of lordosis is present in combination with stenosis, an anterior approach can accomplish two goals, direct decompression and deformity correction.[7] When more than three levels need to be decompressed, supplemental posterior fixation must be considered.[7] Gok was able to show similar complication rates when comparing anterior alone versus anterior with combined posterior fixation. An oblique corpectomy without fusion could be considered in this patient; however, the presence of multiple subluxations is indicative of some spinal instability which is a relative contraindication to this procedure.[10] The MRI demonstrates compression on both sides of the cord as well.

The patient's age must also be taken into consideration when contemplating care. No statistical difference has been shown between the recovery rate and complication rate in elderly patients and controls.[11] Though this patient has none, preoperative comorbidities must also be taken into account when considered anterior versus posterior surgery. Those patients with dysphasia, history of dysphonia, or other poor aspiration control may not be candidates for anterior procedures.

The patient has a mild kyphosis and multiple subluxations or degenerative cervical spondylolisthesis. Only a few studies have studied this presentation.[9,4] The majority of patients found in these studies are also myelopathic and were treated with mostly anterior procedures. One of the studies is retrospective and the other is a case series. They both suggest focusing on spinal cord decompression, deformity correction, and fusion. Anterior decompression and fusion yield very high fusion rates and improvement in neurologic status in patients with cervical stenosis and multiple subluxations.[9,4]

Cervical Disc Arthroplasty

The United States Food and Drug Administration's Investigational Device Exemption studies provide very good data on the treatment of myelopathy.[12–15] However, these studies excluded patients with significant spondylosis, decreased segmental motion, significant disc space narrowing, cervical kyphosis, instability, or spondylolisthesis. Although these studies show equivalency between anterior cervical decompression and fusion and cervical disc arthroplasty for neurologic and gait improvement at 2 years follow-up, the current patient's clinical scenario has not been included in these trials. The current patient exhibits advanced age, multiple subluxation, and multiple levels of stenosis. These characteristics would have excluded the patient from these studies. Therefore, current data does not support the use of cervical disc arthroplasty in this patient.

Laminectomy and Fusion

Laminectomy has been employed in the treatment of myelopathy for many years. The advantages of laminectomy are well known: less surgically demanding, do not require stabilization or fusion, little risk to ventral structures, no dysphagia, direct visualization of the nerve roots. The disadvantages are also well known: postoperative neck pain, development of postlaminectomy kyphosis, inability to access ventral pathology. Preoperative subluxation with hypermobility is a risk factor for postoperative destabilization.[16] Guigui followed 58 patients after multilevel laminectomy without fusion for myelopathy for more than 3 years. Thirty percent changed curvature after laminectomy. These patients had mean improvement rates that were significantly less than those with stable cervical curvature.

Considering the patients segmental instability and mild kyphosis, he may be at increased risk for development of postoperative kyphosis after laminectomy alone.[17,18] Therefore, in this setting a fusion should be considered.

Though it has been used for many years, few well-designed studies exist assessing laminectomy and fusion for myelopathy. The best data available are retrospective or consecutive case series. The consensus from these studies is that outcomes are very good for most patients, sagittal balance remains constant, and complications are few.[17,18]

Laminoplasty

The patient's kyphosis is mild and a consideration of a posterior approach must be considered. Dynamic radiographs are lacking; therefore it is unknown as to whether neck extension can help correct the patient's lordosis with neck extension. Studies have shown that posterior procedures offer low complication rates and neurologic significant improvement.[11]

Laminoplasty can provide a multilevel decompression while maintaining posterior structures in order to prevent iatrogenic kyphosis. Considering the patient's age, a review of laminoplasty in the elderly is important. Kawaguchi et al. retrospectively compared patients older than 70 years with those younger than seventy. No statistical differences existed between the groups preoperatively. Their respective JOA (Japanese Orthopaedic Association) scores, preoperative and postoperative, as well as their recovery rates, were not statically different.[19] A majority of the elderly patients demonstrated spondylolisthesis. This had no effect on JOA score. The controls and the elderly both showed significant improvements in their JOA scores. This is consistent with other studies; both groups experienced a decreased postoperative range of motion and slightly increased kyphosis. No patients in either group developed postoperative instability.[19]

Three studies have evaluated the biomechanics of laminoplasty.[20–22] Matsumoto conducted a retrospective study to assess the risk factors for closure of lamina after open-door laminoplasty. From a review of 82 patients, they were able to conclude two things. First, closure of the laminoplasty was associated with preoperative cervical kyphosis. Secondly, patients with and without closure of greater than one level of laminoplasty experienced similar recovery.[20] In one of the few prospective studies, Sakai followed 76 patients to assess the effect of preoperative spondylolisthesis on postoperative stability after laminoplasty.[21] Preoperative spondylolisthesis decreased or disappeared in 85% of their patients on neutral radiographs. The recovery rate for those with posterior spondylolisthesis was significantly less. The authors suggest that preoperative posterior spondylolisthesis represents more significant spinal cord compression thus decreased recovery rates. Overall, they demonstrate that laminoplasty can be performed in the presence of multiple subluxations with good clinical outcomes.[21] Suk et al.[22] further delineates the issues of alignment after laminoplasty; retrospectively reviewed 85 patients and followed them for 2 years. As with several other studies, ROM was shown to decrease significantly after laminoplasty. Postoperative kyphosis developed in 10% of their patients. Analysis revealed that cervical spondylosis, neutral lordosis of <10 degrees, and flexion kyphosis that is greater than extension lordosis are factors associated with the development of postoperative kyphosis.[22] Long-term improvement in neurologic symptoms are maintained in 70% to 80% of patients at 10 years.[23,24] Considering these studies, the current patient would seem to be a candidate for laminoplasty.

Anterior and Posterior Combined

A combined anterior and posterior approach is sometimes required. This may be necessary when the patient has postlaminectomy kyphosis or a fixed sagittal kyphosis is present.[25,26] The current patient has a mild kyphotic deformity. Correction of kyphosis to neutral or lordosis significantly improves neurologic outcomes.[25,26] Revision procedures may sometimes require a circumferential approach. This may be because of sagittal imbalance, segmental instability from previous procedures, progressive myelopathy, or pseudoarthrosis. However, successful outcomes can be achieved.[27] Patients with significant osteoporosis should be considered for combined procedures when long constructs are necessary because of an increased risk of end plate fracture and hardware failure.[28,29] It has been shown that corpectomies at three of more levels warrant posterior fixation to increase fusion rates and decrease hardware related complications.[30,31] Significant circumferential compression is also an indication for a combined procedure when unilateral decompression and stabilization alone do not meet the surgical goals.[32] Significant improvements in neurologic outcomes can be expected with a combined anterior and posterior procedure.[32–34] A circumferential decompression and fusion reestablishes sagittal balance, provides a stable biomechanical construct, and extensively decompresses the entire spinal cord.[33] When performed in a single stage, the complications are not significantly higher than in unilateral procedures.[34] Our patient has anterior and posterior compression; however, a majority of his pathology is anterior.

Literature Inconsistencies

Several authors have reported that surgical outcomes do not exceed conservative measures.[35–37] A controlled prospective, randomized study by Kadanka compared conservative and operative treatment for cervical myelopathy.[35] After an average of 24 months'

follow-up, surgical and conservative outcomes were not significantly different. No significant differences in modified JOA or gait were found between the groups. Our patient has progressive disease with significant disability and gait changes. Kadanka et al. studied patients with mild to moderate disease averaging 6 years of symptoms before enrollment. Eighty-eight percent of their patients exhibited less than three level disease and all had fairly high mJOA scores preoperatively. Therefore, Kadanka data cannot be used in the evaluation of our patient.

EVIDENTIARY TABLE AND SELECTION OF TREATMENT METHOD

The best available evidence dictates that the current patent should be treated operatively. We critically examined articles focusing on surgical treatment of cervical myelopathy with multiple subluxations. These results are summarized in Table 1.1.

Anterior or Posterior

The patient demonstrates cervical stenosis with multiple subluxations. The patient in the clinical scenario fits well into multiple studies.[3,22,38] An analysis of the long-term results of anterior versus posterior techniques gives insight into which is more appropriate for this patient. Two studies have looked at the long-term results of anterior versus posterior procedures. Both studies followed patients for at least 10 years after anterior spinal fusion or laminoplasty for meylopathy.[8,39] The neurologic improvement was equal and maintained in both groups throughout the follow-up period. However, the anterior groups experienced higher postoperative complications. Bapat prospectively followed 129 patients that were treated with posterior or anterior procedures.[40] Those patients with three-level disease who underwent anterior decompression and fusion had significantly higher neurologic function postoperatively. A 10-year prospective outcome analysis by Chagas revealed patient satisfaction rates of more than 80% for anterior decompression and fusion for myelopathy.[41] It is reasonable to assume from the reviewed studies that anterior and posterior procedures both would offer the patient good long improvement in his symptoms.

Vascular factors have been shown to play a role in the pathophysiology of cervical myelopathy.[42] A majority of the blood supply to the spinal cord comes from the anterior blood supply, thus an anterior procedure provides the benefit of direct decompression of the spinal cord and the anterior vessels.[38,43]

Anterior decompression and fusion allows reduction of the subluxations and correction of the kyphotic deformity.[44] Posterior procedures require a lordotic

TABLE 1.1 Evidentiary Table.

Paper Author (Year)	Description	Summary of Results	Quality of Evidence
Emery et al. (1998)	Retrospective, case series	108 patients with cervical myelopathy were treated with anterior decompression and fusion. Significant improvement of 1.2 Nurick grades. Older age predicted more severe preoperative myelopathy. Preoperative neurologic function predicted postoperative neuroligic function. Unsatisfactory outcome was associated with pseudoarthrosis.	Very low
Dean et al. (2008)	Retrospective, case series	58 patients with degenerative spondylolithesis and myelopathy were treated with anterior decompression and fusion. 92% fusion rate Average Nurick grade improved 1.5.	Very low
Woiciechowsky et al. (2004)	Retrospective, case series	16 patients with degenreative spondylolethsis and myelopathy were treated with anterior decompression and fusion. All patients fused. Neurologic improvement in 10/13. No neck pain in 3/3 with preop neck pain. 81% satisfactory of better outcome according to Odom's criteria. No validated outcome score.	Very low

alignment to allow the spinal cord to move back away from anterior compression after posterior decompression.[45] Kyphosis can have a negative effect on outcomes.[46] Considering the patient's age, a combined anterior and posterior procedure would add increased morbidity and mortality risk. The patient's deformity is mild and a less invasive approach would be reasonable. If he continued to decline neurologically after an anterior procedure, a second posterior procedure would still be an option. Therefore, the advantages of increased blood flow, kyphosis correction, and good long-term results make an anterior decompression more desirable in this clinical scenario.

Corpectomy or Multilevel Discectomy or Hybrid Construct

Corpectomy and multilevel discectomy have both been shown to offer good clinical outcomes in the treatment of myelopathy.[47–49] Discectomy addresses pathology at the disc level while corpectomy address pathology behind the vertebral body. Wang et al.[50] demonstrated similar fusion and complication rates between a single-level corpectomy and a double-level discetomy. Anterior cervical corpectomy with plating has a very high fusion rate and a low complication rate.[47,51] A corpectomy offers the advantage of decreasing the number of surfaces needed to fuse. When compared to multilevel discectomies in a long construct, corpectomies have a significantly higher fusion rate.[52]

Hybrid decompression fixation technique involves a combined discotomy and corpectomy with fusion and plating. The advantages of both are utilized. The discectomy and fusion allows restoration of lordosis. The addition of the corpectomy decreases the number of bone surfaces to be fused. Ashkenazi et al.[53] has shown that this construct provides significant improvements in neuorlogic outcomes and a fusion rate of >95%.

DEFINITIVE TREATMENT PLAN

Operative intervention should be undertaken in this patient considering the progressive nature of his cervical myelopathy. The patient should be positioned on a regular table with mild neck hyperextension as to prevent further compression upon his spinal cord. A left sided longitudinal incision should be used. Discectomies of C3-4, C4-5, and C5-6 would be performed first. A corpectomy of C4 would be the next step to give the cord more room to float forward away from the compression posteriorly at C3-4. This decompression would help restore blood flow to the spinal cord. Bilateral foraminotomies would be performed at each level to decompress the roots. A fibular strut graft would then be placed at C4. A fibular wedge would then be placed at C5-6 to help restore lordosis.[54,55] An anterior plate would be placed from C3-6. The role of a static versus a dynamic plate is still unclear.[56,57]

A plate decreases the risk of graft related complications and contributes to construct rigidity.[31,58] Screws would be placed in C3, C5, and C6 to provide more points of fixation to improve stability.[59] The construct would allow immediate mobilization in a collar.

Grading the Evidence for this Plan

The evidence to support the technical aspects of this treatment is considered very low because it comes from retrospective case series. Our treatment goals have been met in the articles found in Table 1.1. Anterior decompression and fusion are shown to provide good outcomes for myelopathy with multiple subluxations. In accordance with the method of grading recommendations set forth by Schunemann et al.[60] our proposed treatment would be considered a **strong recommendation** with low quality evidence. Overall, very good fusion rates, symptomatic improvement, and few complications are associated with multilevel anterior cervical surgery for myelopathy.[7,11,48]

PREDICTING OUTCOMES

Multiple outcome instruments exist for cervical myelopathy such as the Nurick, Japanese Orthopaedic Association scale, and the SF-36. Whether, disease specific or generalized, they all seem to exert relative strengths and weaknesseses.[61] For this reason, no study has defined any particular outcome measure as the gold standard for outcome of treatment for cervical myelopathy. Therefore, it is difficult to predict out patient's outcome based on a single outcome measure though this would be ideal.

Multiple studies have sought to predict outcome. Yamazaki et al.[62] followed elderly patients and controls that underwent surgical treatment for spondylotic myelopathy for an average of 40 months. Multivariate analysis revealed that age, preoperative Japanese Orthopaedic Association score, canal diameter, and an intensity change on the spinal cord were not predictive of outcome. Their data suggest that an excellent neurologic improvement can be obtained in elderly patients with symptom duration of <12 months. An excellent recovery was obtained in both groups when the transverse area of the spinal cord was >30 mm[34] at the level of maximal compression. The duration of our patient's symptoms is unknown in this scenario but could be assessed in real life. The MRI demonstrates the most significant compression at C3-4, but the original film would be necessary to transverse measure area. Several studies have suggested that T2 MRI signal changes predict less favorable outcomes.[63,64] Yukawa et al.[64] prospectively studied patients with cervical myelopathy to assess the relationship between MRI increased signal intensity and severity of disease and outcome. Patient

age, duration of disease, postoperative JOA score, recovery rate, all correlated with preoperative T2 MRI increased signal intensity. They went on to conclude that once intense T2 MRI changes occur that outcomes were worse. Our patient demonstrates intense T2 signal intensity at C3-4. This may suggest a less favorable outcome.

Ultimately, the surgeon must now take into account his own technical skill, his comfort level with each procedure, and the patient's wishes.[61] The patient's must be made fully aware of the severity of his disease and its natural history. Cervical myelopathy is a progressive disorder and his symptoms may digress, arrest, or progress regardless of surgical or conservative treatment. He must understand that no treatment is without risk or benefit and that no promises or guarantees can made. These results are consistent with my experience as a spine surgeon. A meticulous assessment of the entire clinical scenario and a careful education of the patient will provide the foundation for making the treatment plan.

SUMMARY

The clinical scenario involves a 81-year-old male with cervical myelopathy and multiple subluxations. He has significant stenosis with anterior and posterior compression. A hybrid construct of anterior C4 corpectomy and C5-6 discectomy and fusion with plating provides the spinal cord with the best opportunity to reperfuse and allows correction of the mild kyphotic deformity. He can expect some improvement in his condition without progression of his symptoms.

REFERENCES

1. Hoppenfeld S, ed. *Physical Examination of the Spine and Extremities*. New York, NY: Appleton-Century-Crofts, 1976.
2. Houten JK, Noce LA. Clinical correlations of cervical myelopathy and the Hoffmann sign. *J Neurosurg Spine*. 2008;9(3):237–242.
3. Dean CL, Gabriel JP, Cassinelli EH, et al. Degenerative spondylolisthesis of the cervical spine: analysis of 58 patients treated with anterior cervical decompression and fusion. *Spine J*. 2009;9(6):439–446.
4. Woiciechowsky C, Thomale UW, Kroppenstedt SN. Degenerative spondylolisthesis of the cervical spine– symptoms and surgical strategies depending on disease progress. *Eur Spine J*. 2004;13(8):680–684.
5. Clarke E, Robinson PK. Cervical myelopathy: a complication of cervical spondylosis. *Brain*. 1956;79(3): 483–510.
6. Sampath P, Bendebba M, Davis JD, et al. Outcome of patients treated for cervical myelopathy. A prospective,

multicenter study with independent clinical review. *Spine*. 2000;25(6):670–676.

7. Gok B, Sciubba DM, McLoughlin GS, et al. Surgical treatment of cervical spondylotic myelopathy with anterior compression: a review of 67 cases. *J Neurosurg Spine*. 2008;9(2):152–157.

8. Sakaura H, Hosono N, Mukai Y, et al. Long-term outcome of laminoplasty for cervical myelopathy due to disc herniation: a comparative study of laminoplasty and anterior spinal fusion. *Spine*. 2005;30(7):756–759.

9. Emery SE, Bohlman HH, Bolesta MJ, et al. Anterior cervical decompression and arthrodesis for the treatment of cervical spondylotic myelopathy. Two to seventeen-year follow-up. *J Bone Joint Surg Am*. 1998;80(7): 941–951.

10. Kiris T, Kilincer C. Cervical spondylotic myelopathy treated by oblique corpectomy: a prospective study. *Neurosurgery*. 2008;62(3):674–682; discussion 674–682.

11. Lu KW, Jin DD, Wang J, et al. Analysis of the long-term outcome of anterior approach surgery on cervical spondylotic myelopathy. *Zhonghua Wai Ke Za Zhi*. 2006;44(16):1091–1093.

12. Lafuente J, Casey AT, Petzold A, et al. The Bryan cervical disc prosthesis as an alternative to arthrodesis in the treatment of cervical spondylosis: 46 consecutive cases. *J Bone Joint Surg Br*. 2005;87(4):508–512.

13. Pimenta L, McAfee PC, Cappuccino A, et al. Superiority of multilevel cervical arthroplasty outcomes versus single-level outcomes: 229 consecutive PCM prostheses. *Spine*. 2007;32(12):1337–1344.

14. Riew KD, Buchowski JM, Sasso R, et al. Cervical disc arthroplasty compared with arthrodesis for the treatment of myelopathy. *J Bone Joint Surg Am*. 2008;90(11): 2354–2364.

15. Sekhon LH. Two-level artificial disc placement for spondylotic cervical myelopathy. *J Clin Neurosci*. 2004;11(4):412–415.

16. Guigui P, Benoist M, Deburge A. Spinal deformity and instability after multilevel cervical laminectomy for spondylotic myelopathy. *Spine*. 1998;23(4):440–447.

17. Huang RC, Girardi FP, Poynton AR, et al. Treatment of multilevel cervical spondylotic myeloradiculopathy with posterior decompression and fusion with lateral mass plate fixation and local bone graft. *J Spinal Disord Tech*. 2003;16(2):123–129.

18. Sekhon LH. Posterior cervical decompression and fusion for circumferential spondylotic cervical stenosis: review of 50 consecutive cases. *J Clin Neurosci*. 2006;13(1):23–30.

19. Kawaguchi Y, Kanamori M, Ishihara H, et al. Pathomechanism of myelopathy and surgical results of laminoplasty in elderly patients with cervical spondylosis. *Spine*. 2003;28(19):2209–2214.

20. Matsumoto M, Watanabe K, Tsuji T, et al. Risk factors for closure of lamina after open-door laminoplasty. *J Neurosurg Spine*. 2008;9(6):530–537.

21. Sakai Y, Matsuyama Y, Inoue K, et al. Postoperative instability after laminoplasty for cervical myelopathy with spondylolisthesis. *J Spinal Disord Tech*. 2005;18(1):1–5.

22. Suk KS, Kim KT, Lee JH, et al. Sagittal alignment of the cervical spine after the laminoplasty. *Spine*. 2007;32(23):E656–E660.

23. Chiba K, Ogawa Y, Ishii K, et al. Long-term results of expansive open-door laminoplasty for cervical myelopathy–average 14-year follow-up study. *Spine*. 2006;31(26):2998–3005.

24. Seichi A, Takeshita K, Ohishi I, et al. Long-term results of double-door laminoplasty for cervical stenotic myelopathy. *Spine*. 2001;26(5):479–487.

25. Ferch RD, Shad A, Cadoux-Hudson TA, et al. Anterior correction of cervical kyphotic deformity: effects on myelopathy, neck pain, and sagittal alignment. *J Neurosurg*. 2004;100(1 suppl Spine):13–19.

26. O'Shaughnessy BA, Liu JC, Hsieh PC, et al. Surgical treatment of fixed cervical kyphosis with myelopathy. *Spine*. 2008;33(7):771–778.

27. Gok B, Sciubba DM, McLoughlin GS, et al. Revision surgery for cervical spondylotic myelopathy: surgical results and outcome. *Neurosurgery*. 2008;63(2):292–298; discussion 298.

28. Emery SE. Cervical spondylotic myelopathy: diagnosis and treatment. *J Am Acad Orthop Surg*. 2001;9(6):376–388.

29. Hee HT, Majd ME, Holt RT, et al. Complications of multilevel cervical corpectomies and reconstruction with titanium cages and anterior plating. *J Spinal Disord Tech*. 2003;16(1):1–8; discussion 8–9.

30. Isomi T, Panjabi MM, Wang JL, et al. Stabilizing potential of anterior cervical plates in multilevel corpectomies. *Spine*. 1999;24(21):2219–2223.

31. Vaccaro AR, Falatyn SP, Scuderi GJ, et al. Early failure of long segment anterior cervical plate fixation. *J Spinal Disord*. 1998;11(5):410–415.

32. Kim PK, Alexander JT. Indications for circumferential surgery for cervical spondylotic myelopathy. *Spine J*. 2006;6(6 suppl):299S–2307S.

33. Acosta FL Jr, Aryan HE, Chou D, et al. Long-term biomechanical stability and clinical improvement after extended multilevel corpectomy and circumferential reconstruction of the cervical spine using titanium mesh cages. *J Spinal Disord Tech*. 2008;21(3):165–174.

34. Aryan HE, Sanchez-Mejia RO, Ben-Haim S, et al. Successful treatment of cervical myelopathy with minimal morbidity by circumferential decompression and fusion. *Eur Spine J*. 2007;16(9):1401–1409.

35. Kadanka Z, et al. Conservative treatment versus surgery in spondylotic cervical myelopathy: a prospective randomised study. *Eur Spine J*. 2000;9(6):538–544.

36. Long DM. Lumbar and cervical spondylosis and spondylotic myelopathy. *Curr Opin Neurol Neurosurg*. 1993;6(4):576–580.

37. Rowland LP. Surgical treatment of cervical spondylotic myelopathy: time for a controlled trial. *Neurology*. 1992;42(1):5–13.

38. Dommisse GF. The blood supply of the spinal cord. A critical vascular zone in spinal surgery. *J Bone Joint Surg Br*. 1974;56(2):225–235.

39. Wada E, Suzuki S, Kanazawa A, et al. Subtotal corpectomy versus laminoplasty for multilevel cervical spondylotic myelopathy: a long-term follow-up study over 10 years. *Spine*. 2001;26(13):1443–1447; discussion 1448.

40. Bapat MR, Chaudhary K, Sharma A, et al. Surgical approach to cervical spondylotic myelopathy on the basis of radiological patterns of compression:

prospective analysis of 129 cases. *Eur Spine J.* 2008;17(12): 1651–1663.

41. Chagas H, Domingues F, Aversa A, et al. Cervical spondylotic myelopathy: 10 years of prospective outcome analysis of anterior decompression and fusion. *Surg Neurol.* 2005;64(suppl 1):S1:30–35; discussion 35–36.

42. Taylor AR. Vascular factors in the myelopathy associated with cervical spondylosis. *Neurology.* 1964;14:62–68.

43. Schweighofer F, Anderhuber F, Zolss C, et al. Blood supply to the cervical spinal cord and possible therapeutic consequences in cervical spinal cord injuries. *Unfallchirurg.* 1993;96(3):134–137.

44. Hillard VH, Apfelbaum RI. Surgical management of cervical myelopathy: indications and techniques for multilevel cervical discectomy. *Spine J.* 2006;6(6 suppl): 242S–251S.

45. Batzdorf U, Batzdorff A. Analysis of cervical spine curvature in patients with cervical spondylosis. *Neurosurgery.* 1988;22(5):827–836.

46. Satomi K, Nishu Y, Kohno T, et al. Long-term follow-up studies of open-door expansive laminoplasty for cervical stenotic myelopathy. *Spine.* 1994;19(5):507–510.

47. Macdonald RL, Fehlings MG, Tator CH, et al. Multilevel anterior cervical corpectomy and fibular allograft fusion for cervical myelopathy. *J Neurosurg.* 1997;86(6):990–997.

48. Mayr MT, Subach BR, Comey CH, et al. Cervical spinal stenosis: outcome after anterior corpectomy, allograft reconstruction, and instrumentation. *J Neurosurg.* 2002;96(1 suppl):10–16.

49. Sevki K, Mehmet T, Ufuk T, et al. Results of surgical treatment for degenerative cervical myelopathy: anterior cervical corpectomy and stabilization. *Spine.* 2004;29(22):2493–2500.

50. Wang JC, McDonough PW, Endow KK, et al. A comparison of fusion rates between single-level cervical corpectomy and two-level discectomy and fusion. *J Spinal Disord.* 2001;14(3):222–225.

51. Eleraky MA, Llanos C, Sonntag VK. Cervical corpectomy: report of 185 cases and review of the literature. *J Neurosurg.* 1999;90(1 suppl):35–41.

52. Hilibrand AS, Fye MA, Emery SE, et al. Increased rate of arthrodesis with strut grafting after multilevel anterior cervical decompression. *Spine.* 2002;27(2):146–151.

53. Ashkenazi E, Smorgick Y, Rand N, et al. Anterior decompression combined with corpectomies and discectomies in the management of multilevel cervical myelopathy: a hybrid decompression and fixation technique. *J Neurosurg Spine.* 2005;3(3):205–209.

54. Herrmann AM, Geisler FH. Geometric results of anterior cervical plate stabilization in degenerative disease. *Spine.* 2004;29(11):1226–1234.

55. Wang JC, McDonough PW, Endow K, et al. The effect of cervical plating on single-level anterior cervical discectomy and fusion. *J Spinal Disord.* 1999;12(6):467–471.

56. DuBois CM, Bolt PM, Todd AG, et al. Static versus dynamic plating for multilevel anterior cervical discectomy and fusion. *Spine J.* 2007;7(2):188–193.

57. Nunley PD, Jawahar A, Kerr EJ III, et al. Choice of plate may affect outcomes for single versus multilevel ACDF: results of a prospective randomized single-blind trial. *Spine J.* 2009;9(2):121–127.

58. Kanayama M, Cunningham BW, Weis JC, et al. The effects of rigid spinal instrumentation and solid bony fusion on spinal kinematics. A posterolateral spinal arthrodesis model. *Spine.* 1998;23(7):767–773.

59. Zdeblick TA, Ducker TB. The use of freeze-dried allograft bone for anterior cervical fusions. *Spine.* 1991;16(7): 726–729.

60. Schunemann HJ, et al. An official ATS statement: grading the quality of evidence and strength of recommendations in ATS guidelines and recommendations. *Am J Respir Crit Care Med.* 2006;174(5):605–614.

61. Jankowitz BT, Gerszten PC. Decompression for cervical myelopathy. *Spine J.* 2006;6(6 suppl):317S–322S.

62. Yamazaki T, Yanaka K, Sato H, et al. Cervical spondylotic myelopathy: surgical results and factors affecting outcome with special reference to age differences. *Neurosurgery.* 2003;52(1):122–126; discussion 126.

63. Wada E, Yonenobu K, Suzuki S, et al. Can intramedullary signal change on magnetic resonance imaging predict surgical outcome in cervical spondylotic myelopathy? *Spine.* 1999;24(5):455–461; discussion 462.

64. Yukawa Y, Kato F, Yoshihara H, et al. MR T2 image classification in cervical compression myelopathy: predictor of surgical outcomes. *Spine.* 2007;32(15):1675–1678; discussion 1679.

2

Multilevel Cervical Stenosis with Straight Spine

CHRISTOPHER C. HARROD, MD, ANDREW P. WHITE, MD,
AND KEVIN J. MCGUIRE, MD, MS

EDITORS' CASE PRESENTATION

A 58-year-old woman presents with bilateral upper extremity numbness and tingling from the forearms down to the fingers. She has been in this state for approximately 3 weeks. She does not have any complaints of imbalance or of subjective weakness in the lower extremities. She does indicate bilateral weakness in the hands, right greater than the left.

Physical examination demonstrates that she has decreased sensation in the bilateral C6, C7, and C8 distribution. She also has decreased grip strength bilaterally as well as decreased strength with wrist flexion, wrist extension, biceps and triceps bilaterally. The patient has a positive Hoffmann reflex bilaterally along and a positive inverted radial reflex on the right side. She has a negative Lhermitte test. Her balance with walking appears to be generally preserved. Her range of motion is nearly full with flexion and extension. Examination of the lower extremities shows that she has full strength, intact sensation, and normal reflexes.

Radiographic imaging studies are shown in Figures 2.1 and 2.2.

INTERPRETATION OF CLINICAL PRESENTATION

The clinical scenario describes a middle-aged woman with subacute neurologic symptoms without a history of trauma. The chief complaints of painless bilateral upper extremity sensory and motor dysfunction can be the result of cervical spinal cord compression and may be consistent with myelopathy. The approach to this patient must consider the full array of possible etiologies, however, including trauma, degenerative conditions of the cervical spine including spondylosis and herniated disks, congential defects, transverse myelitis, multiple sclerosis, adrenomyeloneuropathy, infection, postinfectious syndrome, or postvaccination myelitis, arachnoiditis, epidural abscess, connective tissue disorders including rheumatoid arthritis and systemic lupus erthythematosus and other medical entities such as sarcoid, paraneoplastic or ulcerative colitis-induced myelopathy. Toxins, electrical injury, radiation injury, and metabolic conditions including vitamin B_{12} deficiency, liver disease, thyroid or parathyroid disease can cause a presentation similar to myelopathy. Other etiologies more likely to mimic cervical myelopathy include syringomyelia, motor neuron disease, subacute combined degeneration, Arnold-Chiari malformation, intracranial and intraspinal tumors, vertebrobasilar ischemia, and peripheral neuropathy including Guillain-Barré syndrome, compression peripheral neuropathies, and arthritis.

A diagnosis of cervical myelopathy is considered based on the typical history of neurologic symptoms involving the upper more than the lower extremities with physical examination findings reflecting cervical spine involvement. Nonetheless, it may be beneficial to rule out thoracic and lumbar spinal compression if lower extremity symptoms coexist or predominate. Cervical spondylotic myelopathy should be strongly suspected, and not simply by exclusion of other diagnoses. It afflicts approximately one-fourth of patients with nontraumatic spastic paraparesis and tetraparesis.[1] Weakness in the hands helps to localize the level

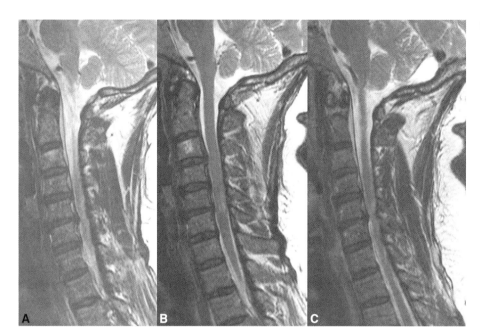

Figure 2.1.

of neurologic involvement. Patients <60 years old are more likely to exhibit C5-6 and C6-7 involvement while patients over 70 are more likely to show C3-4 and C4-5 involvement.[2] Symptoms for only 3 weeks in addition to no gait, lower extremity, or bladder dysfunction suggest an early stage in the course of cervical myelopathy.

The natural history of cervical spondylotic myelopathy is not benign. Up to one third of patients symptomatically improve, approximately one third remain stable, and more than one third of patients deteriorate.[3–5] The overall duration of symptoms has prognostic significance. There appears to be agreement that patients with symptoms for <2 years are more likely to clinically improve.[6,7]

This patients' decreased sensation in bilateral C6-8 nerve root distribution may correspond either to dermatomal sensory loss in the upper extremities secondary to compression of the dorsal nerve roots and/or the anterior spinothalamic tracts. Typically,

the array of motor weakness corresponds to the spinal segments being compressed, causing lower motor neuron involvement at the levels of the lesion in the cervical cord. Weak biceps and wrist extensors in this example corresponds to C6 nerve root and/or corticospinal tract compression whereas weak triceps and wrist flexion corresponds to C7 and weak grip strength corresponds to C8 compression. Preserved strength in the lower extremities is characteristic of early myelopathy. Lower motor neuron findings are typically present at the involved levels in the cervical myotomes while upper motor neuron findings are typically present below the site of compression. The motor and sensory findings are related to the anatomic sites, degree of compression, and number of levels compressed in the cervical cord.[8]

The positive Hoffmann sign and the inverted radial reflex found in this patient are pathologic reflexes that suggest compression of the corticospinal tract. The Hoffmann reflex is elicited by flicking the nail of the

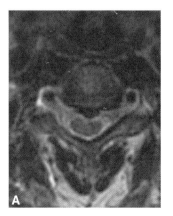
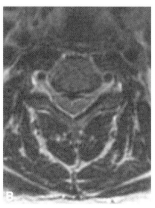
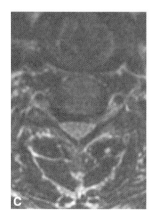
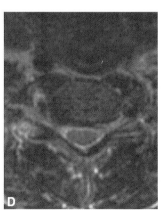

Figure 2.2.

third or fourth digit with resultant flexion of the thumb or adjacent digits. This monosynaptic reflex occurs because of the absence of normal inhibitory descending input to the Rexed Lamina IX.[9] The positive inverted radial reflex can signify cord or nerve root compression at the C6 level. Upon testing the brachioradialis reflex, a pathologic reflex contraction of the spastic finger flexors is noted as well as a relative decrease in the normal reflex of the brachioradialis. Normal lower extremity reflexes observed in this patient are consistent with the wide array of clinical variations seen in myelopathic patients. This substantial degree of variability emphasizes the high suspicion needed to effectively identify myelopathy. Distribution of physical findings varies greatly. Hoffmann reflex and Babinski sign is noted to be positive in less than one fifth of patients while Lhermitte sign and neck pain are often absent.[10] This patient's preservation of balance with normal gait may be related to a lack of dorsal compression of the posterior funiculi. In severely myelopathic patients, gait can be broad-based, hesitant, and jerky. It is often termed a "scissor gait," as the legs are flexed slightly at both hips and knees yielding a crouched appearance with knees and thighs hitting or crossing in scissors-like movements. In early myelopathy, as in this case, balance and proprioceptive problems are often more subtle and diagnosed more by subjective history (often noted by family members) or specific tests such as the Rhomberg test or an inability to perform tandem gait.

The cervical spine magnetic resonance images (MRI) of this patient include two T2 parasagittal images, a midline sagittal T2 image, and four T2 axial images through the C3-4, C4-5, C5-6, C6-7 disc spaces. Figure 2.1 demonstrates a loss of the normal sagittal cervical lordosis (normal is 30 degrees) but without significant kyphosis (<10 degrees). This can be demonstrated by measuring a Cobb angle from the C3 to the T1 endplate. Flexion and extension radiographs are not available for review but could be considered to demonstrate the extent of possible motion. Given that the patient has full range of motion on exam, particularly in extension without worsening of her symptoms, the demonstrated alignment is unlikely to be compensatory/postural. The sagittal MRIs demonstrate multilevel posterior disc protrusions with adjacent osteophytes, most significantly at C3-4, C4-5, C5-6, with some spondylotic changes also at C6-7. Ligamentous hypertrophy is imaged on the right side at C5-6 (Fig. 2.1C). Mild cord signal changes are seen in Figure 2.1B and C at the C5-6 level, which are most likely consistent with myelomalacia. An MRI with contrast could be considered, however, to rule out an intraspinal lesion even in severe stenosis.

Axial T2 weighted images (Fig. 2.2) confirm the local compression seen on sagittal images. At C3-4

(Fig. 2.2A) a central disc protrusion indents the thecal sac but spinal fluid remains circumferentially around the spinal cord. At C4-5 (Fig. 2.2B) there is effacement of the thecal sac with loss of circumferential spinal fluid and compression of the spinal cord, but no significant foraminal stenosis. At C5-6 (Fig. 2.2C) there is significant paracentral and central thecal sac compression related to disk and osteophyte as well as posterior left greater than right ligamentous hypertrophy and significant right greater than left foraminal stenosis. At C6-7 (Fig. 2.2D) there is no significant central stenosis but moderate right foraminal stenosis from an anterior disk and osteophyte complex.

DECLARATION OF SPECIFIC DIAGNOSIS

This patient has cervical spondylotic myelopathy with central compression from C3-7 with a straight cervical spine.

BRAINSTORMING: WHAT ARE THE TREATMENT GOALS AND SURGICAL OPTIONS?

The treatment goals are

1. Halting progression of neurologic symptoms
2. Decompression of the spinal cord via direct or indirect measures
3. Decompression of nerve roots
4. Maintenance or improvement of spinal sagittal alignment
5. Maintenance of spinal stability
6. Early mobilization
7. Rehabilitation and healing

The treatment options are

1. Conservative measures including: cervical orthosis (soft collar), nonsteroidal or steroidal anti-inflammatory medication, epidural steroid injections, biofeedback, physiotherapy, halter traction
2. Multilevel anterior cervical discectomy (±C3-4, C4-5, C5-6, ±C6-7) and fusion (ACDF)
3. Multilevel (C4, C5, ±C6) anterior cervical corpectomy and instrumented fusion
4. Hybrid surgery: Single-level ACDF above or below with single anterior corpectomy and instrumented fusion (either C3-4 ACDF with C5 corpectomy or C4 corpectomy with C5-6 ■ ACDF)

5. Multilevel (C3-6 or C3-7) laminoplasty
6. Multilevel laminectomy with instrumented fusion
7. C4 and C6 skip laminectomy

EVALUATION OF THE LITERATURE

To identify relevant publications on cervical spondylotic myelopathy, a Pubmed search for cervical spondylosis "AND" myelopathy was performed from 1950 to 2008, which yielded 843 abstracts. Publications within the English language with subsets listed in Medline yielded 660 publications. Comparative studies regarding management were given highest priority. Further, these results were cross referenced to bibliographies from appropriate, most recent editions of texts covering cervical myelopathy diagnosis and management to ensure the identification of pertinent classic and recent articles. One-hundred twenty-five English abstracts were viewed electronically or via hand-searched journals. Forty-one full text articles were reviewed in detail.

DETAILED REVIEW OF PERTINENT ARTICLES

Operative or Nonoperative Treatment

While a review of the literature regarding cervical spondylotic myelopathy did reveal many relevant studies, only one recent prospective study and no prospective randomized controlled trials were found which compare nonsurgical and surgical treatment of cervical spondylotic myelopathy. Five retrospective studies compared results of anterior diskectomy or corpectomy with laminoplasty.[11–15] One prospective randomized clinical trial and two retrospective studies compared laminoplasty with skip laminectomy and laminectomy with instrumented fusion.[16–18] Laminectomy without fusion was once considered the standard treatment for multilevel disease. However, experimental rabbit and goat prospective randomized studies have demonstrated biomechanical, radiographic, and clinical superiority of laminoplasty over laminectomy without fusion in addition to less risk for instability, postoperative kyphosis, and late neurologic deterioration.[19,20] While there is evidence that operative treatment is indicated for patients with severe cervical spondylotic myelopathy, nonoperative measures have been successful in mild cases. In a prospective randomized trial, Kadanka et al.[21] reported similar outcomes in nonsurgical and surgical treatment of mild cervical myelopathy with 3-year follow-up. Conservative measures included soft collar immobilization; anti-inflammatory medications; bed rest; avoidance of risky activities and environments including cold, physically demanding situations; movement on slippery surfaces; manipulation therapies; and vigorous or sustained head flexion. These studies, in addition to numerous case series, represent the best available evidence.

A combination of clinical signs and symptoms in addition to imaging evidence of spinal stenosis, with or without signal changes in the cord, favor operative treatment of myelopathy. Our patient demonstrates upper extremity sensory and motor changes with decreased function for a short duration with evidence of long tract dysfunction with corresponding radiographic imaging. Most authors tend to use a combination of neurologic symptoms, preoperative functional scoring utilizing the modified Japanese Orthopaedic Association (JOA) system and radiographic findings to determine the need for operative treatment. The JOA myelopathy scale has been found to have high interobserver and intraobserver reliability and is widely used for grading severity. It assesses motor and sensory dysfunction in the upper and lower extremities and trunk in addition to bladder function.[18,22] The upper extremity function receives likely one or two points due to loss of bilateral finger dexterity and upper extremity weakness, four points for normal lower extremity function, three points for normal bladder function, two points each for normal trunk and lower extremity sensation and zero points for upper extremity sensory loss. For a score of <13 with evidence of spinal cord compression on imaging studies, operative management is typically recommended. According to the modified JOA scale, our patient would likely receive a total of 12 or 13 points. Fujiwara et al.[23] and Koyanagi et al.[24] noted positive prognostic indicators for surgery to include larger transverse cord area, shorter duration of symptoms, younger age at presentation, and single rather than multiple levels of involvement. Results of operative treatment were found to be better in individuals undergoing surgical decompression early as compared to late. Suri et al. reported that in a prospective randomized trial, 146 patients who were symptomatic <1 year showed significantly greater motor recovery[25–27] after surgery. In summary, the literature offers ambiguous evidence—those with early myelopathy will do well with conservative measures as well as surgical intervention. The lack of a randomized controlled trial, therefore, leaves this question unanswered. Nonetheless, in this patient who is younger than 60 and exhibits significant neurologic symptoms and deficits in function and a relatively preserved transverse cord area, surgical decompression should be considered a reasonable option.

Management of this patient is best achieved by an integration of patient aspects, critical appraisal of the pertinent literature, and self-derived clinical expertise with the latter guiding decision-making regarding controversial or near equivalent data between surgical methods and postoperative management. Given the primary neurologic complaints and signs, an adequate decompression is the primary technical goal of surgical intervention. The primary factors guiding decision-making regarding anterior versus posterior approaches for decompression of the cervical cord and roots include: (a) spinal sagittal alignment, (b) location of the greatest compressive pathology, (c) extent of pathology, (d) history of previous operations, and (e) preoperative neck pain.

Spinal Sagittal Alignment. This patient has a neutral spine with loss of normal lordosis yet lack of frank kyphosis. Great controversy hinges on this point in the literature. Direct decompression of neural structures and arthrodesis of bony segments with restoration of sagittal alignment is possible via multilevel discectomy or anterior corpectomy operations whereas posterior options such as laminoplasty and laminectomy rely on indirect posterior translation of neural elements from compressive anterior structures. Sodeyama et al.'s[28] work supports this rationale as the expected dorsal translation was found to be greatest in lordotic (3.1 mm peak shift) spines compared to neutral (2.8 mm) or kyphotic spines (<2 mm). Mean spinal cord shift of 3 mm was associated with good outcomes after enlargement laminoplasty which supports Itoh and Tsuji's assertion that 4 mm is an ideal enlargement.[29] Though retrospective, Suda et al.'s[30] incorporation of the presence/absence of signal intensity change in the spinal cord with the degree of lordosis and kyphosis angle calculates the predictive probability of a poor outcome (defined as a JOA recovery rate of <50%). This patient has a local kyphosis angle of near zero degrees with the presence of signal intensity change. Suda et al.'s work predicts good clinical outcomes in patients with and without signal change with kyphosis angles up to 5 and 13 degrees respectively. Contrastingly, Kawakami et al. assert that preoperative and postoperative sagittal alignment have no bearing on neurologic recovery in myelopathic patients whether pathology is disc or spondylotic related. Instead, they contend that anterior discectomy and fusions for patients with one- or two-level disease without congenital stenosis and laminoplasty for patients with three or more levels or congenital (AP diameter < 13 mm) stenosis predict good outcomes.[31] Additionally, Chiba et al.[32] suggest that spinal cord slack by decreased disc height allows acceptable recovery rate even in straight or kyphotic spines.

Location of Compressive Pathology. Anterior or posterior surgery should consider the anatomic location of compression. Anterior central disc herniations are best directly approached via anterior approaches whereas posterior ligamentum flavum hypertrophy

or lamina shingling is reliably addressed via posterior approaches. This patient has a combination of anterior and posterior pathology particularly at C5-6 thereby shifting greater importance to other decision-making factors.

Extent of Pathology. Although the C5-6 level is the most severe, the patient has three-level pathology at C3-4, C4-5, and C5-6. Disease involving one or two levels is typically approached via anterior procedures, either discectomy or corpectomy, while involvement of four or more levels is well managed posteriorly via laminoplasty or laminectomy.[11,31] Three-level pathology can be managed by any of the three techniques, though in one study functional gain was demonstrated to be maintained best by corpectomy when three-level involvement occurred.[11] Corpectomy was deemed superior in patients with (a) congenital stenosis (AP diameter <13 mm), (b) a free extruded disc posterior to a vertebral body, or (c) excessively large posterior osteophytes adjacent to endplates.[11] None of these exist in our patient.

History of Previous Operations. This is not present in our patient. This may be an important consideration, however, when there may be adhesions secondary to scar tissue with increased risk of inadvertent durotomy. Additionally, prior anterior surgery may be associated with an increased risk of dysphonia and vocal cord paralysis and can make the alternative posterior approach more desirable than revision anterior. If a revision anterior approach is required, then it may be advantageous to use the contralateral side to the prior operation, but only after direct laryngoscopy has demonstrated normal and symmetric vocal cord function to rule out occult iatrogenic, unilateral dysfunction.

Preoperative Neck Pain. Our patient does not have preoperative neck pain. Laminoplasty is relatively contraindicated in patients with preoperative neck pain secondary to disruption of the posterior extensor musculature and maintenance of motion in a spondylotic spine. Reported rates of neck pain range from 6% to 60% following this procedure. Laminoplasty from C3 to C6 has, however, been demonstrated in a prospective nonrandomized trial in lordotic spines to significantly reduce neck pain from 30% to 5%.[33,34]

Shared decision-making occurs as patient characteristics and personal opinion is melded with the surgeon's knowledge of pertinent components of the literature to create an individualized definitive treatment plan. Unfortunately, no prospective studies are available regarding the management of three-level cervical spondylotic myelopathy (with slightly more ventral than dorsal cord compression) in patients with a neutral spine. There are no retrospective matched studies that compare the three surgical techniques, namely anterior cervical decompression and fusion, laminoplasty, and laminectomy with modern instrumented fusion. One prospective randomized study is available for comparison of motion, neck pain, and surgical outcomes in laminoplasty and skip laminectomy. Four retrospective studies exist comparing anterior decompression and arthrodesis (predominately subtotal corpectomy) with laminoplasty while two retrospective studies compare laminectomy with and without fusion with laminoplasty.[12–17] An adjunct to analyze available studies is utilized from the literature by Schunemann et al.[35]

In order to obtain appropriate recommendations while evaluating risks and benefits of surgical treatments for this individual patient, the quality of each study must be examined. The best articles comparing treatment options are shown in Tables 2.1 and 2.2, which demonstrate that each of the surgical treatments results in acceptable disease-specific outcome scores with regard to neurologic improvement. In general, the articles tend to evaluate not only clinical outcome variables but also preoperative and postoperative radiographic data, which are in general acceptable in comparison to the previous catastrophic failures of laminectomy alone. Surgical complications specific to each treatment differ markedly, however, and distinguish operative treatments. Large prospective trials have shown nonoperative treatment to have an unpredictable course and also typically with lack of neurologic improvement and neurologic deterioration.[3–7] For this particular patient, operative treatment is selected because of reliable ability to arrest neurologic deterioration in addition to providing a reasonable expectation of improved but not necessarily full neurologic including motor recovery at her stage due to her age, relatively short duration of symptoms, and preservation of transverse cord area.[23–27]

Literature Inconsistencies

The key components of this case hinge on the best treatment available for multilevel cervical myelopathy in the sagittally neutral spine. The major literature inconsistencies surround fusion rates and graft-related complications regarding anterior approaches for three or more level pathology. The optimal operative approach for three-level pathology in a straight or neutral lordosis spine is another broadly contested topic. Lastly, the amount of postoperative neck pain developed in patients undergoing laminoplasty has wide-ranging estimates.

EVIDENTIARY TABLE AND SELECTION OF TREATMENT METHOD

The best available evidence dictates that the patient presented in the clinical scenario would be best treated operatively. In order to evaluate the most appropriate surgical treatment, only articles pertaining to adult patients with cervical spondylotic myelopathy comparing outcomes between anterior decompression and arthrodesis with posterior decompressive techniques including laminoplasty, skip laminectomy, and laminectomy with instrumented arthrodesis were critically evaluated. These results are summarized in Tables 2.1 and 2.2.

Corpectomy Versus Laminoplasty. Careful analysis of the five retrospective studies comparing anterior decompression and fusion with laminoplasty indicates no difference in neurologic improvement by measurement of JOA and Nurick grades in studies by Sakaura et al., Wada et al., and Hukuda et al.[11,13,15] Alternatively, Edwards et al. found that laminoplasty resulted in slightly better neurologic outcomes while Yonenobu et al. found that subtotal corpectomy with strut grafting (SCS) resulted in similar (not statistically different) JOA scores and recovery rates as laminoplasty, though it had more durable (higher final JOA scores) recovery results.[12,14] In regards to radiographic measurements, SCS was consistently found to have high rates of adjacent-level degeneration with a pseudarthrosis rate of 26%.[13] Edwards et al. noted laminoplasty to have less loss of lordosis while Yonenobu et al. noted a higher rate of sagittal spinal malalignment.[12,14] Complications were noted to be consistently rare with low reoperation rates in the laminoplasty groups with the exception of axial neck pain, which ranged from 28% to 40% in a previous study. Yonenobu et al. noted axial neck pain to be 60%. Notable laminoplasty neurologic complications were limited to transient C5 palsies with the exception of a single hyperextension injury in Edwards et al.'s[14] cohort. SCS or anterior decompression cohorts were noted to have reoperation rates as high as 20% in Sakaura's group while Wada reported 26% need for posterior wiring and fusion for pseudarthrosis. Overall, SCS complications included nonunion, dysphagia, dysphonia, progressive myelopathy, and esophageal fistula, with graft-related complications the most common. Hukuda et al. makes no assertion regarding a superior surgical approach. Wada et al. used either anterior techniques or laminoplasty for one or two levels while favoring laminoplasty for three or more levels. Edwards et al., Yonenobu et al., and Sakaura et al. concluded that laminoplasty was their technique of choice.

Laminoplasty Versus Laminectomy and Fusion or Skip Laminectomy. In regards to laminoplasty versus laminectomy with instrumented arthrodesis, Heller et al.[16] has the only comparative study. The primary weakness of the study remains the paucity of subjects in addition to the preoperative kyphosis being greater in the laminectomy with fusion group. His conclusions, however, were that the laminoplasty group experienced greater subjective and objective (Nurick)

TABLE 2.1	Evidentiary Table: A Summary of the Quality of Evidence for Comparison of Primarily Anterior Corpectomy Versus Laminoplasty for Multilevel Cervical Spondylotic Myelopathy.

Paper Author (Year)	Description	Summary of Results	Quality of Evidence
Sakaura et al. (2005)	Retrospective cohort study Herniated discs only—average levels 1.3. Old ASF grafting techniques without plating. Matched pre-op prognostic factors—not sagittal alignment. Small patient numbers.	15 patients treated with ASF (10 single-level ACDF, 5 single-level SCS) vs. 18 C3-7 lamino (Itoh tech). 15 (ASF) and 10 (lamino) y f/u. Equal neurologic improvement (JOA), postoperative kyphosis (20% vs. 22%) and ROM (65% and 64% pre-op). ASF—40% early comp, 20% reop, 73% adjacent-level degeneration. Lamino—6% early comp, 0% reop, 28% neck pain.	Low
Edwards et al. (2002)	Retrospective cohort study Three-level pathology. Matched pre-op prognostic factors including sagittal alignment. Small patient numbers.	13 patients each were treated with multilevel corpectomy and C3-7[12] and C3-6[1] lamino. 49 and 40 mo f/u. Similar subjective strength, dexterity, sensation, pain, and gait. Greater functional improvement (1.6 vs. 0.9 Nurick grades), less pain, less loss of lordosis in lamino Complications of lamino—1 HNP, 1 reop. Corpectomy—1 nonunion, 1 subjacent ankylosis, 4 persistent dysphagia, 2 persistent dysphonia, 1 progressive myelopathy, no reop.	Low
Wada et al. (2001)	Retrospective cohort study Average 2.4 level pathology. Small patient numbers.	23 patients treated with SCS and 24 with C3-7 lamino (modified Itoh—open door)—10–14 y f/u. No significant difference in early or late neurologic recovery (JOA) Complications of lamino—40% axial pain, 6% kyphosis, 40% C2/3 spontaneous fusion, 1 hyperextension neurologic injury. SCS—15% axial pain, 38% and 54% adjacent-level degeneration, 26% pseudarthrosis—reop with post wiring.	Low
Yonenobu et al. (1992)	Retrospective cohort study Multiple level spondylosis. Matched pre-op prognostic factors—not sagittal alignment. Old ant. grafting techniques without plating.	41 patients were treated with multilevel SCS and 42 with C3-7 lamino with >2 y f/u. Similar JOA scores and recovery rates but slightly more durable results with SCS. SCS—29.3% comp, 10 graft related, 1 esophageal fistula, one retrolisthesis, 4 neuro deterioration, 5/41 adjacent segment spondylotic changes Lamino—7.1% compl, all transient C5 nerve root palsies, 6/42 developed spinal malalignment, 60% axial neck pain in previous laminoplasty study.	Low
Hukuda et al. (1985)	Retrospective Unmatched prognostic factors Mult procedures (3 anterior—ACDF, 3 post—lamino and laminectomy)	191 patients treated with 151 anterior, 25 posterior, and 15 combined approaches. 1–12-y follow-up. No single anterior or posterior procedure proved superior. Recurrence of symptoms in 5% anterior and 10.5% posterior treated patients.	Very low

ACDF, anterior cervical discectomy and fusion; ASF, anterior spinal fusion; HNP, herniated nucleus propulsus; JOA, Japanese Orthopaedic Association Scale; Lamino, laminoplasty; ROM, range of motion; SCS, subtotal corpectomy with strut grafting.

TABLE 2.2	Evidentiary Table: A Summary of the Quality of Evidence for Comparison of Laminoplasty Versus Skip Laminectomy or Laminectomy and Fusion for Multilevel Cervical Spondylotic Myelopathy.

Paper Author (Year)	Description	Summary of Results	Quality of Evidence
Yukawa et al. (2007)	Prospective Randomized Clinical Trial Exclusion: Congenital stenosis and OPLL. Short follow-up. Unknown long-term outcomes of skip. Small numbers.	41 pts randomized according to birth month (even—Lamino, odd—skip) with average 28 mo f/u. C4 and C6 Skip and C3-6 lamino (modified Kurokawa double door) No significant difference in post-op ROM, pain (VAS), and neurologic outcomes (JOA) Narrow indications for skip (15% CSM patients—all lamino candidates)	Moderate
Shiraishi et al. (2003)	Retrospective matched cohort study OPLL and congenital stenosis patients included. Variable level skip operative technique	43 skip and 51 lamino patients followed for average 30 mo Similar neurologic recovery rates (59% and 60% by JOA) with skip pts having less axial pain (2% vs. 66%) and more post-op ROM (98% vs. 61%) Skip had 2 CSF leaks, 3 preserved laminar fractures, no neuro compl. Lamino had 4 C5 palsies, 2 full recoveries, 1 partial.	Low
Heller et al. (2001)	Retrospective cohort study Small numbers Lamifuse group had increased pre-op kyphosis compared with lamino group Short follow-up	13 patients each in lamino and lamifuse group with average 26 mo f/u Objective (Nurick) and subjective strength, dexterity, sensation, pain, and gait were greater in lamino group. Lamino—zero comps/reops. Lamifuse—14 complications in 9 pts—2 myelopathic progression, 11% pseudarthrosis, 2 broken screws, subjacent spondylosis (ACDF reop), 1 deep infection, iliac harvest pain, and cervical kyphosis	Low

ACDF, anterior cervical discectomy and fusion; CSM, cervical spondylotic myelopathy; JOA, Japanese Orthopaedic Association Scale; Lamifuse, laminectomy and fusion with lateral mass instrumentation; Lamino, laminoplasty; OPLL, ossification of the posterior longitudinal ligament; ROM, range of motion; Skip, skip laminectomy (mostly C4 and C6); VAS, Visual Analogue Scale.

neurologic improvements. Remarkably, they reported no complications in this select group of laminoplasty patients while the laminectomy and fusion group had 14 complications in nine patients including two cases of progressive myelopathy, 11% pseudarthrosis, broken hardware, subjacent spondylosis requiring reoperation with ACDF, deep infection treated nonoperatively, graft donor site pain, and significant cervical kyphosis.[16]

The only prospective study in the literature compares laminoplasty and skip laminectomy, which is a relatively new decompressive technique developed to spare cervical extensor musculature while simultaneously preserving motion and adequately decompressing up to four levels typically by performing C4 and C6 laminectomies. This trial's primary weakness lies in the small numbers of patients in addition to the quite narrow indications for skip laminectomy. Only 15% of cervical spondylotic myelopathy patients were candidates in the author's assessment while all patients were considered to be laminoplasty candidates.[18] Outcomes between the two groups were not significantly different in respect to the postoperative range of motion, pain, and neurologic outcomes. Shiraishi et al. notes significantly less axial neck pain (2%) in his skip laminectomy group, however, than in laminoplasty patients (66%) while simultaneously maintaining much better range of motion (98% vs. 61%), although neurologic outcomes were no different.[17] Another notable weakness to the study is the variable operative techniques utilized in his skip laminectomy cohort, which uniformly employed a C5 cephalad laminotomy that resulted in two cerebrospinal fluid leaks and three laminar fractures in the skip group. Interestingly, no neurologic complications were noted in the skip cohort while four C5 palsies were observed in the laminoplasty group with all but one gaining full recovery. Analysis of the three posterior techniques is quite limited in comparative studies. However, laminoplasty seems to be favored over laminectomy with arthrodesis while skip laminectomy is favored in Yukawa et al.'s group, though this is admittedly applicable to a very small group of CSM patients. Until further data is available regarding performance of skip laminectomy, laminoplasty would still be favored.

Sagittal Alignment. Notwithstanding the higher rate of severe complications evidenced in the above chosen studies and the literature in general, a key determining characteristic for choosing an operative technique is sagittal alignment. General agreement exists in the literature that three-level cervical spondylotic myelopathy with fixed kyphosis is best treated via an anterior decompressive approach. Lordotic sagittal alignment with the same compression, however, is arguably better treated via a posterior approach due to excessive increase in pseudarthrosis and graft-related complications with anterior procedures while anterior compression can be relieved due to posterior cord float with posterior decompression with this alignment. Our patient's scenario, with three-level pathology in a straight spine, is controversial. The final decision is determined by the patient and surgeon's balance of risks versus benefits of each approach. Suda has predicted, however, good clinical outcomes in patients with and without signal change with kyphosis angles up to 13 degrees. As noted before, Kawakami et al. assert that preoperative and postoperative sagittal alignment have no bearing on neurologic recovery in myelopathic patients whether pathology is disk or osteophyte-related. Instead, they contend that anterior discectomy and fusion for patients with one or two-level disease without congenital stenosis and laminoplasty for patients with three or more levels or congenital (AP diameter <13 mm) stenosis have better outcomes.[31] Additionally, Chiba et al. suggest that spinal cord slack by decreased disc height allows acceptable recovery even in straight or kyphotic spines.[32] Kawakami et al. retrospectively compared anterior decompression and fusion in one- and two-level pathology CSM patients with three-level CSM pathology treated with laminoplasty and noted improved neurologic recovery rates in laminoplasty (59%–49%) patients while interestingly noting that patients with preoperative kyphotic or straight spines had no significant differences in sagittal alignment. They concluded that preoperative and postoperative sagittal alignment did not influence the neurologic recovery rates of either group.[36] Conversely,

Suk et al. in a prospective study contend that the preoperative factors that affect sagittal alignment postlaminoplasty include (a) diagnosis of CSM, (b) lordosis angle <10 degrees, and (c) a kyphotic angle during flexion larger than a lordotic angle during extension.[37] Clearly the most controversial aspect of management of this patient involves the approach as dictated by the sagittal alignment. The merits of each of the above studies is noted. Although controversies do abound on this topic in the literature, the data support treatment of three-level pathology in CSM patients with straight spines with laminoplasty. We favor this technique due to the increased risks of significant complications with three-level ACDF or three-level corpectomy.

Length of Decompression. We would plan a C3-6 laminoplasty. We believe that the minimal compression at C6-7 on imaging supports this plan. In support, Hosono et al. demonstrated in a prospective trial that reducing the range of laminoplasty from five (C3-7) to four (C3-6) had no effect on neurologic gain, radiographic changes, or postoperative MRI, which demonstrated sufficient expansion of the dura and spinal cord (43). In addition, significantly shorter operating times, wound length, and, most importantly, decreased postoperative axial neck pain (29% vs. 5%) was seen in the four-level group.

DEFINITIVE TREATMENT PLAN

The patient in this clinical scenario should be managed with operative intervention primarily because of the significant neurologic deficits and the unpredictable nature of nonoperative treatment with respect to neurological deterioration. By giving careful attention to detail, complications can be minimized and efficacy maximized. The patient's safe preoperative range of motion is established with neck flexion and extension measurements recorded. The limits at which symptoms are aggravated are noted as to avoid precipitating neurologic decline during intubation, positioning, and surgery.

After induction and intubation, the patient is placed prone on a radiolucent Jackson frame with the head secured via a three-point Mayfield tong application. The neck is secured in a neutral to gently flexed position, the so-called Soldiers or Military Tuck position. Extremities are carefully padded to ensure minimal pressure points over the iliac crests, elbows, and knees. The head of the operating table is raised 30 degrees angle to minimize venous congestion and airway and facial edema. The eyes should be without external pressure. Taping both shoulders can facilitate improved intraoperative imaging.

A midline incision is made through the skin and down through the nuchal ligament (ligamentum nuchae) to the spinous processes with paraspinal muscle dissection from posterior elements only at levels of decompression. Care should be taken to preserve muscle attachments to the C2 spinous process. The junction of the medial aspect of the lateral mass with the lateral portion of the lamina is identified at each level planned in the decompression. Care is taken to maintain the integrity of the facet capsules at each level. Open door laminoplasty is then undertaken.

The "open side" would be on the right as standard bilateral C5-6 and right sided C6-7 keyhole foraminotomies for nerve root decompression are performed in addition to standard laminoplasty. The "open side" trough is prepared at the junction of the lamina and the lateral mass utilizing a 4.0-mm oval cutting burr with low-aggression teeth (some may prefer either an AM-8 tip or a 4.0-mm extracoarse diamond burr). Once the burr has penetrated to a depth equivalent to its diameter, the pressure and working direction are directed medially to prevent lateral facet encroachment. The inner cortex is removed completely on the open side whereas it is only thinned enough to form a "greenstick hinge" on the opposite side. Opening the laminoplasty is done with great attention to the location and branching of the epidural veins as they are often empty and not easily seen in stenotic canals. They are coagulated and divided for the length of the lateral gutter. This is facilitated by applying a gentle traction force with a nerve hook or angled curette as bipolar forceps coagulate and divide the veins.

The author's preferred method is to apply appropriate-size laminoplasty plates for each level which are selected with plate insertion by fitting the cut edge of the lamina into its "mouth" and then seating the lateral portion (ventral prong) of the plate down onto the edge of the lateral mass. Plate adjustment should err towards the superior aspect of the lateral mass to avoid screw penetration into the subjacent facet joint. A 2.0-mm depth-stopped drill bit created each lateral mass screw hole and self-tapping screws anchor the plate to the lateral mass. Closure in layers is standard.

The role for postoperative bracing is supported by most but for varying lengths of time with both hard and soft collars utilized from day 1 to 3 months. She will remain in a soft collar for 2 weeks.

Grading the Evidence for this Plan

The evidence to support the technical aspects of our treatment selection would be considered low as it is derived predominately from observational studies of moderate quality in addition to one randomized clinical trial with lack of uniform patient population. The treatment goals have been met in the three studies found in Table 2.1. Laminoplasty has clearly been shown to result in predictably good results in regard to halting neurologic deterioration with most cases

experiencing improvement based on modified JOA or Nurick grading scales in the short-term.

Our proposed treatment would be considered a strong recommendation in accordance with the method of grading recommendations set forth by Schunemann et al.[35] The grading model employed is relevant because it not only considers the quality of evidence but also emphasizes the benefits, harms and burdens of the proposed interventions. The benefits of laminoplasty in regard to neurologic outcomes are similar to other proposed surgical options. However, the complications in general are significantly less when compared to anterior decompression and fusion and laminectomy with and without arthrodesis.[12,16,38]

PREDICTING OUTCOMES

To adequately predict outcomes and counsel patients with this disease, one has to rely on validated outcome measures, since radiographic outcomes rarely correlate with patient satisfaction.[11,39] We can expect a favorable outcome given that our patient is relatively young, is early in the course of disease, has limited gait involvement, lack of bladder dysfunction, and has a relatively preserved transverse cord area.[23–27,40] The signal abnormality in the cord can represent cord edema or irreversible changes such as gliosis or microcavitation. Although some authors insist no correlation with myelopathy severity, consensus supports better recovery in patients not demonstrating these signal changes.[27,41,42] In some patients, preoperative function can be affected by lumbar canal stenosis, hip osteoarthritis, and cardiac dysfunction, which can all contribute to overall disability, impaired walking ability, and a worsening Nurick grade.[39] Per Sodeyama et al., an expected peak dorsal translation of the cord in this patient's neutral spine (2.8 mm) is less than the 3 mm, which was associated with good outcomes after enlargement laminoplasty. Perhaps the best predictor is derived from Suda et al.'s[30] incorporation of the presence or absence of signal intensity change in the spinal cord with the degree of lordosis and kyphosis angle by which they calculated the predictive probability of a poor outcome (defined as a JOA recovery rate of <50%). This patient's presence of a local kyphosis angle of near zero degrees with the presence of signal intensity change would predict a JOA score of around 28%, signifying a good clinical outcome. Suda et al. predicts good clinical outcomes in patients with and without signal change with kyphosis angles up to 5 and 13 degrees, respectively.

Evidence-based medicine is instrumental in playing a role in the decision-making process for clinical problems. However, the surgeon must not forget the profound role that the patient plays. Shared decision making with the surgeon after honest and pointed preoperative counseling of the treatment options and the innate risks, benefits, and potential outcomes is both expected and appreciated. The information conveyed must contain the best available evidence and expert opinion so that the patient can make an informed choice.

SUMMARY

We are presented with a 58-year old woman with subacute atraumatic painless neurologic deficits with clinical and radiographic findings consistent with multilevel cervical spondylotic myelopathy. Based on the existing literature, well-documented natural history, and comparative conservative and operative reports, we feel the most appropriate treatment for this patient's disease consists of operative decompression with a modified four-level laminoplasty from C3 to C6 with appropriate correlating foraminotomies. Reasonable expectations include the halting of neurologic progression with modest expectation of improvement in neurologic function. Besides peak sustained neurologic recovery, her functional outcome and morbidity will likely be dependent on the severity of her postoperative axial neck pain.

REFERENCES

1. Moore AP, Blumhardt LD. A prospective survey of the causes of non-traumatic spastic paraparesis and tetraparesis in 585 patients. *Spinal Cord*. 1997;35:361–367.
2. Tani T, Ushida T, Tanigachi S, et al. Age related shift in the primary sites of involvement in cervical spondylotic myelopathy from lower to upper levels. *J Neurol Neurosurg Psychiatry*. 2002;73:316–318.
3. Epstein JA, Epstein WE. The surgical management of cervical spinal stenosis, spondylosis, and myeloradiculopathy by means of the posterior approach. In: *Cervical Spine Research Society: The Cervical Spine*. Philadelphia, PA: JB Lippincott, 1989.
4. Clark E, Robinson PK. Cervical myelopathy: a complication of cervical spondylosis. *Brain*. 1956;79:483.
5. Symon L, Lavender P. The surgical treatment of cervical spondylotic myelopathy. *Neurology*. 1967;17:117–127.
6. Phillips DG. Surgical treatment of myelopathy with cervical spondylosis. *J Neurol Neurosurg Psychiatry*. 1973;36:879–884.
7. Campbell AM, Phillips DG. Cervical disk lesion with neurological disorder. *Br Med J*. 1960;5197:481–485.
8. Clark CR. Cervical spondylotic myelopathy: History and physical findings. *Spine*. 1988;13:847–849.
9. Harrop JS, Hanna A, Silva MT, et al. Neurological manifestations of cervical spondylosis: an overview of signs, symptoms, and pathophysiology. *Neurosurgery*. 2007;60 (1 suppl 1):S14–S20.
10. Lunsford LD, Bissonette D, Zorub D. Anterior surgery for cervical disc disease: II. *J Neurosurg*. 1980;53:12–19.
11. Hukuda S, Mochizuki T, Ogata M, et al. Operations for cervical spondylotic myelopathy. A comparison of the results of anterior and posterior procedures. *J Bone Joint Surg Br*. 1985;67:609–615.
12. Yonenobu K, Hosono N, Iwasaki M, et al. Laminoplasty versus subtotal corpectomy. A comparative study of results in multisegmental cervical spondylotic myelopathy. *Spine*. 1992;17:1281–1284.
13. Wada E, Suzuki S, Kanazawa A, et al. Subtotal corpectomy versus laminoplasty for multilevel cervical spondylotic myelopathy: a long-term follow-up study over 10 years. *Spine*. 2001;26:1443–1448.
14. Edwards CC, Heller JG, Murakami H. Corpectomy versus laminoplasty for multilevel cervical myelopathy: an independent matched-cohort analysis. *Spine*. 2002;11:1168–1175.
15. Sakaura H, Hosono N, Mukai Y, et al. Long-term outcome of laminoplasty for cervical myelopathy due to disc herniation: a comparative study of laminoplasty and anterior spinal fusion. *Spine*. 2005;30:756–759.
16. Heller JG, Edwards CC II, Murakami H, et al. Laminoplasty versus laminectomy and fusion for multilevel cervical myelopathy: an independent matched cohort analysis. *Spine*. 2001;26:1330–1336.
17. Shiraishi T, Fukuda K, Yato Y, et al. Results of skip laminectomy- minimum 2-year follow-up study compared with open-door laminoplasty. *Spine*. 2003;28:2667–2672.
18. Yukawa Y, Kato F, Ito K, et al. Laminoplasty and skip laminectomy for cervical compressive myelopathy: range of motion, postoperative neck pain, and surgical outcomes in a randomized prospective study. *Spine*. 2007;18:1980–1985.
19. Fields MJ, Hoshijima K, Feng AHP, et al. A biomechanical, radiologic, and clinical comparison of outcome after multilevel cervical laminectomy or laminoplasty in the rabbit. *Spine*. 2000;22:2925–2931.
20. Baisden J, Voo LM, Cusick JF, et al. Evaluation of cervical laminectomy and laminoplasty: a longitudinal study in the goat model. *Spine*. 1999;24(13):1283–1288; discussion 1288–1289.
21. Kadanka Z, Mares M, Bednanik J, et al. Approaches to spondylotic cervical myelopathy: conservative versus surgical results in a 3-year follow-up study. *Spine*. 2002;27:2205–2211.
22. Yonenobu K, Mocchizuki T, Ogata M, et al. Interobserver and intraobserver reliability of the Japanese orthopaedic association scoring system for evaluation of cervical compression myelopathy. *Spine*. 2001;26:1890–1894; discussion 1895.
23. Fujiwara K, Yonenobu K, Evara S, et al. The prognosis of surgery of cervical compression myelopathy: an analysis of the factors involved. *J Bone Joint Surg Br*. 1989;71:393–398.
24. Koyanagi T, Hirabayashi K, Satomi K, et al. Predictability of operative results of cervical compression myelopathy based on preoperative computed tomographic myelopathy. *Spine*. 1993;18:1958–1963.
25. Tanaka J, Seki N, Tokimura F, et al. Operative results of canal expansive laminoplasty for cervical spondylotic myelopathy in elderly patients. *Spine*. 1999;24:2308–2312.

26. Lee TT, Manzano GR, Green BA. Modified open-door cervical expansive laminoplasty for spondylotic myelopathy: operative technique, outcome, and predictors for gait improvement. *J Neurosurg*. 1997;86:64–68.
27. Suri A, Chabbra RP, Mehta VS, et al. Effect of intramedullary signal changes on the surgical outcome of patients with cervical spondylotic myelopathy. *Spine J*. 2003;3:33–45.
28. Sodeyama T, Goto S, Mochizuki M, et al. Effect of decompression enlargement laminoplasty for posterior shifting of the spinal cord. *Spine*. 1999;24:1527–1532.
29. Itoh K, Tsuji H. Technical improvements and results of laminoplasty for compressive myelopathy in the cervical spine. *Spine*. 1985;10:729–736.
30. Suda K, Abumi K, Ito M, et al. Local kyphosis reduces surgical outcomes of expansive open-door laminoplasty for cervical spondylotic myelopathy. *Spine*. 2003;28:1258–1262.
31. Kawakami M, Tamaki T, Iwasaki H, et al. A comparative study of surgical approaches for cervical compressive myelopathy. *Clin Orthop Relat Res*. 2000;381:129–136.
32. Chiba K, Toyama Y, Watanabe M, et al. Impact of longitudinal distance of the cervical spine on the results of expansive open-door laminoplasty. *Spine*. 2000;25:2893–2898.
33. Ratliff JK, Cooper PR. Cervical laminoplasty: a critical review. *J Neurosurg*. 2003;98(3 suppl):230–238.
34. Hosono N, Sakaura H, Mukai Y, et al. C3-6 Laminoplasty takes C3-7 laminoplasty with significantly lower incidence of axial neck pain. *Eur Spine J*. 2006;15(9):1375–1379.
35. Schunemann HJ, Jaeschke R, Cook DJ, et al. ATS Documents Development and Implementation Committee. An official ATS statement: grading the quality of evidence and strength of recommendations in ATS guidelines and recommendations. *Am J Respir Crit Care Med*. 2006;174:605–614.
36. Kawakami M, Tamaki T, Iwasaki H, et al. A comparative study of surgical approaches for cervical compressive myelopathy. *Clin Orthop Rel Res*. 2000;381:129–136.
37. Suk K, Kim K, Lee J, et al. Sagittal alignment of the cervical spine after the laminoplasty. *Spine*. 2007;23:E656–E660.
38. Herkowitz HN. A comparison of anterior cervical fusion, cervical laminectomy, and cervical laminoplasty for the surgical management of multiple level spondylotic radiculopathy. *Spine*. 1988;13:774–780.
39. Nurick S. The natural history and the results of surgical treatment of the spinal cord disorder associated with cervical spondylosis. *Brain*. 1972;95:101–108.
40. Kawaguchi Y, Kanamori M, Ishihara H, et al. Pathomechanism of myelopathy and surgical results of laminoplasty in elderly patients with cervical spondylosis. *Spine*. 2003;28:2209–2214.
41. Morio Y, Teshima R, Nagashima H, et al. Correlation between operative outcomes of cervical compression myelopathy and mri of the spinal cord. *Spine*. 2001;26:1238–1245.
42. Matsuda Y, Miyazaki K, Tada K, et al. Increased MR signal intensity due to cervical myelopathy. Analysis of 29 surgical cases. *J Neurosurg*. 1991;74:887–892.

3

Cervical Disc Disease with Radiculopathy

JOHN M. RHEE, MD

EDITORS' CASE PRESENTATION

A 36-year-old man presents with a complaint of right-sided neck pain with radiation into the posterior aspect of his right arm. He indicates that this pain has been present for approximately 2 years, precipitated by a car accident. He has numbness and tingling primarily in the right hand and also some in his left hand. He is unable to localize these symptoms to one particular location of the hand. He has had two epidural injections without relief, though he does not know the location of these injections. In addition, he has had physical therapy as part of a long course of conservative treatment. He does not have any dexterity complaints, his balance is unaffected, and he does not have any bowel or bladder complaints.

The patient's physical examination demonstrates a positive Spurling test with rotation toward the right side. Forward flexion of the neck reproduces neck pain. Sensation is slightly decreased on the right side somewhat in the C6 distribution, though it is not completely in a dermatomal pattern, with the hand more affected than the arm. He demonstrates some mild decrease of strength in the biceps and triceps on the right side compared to the left side. Otherwise, he has intact grip strength and shoulder abduction that is equal bilaterally. Reflexes are 1+ bilaterally. He has a negative Hoffman reflex and a negative inverted radial reflex. Lower extremity examination is normal.

Radiographic imaging studies are shown in Figure 3.1A–F.

INTERPRETATION OF CLINICAL PRESENTATION

The case describes a patient with neck and arm pain. It appears to have been precipitated by a motor vehicle accident, and it persists despite 2 years of observation and nonoperative management. The symptoms are bilateral in that there is some numbness and tingling in the left hand, but the majority of symptoms are on the right. He denies any symptoms of myelopathy. The distribution of neck versus arm pain is unclear, but the patient complains of unilateral neck pain that is ipsilateral to the side of the radicular symptoms, which makes the clinical diagnosis more likely to be cervical radiculopathy rather than axial pain or degenerative disc disease. The distribution of pain is not in a clear-cut dermatomal pattern. Often, patients with radiculopathy do not have classic dermatomal symptoms. Overlap between adjacent dermatomes is not uncommon (e.g., a patient with C6 radiculopathy can complain of symptoms that include the ulnar digits), and patients with radiculopathy involving the C4, C5, C6, or C7 roots may only have pain in the shoulder and scapular regions.

The presence of a positive Spurling sign is consistent with radiculopathy, helping to make peripheral causes such as carpal or cubital tunnel less likely. The examination findings focus the root level toward C6, based on the sensory evaluation and the decrease in motor strength of muscles that are usually innervated at least in part by C6 (i.e., biceps and triceps). Weakness in supination would further assist in localizing the root level to C6, but this information is not provided.[1] Normal deltoid and grip strength make C5 and C8 levels less likely to be involved. However, just as patients may not present with classic dermatomal pain or numbness complaints, they may also not present with physical findings that are entirely consistent with a specific root-level diagnosis. The absence of hyperreflexia, a Hoffmann sign, or an inverted radial reflex is consistent with this patient's diagnosis being more likely to be radiculopathy rather than myelopathy. However, it is important to keep in mind that physical signs may be absent in approximately 21% of patients who are myelopathic.[2] A normal lower extremity examination again focuses the diagnosis on root- rather than cord-level compression in the cervical spine.

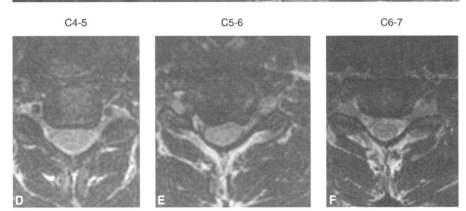

Figure 3.1.

C4-5   C5-6   C6-7

Thus, on the basis of history and physical examination alone, the most likely diagnosis would be C6 radiculopathy. The sagittal MRI scans demonstrate degenerative changes mostly at the C5-6 level. There is some loss of anterior disc height at C5-6 versus the adjacent levels. The paramedian images demonstrate bulging laterally at the C5-6 level only. There is a mild amount of segmental kyphosis at the C5-6 level, and the overall alignment of the cervical spine is straight, keeping in mind that this is a supine MRI rather than an upright x-ray, which is needed to definitively determine alignment. There may be a mild retrolisthesis, which again would need plain x-ray confirmation. There appears to be some spurring anteriorly at the bottom of C5 and the top of C6.

The axial MR images show the absence of significant spinal cord deformation, although there is a very mild amount of flattening of the cord on both sides at C5-6 in the uncovertebral regions but not centrally. At C5-6, there is narrowing of the entry zone of both the left and right C6 roots at the uncovertebral

region, which may be due to small disc herniations or spondylotic spurs. Plain oblique x-rays or a CT scan would be helpful in making this differentiation if it were clinically indicated to do so. The neuroforaminae at C4-5 and C6-7 appear patent.

DECLARATION OF SPECIFIC DIAGNOSIS

This patient's diagnosis is C6 radiculopathy, right greater than left, arising from the C5-6 level.

BRAINSTORMING: WHAT ARE THE TREATMENT GOALS AND THE SURGICAL OPTIONS?

In the classic study by Lees and Turner,[3] the natural history of cervical radiculopathy was demonstrated to be generally favorable. Of 51 patients with radiculopathy and long-term follow-up (2–19 years), 45% had only a single episode of pain without recurrence, 30% had mild symptoms, and only 25% had persistent or worsening symptoms. No patients progressed to myelopathy in this series.

Because the natural history seems to favor resolution in the majority of cases, nonoperative treatment is advocated as the initial treatment of choice in most situations. Accordingly, our patient has had a course of nonoperative care, but it has not been effective in relieving his symptoms. Furthermore, whereas surgery can alter the natural history of cervical radiculopathy, commonly utilized nonoperative treatments, such as physical therapy, medications, and injections, have not been shown to do so. The benefit of nonoperative therapies such as these lies in controlling symptoms as the natural history runs its course. Thus, further conservative care could be chosen but is unlikely to be of long-term benefit to the patient at this point in the course of his disorder.

In patients such as this one who are not myelopathic and do not have major or progressive neurologic deficit, the decision to proceed with surgery should be made by the informed consent of the patient primarily based on his level of pain and disability. The primary goals of treatment in this patient are to

1. Relieve pain by
2. Decompressing the nerve root

Popular surgical options as of 2009 to achieve these goals include

1. Anterior cervical discectomy and fusion (ACDF)
2. Anterior cervical discectomy and total disc replacement
3. Posterior laminoforaminotomy

EVALUATION OF THE LITERATURE

A PubMed search with the keywords "cervical spine," "radiculopathy," and "surgery" elicited 637 results. The results were then hand searched in order to find pertinent articles. Forty-eight articles were reviewed.

DETAILED REVIEW OF PERTINENT ARTICLES AND EVIDENTIARY TABLE

Anterior Cervical Discectomy and Fusion

ACDF is currently the most common procedure used in the operative treatment of cervical radiculopathy. Reported outcomes for relief of arm pain as well as improvements in motor and sensory function are typically in the 80% to 90% range.[4] Benefits of ACDF include the direct removal of most lesions causing cervical radiculopathy (e.g., herniated discs, uncovertebral spurs) without requiring intraoperative neural retraction, restoration or improvement in overall cervical alignment, indirect foraminal decompression resulting from restoration of interbody height with the graft, improvement in spondylotic neck pain with fusion, extremely low rates of infection or wound complications, cosmetically acceptable scars compared to posterior incisions, and mild perioperative pain in most cases. Potential downsides include pseudarthrosis, with rates varying widely according to graft type and use of plate though modern data report it to be around 5% to 10% for a single-level surgery,[5-7] persistent speech and swallowing complications associated with the anterior approach,[8,9] and the potential for accelerated adjacent segment degeneration with fusion.

Biomechanical studies have demonstrated increased disc pressures[10] and motion[11] at segments adjacent to ACDF, suggesting greater adjacent segment wear over time adjacent to a fusion. Clinically, the rate of symptomatic adjacent-level disease requiring adjacent-level surgery in patients after anterior cervical fusion has been estimated to be about 3% per year over a 10-year follow-up period.[12] However, it has yet to be proved that this rate is actually accelerated in those who have undergone fusion versus being a manifestation of such patients' propensity toward spondylosis not only at the index but also adjacent segments over time. In fact, the currently available evidence, most of which is admittedly nonrandomized and retrospective, suggests that symptomatic adjacent segment disease occurs at a rate of about 3% per year regardless of whether the index operation for radiculopathy was anterior discectomy with fusion,[12] anterior discectomy without fusion,[13] or posterior foraminotomy[14] without fusion. Contrasting data come from a short-term (2-year) follow-up study comparing two independent clinical trials of ACDF with a cage versus Bryan total disc replacement, which reported statistically lower rates of symptomatic adjacent-level disease with arthroplasty versus fusion at 2-year follow-up.[15] However, it is important to note that this was not a randomized trial comparing the two groups, but rather a post hoc comparison of two different clinical series. Furthermore, because the decision to operate on an adjacent segment is not without potential bias, these results need to be viewed cautiously and validated by further studies.

Anterior Cervical Discectomy without Fusion

Anterior cervical discectomy without fusion was historically popular but has generally fallen out of favor due to the potential for local kyphosis and worsening neck pain in the absence of fusion.[16]

Anterior Cervical Discectomy and Total Disc Arthroplasty

Currently, three cervical disc replacements have been FDA approved for the surgical management of cervical radiculopathy (Prestige, Bryan, and Prodisc). Several other designs are in investigational device exemption (IDE) randomized trials. Proposed advantages of arthroplasty over fusion include maintenance of motion, avoiding nonunions, and avoiding plate and screw complications such as backout, esophageal erosion, and periplate ossification. As mentioned above, the major long-term benefit may be the as-yet-unproven potential to reduce the incidence of adjacent segment degeneration. Clinical outcomes at 2-year follow-up for total disc replacement in single-level disease have been excellent. The Prestige IDE trial[17] was a large ($n = 541$ total patients), prospective, randomized trial comparing arthroplasty to a plated ACDF with allograft as a control. Both the Prestige and ACDF control groups had similar results at 2-year follow-up with no significant differences in NDI score, VAS score for neck or arm pain, and SF-36 scores. However, when the criteria of so-called overall success were defined as a minimum 15-point improvement in NDI, no worsening of neurologic status, no serious implant-related adverse events, and no second surgeries for failure, the Prestige had significantly better "overall success" than ACDF (79% vs. 68%, $p = 0.004$). The Prestige also had significantly lower rates of secondary surgeries at both the treated and adjacent levels than ACDF.

Although these results are promising, it should be kept in mind that a greater potential for bias exists in the setting of randomized but not blinded surgical trials like these as opposed to double-blinded drug trials. For example, patients who enter nonblinded surgical trials with the intent to be randomized to the "latest and greatest" treatment (i.e., arthroplasty) may be disappointed with randomization to fusion and not be as positive when answering postoperative questionnaires, tending to focus on any residual symptoms or imperfections and attributing these shortcomings as a direct result of not having had the most technologically up-to-date treatment. Conversely, those who are randomized to their procedure of choice (whether it be fusion or arthroplasty) may have a more sanguine outlook on their postoperative conditions and not think that the grass is greener on the other side. A subtler but potentially important bias is also present in seemingly objective outcomes such as the postoperative neurologic assessment, because determining sensory, motor, and reflex grades is not entirely objective from the standpoint of either the surgeon or the patient. These and other biases, large and small, can add up to skew results, particularly when amalgamated outcomes such as "overall success" are examined, because small declines in one or more of the four subcriteria that make up "overall success" may not be clinically relevant yet, when taken together, result in treatment data appearing statistically inferior. Furthermore, when considering outcomes such as repeat operations, it must be kept in mind that recommendations by surgeons for revision surgery for reasons other than catastrophic problems (e.g., for persistent pain, nonunion, etc.) as well as decisions by patients to pursue additional surgery are also neither objective nor without bias. Thus, in the author's opinion, data from IDE trials such as these are extremely valuable but do not necessarily represent gospel truth simply because their study designs were "randomized," "controlled," and "prospective."

The Bryan disc replacement trial[18] also demonstrated excellent results at 2-year follow-up. There were no differences in visual analog scale (VAS) for arm pain or SF-36 between the Bryan disc versus ACDF. However, the Bryan disc had statistically significant better NDI and VAS neck pain scores at 2 years versus fusion, although the numerical differences between the groups were small and of unclear clinical significance. The Prodisc C also demonstrated excellent outcomes,[19] with VAS for neck and arm pain significantly better than preoperative values at all timepoints but not different from control patients. Secondary surgeries were performed in 8.5% of control patients versus 1.8% of Prodisc-C patients ($p = 0.033$). Prodisc-C patients were also significantly less likely to be taking narcotics than controls (90% vs. 82%) at 24 months postoperative.

Taken together, the IDE trials for several total disc replacements suggest that clinical outcomes are excellent and similar for both fusion and arthroplasty at 2-year follow-up. Arthroplasty may have an advantage with respect to fewer repeat operations, keeping in mind the aforementioned potential sources of bias inherent in these studies. However, long-term durability data on arthroplasty are not available, whereas it is known that once a fusion is solid, repeat symptoms rarely occur at the fused level.

Posterior Cervical Laminoforaminotomy

Benefits of laminoforaminotomy include complete avoidance of fusion or placement of an artificial disc and their attendant risks, as well as speech and swallowing issues related to anterior surgery. Potential downsides include instability with overly aggressive facet resection, persistent symptoms in the face of remaining anterior impinging structures, persistent spondylotic neck pain, air embolism (rare but possible) if the seated approach is used, and the need to retract neural elements if it is elected to remove anterior structures such as disc herniations and osteophytes through a dorsal approach. Despite these potential limitations, cervical laminoforaminotomy has been reported to be effective in the treatment of cervical radiculopathy. Large series have reported arm pain relief in 90% to 97% of patients.[14,20] In a randomized trial of 44 patients, there were no statistical differences in outcomes between posterior laminoforaminotomy versus ACDF (unplated with autograft), although ACDF yielded better long-term results.[21] Laminoforaminotomy also lends itself to a minimally invasive approach, and microendoscopic laminoforaminotomy has demonstrated good or excellent clinical results in 97% of patients.[22]

EVIDENTIARY TABLE AND SELECTION OF TREATMENT METHOD

The best evidence, summarized in Table 3.1, suggests that this patient would benefit from surgical treatment. Of the surgical options discussed above, the literature can be used to support treatment with ACDF, disc arthroplasty, or laminoforaminotomy, with no clear-cut superiority of one treatment option versus the others. However, in this particular patient, as there may be a mild amount of segmental kyphosis (albeit on MRI only), a mild amount of cord flattening bilaterally, and bilateral foraminal compression with symptoms to a certain extent in both arms, the author would prefer an anterior rather than a posterior approach. Furthermore, because there are few long-term data currently available for disc arthroplasty, the author would favor an ACDF, which has a proven track record as well as relatively manageable long-term sequelae over a follow-up period spanning more than 50 years.[23]

DEFINITIVE TREATMENT PLAN

The patient is placed supine on a standard operating table with the neck in a gentle amount of extension. The shoulders are lightly taped down to facilitate

TABLE 3.1 Evidentiary Table: A Summary of the Quality of Evidence for ACDF in the Treatment of Cervical Radiculopathy.

Paper Author (Year)	Description	Summary of Results	Quality of Evidence
Bohlman et al. (1993)	Prospective cohort study of clinical outcomes of ACDF No control group Mean 6-y follow-up (2–15 y) All treated with Robinson ACDF (iliac crest bone graft [ICBG] and no plate)	122 patients with cervical radiculopathy with long-term follow-up after ACDF 108/122 (89%): no impairment in function, able to return to work, and activities of daily living 81/122 (67%): no neck or arm pain at all 53/55 (96%): complete recovery of motor deficits 71/77 (92%): improvement in sensory disturbance No neurologic worsening in any patient 171/195 (88%): solid fusion Summary: ACDF has satisfactory long-term clinical outcomes.	Low
Herkowitz et al. (1990)	Prospective randomized trial of ACDF vs. posterior laminoforaminotomy Clinical outcomes assessed by a different (i.e., not the treating) surgeon, and graded as excellent, good, fair, or poor Mean 4.2-y follow-up (1.6–8.2 y)	33 patients with cervical radiculopathy due to soft disc herniation 17 treated with Robinson ACDF (autograft ICBG and no plate) vs. 16 treated with laminoforaminotomy 94% good/excellent outcomes with ACDF, vs. 75% for laminoforaminotomy ($p < 0.175$, not significant) Summary: ACDF may have better clinical outcomes vs. laminoforaminotomy for cervical radiculopathy due to soft disc herniation, although this finding was not statistically significant.	Low

(Continued)

TABLE 3.1 Evidentiary Table: A Summary of the Quality of Evidence for ACDF in the Treatment of Cervical Radiculopathy. *(Continued)*

Paper Author (Year)	Description	Summary of Results	Quality of Evidence
Wang et al. (1999)	Retrospective case-control series of 80 patients looking at the effect of cervical plating on single-level ACDF ACDF with ICBG and plate ($n = 44$) or no plate ($n = 36$) Mean 2.3-y follow-up	Pseudarthrosis: 4.5% (plate) vs. 8.3%(no plate), $p > 0.05$ Graft collapse: 0.75 mm (plate) vs. 1.5 mm (no plate), $p = 0.03$ Segmental kyphosis: 1.2 degrees (plate) vs. 1.9 degrees (no plate), $p > 0.05$ Plating not associated with higher complications Summary: there is less collapse and kyphosis with plated vs. nonplated single-level ACDF.	Low
Samartzis et al. (2005)	Retrospective case-control series of 66 patients undergoing single-level ACDF with a rigid plate and autograft ICBG ($n = 31$) or fresh frozen allograft ($n = 35$) Graft type chosen by patient Independent radiographic review at 12 mo	Fusion: 100% (allograft) vs. 90% (ICBG), $p > 0.05$ No statistically significant difference was noted between the type of graft or the presence of smoking and fusion Summary: the fusion rate for single-level rigidly plated ACDF is the same whether fresh-frozen allograft or ICBG is used.	Low

intraoperative x-ray imaging. A small bump is placed under the shoulders. The literature does not mandate the use of intraoperative neural monitoring for ACDFs done for radiculopathy in patients without spinal cord compression. The use of neural monitoring for such procedures is generally based on local standards. The author uses neural monitoring for myelopathic patients but not necessarily for those with only radiculopathy.

Either a left- or a right-sided Smith-Robinson approach can be taken; despite arguments suggesting a higher rate of recurrent laryngeal nerve injury from a right-sided approach due to the potential for nonrecurrent nerves, the literature is not conclusive on that point. A complete discectomy is performed from uncus to uncus. Parallel endplate decortication is achieved with a combination of a high-speed burr and curettes. The current author prefers to remove the posterior longitudinal ligament (PLL) in all cases under the operative microscope and then perform bilateral foraminotomies, although the literature suggests that direct removal of uncovertebral osteophytes may not be necessary to achieve equivalent outcomes in the setting of disc space distraction with a graft and spinal fusion.[24] The removal of the PLL and inspection of the dura and roots helps to ensure complete decompression.

After satisfactory decompression, the interspace is sized under gentle distraction. An allograft spacer of the appropriate size is inserted. If the patient is a smoker, iliac autograft may be considered to increase fusion rates, though a yet-unpublished study by the Cervical Spine Research Society suggests that the fusion rate in smokers for single-level ACDF may be no different with allograft versus autograft. Although the use of rhBMP-2 in the anterior cervical spine has been reported with success,[25] other series have demonstrated high rates of soft-tissue swelling complications.[26,27] Given the overall high fusion rates associated with single-level ACDF, the routine use of BMP in such cases does not appear warranted at the present time, until issues related to proper dosing and containment of the protein can be determined.

A plate is then applied after decompression. Plated ACDFs are less likely to settle into segmental kyphosis or subside and probably lead to higher fusion rates than unplated ACDFs when allograft is used. The literature does not support the superiority of either dynamic or rigid plates.[28] If a dynamic plate is chosen, however, it should be inserted so as to stay at least 5 mm away from the adjacent disc spaces in the fully settled position.[29] The necessity of postoperative bracing has not been determined in the literature, although a recent study suggests that bracing may not influence the fusion rate in plated one-level ACDF with allograft.[30] The author prefers to use hard collars (e.g., Aspen, Philadelphia, etc.) if plate fixation was suboptimal but provide a soft collar if the fixation was strong.

Grading the Evidence for this Plan

In accordance with the method of grading recommendations set forth by Schunemann et al.,[31] the proposed treatment would be considered a strong recommendation. The benefits to the patient at this point in the course of his disorder clearly outweigh the harms and burdens. The recommendation for surgery versus currently available nonoperative care (physical therapy, medications, injections) in a patient such as the one described is unlikely to change based on the outcomes of further research. The recommendation for ACDF versus arthroplasty may change based on long-term follow-up studies from multiple sources, notwithstanding the manufacturer-supported IDE trials, if arthoplasty is demonstrated to (a) be durable, (b) continue to maintain similar or better arm and neck pain outcomes, and (c) have lower rates of index and adjacent-level reoperations.

PREDICTING OUTCOMES

In the author's practice, patients are counseled that ACDF has approximately an 80% to 90% likelihood of significantly improving radicular pain. In actuality, almost 100% of properly selected patients experience significant improvement in arm pain. Unilateral neck pain may fall into that category as well, but midline axial pain may not, as patients are extensively counseled that the primary goal is relief of radicular rather than axial spondylotic pain. Weakness typically improves in most cases, but may not improve quite as reliably or completely as radicular pain, particularly with higher grades of preoperative weakness (i.e., less than grade 2 strength). Intermittent numbness and tingling also significantly improve almost 100% of the time.

On the other hand, numbness that has been present constantly (i.e., 24 h/d) may not improve significantly, especially if it has been constant for more than 3 to 6 months. If that type of numbness does improve, it may take up to a year or more to do so. The most frequent complication is transient dysphagia, which almost always resolves with time. In the author's experience, the vast majority of patients undergoing one-level ACDF do not report more than a few days to few weeks at most of clinically relevant dysphagia. Overall, patients tolerate single-level ACDF extremely well with excellent outcomes and mild morbidity. Although nonunions clearly do occur, symptomatic nonunions are very rare for single-level plated ACDF, making allograft usage popular. If allografts are used, it should be kept in mind that freeze-dried cortical[6] and fresh-frozen tricortical[7] allografts likely have better radiographic outcomes than dense cancellous allografts, which tend to resorb[32] and are therefore not recommended.

REFERENCES

1. Rainville J, Noto DJ, Jouve C, et al. Assessment of forearm pronation strength in C6 and C7 radiculopathies. *Spine*. 2007;32:72–75.
2. Rhee JM, Hamasaki T, Heflin JA, et al. Prevalence of physical signs in cervical myelopathy: a controlled, prospective study. *Spine*. 2009;34.
3. Lees F, Turner JW. Natural history and prognosis of cervical spondylosis. *Br Med J*. 1963;2:1607–1610.
4. Bohlman HH, Emery SE, Goodfellow DB, et al. Robinson anterior cervical discectomy and arthrodesis for cervical radiculopathy. Long-term follow-up of one hundred and twenty-two patients. *J Bone Joint Surg Am*. 1993;75:1298–1307.
5. Wang JC, McDonough PW, Endow K, et al. The effect of cervical plating on single-level anterior cervical discectomy and fusion. *J Spinal Disord*. 1999;12:467–471.
6. Martin GJ Jr, Haid RW Jr, MacMillan M, et al. Anterior cervical discectomy with freeze-dried fibula allograft. Overview of 317 cases and literature review. *Spine*. 1999;24:852–858; discussion 8–9.
7. Samartzis D, Shen FH, Goldberg EJ, et al. Is autograft the gold standard in achieving radiographic fusion in one-level anterior cervical discectomy and fusion with rigid anterior plate fixation? *Spine*. 2005;30:1756–1761.
8. Bazaz R, Lee MJ, Yoo JU. Incidence of dysphagia after anterior cervical spine surgery: a prospective study. *Spine*. 2002;27:2453–2458.
9. Winslow CP, Winslow TJ, Wax MK. Dysphonia and dysphagia following the anterior approach to the cervical spine. *Arch Otolaryngol Head Neck Surg*. 2001;127:51–55.
10. Eck JC, Humphreys SC, Lim TH, et al. Biomechanical study on the effect of cervical spine fusion on adjacent-level intradiscal pressure and segmental motion. *Spine*. 2002;27:2431–2434.
11. DiAngelo DJ, Roberston JT, Metcalf NH, et al. Biomechanical testing of an artificial cervical joint and an anterior cervical plate. *J Spinal Disord Tech*. 2003;16:314–323.
12. Hilibrand AS, Carlson GD, Palumbo MA, et al. Radiculopathy and myelopathy at segments adjacent to the site of a previous anterior cervical arthrodesis. *J Bone Joint Surg Am*. 1999;81:519–528.
13. Lunsford LD, Bissonette DJ, Jannetta PJ, et al. Anterior surgery for cervical disc disease. Part 1: treatment of lateral cervical disc herniation in 253 cases. *J Neurosurg*. 1980;53:1–11.
14. Henderson CM, Hennessy RG, Shuey HM Jr, et al. Posterior-lateral foraminotomy as an exclusive operative technique for cervical radiculopathy: a review of 846 consecutively operated cases. *Neurosurgery*. 1983;13:504–512.
15. Robertson JT, Papadopoulos SM, Traynelis VC. Assessment of adjacent-segment disease in patients treated with cervical fusion or arthroplasty: a prospective 2-year study. *J Neurosurg Spine*. 2005;3:417–423.
16. Watters WC III, Levinthal R. Anterior cervical discectomy with and without fusion. Results, complications, and long-term follow-up. *Spine*. 1994;19:2343–2347.

17. Mummaneni PV, Burkus JK, Haid RW, et al. Clinical and radiographic analysis of cervical disc arthroplasty compared with allograft fusion: a randomized controlled clinical trial. *J Neurosurg Spine*. 2007;6:198–209.

18. Heller JG, Sasso RC, Papadopoulos SM, et al. Comparison of BRYAN cervical disc arthroplasty with anterior cervical decompression and fusion: clinical and radiographic results of a randomized, controlled, clinical trial. *Spine (Phila Pa 1976)*. 2009;34:1740.

19. Murrey D, Janssen M, Delamarter R, et al. Results of the prospective, randomized, controlled multicenter Food and Drug Administration investigational device exemption study of the ProDisc-C total disc replacement versus anterior discectomy and fusion for the treatment of 1-level symptomatic cervical disc disease. *J Bone Joint Surg Am*. 2009;91:2748.

20. Zeidman SM, Ducker TB. Posterior cervical laminoforaminotomy for radiculopathy: review of 172 cases. *Neurosurgery*. 1993;33:356–362.

21. Herkowitz HN, Kurz LT, Overholt DP. Surgical management of cervical soft disc herniation. A comparison between the anterior and posterior approach. *Spine*. 1990;15:1026–1030.

22. Adamson TE. Microendoscopic posterior cervical laminoforaminotomy for unilateral radiculopathy: results of a new technique in 100 cases. *J Neurosurg*. 2001;95:51–57.

23. Robinson RA, Smith GW. Anterolateral cervical disc removal and interbody fusion for cervical disc syndrome. *Bull Johns Hopkins Hosp*. 1955;96:223–224.

24. Shen FH, Samartzis D, Khanna N, et al. Comparison of clinical and radiographic outcome in instrumented anterior cervical discectomy and fusion with or without direct uncovertebral joint decompression. *Spine J*. 2004;4:629–635.

25. Baskin DS, Ryan P, Sonntag V, et al. A prospective, randomized, controlled cervical fusion study using recombinant human bone morphogenetic protein-2 with the CORNERSTONE-SR allograft ring and the ATLANTIS anterior cervical plate. *Spine*. 2003;28:1219–1224; discussion 25.

26. Smucker JD, Rhee JM, Singh K, et al. Increased swelling complications associated with off-label usage of rhBMP-2 in the anterior cervical spine. *Spine*. 2006;31:2813–2819.

27. Shields LB, Raque GH, Glassman SD, et al. Adverse effects associated with high-dose recombinant human bone morphogenetic protein-2 use in anterior cervical spine fusion. *Spine*. 2006;31:542–547.

28. Rhee JM, Riew KD. Dynamic anterior cervical plates. *J Am Acad Orthop Surg*. 2007;15:640–646.

29. Park JB, Cho YS, Riew KD. Development of adjacent-level ossification in patients with an anterior cervical plate. *J Bone Joint Surg Am*. 2005;87:558–563.

30. Campbell MJ, Carreon LY, Traynelis V, et al. Use of cervical collar after single-level anterior cervical fusion with plate: is it necessary? *Spine*. 2009;34:43–48.

31. Schunemann HJ, Jaeschke R, Cook DJ, et al. An official ATS statement: Grading the quality of evidence and strength of recommendations in ATS guidelines and recommendations. *Am J Respir Crit Care Med*. 2006;174:605–614.

32. Rhee JM, Patel N, Yoon ST, et al. High graft resorption rates with dense cancellous allograft in anterior cervical discectomy and fusion. *Spine*. 2007;32:2980–2984.

Cervical Degeneration with C8 Radiculopathy

CHINTAN SAMPAT, MD AND DAVID H. KIM, MD

■ EDITORS' CASE PRESENTATION

A 73-year-old man with a history of multiple myeloma presents with right upper extremity pain that radiates into the medial aspect of the forearm and the ulnar two digits. Initially worked up for cubital tunnel syndrome, he had undergone an electromyogram (EMG) that demonstrated right-sided C8 involvement. He has no complaints of neck pain, clumsiness, or balance difficulty. He subjectively complains of some weakness on the right side compared to the left side.

Upon physical examination, he has mild intrinsic wasting of the right hand. The patient demonstrates sensation that is equal bilaterally. Finger abduction and grip strength is mildly decreased on the right side. He has a negative Spurling test and negative Lhermitte sign. Reflexes are also equal bilaterally. Range of motion of the neck is full and painless.

Radiographic imaging studies are shown in Figures 4.1 to 4.3.

INTERPRETATION OF CLINICAL PRESENTATION

The clinical scenario describes an older man presenting with unilateral right forearm/hand pain and weakness in the right ulnar nerve distribution. The differential diagnoses include compression of the spinal cord, C8 nerve root, brachial plexus, ulnar nerve, or a combination of these structures (so-called double crush syndrome). Additional diagnostic possibilities include thoracic outlet syndrome (TOS), brachial neuritis, and tendinosis of the common flexor tendon (i.e., golfer's elbow).

The history involves unilateral involvement of the right upper extremity with pain and subjective weakness. There are no complaints of clumsiness or difficulty with balance. The additional history of multiple myeloma in this case makes it particularly important to consider spinal cord or nerve root compression, as up to 5% of these patients may present with myelopathic or radicular findings during their lifetime secondary to tumor involvement of the spine.[1] The physical examination reveals peripheral muscle atrophy and weakness in the C8 distribution, no Lhermitte sign, and equal deep tendon reflexes. These findings suggest neurocompression distal to the spinal cord. Cervical radiculopathy is possible despite a negative Spurling test, as this test is 93% specific but only 30% sensitive in identifying anatomic cervical nerve root compression.[2] An additional and potentially useful physical exam maneuver for cervical radiculopathy not described here is the shoulder abduction sign, which results in relief of radicular pain with abduction of the shoulder.[3] This test is between 80% and 100% specific but only 43% to 50% sensitive for cervical nerve root compression.[4]

The EMG demonstrates evidence of a right C8 radiculopathy without evidence of compression of the ulnar nerve in the cubital tunnel or Guyon canal. Additionally, the EMG findings decrease the likelihood of entrapment of the anterior interosseous nerve, which can mimic C8 radiculopathy. Finally, the EMG results make the existence of a double-crush syndrome less likely. In general, a double crush syndrome is considered very rare in the ulnar nerve distribution.[5] The potential sources of anatomic C8 nerve root compression within or in proximity to the C7-T1 neuroforamen include a C7-T1 disc herniation, spondylotic foraminal stenosis, epidural arteriovenous malformation, neoplastic involvement of the nerve sheath or nerve root, pathologic vertebral fracture, or direct pressure by a vertebral neoplasm or Pancoast apical lung tumor.[1,6–8]

TOS may also lead to similar symptoms. The prevalence and incidence of TOS are unknown due to controversy regarding the symptoms and etiology

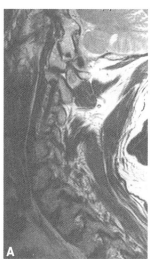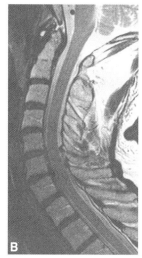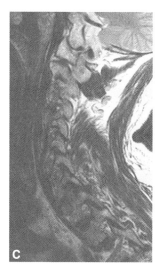

Figure 4.1.

of the disease. The sources of compression in TOS include a prominent C7 transverse process, cervical rib, congenital fibrous bands, or anomalous anterior scalene musculature.[9] TOS typically leads to worsening symptoms with Adson maneuver (arm along the side, neck hyperextension, and ipsilateral head turning) or Wright maneuver (arm abduction and external rotation of the shoulder). These findings are not described in this patient. EMG has not been shown to provide reliable information regarding this diagnosis.[9] This patient's MRI scan does not show any abnormal anatomic structures suggestive of TOS.

Brachial neuritis, also known as Parsonage-Turner syndrome, is an idiopathic condition that can produce sudden, unilateral arm pain, often followed by significant arm weakness.[10,11] The etiology is hypothesized to involve a postviral or autoimmune neuritis although this remains unclear. Typically, the syndrome involves the upper trunk of the brachial plexus. However, lesions of the ulnar nerve have been described, which may lead to findings similar to those of our

patient. This diagnosis is one of exclusion and should be considered when findings of advanced imaging studies do not correlate with the history and physical examination.

The MRI scan images include two T1-weighted paramedian cuts (Fig. 4.1A and C) and a midline sagittal cut (Fig. 4.1B). Figure 4.1A shows potentially significant stenosis of the right C7-T1 neuroforamen with hypertrophy of the facet joint synovium and absence of the normal fat signal around the exiting C8 nerve root. Figure 4.1B shows a small (<15%) anterolisthesis of C7 upon T1. Of note, there is also mild degeneration of the C6-7 disc (Fig. 4.1B) with a small posterior disc bulge.

Axial T1-weighted images show a broad-based left-sided posterolateral disc bulge at C6-7 (Fig. 4.2C) and right-sided foraminal stenosis at the C7-T1 level again with absence of the normal fat signal around the exiting C8 nerve root (Fig 4.2D). Hypertrophy of the ligamentum flavum and right C7-T1 facet joint synovium is again visualized. The C7-T1 disc is not visualized. Of

C4-5	C5-6	C6-7	C7-T1

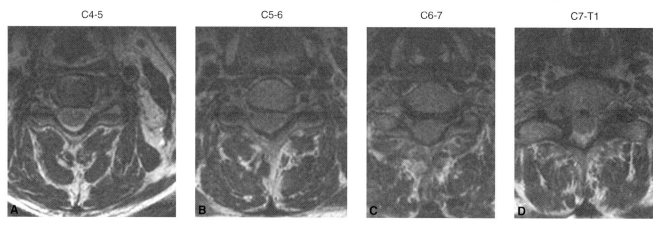

Figure 4.2.

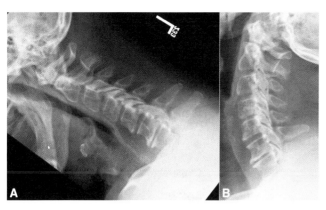

Figure 4.3.

note, this patient does not appear to exhibit symptoms specifically referable to the C6-7 spondylosis and disc degeneration seen on imaging. He lacks axial neck pain, and has no signs or symptoms of C7 nerve root impingement.

The MRI scan does not show any signal change within the spinal cord or any evidence of neoplasm. The lateral radiographs, including flexion (Fig. 4.3A) and extension (Fig. 4.3B) views, show maintenance of normal cervical alignment. Spondylotic degeneration is again observed at the C6-7 level with decreased disc space height and ventral osteophyte formation between vertebral bodies. The cervicothoracic junction is poorly visualized with the shoulders obscuring the C7-T1 level. Importantly, there is no evidence of increased instability with flexion and extension at the C7-T1 level despite the mild anterolisthesis seen on MRI. There are no fractures or pathologic lesions seen on the radiographs.

DECLARATION OF SPECIFIC DIAGNOSIS

This patient has symptomatic right-sided C8 nerve root compression in the neuroforamen secondary to spondylosis with hypertrophic ligamentum flavum and synovial tissue at the C7-T1 facet joint. There exists mild C7-T1 anterolisthesis without segmental instability. There exists mild, apparently asymptomatic, spondylosis and disc degeneration at the adjacent C6-7 level.

BRAINSTORMING: WHAT ARE THE TREATMENT GOALS AND SURGICAL OPTIONS?

The treatment goals are

1. Relieve the compression and/or irritation of the right C8 nerve root
2. Maintain spinal stability

3. Facilitate early mobilization
4. Rehabilitation and healing
5. Minimize the risk of adjacent segment degeneration

The treatment options are

1. Nonsurgical and noninvasive management with anti-inflammatory/analgesic medications, traction, bracing, and activity modification
2. Corticosteroid cervical spinal injection, including cervical epidural, transforaminal selective C8 nerve root injection (diagnostic and therapeutic)
3. Anterior cervical discectomy and fusion
4. Anterior cervical foraminotomy
5. Posterior cervical foraminotomy

EVALUATION OF THE LITERATURE

A search was performed in the PubMed database to identify relevant publications on C8 radiculopathy and cervicothoracic degeneration. Key words for the search included "cervicothoracic," "C8 and radiculopathy," "cervical and degeneration," "cervical and radiculopathy," "cervical and spondylosis," and "radiculopathy and natural history." A similar search was performed in the MedLine database. Journals were hand searched and references were reviewed to identify pertinent articles. The search was limited to English language articles. There were 74 abstracts that were reviewed and 38 full text articles were read in detail.

DETAILED REVIEW OF PERTINENT ARTICLES

Natural History of Cervical Radiculopathy

There is a paucity of literature describing the natural history of cervical radiculopathy.[8] Lees and Turner[12] reported their experience with 51 nonmyelopathic patients with cervical spondylosis with complaints of pain in the neck, shoulder, arm, or hand. Nonoperative treatment was associated with rapid and complete resolution of symptoms in 45% of patients, while the remaining patients continued to experience minor or moderate symptoms. No patient developed myelopathy in follow-up up to 19 years. Gore et al.[13] reported similar findings in a study of 205 patients with cervical spondylosis and axial neck pain or upper extremity radiculopathy. At 10- to

25-year follow-up, 43% of 161 patients had resolution of pain with conservative management involving rest, traction, a collar, medications, or combinations of these treatments. The remaining 57% of patients continued to experience mild to severe pain. Patients with radicular symptoms were found to have a worse prognosis than those with isolated axial neck pain.

Radiculopathy secondary to soft disc herniation has a favorable prognosis with nonoperative treatment because of the likelihood of spontaneous resorption of herniated disc material. On the other hand, radiculopathy secondary to posterior marginal uncovertebral osteophytes, so-called "hard disc herniations," or foraminal stenosis due to hypertrophic ligamentum flavum and synovium tends to worsen with aging, and often continues to be symptomatic.[14]

Nonoperative Versus Operative Treatment

This patient has subjective pain and mild weakness consistent with C8 radiculopathy. The C8 nerve root compression is primarily due to posterior pathology, including hypertrophy of the synovial tissue and ligamentum flavum. The patient appears to be asymptomatic with respect to the C6-7 spondylosis. The favorable natural history of nearly half of affected patients indicates that this patient should initially be treated nonoperatively with activity modification and nonsteroidal or narcotic pain medication as needed for reasonable pain control. The use of a soft collar, traction, and physical therapy is poorly supported by clinical evidence but these are often added to a nonoperative treatment regimen. Early surgery in this patient could be considered for progressive hand weakness or ongoing severe radicular pain that is inadequately controlled by conservative measures. This patient appears to be at very low risk of developing severe myelopathy, which would be the only absolute indication for surgery in this particular case. Other factors to consider in the selection and timing of treatment include specific occupational needs, issues of secondary gain such as on-going litigation or worker's compensation, and specific psychosocial characteristics. Elective surgical treatment becomes an option for this patient if significant radicular symptoms persist despite conservative treatment for a period of approximately 8 to 12 weeks.[15] Overall, the decision of when to operate on this patient is based on evidence of low quality.

Nonoperative Treatment

Nonoperative treatment of cervical radiculopathy may include rest, medications, physical therapy, manipulation, and injections.[16]

Rest. There are no clinical studies specifically addressing the role of bedrest in the treatment of acute cervical radiculopathy. In a prospective randomized trial of acute low back pain, Deyo et al.[17] showed no added benefit of bedrest for 7 days compared with 48 hours and in fact an increased risk of diminished muscle strength and osteopenia associated with longer periods of bedrest.

Medications. No clinical study has demonstrated the ability of any medication to alter the natural history of cervical radiculopathy. Agents are used to treat the symptoms only and include oral medications such as corticosteroids, nonsteroidal anti-inflammatory drugs, muscle relaxants, narcotics, and antidepressants.[16,18] In general, prolonged use of nonsteroidal anti-inflammatory medication can lead to gastric, hepatic, and renal disorders and should be supervised. Narcotic pain medication and benzodiazepines have well-known abuse potential.

Physical Therapy. Physical therapy does not appear to affect the intermediate or long-term natural history of cervical radiculopathy. However, enrolment in physical therapy may maintain paravertebral muscle tone and cervical range of motion in the early phase.[16,19] Similarly, use of cervical traction does not appear to have a significant effect on axial neck pain or radicular symptoms.[19] There is little evidence to support the use of transcutaneous electrical stimulation for cervical radiculopathy.

Manipulation. Manipulation has not been shown to be effective in improving the natural history of cervical radiculopathy. However, there are reports of iatrogenic neurologic injury with high-velocity thrusting maneuvers, and this should be discouraged.[16]

Injection. No clinical study has demonstrated the ability of any medications injected around cervical nerve roots to alter the natural history of cervical radiculopathy. However, selective nerve root blocks may be a useful adjunct to establish the diagnosis of cervical radiculopathy. The potential risks of such injections should be discussed with the patient, including serious complications such as death, epidural hematoma, paralysis, vertebral artery injury, and stroke.[20]

Operative Treatment

Assuming failure of nonoperative treatment of this patient, surgical decompression may be performed from an anterior or posterior approach. Anterior surgical options include anterior cervical discectomy with fusion (ACDF) or anterior cervical foraminotomy. The goal of anterior surgery would be to provide a direct decompression of any disc material and uncovertebral osteophytes compressing the C8 nerve. Additionally, ACDF would provide indirect decompression of the nerve root via distraction at the C7-T1 level, resulting in a taller neural foramen and decreased buckling of the ligamentum flavum. The fusion component of the surgery would provide immediate stabilization of the motion segment and elimination of a majority of any dynamic component of nerve root irritation. Successful healing of the fusion would also remove a majority of the stimulus for ongoing pathological tissue generation such as disc-osteophyte complexes or recurrent disc herniation.

Posterior surgery involves foraminotomy with direct decompression of the hypertrophic synovial tissue and ligamentum flavum. Both anterior and posterior foraminotomy options have the added benefit of avoiding fusion-related complications including those associated with use of bone graft and instrumentation, pseudoarthrosis, and the theoretical issue of accelerated adjacent-level degeneration.

The cervicothoracic junction represents a transition from the relatively stiff, kyphotic thoracic spine to a more mobile, lordotic cervical spine.[21,22] This region therefore represents a natural stress riser when exposed to routine physiologic loading and is particularly vulnerable to destabilization with any surgical approach.[22] The anterior surgical approach to this level is complicated by the proximity of the right brachiocephalic artery, innominate vein, left common carotid artery, sympathetic chain, thoracic duct, recurrent laryngeal nerve, sternum, and thoracic rib cage.[23–26] In some cases, anterior approach to the cervicothoracic junction may require splitting of the sternum, manubrium, or clavicle. Thoracic kyphosis can make visualization of the inferior endplate of C7 particularly difficult from an anterior approach.[25]

Fortunately, disc herniation at the C7-T1 level is relatively rare, accounting for only 4% to 8% of cervical disc herniations.[6,27] The rarity of disc herniations at this level may be due to the relative stiffness of the cervicothoracic junction as compared to the more mobile cephalad cervical levels.[6,21,28] Most disc herniations at the C7-T1 tend to displace laterally, possibly due to the absence of uncovertebral joints which form lateral margins around the disc space at the more cephalad levels.[28] For obvious anatomic reasons, lateral disc herniations are typically associated with radiculopathy as opposed to myelopathy.

The C8 nerve root is longer in the cranial-caudal direction and exits the C7-T1 intervertebral foramen more laterally relative to the more cephalad nerve roots.[29] The C8 nerve root is also uniquely cephalad to the C7-T1 disc, such that the most significant contact with disc herniations occurs at the exit zone of the neural foramen. Therefore, if a posterior foraminotomy is chosen for treatment, a larger C7-T1 facet resection in the lateral and cephalad directions may be required.[20] Decreased torsional stiffness and increased posterior strain with flexion in the cervical spine results from excessive facet resection, and avoidance of >50% resection of an individual facet joint has been recommended to prevent iatrogenic hypermobility.[30]

Outcomes of Surgery in the Literature

Posterior Cervical Foraminotomy. Harrop et al.[26] performed a retrospective review of 19 patients undergoing posterior cervical foraminotomy/discectomy for cervicothoracic radiculopathy resulting from either lateral disc herniation or foraminal stenosis. The follow-up period ranged from 23 to 62 months. The surgical protocol involved an open posterior keyhole laminoforaminotomy with removal of the medial one third of the facet joint. Subsequently, discectomy was performed if a lateral disc herniation was present and significant C8 nerve root compression persisted. Significant improvement in radicular pain was reported from a mean preoperative visual analog scale (VAS range 0–10) score of 7.45 to 0.2 ($p < 0.0001$). Nine of sixteen patients had complete resolution of preoperative numbness, with the remaining seven patients having partial improvement. Preoperative weakness was present in 11 patients. Eight of eleven patients with preoperative weakness had complete recovery of strength postoperatively occurring in <1 week, with the remaining patients having partial recovery. There were no significant surgical complications reported.

Witzmann et al.[31] reported good to excellent outcomes in 94% of 67 patients in a retrospective review of posterior cervical foraminotomy with mean follow-up of 3 years. Three patients in this study had C7-T1 spondylosis. The mean time to recovery of preoperative weakness was 33 weeks in these three patients. One of these three patients had persistent paresthesias despite surgery.

Kumar et al.[32] reported good to excellent outcomes in 95.5% of 89 patients in a retrospective review of posterior cervical foraminotomy at mean follow-up of 8.6 months. Four patients in this study had C8 radiculopathy. Outcomes were favorable in these patients, including resolution of preoperative arm pain in all patients. Furthermore, sensation and strength improved in 75% and 89% of patients, respectively.

All three of these studies are retrospective, cohort observational studies without any control groups. Overall, these studies represent the best available evidence to support the use of posterior cervical foraminotomy for cervical radiculopathy.

Open and minimally invasive endoscopic techniques have been described to perform posterior cervical foraminotomy.[33,34] Potential advantages of the minimally invasive technique include decreased blood loss, shorter hospitalization, and decreased postoperative pain medication requirements.[35] However, the endoscopic technique requires specific training to be performed safely. Furthermore, there are no comparative outcome studies to demonstrate long-term superiority of either technique.

Anterior Cervical Foraminotomy. Johnson et al.[36] performed a retrospective study of anterior cervical foraminotomy for unilateral radiculopathy via the Jho technique. Only one patient was treated at the C7-T1 level. This patient had continued dominant hand weakness postoperatively and was treated with subsequent posterior foraminotomy at the same level. This patient did not have any approach-related complications.

Anterior Cervical Discectomy and Fusion. We did not find any studies in the literature evaluating the outcome of ACDF specifically for a diagnosis of C7-T1 foraminal stenosis without a disc herniation. Post et al.[6] reported the outcomes of ACDF in ten patients with disc herniation at the C7-T1 level. Follow-up ranged from 6 to 99 months. They reported no difficulty in performing the surgery with a standard Smith-Robinson approach. All patients had immediate resolution of radicular pain postoperatively. One patient had transient vocal cord dysfunction, which resolved in 1 month. There were no hardware or graft-related complications.

Boockvar et al.[37] reported a 36% rate of graft-plate failure at the cervicothoracic junction and cited the biomechanical transition from a stiff, kyphotic thoracic spine to a more mobile, lordotic cervical spine as the main reason. Steinmetz et al.[22] also reported on the unique biomechanical stresses present at the cervicothoracic junction, and the potential for failure of fusion constructs. Ruetten et al.[34] reported equivalent outcomes at 2-year follow-up between ACDF and endoscopic posterior foraminotomy for lateral disc

herniation in a prospective, randomized trial. However, the specific cervical levels treated were not described.

EVIDENTIARY TABLE AND SELECTION OF TREATMENT METHOD

The best available evidence dictates that the patient presented in this clinical scenario should be initially treated nonoperatively. These results are summarized in Table 4.1. If symptoms persist for longer than 8 to 12 weeks despite nonoperative treatment, then a posterior cervical foraminotomy should be offered to the patient on an elective basis. The best available evidence for this treatment is summarized in Table 4.2.

DEFINITIVE TREATMENT PLAN

This patient's history and physical examination reveal only unilateral upper extremity radiculopathy without axial neck pain. The imaging studies show C7-T1 foraminal stenosis without a significant disc herniation. He should initially be managed with nonoperative treatment including brief rest, medications, physical therapy, activity modification, and pos-

---

TABLE 4.1 Evidentiary Table: A Summary of the Quality of Evidence for Nonoperative Treatment of Cervical Radiculopathy.

Paper Author (Year)	Description	Summary of Results	Quality of Evidence
Gore et al. (1987)	Prospective cohort study No control group	• 205 patients with cervical spondylosis and axial neck pain or upper extremity radiculopathy • At 10–25 y follow-up, 43% of 161 patients had resolution of pain with conservative management • Remaining 57% had continued mild to severe pain • Patients with radicular symptoms were found to have a worse prognosis than those with isolated axial neck pain	Low
Lees and Turner (1963)	Retrospective cohort study No control group	• 51 nonmyelopathic patients with cervical spondylosis with complaints of pain in the neck, shoulder, arm, or hand • At 2–19-year follow-up, nonoperative treatment resulted in complete resolution of symptoms in 45% of patients • Remaining 55% patients continued to experience minor or moderate symptoms. • No patient developed myelopathy in follow-up up to 19 y.	Low

TABLE 4.2 Evidentiary Table: A Summary of the Quality of Evidence for Posterior Cervical Foraminotomy for Cervical Radiculopathy.

Paper Author (Year)	Description	Summary of Results	Quality of Evidence
Harrop et al. (2003)	Retrospective cohort study No control group	• 19 patients with cervicothoracic radiculopathy secondary to disc herniation or foraminal stenosis • Follow-up 23–62 mo • Significant improvement in pain, numbness, and weakness was found postoperatively	Very low
Witzmann et al. (2000)	Retrospective cohort study No control group	• 67 patients with cervical radiculopathy (3 with C8 radiculopathy) • Mean follow-up 3 years • One of three patients with C7-T1 radiculopathy had persistent paresthesias despite surgery	Very low
Kumar et al. (1998)	Retrospective cohort study No control group	• 89 patients with cervical radiculopathy (4 with C8 radiculopathy) • Good to excellent outcome in 95.5% of patients at mean 8.6 mo follow-up • All four patients with C8 radiculopathy had resolution of arm pain postoperatively	Very low

sible corticosteroid injections. The natural history is favorable with nonoperative treatment. The literature does not guide us in deciding when to offer operative treatment to this patient. Anecdotal evidence suggests surgical treatment may be offered to this patient on an elective basis if the symptoms persist, despite conservative treatment, for longer than 8 to 12 weeks.

The surgical treatment for this patient should be a right-sided posterior cervical laminoforaminotomy. This technique avoids any approach-related complications associated with anterior procedures. The buckled ligamentum flavum and hypertrophic synovial tissue should be removed. The exiting C8 nerve root should be visualized. The decompression should be carried laterally until a small probe can easily be passed lateral to the C7 pedicle in the neural foramen. Care should be taken to avoid resection of >50% of the C7-T1 facet joint to prevent iatrogenic postoperative instability. This procedure may be performed safely by a fellowship-trained spine surgeon.

Grading the Evidence for this Plan

The evidence to support initial nonoperative treatment for our patient would be considered low grade as it is derived from observational cohort studies of low quality without any controls. The evidence to support posterior cervical foraminotomy if the patient has continuing symptoms despite nonoperative treatment would be considered low as it is derived from observational cohort studies of very low quality without any

controls. The treatment goals have been met based on the studies listed in Tables 4.1 and 4.2.

In accordance with the method of grading recommendations set forth by Schünemann et al.[38] our proposed treatment of initial nonoperative treatment would be considered a **strong recommendation**. In the case of persistent symptoms, our treatment with posterior cervical foraminotomy would be considered a **weak recommendation**.

PREDICTING OUTCOMES

The outcome of nonsurgical treatment of this patient is predicted by the natural history studies.[12,13] We expect an approximate 45% chance of complete resolution of symptoms. If he has persistent symptoms, and chooses to undergo posterior laminoforaminotomy, we would expect an approximate 95% chance for a good to excellent outcome, with significant improvement in his radicular pain and weakness.[26,31,32] Prior to any surgical intervention, a thorough and frank discussion should be carried out with the patient regarding the natural history of the disease, as well as the risks and benefits of surgical treatment. This patient must understand that surgical treatment may be carried out on an elective basis.

These outcomes are consistent with our experience. Initial nonoperative treatment of cervical radiculopathy has a good success rate. We offer surgical treatment to patients with symptoms persisting longer than 8 to

12 weeks despite nonoperative treatment or those with progressive neurological deficits.

SUMMARY

We are presented with a 73-year-old man with right-sided C8 radiculopathy secondary to foraminal stenosis due to spondylosis. The most appropriate treatment for this patient would be an initial trial of nonoperative treatment for up to 12 weeks. If symptoms persist, the patient should be offered posterior surgical decompression on an elective basis. An improvement in his pain and weakness is anticipated.

REFERENCES

1. Dispenzieri A, Kyle RA. Neurological aspects of multiple myeloma and related disorders. *Best Prac Res Clin Haematol.* 2005;18:673–688.

2. Tong HC, Haig AJ, Yamakawa K. The Spurling test and radiculopathy. *Spine.* 2002;27:156–159.

3. Davidon RI, Dunn EJ, Metzmaker JN. The shoulder abduction test in the diagnosis of radicular pain in cervical extradural compressive monoradiculopathies. *Spine.* 1981;6:441–446.

4. Viikari-Juntura E, Porras M, Laasonen EM. Validity of clinical tests in the diagnosis of root compression in cervical disease. *Spine.* 1989;14:253–257.

5. Morgan G, Wilbourn AJ. Cervical radiculopathy and coexisting distal entrapment neuropathies—double crush syndromes. *Neurology.* 1998;50:78–83.

6. Post NH, Cooper PR, Frempong-Boadu AK, et al. Unique features of herniated discs at the cervicothoracic junction: clinical presentation, imaging, operative management, and outcome after anterior decompressive operation in 10 patients. *Neurosurgery.* 2006;59:497–501.

7. Vargo MM, Flood KM. Pancoast tumor presenting as cervical radiculopathy. *Arch Phys Med Rehab.* 1990;71:606–609.

8. Rao R. Neck pain, cervical radiculopathy, and cervical myelopathy—Pathophysiology, natural history, and clinical evaluation. *J Bone Joint Surg Am.* 2002;84:1872–1881.

9. Leffert RD. Thoracic outlet syndrome. *J Am Acad Orthop Surg.* 1994;2:317–325.

10. Misamore GW, Lehman DE. Parsonage-Turner syndrome (acute brachial neuritis). *J Bone Joint Surg Am.* 1996;78:1405–1408.

11. Feinberg JH, Doward DA, Gonsalves A. Cervical radiculopathy vs. Parsonage-Turner syndrome: a case report. *HSS J.* 2007;3:106–111.

12. Lees F, Turner JWA. Natural history and prognosis of cervical spondylosis. *Br Med J.* 1963;2:1607–1610.

13. Gore DR, Sepic SB, Gardner GM, et al. Neck pain: a long-term follow-up of 205 patients. *Spine.* 1987;12:1–5.

14. Bush K, Chaudhuri R, Hillier S, et al. The pathomorphologic changes that accompany the resolution of cervical radiculopathy: a prospective study with repeat magnetic resonance imaging. *Spine.* 1997;22:183–186.

15. Fischgrund JS. Surgical management of cervical radiculopathy: anterior procedures. In: Clark CR, ed. *The Cervical Spine.* 4th ed. Philadelphia, PA: Lippincott Williams & Wilkins, 2005:1017–1031.

16. Weber SE, Rechtine G. Nonoperative treatment of radiculopathy and myelopathy. In: Clark CR, ed. *The Cervical Spine.* 4th ed. Philadelphia, PA: Lippincott Williams & Wilkins, 2005:991–994.

17. Deyo RA, Dhihl AK, Rosenthal M. How many days of bed rest for acute low back pain? A randomized clinical trial. *N Engl J Med.* 1986;315:1064–1070.

18. Dillin W, Uppal G. Analysis of medications used in the treatment of cervical disc degeneration. *Orthop Clin North Am.* 1992;23:421–433.

19. Graham N, Gross A, Goldsmith CH, et al. Mechanical traction for neck pain with or without radiculopathy. *Cochrane Database Syst Rev.* 2008;3:CD006408.

20. Wallace MA, Fukui MB, Williams RL, et al. Complications of cervical selective nerve root blocks performed with fluoroscopic guidance. *Am J Roentgenol.* 2007;188:1218–1221.

21. An HS, Vaccaro A, Cotler JM, et al. Spinal disorders at the cervicothoracic junction. *Spine.* 1994;19:2557–2564.

22. Steinmetz MP, Miller J, Warbel A, et al. Regional instability following cervicothoracic junction surgery. *J Neurosurg Spine.* 2006;4:278–284.

23. Luk KD, Cheung KM, Leong JC. Anterior approach to the cervicothoracic junction by unilateral or bilateral manubriotomy. *JBJS Am.* 2002;84A:1013–1017.

24. Ebraheim NA, Lu J, Yang H, et al. Vulnerability of the sympathetic truck during the anterior approach to the lower cervical spine. *Spine.* 2000;25:1603–1606.

25. Gieger M, Roth PA, Wu JK. The anterior cervical approach to the cervicothoracic junction. *Neurosurgery.* 1995;37:704–710.

26. Harrop JS, Silva MT, Sharan AD, et al. Cervicothoracic radiculopathy using a posterior cervical foraminotomy/discectomy. *J Neurosurg Spine.* 2003;98:131–136.

27. Murphey F, Simmons JC, Brunson B. Ruptured cervical discs: 1939 to 1972. *Clin Neurosurg.* 1973;20:9–17.

28. Yamazaki S, Kokubun S, Ishii Y, et al. Courses of cervical disc herniation causing myelopathy and radiculopathy. *Spine.* 2003;28:1171–1175.

29. Tanaka N, Fujimoto Y, An HS, et al. The anatomic relation among the nerve roots, intervertebral foramina, and intervertebral discs of the cervical spine. *Spine.* 2000;25:286–291.

30. Zdeblick TA, Zou D, Warden KE, et al. Cervical stability after foraminotomy: a biomechanical in vitro analysis. *JBJS Am.* 1992;74:22–27.

31. Witzmann A, Hejazi N, Krasznai L. Posterior cervical foraminotomy—a follow-up study of 67 surgically treated patients with compressive radiculopathy. *Neurosurg Rev.* 2000;23:213–217.

32. Kumar GRV, Maurice-Williams RS, Bradford R. Cervical foraminotomy—an effective treatment for cervical spondylotic radiculopathy. *Br J Neurosurg.* 1998;12:563–568.

33. Riew KD, Cheng I, Pimenta L, et al. Posterior cervical spine surgery for radiculopathy. *Neurosurgery.* 2007; 60-S1:57–63.

34. Ruetten S, Komp M, Merck H, et al. Full-endoscopic cervical posterior foraminotomy for the operation of

lateral disc herniations using 5.9 mm endoscopes. *Spine.* 2008;33:940–948.

35. Fessler RG, Knoo LT. Minimally invasive cervical microendoscopic foraminotomy: an initial experience. *J Neurosurg.* 2002;51:S37–S45.

36. Johnson JP, Filler AG, McBride DQ, et al. Anterior cervical foraminotomy for unilateral radicular disease. *Spine.* 2000;25:905–909.

37. Boockvar JA, Philips MF, Telfeian AE, et al. Results and risk factors for anterior cervicothoracic junction surgery. *J Neurosurg Spine.* 2001;94:12–17.

38. Schünemann HJ, Jaeschke R, Cook DJ, et al. An official ATS statement: grading the quality of evidence and strength of recommendations in ATS guidelines and recommendations. *Am J Respir Crit Care Med.* 2006;174: 605–614.

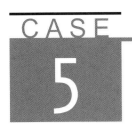

5 Two-Level Degeneration and Radiculopathy

AMY MARCINI, MD, KEVIN J. MCGUIRE, MD, MS, AND ANDREW P. WHITE, MD

EDITORS' CASE PRESENTATION

A 39-year-old man presents with a year and a half of neck and right arm pain. His arm pain is associated with numbness and tingling. The pain radiates down his arm and into the ulnar two digits. His neck pain is significant, however; he categorizes the symptoms as 50% neck and 50% arm. He has no difficulty with dexterity or balance and has no bowel or bladder complaints. He has undergone a prolonged and multimodal course of nonoperative treatment that has included epidural injections as well as physical therapy.

His physical examination demonstrates mildly decreased neck range of motion. His gait is normal. There is decreased sensation in the C7 and C8 distribution on the right side. He has a negative Hoffmann sign, but has an exquisitely positive Spurling sign provoked by rightward rotation. The patient has no Babinski sign, no clonus, and normal reflexes in the upper and lower extremities.

A magnetic resonance imaging (MRI) study was performed; T2-weighted sagittal (Fig. 5.1A–D) and axial (Fig. 5.2A–E) images characterize his disorder.

INTERPRETATION OF CLINICAL PRESENTATION

This patient presents with axial neck pain and equally bothersome unilateral arm pain. Both of these symptoms can be associated with cervical spondylosis; axial neck pain, radiculopathy, myelopathy, or a combination has been observed.[1] Axial neck pain may present in a nondermatomal distribution, radiating posteriorly to the shoulder or periscapular region.[2] In a review

of 736 patients with cervical radiculopathy, 80% of patients reported coincident neck pain.[3]

There is no subjective or objective evidence of cervical myelopathy in this patient. He demonstrates a normal gait, and has normal deep tendon reflex responses in the upper and lower extremities. The described long tract evaluations are normal, as well. With this presentation, clinically significant myelopathy can be considered unlikely.

The patient's arm pain radiates, terminating in the ulnar two digits. Objective physical examination findings include decreased sensation in the C7 and C8 distribution. This correlates with the nerve root level of his subjective radicular pain. Additionally, this patient demonstrates a sensitive Spurling sign, provoking exacerbation of his arm symptoms. In patients with arm pain, the Spurling test can be used to help confirm a cervical radiculopathy, but is not very useful as a screening tool. The Spurling sign was found to be 30% sensitive and 93% specific in predicting abnormalities found on electrodiagnostic testing in 255 consecutive patients referred to an electrodiagnostic clinic.[4]

The MR images include four T2-weighted sagittal images (Fig. 5.1) and T2 weighted axial images for C3-T1 (Fig. 5.2). The axial images at the level of the C3-4 and the C4-5 disks demonstrate no significant foraminal or central stenosis and no significant imaging evidence of spondylosis. There is, however, evidence of desiccation of the C5-6 and the C6-7 nucleus seen with a relative decrease in the T2 signal. There also are mild disk protrusions at C5-6 and C6-7, but with no effacement of the spinal cord. There is an osteophyte seen at the posterior-inferior aspect of C5, and posterior projecting osteophytes from the superior endplate and inferior endplate of C6. There is mild bilateral foraminal stenosis at C5-6. There is a right-sided, paramedian herniated nucleus pulposus at C6-7, encroaching on the C7 exiting nerve root. The C7-T1 level shows no evidence of neural compression and no radiographic spondylosis. There is no abnormal signal evident in the spinal cord.

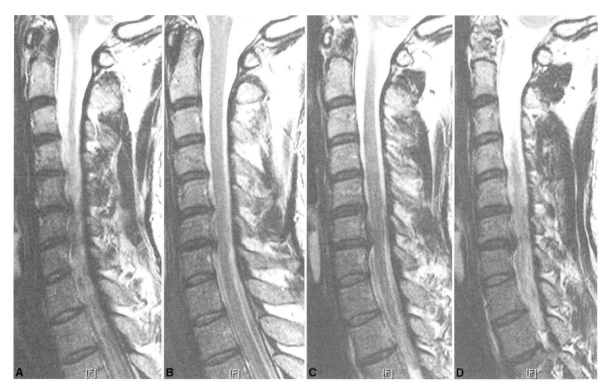

Figure 5.1.

While imaging studies are an important consideration to help reach a diagnosis, correlation of the clinical signs, symptoms, and provocative tests are critical in establishing an accurate diagnosis. It is important to recognize that MRI evidence of nerve root compression has been observed in 19% of asymptomatic individuals, and a reliable diagnosis of radiculopathy is best made by correlating clinical signs and symptoms with radiologic abnormalities.[5]

With regard to the etiology of the patients arm pain, the most significant finding on MRI is a soft disk herniation at C6-7. The patient has decreased sensation in the C7 and C8 distributions, as well as pain that radiates down the arm into the ulnar digits.

This radiculopathy correlates well with right-sided disk herniation, affecting the exiting C7 nerve root.

There is relative uncertainty as to the etiology of the patient's neck pain. The clinical scenario does not describe diagnostic tests that may help to characterize the pain or its cause. The source of pain may be discogenic or be related to the facet joints or other structures. There are radiographic signs of disk degeneration at the C5-6 and C6-7 levels. These spondylotic findings may or may not be incidental, given that pain may or may not be caused by this disorder.

His neck pain may be caused by other conditions entirely, many of which are not associated with imaging abnormalities. In the evidence reviewed by the

C3-4 C4-5 C5-6 C6-7 C7-T1

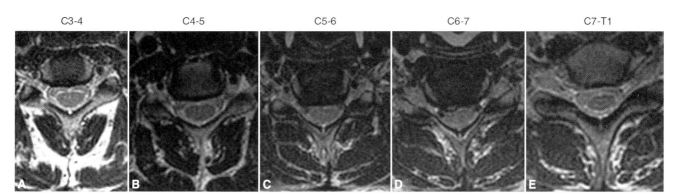

Figure 5.2.

Task Force on Neck Pain, it was determined that neck pain without clear radiculopathy cannot be reasonably ascribed to specific common degenerative changes seen on MRI.[6,18–20] In studies of asymptomatic volunteers, cervical MRI found a high prevalence (up to 78%) of imaging abnormalities, including disk degeneration, disk bulging, narrowing of the disk space, foraminal stenosis, and/or abnormal spinal cord morphology.[7,8] This high prevalence of positive findings in asymptomatic individuals emphasizes that common degenerative findings on MRI imaging cannot be assumed to be the primary cause of the neck pain symptoms in adult patients.

DECLARATION OF SPECIFIC DIAGNOSIS

The diagnosis most consistent with the provided clinical presentation is cervical spondylotic radiculopathy. The patient demonstrates radiographic spondylosis at two intervertebral levels, C5-6 and C6-7, characterized by disk desiccation, loss of disk height, periarticular osteophytes, subchondral sclerosis, as well as a herniated disk at C6-7. His arm pain, concordant side and level of his imaging findings, with concordant sensory deficit, and with sensitive provocation by Spurling maneuver, is most likely attributed to right-sided C7 nerve root compression. His neck pain, however, may or may not be related to his spondylosis.

BRAINSTORMING: WHAT ARE THE TREATMENT GOALS AND SURGICAL OPTIONS?

The treatment goals are

- Effective and efficient resolution or reduction of radicular symptoms
- Effective and efficient resolution or reduction of axial symptoms
- Maintenance or restoration of alignment
- Limitation of short and long-term morbidity

Treatment options include

- Observation
- Activity modifications
- Medications: NSAIDs, steroids, muscle relaxants, narcotics, others (SSRI, etc.)
- Immobilization/bracing
- Physical therapy
- Cervical traction
- Massage therapy
- Manipulation
- Acupuncture
- Epidural corticosteroid injections
- Other injections (trigger point, facet, etc.)
- Anterior cervical diskectomy/diskectomies and fusion
- Anterior cervical corpectomy and fusion
- Anterior cervical diskectomy (ACD) and cervical total disk replacement
- Posterior cervical laminoforaminotomy
- Posterior cervical laminoplasty
- Posterior cervical laminectomy

EVALUATION OF THE LITERATURE

Publications relevant to cervical radiculopathy were reviewed. A Medline search from 1950 to 2008 was performed, using MeSH (medical subject headings) as well as key words, with "human" and "English language" limits. This search strategy revealed 2801 results for "cervical radiculopathy," 8,915 results for "neck pain," 4,059 for "cervical fusion" and 3,271 for "cervical arthrodesis," 332 results for "adjacent segment disease," and 54 results for "multilevel disk disease." The results for "cervical fusion" when combined with "neck pain," yielded 429 results. "Cervical radiculopathy" and "neck pain" were combined for a total of 288 results. "Adjacent segment disease" and "cervical fusion" combined yielded 50 results.

The results were cross referenced to bibliographies from current editions of texts containing information on the assessment and management of cervical radiculopathy. Seventy abstracts in the English language were reviewed and 29 full text articles were read in detail.

DETAILED REVIEW OF PERTINENT ARTICLES

Nonoperative Versus Operative Treatment

A systematic review of pertinent texts and bibliographies was performed in order to determine the best treatment based on the available evidence. In a recent literature review by the Task Force on Neck Pain and Its Associated Disorders, it was determined that relatively rapid and substantial relief of pain and impairment may be reliably achieved following surgery for cervical radiculopathy in the short-term (6–12 weeks). It is not clear, however, that long-term outcomes are better with surgical treatment compared to nonoperative treatment.[6,18–20]

Generally accepted indications for surgical treatment of cervical radiculopathy include (a) persistent or recurrent radicular symptoms unresponsive to nonoperative management for at least 6 weeks, (b) disabling motor weakness of 6 weeks durations or less (i.e., deltoid palsy, wrist drop), (c) progressive neurologic deficit, (d) static neurologic deficit combined with radicular or referred pain, and (e) instability or deformity in combination with radicular symptoms.[9] It is important to recognize that many patient-related factors must also be considered in treatment decision making. For example, speed of recovery and ability to return to activity were found to be important considerations for patients when deciding whether to have surgery.[6,18–20] The most appropriate surgical options for this patient must address the compressed neural elements associated with his symptoms, but also aim to address his axial neck pain.

Surgical treatment of cervical radiculopathy yields excellent early results compared to preoperative status. With anterior cervical decompression, patients generally achieved a 50% or greater reduction in pain and a 60% to 70% improvement in functional scores which were maintained at 1 and 2 year follow-up.[6,18–20] In multiple studies, few subjects have been seen to have more than a moderate residual functional impairment following surgical treatment as determined by validated metrics such as the Neck Disability Index (NDI).[6,10–20] (Hacker, 2005) None of these studies, however, had a nonoperative control group. A randomized trial by Persson and et al.[21] compared a Cloward-type fusion to either physiotherapy or cervical collar for patients with cervical spondylosis and radicular pain. Pain reduction was greater in the fusion group at all time points up to 16 months, but functional scores were similar for operative and nonoperative groups. After 16 months, substantial cross-over between groups was noted, which may have limited the ability of the study to demonstrate a significant difference between groups.

Addressing Neck Pain and Radicular Symptoms

Axial symptoms may be discogenic. If this is the true etiology, and surgical treatment is required, then symptoms may be best addressed by anterior cervical diskectomy and fusion (ACDF) or total disk arthroplasty (TDA) as compared to procedures which preserve the existing articulation.

It has been observed that patients who underwent ACDF for cervical radiculopathy reported improvement in their neck pain.[22] In this prospective study of 38 patients who underwent ACDF for neck pain in the absence of myelopathy or radiculopathy, a significant decrease in pain, significant increase in function, and a high degree of patient satisfaction were reported. Outcomes were unaffected by worker's compensation status or gender. All the patients in the study had painful disks preoperatively, as determined by discography.

All patients who had moderately or severely painful disks based on provocative disk injection were included in the surgery; no one with painless levels underwent surgery. There were 17 patients with painful disks without structural abnormalities. Discography included the disk that was thought to be the pain generator based on MRI, CT, or radiographic results, as well as at least one level above and below. Normal disks served as controls and guided the limits of surgery. Patient function was evaluated with Oswestry Disability Questionnaire and pain level determined by a numerical rating scale. The mean preoperative rating for neck pain was 8.3 (range 3–10) versus 4.1 (range 0–10) postoperatively; this difference was found to be significant ($p < 0.001$). The preoperative score on the Oswestry Disability Questionnaire was 57.5 (range 0–89) and postoperatively 38.9 (range 0–80); also a significant finding ($p < 0.001$). Seventy-nine percent of patients were satisfied with the outcome of ACDF and 21% were not satisfied.[22]

One other study evaluating provocative discography in patients suffering from chronic head/neck pain demonstrated that these patients reported greater pain response on the whole (on a 0–10 scale of pain intensity).[23] Interestingly, 70% of asymptomatic patients in the group had a painful response of at least 4 or 5 on a scale of 0 to 10, showing a high rate of false-positives in provocative discography. In a separate study of false-positives in lumbar spine discography, it was shown that 10% of pain-free control volunteers had false-positive discography. Painful injections were more common in subjects with annular tears, especially in patients with compensation issues, chronic pain, and/or abnormal psychometric testing.[18–20,24]

In a series of 122 patients treated with ACDF for cervical radiculopathy with an average follow-up of 6 years, 81 patients (66%) had no neck pain, 26 patients had mild neck pain, 9 patients had moderate neck pain, 4 patients had mild radicular pain, and 2 patients had a combination of mild radicular pain and moderate neck pain.[16]

Adjacent Segment Disease and the Natural History of Cervical Spondylosis

In planning a cervical fusion, the determination of which and how many levels to treat must be made carefully. For patients with spondylosis at primary or adjacent segments, there is concern that ongoing or accelerated degeneration may become symptomatic in the future. It has been noted that 25% of patients undergoing cervical fusion will have new onset of symptoms within 10 years of cervical fusion. In a popular and typically misrepresented article, Hilibrand et al. presented a large series of patients who had undergone cervical fusion. This article reported the typical incidence of degeneration of segments adjacent to the fused level(s) as approximately 2.9% (range 0.0%–4.8%) per year following the index fusion procedure over the 21 year study period. Importantly, however, when considering the potential relationship between fusion and future adjacent segment disease (ASD), Hilibrand et al. reported an inverse relationship. Specifically, patients who underwent longer fusions were found to have lower incidence of ASD, despite the previously measured increase in forces at the adjacent segment in patients with long cervical fusions. This finding supports the concept that the natural history of spondylosis may be a greater influence on the development of ASD rather than a consequence of arthrodesis.

The prevalence of cervical spondylosis is level-dependent. As demonstrated in a retrospective review of 206 patients which classified radiographic findings according to the Modified Kellgran Scale, degenerative changes were most advanced at C5-6, followed by C6-7, C4-5, C3-4, C2-3.[25] This has been shown in other patient series as well. The prevalence of radiographic degeneration was noted in a series of 374 patients and was related to the level: C2-3 (1.2%), C3-4 (7.6%), C4-5 (9.3%), C5-6 (13.8%), C6-7 (13%).[26] Segments that were felt to be high-risk were those with greater range of motion, as described by White and Panjabi.[27]

Levels C5-6 and C6-7 show the greatest degenerative changes as well as the most common location for symptomatic ASD. This may be a biomechanical phenomenon due to greater mobility rather than a result of adjacent arthrodesis or failure of operative technique. When a multilevel fusion is performed, the segments at high risk for future degeneration may be included, with the fusion ending adjacent to segments typically at lower risk for developing disease. In single-level fusions, patients may have had preexisting spondylosis at the time of surgery, however since the segment was not symptomatic it was not included in the fusion. As a result of their findings, Hilibrand et al. recommends scrutinizing the adjacent segments of the caudal part of the cervical spine for degenerative changes prior to planning a decompression and fusion.

Motion Preservation

Among the surgical options for treating cervical radiculopathy and axial pain, cervical total disk replacement has been developed as an alternate to fusion. Maintenance of motion has also been proposed to provide a benefit in preventing adjacent segment degeneration.[28] In a multicenter, prospective randomized trial of 209 patients, TDA (with ProDisc-C, Synthes Spine Solutions, West Chester, Pennsylvania) was compared to ACDF. The NDI and visual analog scale (VAS) for both arm pain and neck pain were measured. At 24 months following treatment, 78.6% of arthroplasty patients had significant improvement

in neck pain intensity while 75.6% of patients treated with ACDF had improvement in intensity of neck pain (p = 0.7285). Of those patients treated with TDA, 76.5% had improvement in frequency of neck pain, compared to 78.9% of patients in the ACDF group (p = 0.7289). 84.9% of ProDisc-C patients showed clinically significant improvement in NDI compared to 85.9% of ACDF patients at 24 months after surgery. The mean visual analog scale at 24 months was 80.0 for ACDF and 83.4 for ProDisc-C. Both study groups showed high rates of maintenance or improvement of neurological success (motor, sensory, and reflexes) at 24 months; 88% for ACDF and 90.9% for ProDisc-C. ProDisc-C patients had a mean range of motion of 9.4 degrees at 24 months, while most ACDF patients had motion consistent with fusion (mean 0.9 degree). This was a trial of single-level disease only, and strict inclusion criteria needed to be met (approval letter: http://www.fda.gov/cdrh/pdf7/p070001a.pdf). Exclusion criteria for this trial included more than one vertebral level requiring treatment, radiographic facet joint disease or degeneration, severe spondylosis (characterized by bridging osteophytes, loss of disk height >50%, and/or absence of motion (<2 degrees), and neck or arm pain of unknown etiology.

The ideal candidate for cervical disk replacement may be a patient between 18 and 60 years of age affected by single-level disease with neck or arm pain and moderate disability, evidence of herniated nucleus pulposus or mild spondylosis with loss of disk height <50%. They would also have a NDI score ≥15/50 (30%). Other criteria include a failed course of nonoperative management for at least 6 weeks or the presence of progressive neurological deficits.

Studies have shown favorable outcomes of cervical disk replacement in the treatment of single-level disk disease at 2-year follow-up.[29] In one study, following disk replacement, an average of 7.9 degrees of flexion-extension was retained at 2-year follow-up, in contrast to 0.6 degrees of motion in the fusion group (p < 0.006 at all follow-up intervals leading up to 24 months). Also noted were significant differences in the arthroplasty group in the NDI, neck and arm pain Visual Analog Scores, and SF-36 physical component.

One radiographic study has demonstrated no significant kinematic differences at adjacent spinal levels between patients treated with the Bryan Cervical Disc (Medtronic Sofamor Danek, Memphis, Tennessee) or ACDF at 24-month follow-up. Rabin.[30] There were ten patients in the ACDF group and ten patients in the disk replacement group. Results from this study, which examined kinematics exclusively, seem to dispute the findings elsewhere in the literature, where a 34.6% rate of ASD after arthrodesis versus 17.5% after arthroplasty has been reported at 24 months. This was acknowledged to be a pilot study without enough statistical power, reiterating that larger sample sizes and longer follow-up periods are needed before any conclusions can be drawn on the effect of motion preservation on ASD. There is not enough evidence at this time to support the concept that cervical disk arthroplasty will decrease the incidence of ASD.

EVIDENTIARY TABLE AND SELECTION OF TREATMENT METHOD

Treatment goals for this patient are to alleviate the radicular and axial symptoms to the greatest extent possible and with the lowest risk of complications. A well defined syndrome which is refractory to 18 months of directed and multimodal nonoperative treatment warrants consideration for surgical treatment. The most appropriate surgical options for this patient must address the compressed neural elements associated with his symptoms, but also aim to address his axial neck pain. In selecting the most appropriate surgical treatment, literature addressing multilevel cervical radiculopathy with associated axial neck pain was scrutinized. The best evidence is summarized in Tables 5.1 to 5.3.

Anterior Cervical Diskectomy Alone

With ACD alone, several series have shown good initial outcomes. Both ACD and ACDF, at least in the short term, are rated as "likely helpful" and "worth considering" for neck pain with cervical radiculopathy. Rosenorn et al. compared ACD alone to modified Cloward-type fusion using freeze-dried allograft in 63 subjects with radicular pain (Table 5.1). No baseline data were compared, only nonvalidated global assessment postoperative data were compared. There seemed to be better subjective improvement in ACD alone (at 1-year follow-up). ACD alone has less perioperative morbidity (blood loss, hospital stay, and work loss) compared to ACDF. However, Abd-Alrahman[34] compared one- or two-level ACD alone (n = 40) to ACDF (n = 50) using Smith-Robinson technique (Iliac Crest Bone Graft [ICBG] and no instrumentation) in an RCT.[35] At 6-month follow-up, there was no difference in neck or arm complaints between groups, but postoperative kyphosis was more common in the ACD group than in the ACDF group(55% vs. 26%). In addition, ACD without fusion has been shown to result in higher prevalence of postoperative neck pain, as well as decrease in neuroforaminal area, both of which are contrary to the treatment goals.[28] Patients who underwent ACDF for cervical radiculopathy reported improvement in the axial component of their pain.[17]

Anterior Cervical Diskectomy and Fusion

The evidence regarding ACD without fusion lends compelling support to perform a fusion with the decompression. This seems to be common practice; ACD alone is rarely performed currently. By 1999 the proportion of cervical diskectomies associated with a fusion procedure approached 90% nationwide.[36] In our patient, we recommend fusing both levels to avoid the risk of developing kyphosis, and to address his neck pain.

TABLE 5.1 **Evidentiary Table: The Quality of Evidence Supporting ACDF Versus ACD Alone for Two-level Cervical Radiculopathy.**

Paper Author (Year)	Description	Summary of Results	Quality of Evidence
Abd-Alrahman et al. (1999)	Randomized Clinical Trial Included radiculopathy, myelopathy, or both	Compared one- or two-level ACD alone (n = 40) to ACDF (n = 50) by the Smith-Robinson method without instrumentation, using ICBG. Using Odon criteria for outcome success, 80%–90% of each group had "excellent" or "good" outcomes. Postoperative kyphosis was more common in ACD alone group (55% vs. 26% in ACDF group)	Moderate
Rosenorn et al. (1983)[31]	Randomized Clinical Trial Included subjects with radicular pain and confirmed cervical disk herniation Did not compare baseline characteristics	63 patients randomized to either ACD alone or modified Cloward-type fusion (freeze-dried allograft) Only nonvalidated global assessments followed after surgery Somewhat better subjective improvement in the diskectomy alone group Only 1 y of postoperative follow-up	Low

TABLE 5.2 **Evidentiary Table: The Quality of Evidence Supporting ACDF with Plating.**

Paper Author (Year)	Description	Summary of Results	Quality of Evidence
Kaiser et al. (2002)	Retrospective review Compared to control group (ACDF without plate) from previously published data Used cortical allograft bone Follow-up data ranging from 9 mo to 3.6 y	251 patients, one- or two-level ACDF with plate, compared to control group of 289 patients without plates; 233 patients in study group available for follow-up Fusion rate with plate: one-level 96%, two-level 91% Fusion rate without plate: one-level 90%, two-level 72%	Low
Wang et al. (2000)	Retrospective review All patients had disk herniation at two levels refractory to conservative treatment Single surgeon; average follow-up 2.7 y Autologous iliac crest bone graft	60 patients: 32 had cervical plates, 28 noninstrumented Pseudarthrosis rate 0% for plated group, 25% for the nonplated group ($p = 0.003$) 0.4 degree kyphosis in plated group, 4.9 degrees in those without plating who developed kyphosis ($p = 0.0001$) No significant increase in complication rates	Low

Cervical fusion constructs vary and many have been compared in randomized trials.[13,18–20,37–39] Despite these important studies the literature remains unclear as to whether the more complex operation provides any better clinical improvement over time.[6,18–20]

Autologous bone harvested from the iliac crest (ICBG) is thought to be ideal for its osteoconductive, osteogenic, and mild osteoinductive properties compared to allograft (which is only osteoconductive). Donor site complications of ICBG in 10% or more of

TABLE 5.3 **Evidentiary Table: The Quality of Evidence Supporting Allograft Versus Iliac Crest Autograft in Anterior Cervical Diskectomy, Fusion, and Plating.**

Paper Author (Year)	Description	Summary of Results	Quality of Evidence
Samartzis et al. (2005)	Retrospective review Compared fusion rates of allograft to autograft with rigidly fixed anterior cervical plates Mean radiographic follow-up 12 mo, mean clinical outcome follow-up 17 mo	66 patients, 31 autograft, 35 allograft 33% of patients were smokers Fusion in 100% allografts, 90.3% autografts Satisfactory clinical outcome was noted in all nonunion patients Smoking no significant influence on fusion or clinical outcome in this series ($p < 0.05$)	Low
Samartzis et al. (2003)	Retrospective radiographic and clinical review	45 patients tricortical ICBG, 35 patients tricortical allograft Rigid anterior plate fixation Single institution Soft collar 3–4 wk Mean radiographic follow-up 16 mo, clinical outcome follow-up 20 mo 78 out of 80 patients achieved solid union (2 pseudarthroses were in the allograft group: 1 two-level and 1 three-level fusion; this number was not statistically significant) 88.8% excellent or good clinical results	Low

patients have been reported, thus prompting surgeons to explore other options.[40–42] Silber, 2003 The use of allograft would avoid the morbidity of iliac crest bone graft harvest. It has been demonstrated that excellent clinical and radiographic results can be achieved using tricortical allograft and rigid plate fixation.[32] Fusion rates comparable to ICBG have been demonstrated, thus avoiding donor site morbidity (Table 5.3).

Intervertebral carbon fiber cages have been used for cervical interbody instrumentation, with or without plating. A potential benefit of the stand-alone cage is a decrease in operative time; however, the cost of the cages is to be taken into consideration. In a prospective randomized study comparing a stand-alone carbon fiber cage to the Smith-Robinson technique with allograft and plating, Ryu et al.[43] presented data from 24 months of follow-up on 40 consecutive patients. Clinical pain and disability were similar for the cage group and the allograft and plate group at all time intervals, as determined by SF-36 and NDI scores. They reported 100% fusion rates in both groups and no differences in complication rates. This may or may not become a more commonly performed procedure depending on the results of long-term follow-up data.

Anterior Cervical Diskectomy and Fusion with Instrumentation

The addition of a plate has been demonstrated to prevent graft subsidence and kyphosis at the operated level. In a retrospective review of 60 patients treated with two-level ACDF with an average of 6 years of follow-up, there was less graft collapse, pseudarthrosis, and kyphotic deformity in patients treated with plate fixation (n = 32) compared to nonplated fusions (n = 28).[44] Of the 60 patients, 7 had pseudarthrosis (all occurring in nonplated fusions). The overall rate of pseudarthrosis was 0% of patients with anterior cervical plates and 25% of patients without a cervical plate. This was statistically significant (p = 0.003). Comparing the amount of kyphotic deformity in the patients who have successfully fused, the average kyphosis per treated segment was 0.4 degree for those with cervical plates and 0.5 degree for those without plates, which was not significant (p = 0.459). For patients without plates who developed pseudoarthrosis, the average amount of kyphosis was 4.9 degrees. Comparing this amount of kyphosis to that of patients with plates and successful fusions (0.4 degree), the difference was found to be statistically significant (p = 0.0001). It appears that a successful union may better preserve the normal lordotic alignment.

Other benefits of plating include immediate rigidity, no need for external orthosis, earlier mobilization, and potentially shorter recovery time. Cervical plates have allowed for early mobilization from a cervical orthosis.[45–51] The literature was reviewed for evidence to support the use of a cervical plate over an uninstrumented fusion (Table 5.2). Anterior cervical plate use has been demonstrated to reduce the risk of graft extrusion and the development of kyphosis following single-level diskectomy.[2]

While the plate is effective in protecting the graft, there is a potential for a higher complication rate intrinsic to the nature of implanted hardware. Use of an anterior cervical plate may be associated with an increased risk of postoperative dysphagia. This may be related to plate prominence or the requirement for greater exposure of the anterior aspect of the vertebrae. The pathophysiology of dysphagia following anterior cervical surgery is not well understood. Several variables have been proposed to be independent risk factors, including the prominence of the cervical plate. In a prospective radiographic and clinical analysis by Chin et al.[53] the role of plate thickness in the rate of dysphagia was compared along with the height of preoperative osteophytes. There was no difference in long-term dysphagia rate if the cervical plate was thicker than preoperative osteophyte, within the range of 3 to 7 mm of prominence. This study did report higher rates of dysphagia in plates at C3 and in shorter cervical constructs, but this was not found to be statistically significant. The authors recommended avoiding plate prominence >7 mm, using a larger incision for better visualization, removing osteophytes to allow the plate to sit flush against the vertebral body, and trying to limit time of surgery to under 175 minutes.[53]

Anterior cervical instrumentation technique has also been seen to be associated with radiographic changes at adjacent segments. Riew et al. reported that plates placed too close to adjacent-level annulus were associated with an increased risk of ossification in that annulus. The rate of adjacent-level ossification was 59% in the group with plate-to-disk distance <5 mm, and 29% in the group with plate-to-disk distance of ≥5 mm. They recommend placing the plate at least 5 mm away from the adjacent disk spaces.[54]

The effect of various plate configurations has been determined by biomechanical testing. In a study by Spivak et al.[55] comparing locked to unlocked screws and unicortical versus bicortical fixation, rigidity of the fixation and pull-out strength were tested. Locking screws were shown to significantly increase the rigidity of the unicortical screw-plate system both initially and after cyclic loading. While better performance was shown with bicortical fixation, unicortical fixation may be preferred to avoid the risk of screw misplacement and resultant spinal cord injury. Comparing static to dynamic plates in a separate biomechanical study by Brodke et al.[56] it was demonstrated that both rotationally and translationally dynamic plates maintain load-sharing and stiffness despite simulated subsidence. By comparison static plates with fixed-angle screws lost nearly 70% of load-sharing capability in single-level corpectomy. Static plates allowed significantly more motion in flexion-extension than either dynamic plate constructs following simulated subsidence testing.

A cost-effectiveness analysis has been performed to compare allograft with autograft, and plated with nonplated ACDF procedures.[47] A group of 78 patients who underwent single-level ACDF had retrospective measurement of quality-adjusted life years (QALYs) over a 5-year period. It was demonstrated that ACDF with allograft offers a benefit over ACDF with autograft at a cost of $496 per QALY. ACDF with allograft and plating was shown to have a benefit over ACDF with allograft and no plate at a cost of $32,560 per QALY. Essentially, these figures took into account differences in postoperative recovery, time to return-to-work, additional outcomes measures, as well as base case analysis. The model did not take into account fusion status. As determined in their review of the literature at the time, there are no published data that can be used to correlate fusion rates with the rates of clinical improvement. There may be asymptomatic pseudarthroses that do not require reoperation.

Corpectomy and Strut Graft

There is a concept that fusion success may be reduced with each additional fusion surface. For example, a two-level ACDF with four fusion surfaces between host bone and graft may be different than a single-level corpectomy with two fusion surfaces between host bone and graft. This has been evaluated in a comparison of multilevel interbody grafts versus corpectomy and strut grafting. In a 20-year retrospective series of 190 patients,[57] fusion rates were compared following anterior cervical decompression (for radiculopathy or myelopathy from degenerative spondylosis, herniated disk, deformity or iatrogenic pathology), with patients undergoing either multilevel ACDF or corpectomy and fusion. For patients with multilevel disease and moderate to severe spondylosis, herniated disk, or spinal canal stenosis behind the vertebral body, a single or multilevel corpectomy was performed. There were 98 patients treated with two-level ACDF and 33 patients treated with three-level ACDF. In the corpectomy group, there were 16 one-level, 21 two-level, 20 three-level, and 2 four-level cases. No internal fixation was applied. For multilevel disease, corpectomy and strut graft was shown to have greater success rates of arthrodesis than multilevel interbody fusions. This was also demonstrated for one-level corpectomy compared to two-level interbody grafting. Of the multilevel ACDF patients, 66% achieved solid arthrodesis compared to 93% of patients who underwent corpectomy with strut grafting. Fusion was determined by two criteria: (1) no more than 1 mm of change in the interspinous distance across a fused segment between flexion and extension views, and (2) continuous bony trabeculation without any intervertebral lucency at the disc space. Established pseudarthrosis was associated with a poorer clinical outcome in this study ($p < 0.0001$). Clinical outcomes were measured by severity of pain, need for pain medication, work status, and activity level. A successful result was defined as excellent or good outcome and significant pain relief. Among the ACDF patients, 84% had successful clinical results compared to 88% of corpectomy patients. Of the patients who were demonstrated to be radiographically solid, 94% of ACDF patients had successful clinical results versus 88% of corpectomy patients. Corpectomy and strut graft was associated with higher complication rates in this series, specifically extrusion of the graft (10% among patients treated with multilevel corpectomy). These results must be carefully interpreted in historical context; the authors state that anterior plates were not used in this 20-year period. A modern comparison between these groups may yield different results if internal fixation with anterior plates were to be performed.

In a biomechanical study by An et al., increased rigidity was demonstrated using segmental plate fixation for long anterior cervical reconstructions compared to end-construct plate fixation in three-level diskectomy, single corpectomy and diskectomy, and two-level corpectomy. The conclusion was that an end-construct spanning the strut graft(s) had an increased moment arm, potentially leading to plate migration or dislodgement.[58]

Corpectomy is often used to treat patients with multilevel disease and moderate to severe spondylosis, particularly when there is significant cord compression behind the vertebral body. Removal of posterior osteophytes increases the risk of injury to the cord during ACDF, and corpectomy is recommended for safer removal of large osteophytes.[28] Patients who require corpectomy often have myelopathy.[6,18–20] Our patient does not have symptoms or exam findings of cervical myelopathy and does not have significant compression that cannot be relieved at the level of the disk.

Cervical Total Disc Arthroplasty

With the theoretical benefit of reducing the risk of adjacent segment degeneration, cervical disk replacement may be considered an alternative to ACDF. According to the best evidence summary from the Task Force on Neck Pain in 2008, single-level disk replacement is listed as "possibly helpful/might consider" for treatment of cervical radiculopathy with neck pain based on short-term results. In a prospective, randomized study, favorable outcomes were shown at 2 years of follow-up as compared to the "gold standard" ACDF for a single cervical level.[29] Multilevel cervical disk replacement for the same indication is listed by the Task Force as "not enough evidence to make determination," because of lack of long-term efficacy and safety data.[6,18–20] Long-term follow-up should help to better define the appropriate indications and the role for cervical arthroplasty. Under current FDA guidelines, multilevel disease is listed as an excluding factor for cervical disk replacement. At least at this point in time, our patient does not fit the criteria for TDA, having radiographic evidence of two-level disease.

Posterior Laminoforaminotomy

Several factors may determine whether or not a keyhole foraminotomy is a reasonable option. For example, a patient with severe axial neck pain and segmental kyphosis is best treated with an anterior procedure, as a posterior procedure is potentially destabilizing. If the radiculopathy is due to degenerative changes and hard disk disease, an anterior approach would be the better choice, as it facilitates removal of disk material and safe removal of osteophytes anterior to the nerve root. Posterior laminoforaminotomy does offer the advantage of direct decompression of neural elements and avoidance of fusion and the associated complications.[9] The ideal patient for a posterior laminoforaminotomy would have a unilateral, single-level soft disk herniation and predominant arm pain. To the best of our knowledge, there is no evidence in the literature that supports laminoforaminotomy for the relief of axial neck pain. This is not an ideal operation for this patient, given his symptoms or equivalent arm and neck pain and with his specific imaging findings.

Cervical Laminectomy and Laminoplasty

Laminectomy or laminoplasty is indicated for a patient requiring decompression at four or more segments, for a congenitally narrow canal, or for a patient in whom the anterior column is already fused. A prerequisite is cervical lordosis, as the cord can migrate dorsally following decompression.[2] In addition to lacking the appropriate indications, our patient would be better treated with an anterior cervical diskectomy and fusion, as ACDF is recommended for patients with a substantial component of axial neck pain associated with radicular symptoms.

DEFINITIVE TREATMENT PLAN

This patient may be offered surgical treatment as non-operative management has not provided relief of his symptoms. Based on recommendations in the literature, our own clinical experience and patient factors, we would offer our patient an ACDF with tricortical allograft and cervical plate. In accordance with the method of grading recommendations set forth by Schunemann et al., our proposed treatment would be considered a strong recommendation.

The best evidence available favors two-level ACDF, using tricortical allograft and plating with variable angle screw fixation. Fixed angled screws may be used in the central vertebral body to limit the potential plate migration to the cranial or caudal disk, respectively. With all factors in consideration, fusion of the degenerative segments may reduce his neck pain. The use of a plate for a two-level ACDF has been demonstrated to have a lower rate of pseudarthrosis and better preservation of alignment, as described by Wang et al.[44]

Preoperative planning would take into account the size of the vertebral bodies, as well as the patient's overall cervical alignment, as it is prudent to have proper allograft selections available. Following exposure to the anterior cervical spine via the Southwick-Smith-Robinson approach, proper level is documented radiographically using a radiopaque marker, such as a small gauge spinal needle placed in the disk space. A foraminotomy with removal of the posterior uncus at C6-7 on the right would complement decompression of the exiting C7 nerve root, as there is MRI evidence of foraminal stenosis at this level. Additionally, the patency of the C5-6 foramen (particularly on the right side) would be scrutinized, in accordance with the patient's preoperative symptoms of pain radiating down the right arm. Endplate preparation is carried out to create an optimal surface for graft fusion, while taking care not to remove too much endplate and risking subsidence.

In choosing the size of the plate, we maintain at least a 5 mm distance from either disk space, to lessen the risk of adjacent segment ossification due to close proximity of the plate. The operative field is inspected prior to closure for hemostasis, and the esophagus is carefully inspected as well. Radiographs are taken intraoperatively to evaluate the graft and hardware. Rigid internal fixation would eliminate the need for postoperative cervical orthosis. If the patient were a smoker or has other independent risk factors for pseudarthrosis, a collar may be considered.[59] A cervical collar was not shown to improve the fusion rate or clinical outcome in patients undergoing single-level ACDF with plating, although the study did not look at multilevel ACDF.[60]

The options for cervical fusion constructs vary and many have been compared in randomized controlled studies.[13,18–20,37–39] In the review of current evidence by Carragee et al.,[6] there does not appear to be large advantages in outcome with fusion versus decompression, with decompression and fusion versus cervical disk arthroplasty, or with the use of various fusion-adjuvant measures among carefully selected patients, according to the authors. The best evidence available supports treating our patient with ACDF, using an allograft and an anterior plate, taking care to use techniques to reduce the risk of hardware prominence, injury to adjacent segments, and nonunion, as described by Samartzis et al.[61] Park et al.[54] and others.

Grading the Evidence for this Plan

Most of the evidence to support our proposed treatment plan would be considered low, as it has been derived from retrospective case series. Of the two randomized trials that were selected, one was assigned a moderate level,[34] while the other study was down-graded to a low level,[62] due to a lack of comparison of baseline patient characteristics. In accordance with the method of grading recommendations set forth by Schunemann et al.[63] our choice of treatment would be considered a strong recommendation, as the benefits clearly outweigh harms and burdens and the treatment applies to most patients under most circumstances.

PREDICTING OUTCOMES

ACDF is generally successful in the treatment of radiculopathy due to soft disk herniation, where symptoms correlate with imaging findings, physical exam, or other diagnostic modalities. Relatively rapid and considerable pain relief and relief of impairment are shown to be reliably achieved with this operative treatment.

The often-cited statistic is that 90% of patients undergoing surgery for cervical radiculopathy will experience excellent results. However the best scientific evidence shows a significant proportion (20%–30%) will experience only modest or no real improvement. The best evidence available supports surgical treatment of our patient for his ongoing pain and disability which has not responded to an 18-month trial of nonoperative therapy, for at least short-term improvement of symptoms and return to functionality.

The treatment of neck pain, per se, does not share the consistent clinical outcomes using current surgical strategies. According to Garvey et al., good or excellent results were reported in 82% of patients who underwent ACDF for dominant complaint of neck pain, a statistic that did not change after an average follow-up of 4.4 years. Average VAS score improved from 8.4 preoperatively to 3.8 after surgery. Self-rated functional scores improved by an average of 50% on both Oswestry and the modified Roland-Morris disability indices.[64]

In a review of the literature by Carragee et al.[6] higher levels of evidence, beyond what is normally produced by case series and uncontrolled cohort designs, are needed to determine whether clinical changes seen after surgical interventions are attributed to a spontaneous variation of the disease, the nonspecific effects of applying any intervention, the result of changes in

patients' social support or expectations, or possibly an effect of the surgery itself.

Some authors suggest that the best predictor of functional outcome after ACDF may be preoperative psychometric testing. The following factors are independently associated with better outcomes according to Peolsson et al.[65]—male gender, greater kyphotic deformity (prior to arthrodesis), and less reported preoperative functional impairment.

Our patient is likely to have a good outcome, but he still needs to be counseled that his symptoms have been going on for a considerable length of time and he may only show modest improvement. In our experience, a young individual with radicular symptoms showing a close correlation with exam and imaging findings will notice an improvement in some of the symptoms shortly after the operation. We would counsel him preoperatively that cervical fusion may help reduce the symptoms of neck pain by obliterating painful motion segments, with approximately 80% of patients experiencing good to excellent results in terms of functional improvement and pain relief.[64]

SUMMARY

This is a case of a 39-year-old man with cervical radiculopathy and neck pain, with signs and symptoms correlating to MRI findings of cervical spondylosis primarily at two levels. We recommend two-level ACDF at C5-6 and C6-7, based on current evidence in the literature. The goals of surgical treatment are decompression of the neural foramina with the expectation of improvement of his arm pain, numbness and tingling. It should be addressed in preoperative discussions, however, that his neck pain may or may not improve following the fusion, and that the primary objective of surgery is to preserve or improve neurological function and to relieve the arm pain associated with nerve compression.[54,58]

REFERENCES

1. Rao R. Neck pain, cervical radiculopathy, and cervical myelopathy: pathophysiology, natural history, and clinical evaluation. *Instr Course Lect.* 2003;52:479–488.
2. Rao RD, Currier BL, Albert TJ, et al. Degenerative cervical spondylosis: clinical syndromes, pathogenesis, and management. *J Bone Joint Surg Am.* 2007;89:1360–1378.
3. Henderson CM, Hennessy RG, Shuey HM Jr, et al. Posteriorlateral foraminotomy as an exclusive operative technique for cervical radiculopathy: a review of 846 consecutively operated cases. *Neurosurgery.* 1983;13:504–512.
4. Tong HC, Haig AJ, Yamakawa K. The spurling test and cervical radiculopathy. *Spine.* 2002;27:156–159.

5. Rhee JM, Yoon T, Riew KD. Cervical radiculopathy. *J Am Acad Orthop Surg*. 2007;15:486–494.

6. Carragee EJ, Hurwitz EL, Cheng I, et al. Treatment of neck pain, injections and surgical intervention: results of the Bone and Join Decade 2000–2010 Task Force on Neck Pain and its Associated Disorders. Spine 2008;33: S153–S169.

7. Matsumoto M, Fujimura Y, Suzuki N, et al. MRI of cervical intervertebral discs in asymptomatic subjects. *J Bone Joint Surg Br*. 1998;80(1):19–24.

8. Boden SD, McCowin PR, Davis DO, et al. Abnormal magnetic-resonance scans of the cervical spine in asymptomatic subjects. A prospective investigation. *J Bone Joint Surg*. 1990;72(8):1178–1184.

9. Albert TJ, Murrell SE. Surgical management of cervical radiculopathy. *J Am Acad Orthop Surg*. 1999;7:368–376.

10. Connolly ES, Seymour RJ, Adams JE. Clinical evaluation of anterior cervical fusion for degenerative cervical disc disease. *J Neurosurg*. 1965;23:431–437.

11. DePalma AF, Rothman RH, Lewinnek GE, et al. Anterior interbody fusion for severe cervical disc degeneration. *Surg Gynecol Obstet*. 1972;134:755–758.

12. Gore DR, Sepic SB. Anterior cervical fusion for degenerated or protruded discs. A review of one hundred forty-six patients. *Spine*. 1984;9:667–671.

13. Hacker RJ. A randomized prospective study of an anterior cervical interbody fusion device with a minimum of 2 years of follow-up results. *J Neurosurg*. 2000;93:222–226.

14. Herkowitz HN, Kurz LT, Overholt DP. Surgical management of cervical soft disc herniation. *Spine*. 1990;15: 1026–1030.

15. White AA, Southwick WO, Deponte RJ, et al. Relief of pain by anterior cervical spine fusion for spondylosis. *J Bone Joint Surg Am*. 1973;55:525–534.

16. Bohlman HH, Emery SE, Goodfellow DB, et al. Robinson anterior cervical discectomy and arthrodesis for cervical radiculopathy. *J Bone Joint Surg Am*.1993;75:1298–1307.

17. Fouyas IP, Statham P, Sandercock P. Cochrane review on the role of surgery in cervical spondylotic radiculomyelopathy. *Spine*. 2002;27:736–747.

18. Baskin DS, Ryan P, Sonntag V, et al. A prospective, randomized, controlled cervical fusion study using recombinant human bone morphogenetic protein 2 with the Cornerstone-SR allograft ring and the Atlantis anterior cervical plate. *Spine*. 2003;28:1219–1225.

19. Hacker RJ. Cervical disc arthroplasty: a controlled randomized prospective study with intermediate follow-up results. Invite submission from the joint section on disorders of the spine and peripheral nerves. *J Neurosurg Spine*. 2005;3:424–428.

20. Coric D, Finger F, Boltes P. Prospective randomized controlled study of the Bryan Cervical Disc: early clinical results from a single investigational site. *J Neurosurg Spine*. 2006;4:31–35.

21. Persson LC, Carlsson CA, Carlsson JY. Long-lasting cervical radicular pain manage with surgery, physiotherapy, or a cervical collar. A prospective, randomized study. *Spine*. 1997;22:751–758.

22. Palit M, Schofferman J, Goldthwaite N, et al. Anterior discectomy and fusion for the management of neck pain. *Spine*. 1999;24:2224–2228.

23. Schellhas KP, Smith M, Gundry CR, et al. Cervical discogenic pain: prospective correlation of magnetic resonance imaging and discography in asymptomatic subjects and pain sufferers. *Spine*. 1996;21(3):300–311.

24. Carragee EJ, Chen Y, Tanner C, et al. Can discography cause long term back symptoms in previously asymptomatic subjects? *Spine*. 2000;25(14):1803–1808.

25. White AP, Biswas, Smart LR, et al. Utility of flexion-extension radiographs in evaluating the degenerative cervical spine. *Spine*. 2007;32(9):975–979.

26. Hilibrand AS, Carlson GD, Palumbo MA, et al. Radiculopathy and myelopathy at segments adjacent to the site of a previous anterior cervical arthrodesis. *J Bone Joint Surg Am*. 1999;81:519–528.

27. White AA, Panjabi MM. *Clinical Biomechanics of the Spine*. 2nd ed. Philadelphia, PA: J.B. Lippincott, 1990:98.

28. Anderson PA, Sasso RC, Riew KD. Comparison of adverse events between the Bryan artificial cervical disc and anterior cervical arthrodesis. *Spine*. 2008;33:1305–1312.

29. Sasso RC, Smucker JD, Hacker RJ, et al. Artificial disc versus fusion. *Spine*. 2007;32:2933–2940.

30. Rabin D, Pickett GE, Bisnaire L, et al. The kinematics of anterior cervical discectomy and fusion versus artificial cervical disc: a pilot study. *Neurosurgery*. 2007;61:100–105.

31. Rosenorn J, Hansen EB, Rosenorn MA. Anterior cervical diskectomy with and without fusion. A prospective study. *J Neurosurg*. 1983;59:252–255.

32. Samartzis D, Shen FH, Goldberg EJ, et al. Is autograft the gold standard in achieving radiographic fusion in one-level anterior cervical discectomy and fusion with rigid anterior plate fixation? *Spine*. 2005;30:1756–1761.

33. Samartzis D, Shen FH, Matthews DK, et al. Comparison of allograft to autograft in multilevel anterior cervical discectomy and fusion with rigid plate fixation. *Spine J*. 2003;3:451–459.

34. Abd-Alrahman N, Dokmak AS, Abou-Madawi A. Anterior cervical discectomy (ACD) versus anterior cervical fusion (ACF), clinical and radiological outcome study. *Acta Neurochir*. 1999;141:1089–1092.

35. Smith GW, Robinson RA. The treatment of certain cervical-spine disorders by anterior removal of the intervertebral disc and interbody fusion. *J Bone Joint Surg Am*. 1958;40:607–624.

36. Angevine PD, Arons RR, McCormick PC. National and regional rates and variation of cervical discectomy with and without anterior fusion, 1990–1999. *Spine*. 2003;28:931–939.

37. Peolsson A, Vavruch L, Hedlund R. Long-term randomized comparison between a carbon fibre cage and the Cloward procedure in the cervical spine. *Eur Spine J*. 2007;16:173–178.

38. Vavruch L, Hedlund R, Javid D, et al. A prospective randomized comparison between the Cloward procedure and a carbon fiber cage in the cervical spine: a clinical and radiologic study. *Spine*. 2002;27:1694–1701.

39. Peolsson A, Hedlund R, Vavruch L, et al. Predictive factors for the outcome of anterior cervical decompression and fusion. *Eur Spine J*. 2003;12:274–280.

40. Arrington ED, Smith WJ, Chambers HG, et al. Complications of iliac crest bone grafting. *Clin Orthop Relat Res*. 1996;329:300–309.

41. Younger EM, Chapman MW. Morbidity at bone graft donor sites. *J Orthop Trauma*. 1989;3:192–195.

42. Silber JS, Anderson G, Daffner SD, et al. Donor site morbidity after anterior iliac crest bone graft harvest for single-level anterior cervical discectomy an fusion. *Spine*. 2003;28(2):134–139.

43. Ryu SI, Mitchell M, Kim DH. A prospective randomized study comparing a cervical carbon fiber cage to the Smith-Robinson technique with allograft and plating: up to 24 months follow-up. *Eur Spine J*. 2006;15:157–164.

44. Wang JC, McDonough PW, Endow KK, et al. Increased fusion rates with cervical plating for two-level anterior cervical discectomy and fusion. *Spine*. 2000;25:41–45.

45. Wang JC, McDonough PW, Endow K, et al. The effect of cervical plating on single-level anterior cervical discectomy and fusion. *J Spinal Disord*. 1999;12:467–471.

46. Zoega B, Karrholm J, Lind B. Plate fixation adds stability to two-level anterior fusion in the cervical spine: a randomized study using radiostereometry. *Eur Spine J*. 1998;7:302–307.

47. Angevine PD, Zivin JG, McCormick PC. Cost-effectiveness of single-level anterior cervical discectomy and fusion for cervical spondylosis. *Spine*. 2005;30:1989–1997.

48. Connolly PJ, Esses SI, Kostuik JP. Anterior cervical fusion: outcome analysis of patients fused with and without anterior cervical plates. *J Spinal Disord*. 1996;9:202–206.

49. Kaiser MG, Haid RW, Subach BR, et al. Anterior Cervical Plating Enhances Arthrodesis after Discectomy and Fusion with Cortical Allograft. Neurosurgery 2002;50(2):229–238.

50. Zoega B, Karrholm J, Lind B. One-level cervical spine fusion. A randomized study, with or without plate fixation, using radiosteriometry. *Eur Spine J*. 1998;69:363–368.

51. Zoega B, Karrholm J, Lind B. Plate fixation adds stability to two-level anterior fusion in the cervical spine: a randomized study using radiostereometry. *Eur Spine J*. 1998;7:302–307.

52. Kaiser MG, Haid RW, Subach BR, et al. Anterior cervical plating enhances arthrodesis after discectomy and fusion with cortical allograft. *Neurosurgery*. 2002;50:229–236.

53. Chin KR, Eiszner JR, Adams SB. Role of plate thickness as a cause of dysphagia after anterior cervical. *Spine*. 2007;32:2585–2590.

54. Park J-B, Cho Y-S, Riew KD. Development of adjacent-level ossification in patients with an anterior cervical plate. *J Bone Joint Surg Am*. 2005;87:558–563.

55. Spivak JM, Chen D, Kummer FJ. The effect of locking fixation screws on the stability of anterior cervical plating. *Spine*. 1999;24:334–338.

56. Brodke DS, Klimo P, Bachus KN, et al. Anterior cervical fixation: analysis of load-sharing and stability with use of static and dynamic plates. *J Bone Joint Surg Am*. 2006;88:1566–1573.

57. Hilibrand AS, Fye MA, Emery SE, et al. Increased rate of arthrodesis with Strut grafting after multilevel anterior cervical decompression. *Spine*. 2002;27:146–151.

58. Singh K, Vaccaro AR, Kim J, et al. Enhancement of stability following anterior cervical corpectomy: a biomechanical study. *Spine*. 2004;29:845–849.

59. Hilibrand AS, Fye MA, Emery SE, et al. Impact of smoking on the outcome of anterior cervical arthrodesis with interbody or strut-grafting. *J Bone Joint Surg Am*. 2001;83:668–673.

60. Campbell MJ, Carreon LY, Traynelis V, et al. Use of cervical collar after single-level anterior cervical fusion with plate: is it necessary? *Spine*. 2009;34(1):43–48.

61. Samartzis D, Shen FH, Lyon C, et al. Does rigid instrumentation increase the fusion rate in one-level anterior cervical discectomy and fusion? *Spine J*. 2004;4:636–643.

62. Rosenorn J, Hansen EB, Rosenorn MA. Anterior cervical discectomy with and without fusion. A prospective study. *J Neurosurg*. 1983;59:252–255

63. Schunemann HJ, Jaeschke R, Cook DJ, et al. ATS Documents Development and Implementation Committee. An official ATS statement: grading the quality of evidence and strength of recommendations in ATS guidelines and recommendations. Am J Respir Crit Care Med. 2006;174:605–614.

64. Garvey TA, Transfeldt EE, Malcolm JR, et al. Outcome of anterior cervical discectomy and fusion as perceived by patients treated for dominant axial-mechanical cervical pain. *Spine*. 2002;27:1887–1895.

65. Peolsson A, Karrholm J, Lind B. Predictive factors for arm pain, neck pain, neck specific disability and health after anterior cervical decompression and fusion. *Acta Neurochi*. 2006;148:167–173.

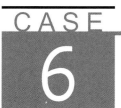

Cervical Stenosis with Kyphosis

JOHN STREET MD, PHD AND BRIAN LENEHAN MD, MCH, FRCS

A 52-year-old woman complains of neck pain along with bilateral numbness and tingling in her hands on the right side more than the left. She feels imbalanced when walking and has decreased dexterity of her hands, also on the right side greater than the left. She has had several previous low back surgeries, with continued low back pain and lower extremity symptoms. She does not have any bowel or bladder complaints.

Physical examination shows a floridly positive Hoffmann reflex bilaterally as well as a positive inverted radial reflex bilaterally. Flexion of the neck reproduces her upper extremity numbness and tingling. She has full strength in the upper and lower extremities; however, there is diffusely decreased sensation in the bilateral upper extremities in a non-dermatomal pattern. Gait is slightly imbalanced in that she deviates to one side while walking down the hallway.

INTERPRETATION OF CLINICAL PRESENTATION

The clinical scenario describes a middle-aged woman with physical symptoms and signs suggestive of cervical spondylotic myelopathy (CSM). Her primary complaints are neck pain, asymmetric non-dermatomal upper extremity numbness, loss of hand dexterity and a gait abnormality. Neck pain is a characteristic symptom of CSM, being absent in only 15% of patients with moderate to severe myelopathy.[1] Sensory disturbance is classically of a non-dermatomal distribution; however, asymmetry, while common, is more usual in the lower

extremities.[2] Loss of manual dexterity is typical[2] and forms an integral component of the Japanese Orthopedic Association (JOA) scoring system for cervical myelopathy.[3] Gait disturbance with spasticity represents one of the subtle signs of early myelopathy and a hallmark of established disease.[1] This forms the basis of the Nurick grading scale for CSM.[4] Five to thirty percent of patients have concomitant symptomatic lumbar and cervical spinal stenosis and this can often lead to diagnostic and therapeutic difficulties given the simultaneous presence of upper and lower motor neuron signs in the lower extremities.[5] Reliance must be placed on history and physical examination when deciding whether the stenosis should be treated surgically at either region in isolation or concomitantly. Loss of sphincter control or frank incontinence is rare; however some patients may complain of mild urinary urgency or hesitancy.[6]

The most typical physical examination findings are suggestive of upper motor dysfunction. In a series of 225 surgically treated patients with CSM, both Hoffman sign and the inverted radial reflex were present in approximately 45% of those with mild disease and over 80% with moderate to severe myelopathy.[7] Lhermitte sign has a low sensitivity (<30%) but a high specificity (about 90%) in the setting of CSM.[8] In terms of the motor examination in the upper extremities, patients with CSM most commonly exhibit triceps and/or hand intrinsic muscle weakness. Wasting of the intrinsic hand musculature is a classical finding in CSM. In the lower extremities however, it is the more proximal muscle groups that are most profoundly affected, further distinguishing the presentation from lumbar spinal stenosis.[1]

Several other conditions may present similar to CSM. Failure to exclude these may explain lack of neurological improvement after surgery. The absence of sensory abnormalities and disproportionate weakness and wasting in the hand muscles should alert one to the possibility of amyotrophic lateral sclerosis. A lack of correlation between sensoromotor findings and spondylotic changes should make one suspicious of a demyelinating process. Other conditions to consider include normal pressure hydrocephalus, subacute combined degeneration (vitamin B_{12} deficiency), tumors, rheumatoid arthritis, and spinal arteriovenous malformations or syringomyelia.

There are five specific CSM outcome scores frequently used to assess the grade of severity and outcome of the disease. These are the Nurick score, the JOA score, the Cooper myelopathy scale, the Prolo score, and the European myelopathy score. All five scores have been validated for qualitative assessment of the clinical characteristics, progression, and outcomes from treatment for cervical myelopathy.[9]

Based on the clinical signs and symptoms, the woman in this case has at least moderate cervical myelopathy. Her functional score as determined by the modified JOA system is in the moderate to severe range.

Representative T2-weighted midsagittal and parasagittal magnetic resonance images are shown in Figure 6.1. Figures 6.1A and C represent right and left parasaggital views respectively. Figure 6.1B represents the midsaggital view. The cervical spine is visualized from the brainstem to the T2/3 disc. The cerebellum, brain stem, and cephalo-medullary angle appear normal. There is no evidence of atlantoaxial disease. There is loss of normal cervical lordosis with 8 to 10 degrees of true kyphosis when measured from the inferior endplate of C2 to the superior endplate of C6. The Torg ratio measures approximately 0.8 at the level of C3. However this ratio, when measured on MRI, has poor correlation with either the space available for the cord or the presence or severity of myelopathy.[10]

There is loss of disc height of more than 50% at C4/5 and C5/6. There are anterior and posterior disc protrusions seen at both levels. The disk protrusions efface the cord with complete loss of CSF at both levels. There is change in the alignment and shape of the cord with associated increased cord signal change, particularly at C5/6. There is no posterior compression of the cord. The discrete pattern of the compression anteriorly is not typical of focal ossification of the posterior longitudinal ligament (OPLL), though if there were a clinical concern a CT would be more appropriate to assess this.

Figure 6.2 shows representative axial T2 weighted images through the levels of the discs from C3 to C7 inclusive. The C3/4 and the C6/7 disc levels are essentially normal (Fig. 6.2A and D). There is a left paracentral disc herniation at C6/7which effaces the thecal sac. At C4/5 and C5/6 there are large broad based disc herniations which displace the thecal sac and cord, resulting in significant change in the shape of the cord. There is associated bilateral neuroforaminal stenosis worse on the left, at both levels (Fig. 6.2B and C). There does not appear to be any posterior compression and there is no aberrant vertebral artery anatomy. The ratio of the dural tube to the spinal canal at the level of the C3/4 disc measures 0.71. This

Figure 6.1.

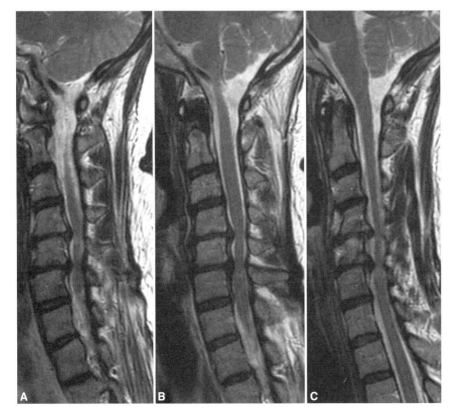

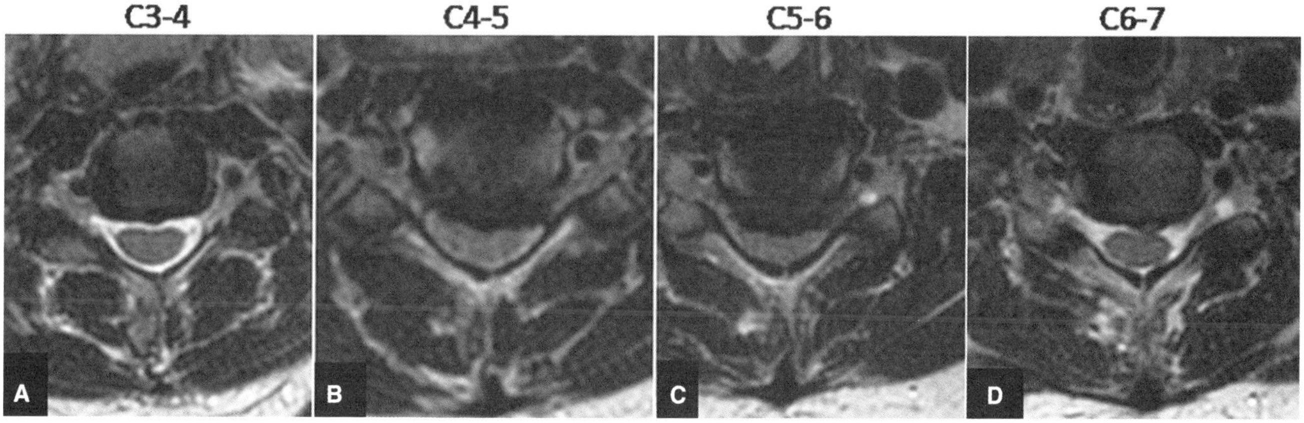

Figure 6.2.

compares to a mean of 0.81 in normal individuals as reported by Okada et al.[11] This study also demonstrated that the canal occupying ratio at nonaffected levels was higher than in age matched non-myelopathic adults. These factors confirm that developmental cervical spinal canal stenosis is contributory to myelopathy as a static factor.

This degree of kyphosis on static supine imaging, particularly as the patient demonstrates Lhermitte phenomena and a positive Spurling sign, mandates, we believe, at least static upright x-rays and perhaps patient controlled flexion and extension views of the cervical spine. Understanding whether this is a static or a dynamic deformity would be critical to the decision making process of the appropriate treatment strategy. A static deformity may suggest that decompression only without stabilization is feasible, while the deformity itself may compromise adequate decompression, for example laminectomy, and not allowing the spinal cord to "float away" from the anterior compression. Similarly, a dynamic deformity probably mandates a stabilizing procedure to augment the decompression. A CT scan would be very helpful in assessing the facet joint complexes, particularly if one was considering cervical disc arthroplasty as a surgical option.

The imaging suggests some coronal deformity also, as the parasaggital cut of the C2 body does not correspond with midline of the spinous processes. Plain x-rays in both coronal and saggital planes would also be helpful.

DECLARATION OF SPECIFIC DIAGNOSIS

This patient has moderate to severe CSM secondary to anterior cord compression from degenerative disk herniations at C4/5 and C5/6 with associated increased cord signal intensity and focal cervical kyphosis.

BRAINSTORMING: WHAT ARE THE TREATMENT GOALS AND OPTIONS?

The treatment goals here are

1. Prevention of neurological deterioration
2. Restoration of normal spinal alignment
3. Ensure continued spinal stability
4. Early mobilization
5. Rehabilitation and long-term maintenance of neurological function

The treatment options are

1. Nonoperative, including immobilization, physical therapy, medications etc.
2. Operative:
   Anterior (a) anterior diskectomy alone
         (b) anterior diskectomy and fusion
         (c) anterior diskectomy and fusion with plate
         (d) anterior vertebrectomy
         (e) cervical disk arthroplasty
   Posterior (a) laminotomy/laminectomy
         (b) laminoplasty
         (c) laminectomy and fusion
         (d) laminectomy and fusion with instrumentation
   Combined anterior and posterior procedures

EVALUATION OF THE LITERATURE

To identify relevant publications on CSM a MEDLINE search from 1950 to January 2009 was performed. Search strategies included the use of MeSH (medical subject headings) and key words. Key Words included "cervical vertebra," "spinal cord diseases," "cervical myelopathy," "cervical stenosis," and "cervical spondylosis." A focused search of "spinal stenosis" with subheadings of natural history, classification, treatment, nonoperative, radiography, prognosis, surgery, and complications was performed. The results of "spinal stenosis" were then combined with "cervical" and "myelopathy" to identify patients with cervical myelopathy within larger heterogeneous studies of spinal stenosis. Journals were hand searched and references were reviewed to identify pertinent articles. Only original clinical studies were included. Basic science studies, biomechanics studies, review articles, editorials, case reports, and letters to the editor were excluded. These strategies revealed 481 potential publications for review. The same search strategy was applied to EMBASE and revealed 252 potential publications. MEDLINE "in process" and non-indexed citations were also searched as was EBM reviews/Cochrane Database. There were a total of 338 English language studies that were reviewed.

DETAILED REVIEW OF PERTINENT ARTICLES

Operative Versus Non-Operative

There are few studies regarding the natural history of CSM and the quality of the evidence available is generally poor. The studies reporting observation or conservative treatment alone include six studies performed prior to 1985, of which four utilized the Nurick five-point scale for outcome and four more recent studies using the JOA scoring system. A summary of these studies is shown in Table 6.1. There are three studies directly comparing operative and nonoperative treatment for CSM. A summary of the results of these studies is shown in Table 6.2.

Although the data from the above studies appears compelling, the data are somewhat inconsistent, the study designs are generally poor (case series or poor observational studies), and many of the observations

TABLE 6.1 Evidentiary Table: Summary of Studies of Conservative Treatment for CSM.

Paper Author (Year)	Description	Summary of Results	Quality of Evidence
Lees and Turner (1963)	Retrospective cohort study	61% with MILD CSM improved clinically. Long periods of stability with short intervals of deterioration observed over 30 y.	Very low quality
Nurick (1972)	Retrospective cohort study	Patients with MILD Nurick grades (I and II) did not deteriorate. Significant association between kyphosis and worse "Nurick grade" on presentation. Age > 60 predicted poorer prognosis.	Very low quality
Clarke and Robinson (1956)	Retrospective cohort study	75% stepwise worsening, 20% slow steady progression, 5% initial worsening then plateau in MODERATE CSM	Very low quality
Roberts (1966)	Retrospective cohort study	Patients with MODERATE or SEVERE CSM continued to deteriorate with conservative treatment	Very low quality
Barnes and Saunders (1984)	Retrospective observational study	Clinical deterioration associated with kyphosis, greater range-of-motion and female gender.	Low quality
Nakamura et al. (1998)	Retrospective observational study	Patients with MODERATE or SEVERE CSM continued to deteriorate with conservative treatment	Low quality
Matsumoto et al. (2000)	Retrospective cohort study	Presence of increased signal intensity on MRI correlated with poorer response to conservative treatment.	Low quality
Matsumoto et al. (2001)	Retrospective cohort study	All patients had MILD disease. 17 improved or plateaued with conservative treatment. 10 patients underwent surgery for deterioration	Low quality
Shimomura et al. (2007)	Prospective observational cohort study	All patients had MILD disease. Circumferential spinal cord compression correlated with poorer outcome with conservative treatment.	Low quality

TABLE 6.2 Evidentiary Table: Summary of Studies of Conservative Versus Operative Treatment for CSM.

Paper Author (Year)	Description	Summary of Results	Quality of Evidence
Bednarik et al. (1999)	Prospective randomized	No difference in modified JOA scores or aggregate EP potentials at 6 and 24 mo	Moderate quality
Sampath et al. (2000)	Prospective multicentre nonrandomized	Functional improvement seen with both treatments but significant in social and work categories with surgery compared with conservative therapy. Neurological improvement seen with surgery but not significant compared to conservative.	Moderate quality
Kadanka et al. (2002)	Prospective randomized	**All patients had MILD CSM, JOA >12** "no significant deterioration in mean JOA score in the 2 groups over the 3-y follow-up period," "the 3-y follow-up study did not show, on the average, that the surgery is superior to conservative treatment" "could mean that the conservative approach can treat CSM with a degree of success similar to that of surgery for at least 3 y."	Moderate quality

are made of patients with mild myelopathic disability only, which does not apply to the patient in this case. The studies of both Nurick[12] and Lees and Turner[13] are consistent with a more benign course than that described by Clarke and Robinson.[14] However the patients in the former study all had mild disease. LaRocca[15] performed a meta-analysis of the nonoperative groups of several other observational and early surgical studies. He noted several studies that demonstrated steady worsening with nonoperative therapy and concluded that only an 18% to 33% improvement was evident with expectant management. He concluded that patients with moderate to severe disease had better outcomes when treated surgically.

From all the data presented above it is important to extract that evidence which is particular to our case in hand. There are four studies of moderate/severe CSM offering very low quality evidence[14,16–18] and three of low quality.[19–21]

Kadanka et al.[22] concluded at a 3-year follow-up that surgery was not superior to conservative treatment for mild to moderate disease. This randomized controlled study, because of the limitations in methodology, must be downgraded to moderate quality evidence. The greatest limitation to this study is that the study design assumed that all forms of spondylotic myelopathy are equivalent with regard to prognosis and response to treatment. Animal models of spondylotic myelopathy suggest that this is not the case, and that multilevel disease carries a worse prognosis. In addition, the study design assumed that all of the operations used for the treatment of spondylotic myelopathy are equally effective. Again, this has not been shown to be true, and is a

subject of ongoing debate. No data are given regarding follow-up studies to determine whether the goals of surgery (decompression, arthrodesis) were achieved. Finally, the cohort in this study only included patients with a JOA of 12 or more. The conclusions of this study, therefore, are not applicable to the patient in our case.

Sampath et al.[23] concluded that surgery improved the social and work categories of function. This was a nonrandomized study. Treatment type was determined by the treating physician. Prior to treatment the surgical group had lower functional status, though this was not statistically significant. Again in this study, the design assumed that all forms of spondylotic myelopathy are equivalent with regard to prognosis and response to treatment. The study design assumed that all the operations used for the treatment of spondylotic myelopathy are equally effective. 16% of the surgical group of patients had a planned fusion only without any decompression. Only 69% of patients were available for follow-up at a mean of 11 months. Validated outcome measures for neurology, functional status, satisfaction or ADLs were not utilized. This study, because of its design represents, at best, low quality evidence.

In Bednarik et al.'s[24] study all patients with severe disease had surgery. Those with mild or moderate disease were randomized to surgery or conservative treatment. It is unclear how this randomization was performed. Those with moderate disease were not identified from those with mild disease and so no conclusions can be made as to the effect of surgery on the moderate group. Knowing the natural history of mild CSM, the potential benefit of surgery in this study for the moderate group may go undetected. However, for those with severe disease, surgery resulted in an improved JOA score at 6, 12 and 24 months. This study represents moderate quality evidence.

The patient in our case has moderate to severe cervical myelopathy with a modified JOA score in the range of 8 to 11. The natural history studies suggest a 95% chance of clinical deterioration for our patient.[14,15] Female gender and the presence of kyphosis are also independent predictors of poor response to conservative treatment.[17]

EVIDENTIARY TABLE AND SELECTION OF TREATMENT METHOD

We conclude that the evidence presented in Tables 6.1 and 6.2 supports the recommendation of surgery in our patient.

Overall the quality of the evidence supporting operative treatment presented in these observational and comparative studies is low/moderate. Given that the natural history of moderate CSM is generally of deterioration, then the benefits of surgery clearly outweigh the burdens. Results of numerous other recent studies demonstrate the ability of surgical procedures to arrest the progression of myelopathy and provide for functional improvement in a majority of patients. Clinical results vary based on the severity of myelopathy at presentation, the extent of the disease process, and numerous patient factors, including saggittal alignment and gender. The rate of neurologic improvement after either anterior or posterior decompressive procedures ranges from 47% to 100%, with most reports indicating some degree of neurologic recovery in more than 90% of patients.[23,25–29]

Thus there is evidence for clinical efficacy with acceptable risk/burden from both observational studies and some randomized controlled trials with important limitations and thus the strength of our recommendation for surgery, in accordance with the method of grading recommendations set forth by Schunemann et al.[30] is strong. This grading paradigm is critical because it not only considers the quality of evidence but also addresses the benefits, harms, and burdens of the proposed interventions.

Choosing Operative Treatment

The best available evidence on the natural history of CSM, as discussed above, dictates that the patient presented in this clinical scenario, with moderate to severe CSM, should be treated operatively. In order to offer a clinical recommendation, the clinician must consider the quality of the evidence available in addition to the perceived benefits, harms, and burdens of the proposed interventions. For each individual scenario,

patient preference will be critical to the interpretation and weighting of the benefits, harms, and burdens. However, without knowing what the patient preferences are in this particular case, the author must take several things into consideration.

Choice of Surgical Approach

In order to evaluate the most appropriate surgical treatment, a number of unique features of this case must be reiterated. The patient has moderate to severe disease, is 52 years of age, has focal loss of normal cervical lordosis, the cord compression is all anterior and at the level of the affected discs only, and there is increased signal intensity in the cord on the T2 weighted MRI.

To summarize, the operative treatment goals here are

1. Decompression of the neural elements and prevention of neurological deterioration
2. Correction of kyphosis with restoration of normal spinal alignment
3. Ensure continued spinal stability with successful fusion
4. Early mobilization
5. Rehabilitation and long-term maintenance of neurological function

Both ventral and dorsal surgical approaches are utilized in the management of CSM. The appropriateness, advantages, and disadvantages of each approach must be considered in each individual case. It is imperative that one determines which patients are most likely to benefit from any given surgical approach while minimizing the risk/benefit ratio. Operative intervention of cervical myelopathy is focused on decompression of the spinal cord to halt neurologic deterioration and promote functional improvement. Appropriate and early decompression restores and improves spinal cord morphology,[31] reverses cord compression,[32,33] and likely improves blood supply to the cord aiding neurological recovery. The secondary goals of operative treatment are to achieve a successful fusion where abnormal segmental mobility may contribute to repeated injury of the cord and to prevent development of late deformity that can compromise the surgical outcome. The decision to use either an anterior or posterior approach and which specific procedure is based on multiple factors, including the source of spinal cord compression, the number of vertebral segments involved in the disease process, cervical alignment, the magnitude of coexisting neck pain, patient comorbidities, and the surgeon's familiarity with various techniques.

An anterior decompressive procedure is ideally suited for the current case in which the stenosing pathology is ventral to the spinal cord at two adjacent levels and is confined to the levels of the intervertebral disc only without significant osteophyte formation. The anterior approach will provide for direct visualization and removal of the offending pathology without manipulation of the cord.[34–38] With a kyphotic cervical sagittal alignment, an anterior procedure will also serve to restore physiologic lordosis. In addition, affording direct anterior decompression restoration of lordosis will allow for shifting of the cord dorsally to diminish the effect of any residual anterior compression. Posterior decompression for the treatment of myelopathy is generally contraindicated for patients who have neutral or kyphotic sagittal alignment of the cervical spinal column.[39] Laminectomy or laminoplasty in our patient with a kyphotic or neutrally aligned spinal column is unlikely to allow posterior translation of the spinal cord away from the anterior compressive abnormality.

Sodeyama et al.[40] showed that the peak postoperative dorsal translation of the spinal cord was greatest (peak shift, 3.1 mm) in patients who had a lordotic spinal curve, and least (peak shift, <2 mm) in patients who had a kyphotic cervical spine. Better recovery of myelopathy has also been reported following laminoplasty in patients without preoperative kyphosis.[41]

After anterior decompression, spinal column stability will need to be restored through segmental arthrodesis. The arthrodesis may also have the added benefit of eliminating painful motion from the spondylotic motion segment, a primary symptom in our patient.

Preoperative neck pain is a relative contraindication to laminoplasty. Disruption of the posterior paraspinal musculature from a posterior approach can aggravate axial neck pain. A review of laminoplasty, reported that the postoperative prevalence of neck pain ranged from 6% to 60% among different series and suggested that the true prevalence may actually be higher as neck pain was frequently not reported in the studies that were reviewed.[42,43] Axial pain is not a major concern following anterior surgery.

A critical component of the decision making in this, and any other, case is the risk/benefit ratio of the procedure options available. We have already demonstrated that an anterior approach can safely and reliably achieve our stated treatment goals. Boakye et al.[44] performed a National Inpatient Sample to identify 58,115 admissions of patients with CSM who underwent spinal fusion in the United States from 1993 to 2002.

The overall in-hospital complication rate was 13.4% and the in-hospital mortality rate for the entire cohort was 0.6%. Overall, 46,562 patients underwent anterior fusion, with a complication rate of 11.35% and mortality rate of 0.5%. A total of 8,112 patients underwent posterior fusion, with a complication rate of 16.4% and a mortality rate of 0.72%. Anterior fusion patients had a mean length of stay (LOS) of 3.4 days and mean hospital charges of $23,209, whereas posterior fusion patients had a mean LOS of 5.74 days with hospital charges of $30,927. Anterior approaches were associated with higher risks of hoarseness (0.21%) and dysphagia (3%), while posterior procedures had significantly higher rates of infection (0.8% vs. 0.2%), hematoma (3.2% vs. 2%) and cardiac and pulmonary complications (6.7% vs. 3.8%).

Choice of Exact Surgical Procedure

Five surgical options deserve consideration:

1. Two-level diskectomy C4/5 and C5/6 with instrumented fusion
2. C5 corpectomy with instrumented reconstruction
3. Circumferential anterior and posterior (ap) fusion
4. Disc arthroplasty
5. Oblique corpectomy

We do not believe circumferential AP Fusion is necessary in this case. Our surgical goals can be achieved from an anterior approach alone. Our patient does not have significant osteophyte formation suggesting a fixed kyphosis, there is no dorsal compression of the cord and anterior decompression is only required at two adjacent levels. Circumferential procedures are associated with higher complication rates, longer in-hospital stay and increased cost.[45]

Disc arthroplasty, while promising, cannot be recommended based on the evidence currently available. Results comparable to fusion have been reported in randomized controlled studies for single-level anterior disease.[46] This study found that patients in both the arthroplasty and arthrodesis groups had improvement following surgery; furthermore, improvement was similar between the groups, with no worsening of myelopathy in the arthroplasty group. The findings at 2 years postoperatively suggest that arthroplasty is equivalent to arthrodesis for the treatment of cervical myelopathy for a single-level anterior abnormality localized to the disc space. A prospective study of cervical arthroplasty reported significantly improved clinical outcomes for multilevel cervical arthroplasty compared with single-level cervical disc replacement for radiculopathy and myelopathy. Outcomes measured included VAS and Odoms.[47] Sekhon[48] reported on a series of 11 patients <55 years of age with anterior cervical decompression treated with a total of 15 artificial disc prostheses with a mean follow-up of 18 months. There were no major complications. There was an improvement in the Nurick grade by 0.91 grades ($p < 0.001$) and in the Oswestry Neck Disability Index by 41.5 percentage points ($p < 0.001$). In one case fusion was attained at 17 months postoperatively and one patient had a transient worsening of preoperative symptoms postoperatively, with focal kyphosis. The spinal cord was decompressed on postoperative imaging in all cases.

Oblique corpectomy as described by George et al.[49] is utilized for patients with anterior compression dorsal to the vertebral body, for example OPLL, and so is not suitable for this case.

There are numerous studies demonstrating the efficacy and safety of either two-level diskectomy and instrumented fusion or corpectomy and reconstruction.[36,50–52] When compared with multilevel ACDF (in which there are two surfaces per level), one hypothesis posits that cervical corpectomy should result in higher fusion rates because there are only two fusion surfaces.[1,53] However, corpectomy has been associated with early hardware failure.[54,55] Fraser showed that regardless of the number of levels fused the use of an anterior cervical plate system significantly increased the rate of fusion over diskectomy alone.[56] For two-level disk disease, as in our case, there was no significant difference between ACDF or corpectomy when a plate system was used.

There have been five studies directly comparing multilevel anterior cervical diskectomy and fusion (ACDF) with corpectomy for multilevel CSM. The results are summarized in Table 6.3.

Swank et al.[57] performed a retrospective study of a single surgeon's series of patients treated by multilevel cervical disc excision (two or three levels), allograft tricortical iliac crest arthrodesis, and anterior instrumentation to compare fusion success and clinical outcome between multilevel Smith-Robinson interbody grafting and tricortical iliac strut graft reconstruction, both supplemented with anterior instrumentation in the cervical spine. Sixty-four consecutive patients underwent allograft tricortical iliac crest reconstruction and anterior cervical plating. The average follow-up was 39 months. There were 38 patients in the discectomy and interbody grafting group and 26 patients in the corpectomy and strut graft reconstruction group. Pseudoarthrosis occurred in 42% of the anterior cervical interbody fusion patients and 31% of the corpectomy patients. Nonunion in two-level interbody fusions occurred in 36% of the patients as compared to 10% for patients with one-level corpectomies; while 54% of patients with three-level interbody fusions and 44% of patients with two-level corpectomies were noted to have pseudoarthrosis. Higher percentages of nonunion were noted in multilevel interbody grafting than in corpectomy with strut grafting and when more vertebral levels were involved. In addition, the authors felt that anterior corpectomy affords decompression of significant osteophytes in a safer and quicker manner than multiple diskectomies.

Wang et al.[58] compared fusion rates between single-level cervical corpectomy and two-level discectomy and fusion. The difference in fusion rates between the two groups was not statistically significant ($p = 0.385$). The clinical results of the surgeries were similar between the groups based on Odom's criteria. The addition of cervical plates to either two-level discectomies or single-level corpectomies yielded similar fusion and complication rates.

In their nonranomized cohort study Hwang et al.[59] evaluated the outcome after anterior corpectomy with iliac bone fusion compared with discectomy with interbody titanium cage fusion for multilevel cervical degenerated disc disease. Both groups demonstrated a significant increase in the JOA scores (preoperatively 11.1 ± 2.1 and 10.4 ± 3.5, postoperatively 14.3 ± 2.4 and 13.9 ± 2.1, respectively) and a significant decrease in

TABLE 6.3 Summary of Studies Comparing Multilevel ACDF and Corpectomy for Multilevel CSM.

Author	Decompression	Fusion Method	Clinical Outcome	Fusion Rate	Hardware Failure
Yonenobu et al. (1985)	Multi-ACDF vs. corpectomy	Autograft	Corpectomy superior	Corpectomy superior	None reported
Swank et al. (1997)	Multi-ACDF vs. corpctomy	Allograft and autograft	Corpectomy superior	Corpectomy superior	Equivalent
Wang et al. (2001)	Multi-ACDF vs. corpctomy	Allograft	Equivalent	Equivalent	Equivalent
Nirala et al. (2004)	Multi-ACDF vs. corpctomy	Autograft	Corpectomy superior	Corpectomy superior	None reported
Hwang (2004)	Multi-ACDF vs. corpctomy	Titanium ca ge vs. iliac crest strut	Equivalent	Equivalent	More in corpectomy group

the visual analog pain scores (preoperatively 8.5 ± 1.1 and 8.7 ± 1.5, postoperatively 2.9 ± 1.8 and 3.0 ± 2.0, respectively). However, there was no significant difference between the groups. Both groups showed a significant increase in the cervical lordosis after operation and reached satisfactory fusion rates (96.3% and 91.4%, respectively). Three patients (2 two-level corpectomies and 1 three-level corpectomy) had construct failures that required a second operation. Eight of thirty-five patients who underwent iliac bone fusion had donor site pain.

While Table 6.3 seems to suggest that corpectomy is superior to multilevel ACDF we must be careful to interpret the results as they pertain to our patient. The patients described by Yonenobu et al.[28] and Nirala et al.[60] underwent decompression/diskectomy/corpectomy without modern instrumentation. In the series described by Swank et al.[57] nonunion in two-level interbody fusions occurred in 36% of the patients as compared to 10% for patients with one-level corpectomies. However all these cases were performed with allograft, and the diagnosis of pseudarthrosis was radiological, with no reference made to the number of cases with symptomatic failure. Based on the studies pertinent to our case two-level diskectomy and fusion is equivalent to single-level corpectomy in terms of clinical outcome and fusion rate. Hardware failure requiring revision is more common with the corpectomy group as described by Hwang et al.[59]

DEFINITIVE TREATMENT PLAN

We propose an anterior surgical approach for the patient in this case. To achieve the surgical goal of neural decompression in this particular case only two-level diskectomy/osteophytectomy is required. Figure 6.1 does not demonstrate any element of compression that is not safely accessible through the interspace. Our patient does not have compression directly behind the vertebral body that would mandate a corpectomy. The evident kyphosis is due to asymmetric disc degeneration. There is no evidence of bony deformity or vertebral body kyphosis and the degree of kyphosis does not warrant an osteotomy or vertebrectomy for correction.

Grading the Evidence for this Plan

Because of the unique anatomical considerations in our case we believe that the specific surgical goals can be safely and adequately achieved with two-level diskectomy and instrumented fusion. The recommendation for multilevel diskectomy over corpectomy would be considered weak with moderate quality of evidence. Unique case specific factors were crucial in choosing multilevel ACDF over corpectomy.

In summary, in accordance with the method of grading recommendation put forward by Schunemann et al.[30] our proposed treatment of anterior decompression and instrumented fusion would be considered a **strong recommendation**. The overall quality of evidence for this recommendation is moderate.

PREDICTING OUTCOMES

The literature as we have synthesized thus far suggests that our patient should anticipate a good to excellent neurological outcome with a low level of morbidity or complication from the recommended surgical intervention. However many of these studies on multilevel ACDF involve three or more levels, many did not utilize modern surgical techniques and many others did not utilize validated outcome measures. Thus to adequately predict outcomes and counsel our patient, we must rely on appropriate and applicable studies of modern surgical techniques utilizing validated outcome measures.

Bapat et al.[38] in 2008 reported a prospective analysis of 129 patients with a subset of 79 patients with moderate myelopathy (mean JOA of 10), mean age 46 years with anterior compression of one or two levels. In this specific group anterior diskectomy and instrumented fusion resulted in a six point increase in the mean JOA score at 36 months follow-up. The mean recovery rate was 82% ± 28%. Complications were odynophagia 45% at 1 month and 0% at 3 months, dysphagia 26% at 1 month and 0% at 3 months, 2.5% asymptomatic pseudarthrosis rate and 3% symptomatic adjacent segment degeneration, all of which settled with conservative treatment. Overall our patient could expect a 96% good to excellent outcome with a near normal postoperative mean JOA score at 3 years' follow-up.

Gok et al.[45] in 2008 reported a retrospective study on a subgroup of 31 consecutive patients with a mean age of 54 years undergoing two-level ACDF for CSM with a mean follow-up of 25 months. The mean preoperative Nurick grade was 2.85, which improved to a mean grade of 1.35 postoperatively ($p = 0.0001$). Forty-three patients (93%) in this group had an improvement in assigned Nurick grade following surgery and 3 patients remained the same. Five patients (10.9%) experienced dysphagia postoperatively with all resolving in <6 weeks. One patient (2.2%) developed a postoperative infection that was successfully treated with a single debridement procedure. One patient (2.2%) underwent reoperation for an epidural hematoma. A total of 4 patients (8.7%) required revision surgery within 4 years, three for symptomatic adjacent-level disease and one for hardware failure.

Wang et al.[58] in 2001 reported on a subgroup of 32 patients with CSM who had two-level discectomies and fusion performed with two tricortical autogenous iliac crest grafts and the use of cervical plates. The average age of the patients was 51.5 years (range: 17–80 years). 88% of patients reported a good to excellent outcome at 3.5 years as determined by Odom's criteria.

Fountas et al.[61] in 2007 reported on the complication rates of ACDF in 1,015 patients, of which 279 underwent two-level anterior cervical diskectomy and instrumented fusion. The mean age was 56 years. Of this subgroup the radiological pseudarthrosis rate was 7.8%. The incidence of postoperative hematoma was 3.2%. Dysphonia was transient in 4.3% and dysphagia in 10%. Two patients had esophageal perforation and two others had an iatrogenic CSF leak.

SUMMARY

In summary, our patient can anticipate approximately a 96% good to excellent outcome with a near normal postoperative mean JOA score at 3 years' follow-up. Major complications are uncommon while transient dysphagia and asymptomatic radiological pseudarthrosis at 2 years occur in approximately 10% of patients. A similar number of patients will require a second surgical procedure within 5 years for either adjacent segment failure or symptomatic pseudarthrosis.

Preoperative counseling of this patient will require a frank discussion of the treatment option recommended and its inherent risks, benefits, potential outcomes, and associated burdens as summarized above. These results are in keeping with my experience as a spine surgeon and should drive the clinician to be selective with surgical treatment.

REFERENCES

1. Emery SE, Bohlman HH, Bolesta MJ, et al. Anterior cervical decompression and arthrodesis for the treatment of cervical spondylotic myelopathy. Two to seventeen-year follow-up. *J Bone Joint Surg Am*. 1998;80(7):941–951.
2. McCormack BM, Weinstein PR. Cervical spondylosis. An update. *West J Med*. 1996;165(1–2):43–51.
3. Hukuda S, Mochizuki T, Ogata M, et al. Operations for cervical spondylotic myelopathy. A comparison of the results of anterior and posterior procedures. *J Bone Joint Surg Br*. 1985;67(4):609–615.
4. Nurick S. The pathogenesis of cervical spondylotic myelopathy. *Acta Neurol Belg*. 1976;76(5–6):274–275.
5. Edwards WC, LaRocca SH. The developmental segmental sagittal diameter in combined cervical and lumbar spondylosis. *Spine*. 1985;10(1):42–49.
6. Young WF. Cervical spondylotic myelopathy: a common cause of spinal cord dysfunction in older persons. *Am Fam Physician*. 2000;62(5):1064–1670, 1073.
7. Houten JK, Cooper PR. Laminectomy and posterior cervical plating for multilevel cervical spondylotic myelopathy and ossification of the posterior longitudinal ligament: effects on cervical alignment, spinal cord compression, and neurological outcome. *Neurosurgery*. 2003;52(5):1081–1087; discussion 1087–1088.
8. Uchihara T, Furukawa T, Tsukagoshi H. Compression of brachial plexus as a diagnostic test of cervical cord lesion. *Spine*. 1994;19(19):2170–2173.
9. Dalitz K, Vitzthum HH. Evaluation of five scoring systems for cervical spondylogenic myelopathy. *Spine J*. 2008.
10. Prasad SS, O'Malley M, Caplan M, et al. MRI measurements of the cervical spine and their correlation to Pavlov's ratio. *Spine*. 2003;28(12):1263–1268.
11. Okada Y, Ikata T, Katoh S, et al. Morphologic analysis of the cervical spinal cord, dural tube, and spinal canal by magnetic resonance imaging in normal adults and patients with cervical spondylotic myelopathy. *Spine*. 1994;19(20):2331–2335.
12. Nurick S. The natural history and the results of surgical treatment of the spinal cord disorder associated with cervical spondylosis. *Brain*. 1972;95(1):101–108.
13. Lees F, Turner JW. Natural history and prognosis of cervical spondylosis. *Br Med J*. 1963;2(5373):1607–1610.
14. Clarke E, Robinson PK. Cervical myelopathy: a complication of cervical spondylosis. *Brain*. 1956;79(3):483–510.
15. LaRocca H. Cervical spondylotic myelopathy: natural history. *Spine*. 1988;13(7):854–855.
16. Roberts A. Myelopathy due to cervical spondylosis. *Neurology*. 1966;16(95):1–4.
17. Barnes MP, Saunders M. The effect of cervical mobility on the natural history of cervical spondylotic myelopathy. *J Neurol Neurosurg Psychiatry*. 1984;47(1):17–20.
18. Nakamura K, Kurokawa T, Hoshino Y, et al. Conservative treatment for cervical spondylotic myelopathy: achievement and sustainability of a level of "no disability". *J Spinal Disord*. 1998;11(2):175–179.
19. Matsumoto M, Toyama Y, Ishikawa M, et al. Increased signal intensity of the spinal cord on magnetic resonance images in cervical compressive myelopathy. Does it predict the outcome of conservative treatment? *Spine*. 2000;25(6):677–682.
20. Matsumoto M, Chiba K, Ishikawa M, et al. Relationships between outcomes of conservative treatment and magnetic resonance imaging findings in patients with mild cervical myelopathy caused by soft disc herniations. *Spine*. 2001;26(14):1592–1598.
21. Shimomura T, Sumi M, Nishida K, et al. Prognostic factors for deterioration of patients with cervical spondylotic myelopathy after nonsurgical treatment. *Spine*. 2007;32(22):2474–2479.
22. Kadanka Z, Mares M, Bednaník J, et al. Approaches to spondylotic cervical myelopathy: conservative versus surgical results in a 3-year follow-up study. *Spine*. 2002;27(20):2205–2210; discussion 2210–2211.
23. Sampath P, Bendebba M, Davis JD, et al. Outcome of patients treated for cervical myelopathy. A prospective, multicenter study with independent clinical review. *Spine*. 2000;25(6):670–676.
24. Bednarik J, Kadanka Z, Vohánka S, et al. The value of somatosensory- and motor-evoked potentials in

predicting and monitoring the effect of therapy in spondylotic cervical myelopathy. Prospective randomized study. *Spine.* 1999;24(15):1593–1598.

25. Edwards CC II, Riew KD, Anderson PA, et al. Cervical myelopathy: current diagnostic and treatment strategies. *Spine J.* 2003;3(1):68–81.

26. Fujiwara K, Yonenobu K, Ebara S, et al. The prognosis of surgery for cervical compression myelopathy. An analysis of the factors involved. *J Bone Joint Surg Br.* 1989;71(3):393–398.

27. Kadanka Z, Bednarík J, Vohánka S, et al. Conservative treatment versus surgery in spondylotic cervical myelopathy: a prospective randomised study. *Eur Spine J.* 2000;9(6):538–544.

28. Yonenobu K, Fuji T, Ono K, et al. Choice of surgical treatment for multisegmental cervical spondylotic myelopathy. *Spine.* 1985;10(8):710–716.

29. Tanaka J, Seki N, Tokimura F, et al. Operative results of canal-expansive laminoplasty for cervical spondylotic myelopathy in elderly patients. *Spine.* 1999;24(22): 2308–2312.

30. Schunemann HJ, Jaeschke R, Cook DJ, et al. An official ATS statement: grading the quality of evidence and strength of recommendations in ATS guidelines and recommendations. *Am J Respir Crit Care Med.* 2006;174(5): 605–614.

31. Fujimura Y, Nishi Y, Nakamura M. Dorsal shift and expansion of the spinal cord after expansive open-door laminoplasty. *J Spinal Disord.* 1997;10(4):282–287.

32. Suri A, Chabbra RP, Mehta VS, et al. Effect of intramedullary signal changes on the surgical outcome of patients with cervical spondylotic myelopathy. *Spine J.* 2003;3(1):33–45.

33. Bucciero A, Vizioli L, Carangelo B, et al. MR signal enhancement in cervical spondylotic myelopathy. Correlation with surgical results in 35 cases. *J Neurosurg Sci.* 1993;37(4):217–222.

34. Ashkenazi E, Smorgick Y, Rand N, et al. Anterior decompression combined with corpectomies and discectomies in the management of multilevel cervical myelopathy: a hybrid decompression and fixation technique. *J Neurosurg Spine.* 2005;3(3):205–209.

35. Ikenaga M, Shikata J, Tanaka C. Radiculopathy of C-5 after anterior decompression for cervical myelopathy. *J Neurosurg Spine.* 2005;3(3):210–217.

36. Ikenaga M, Shikata J, Tanaka C. Long-term results over 10 years of anterior corpectomy and fusion for multilevel cervical myelopathy. *Spine.* 2006;31(14):1568–1574; discussion 1575.

37. Chibbaro S, Benvenuti L, Carnesecchi S, et al. Anterior cervical corpectomy for cervical spondylotic myelopathy: experience and surgical results in a series of 70 consecutive patients. *J Clin Neurosci.* 2006;13(2):233–238.

38. Bapat MR, Chaudhary K, Sharma A, et al. Surgical approach to cervical spondylotic myelopathy on the basis of radiological patterns of compression: prospective analysis of 129 cases. *Eur Spine J.* 2008;17(12): 1651–1663.

39. Rao RD, Gourab K, David KS. Operative treatment of cervical spondylotic myelopathy. *J Bone Joint Surg Am.* 2006;88(7):1619–1640.

40. Sodeyama T, Goto S, Mochizuki M, et al. Effect of decompression enlargement laminoplasty for posterior shifting of the spinal cord. *Spine.* 1999;24(15):1527–1531; discussion 1531–1532.

41. Suda K, Abumi K, Ito M, et al. Local kyphosis reduces surgical outcomes of expansive open-door laminoplasty for cervical spondylotic myelopathy. *Spine.* 2003;28(12):1258–1262.

42. Ratliff JK, Cooper PR. Cervical laminoplasty: a critical review. *J Neurosurg.* 2003;98(3 suppl):230–238.

43. Cooper PR. Cervical spondylotic myelopathy. *J Neurosurg Spine.* 2005;3(3):253–254.

44. Boakye M, Patil CG, Santarelli J, et al. Cervical spondylotic myelopathy: complications and outcomes after spinal fusion. *Neurosurgery.* 2008;62(2):455–461; discussion 461–462.

45. Gok B, Sciubba DM, McLoughlin GS, et al. Surgical treatment of cervical spondylotic myelopathy with anterior compression: a review of 67 cases. *J Neurosurg Spine.* 2008;9(2):152–157.

46. Riew KD, Buchowski JM, Sasso R, et al. Cervical disc arthroplasty compared with arthrodesis for the treatment of myelopathy. *J Bone Joint Surg Am.* 2008;90(11):2354–2364.

47. Pimenta L, McAfee PC, Cappuccino A, et al. Superiority of multilevel cervical arthroplasty outcomes versus single-level outcomes: 229 consecutive PCM prostheses. *Spine.* 2007;32(12):1337–1344.

48. Sekhon LH. Cervical arthroplasty in the management of spondylotic myelopathy: 18-month results. *Neurosurg Focus.* 2004;17(3):E8.

49. George B, Gauthier N, Lot G. Multisegmental cervical spondylotic myelopathy and radiculopathy treated by multilevel oblique corpectomies without fusion. *Neurosurgery.* 1999;44(1):81–90.

50. Eleraky MA, Llanos C, Sonntag VK. Cervical corpectomy: report of 185 cases and review of the literature. *J Neurosurg.* 1999;90(1 suppl):35–41.

51. Herman JM, Sonntag VK. Cervical corpectomy and plate fixation for postlaminectomy kyphosis. *J Neurosurg.* 1994; 80(6):963–970.

52. Mayr MT, Subach BR, Comey CH, et al. Cervical spinal stenosis: outcome after anterior corpectomy, allograft reconstruction, and instrumentation. *J Neurosurg.* 2002; 96(1 suppl):10–16.

53. McAfee PC, Bohlman HH, Ducker TB, et al. One-stage anterior cervical decompression and posterior stabilization. A study of one hundred patients with a minimum of two years of follow-up. *J Bone Joint Surg Am.* 1995;77(12):1791–1800.

54. Sasso RC, Ruggiero RA Jr, Reilly TM, et al. Early reconstruction failures after multilevel cervical corpectomy. *Spine.* 2003;28(2):140–142.

55. Silber JS, Anderson DG, Daffner SD, et al. Donor site morbidity after anterior iliac crest bone harvest for single-level anterior cervical discectomy and fusion. *Spine.* 2003;28(2):134–139.

56. Fraser JF, Hartl R. Anterior approaches to fusion of the cervical spine: a metaanalysis of fusion rates. *J Neurosurg Spine.* 2007;6(4):298–303.

57. Swank ML, Lowery GL, Bhat AL, et al. Anterior cervical allograft arthrodesis and instrumentation: multilevel

interbody grafting or strut graft reconstruction. *Eur Spine J.* 1997;6(2):138–143.

58. Wang JC, McDonough PW, Endow KK, et al. A comparison of fusion rates between single-level cervical corpectomy and two-level discectomy and fusion. *J Spinal Disord.* 2001;14(3):222–225.

59. Hwang SL, Lin CL, Lieu AS, et al. Three-level and four-level anterior cervical discectomies and titanium cage-augmented fusion with and without plate fixation. *J Neurosurg Spine.* 2004;1(2):160–167.

60. Nirala AP, Husain M, Vatsal DK. A retrospective study of multiple interbody grafting and long segment strut grafting following multilevel anterior cervical decompression. *Br J Neurosurg.* 2004;18(3):227–232.

61. Fountas KN, Kapsalaki EZ, Nikolakakos LG, et al. Anterior cervical discectomy and fusion associated complications. *Spine.* 2007;32(21):2310–2317.

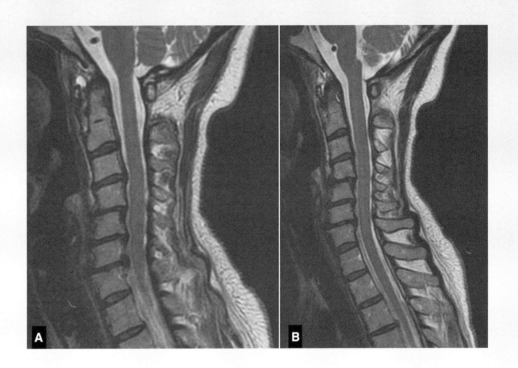

7 Discitis and Osteomyelitis

VINCENT J. DEVLIN, MD, PAUL A. ANDERSON, MD, AND CHRISTOPHER HUME, DO

A 78-year-old man presents with a known history of discitis and osteomyelitis at L5-S1 being treated nonoperatively with antibiotic therapy for the past 12 weeks. Despite treatment, he continues to complain of severe back pain, substantial weight loss (60 pounds), and constitutional symptoms that have worsened over the past 6 months. For a variety of reasons, including imbalance and generalized fatigue, he ambulates with a walker. He has no upper extremity complaints. Medical history includes psoriatic arthritis, diverticulitis (for which he has an ileostomy), prostate adenocarcinoma, hypercholesterolemia, hypertension, and diabetes.

Laboratories have demonstrated mild anemia and persistently elevated ESR and C-reactive protein levels. The patient has 5/5 strength and intact sensation in the upper and lower extremities bilaterally. Reflexes are 0+ at the patella tendon and 1+ at the Achilles tendon. He has a negative straight leg raise test and no tenderness to palpation of the back. He is thin, which, according to his family, represents a profound difference from his usual robust (i.e., a bit rotund) body habitus. Overall alignment of his spine and his extremities appears to be otherwise within normal limits.

Magnetic resonance images of the lumbar spine are shown in Figure 7.1.

INTERPRETATION OF CLINICAL PRESENTATION

The case presentation describes a senior citizen with a history of chronic lumbar discitis and osteomyelitis at the lumbosacral junction. His imaging demonstrates a prior laminectomy in the upper lumbar spine; for the purposes of this discussion, we assume that the prior surgery was not related to the current infection.

The patient's chief complaint is back pain, which is the most common complaint in a patient with pyogenic infection. No information is provided regarding factors that exacerbate or relieve this patient's back pain. Typically, back pain associated with early-stage infection is unrelated to activity and often present at rest. However, when osseous destruction is significant, mechanical symptoms may be evident.

Constitutional symptoms are present (severe weight loss). No history of elevated temperature or signs of systemic sepsis are noted. Although a history of fever is helpful in diagnosing a spinal infection, temperature elevation is present in less than half of all cases. Fever and other signs of inflammatory response such as laboratory tests may be blunted due to the patient's relatively immunocompromised state secondary to psoriasis and cancer.

The history does not elucidate the specific route by which infection entered the spinal column in this patient. Potential mechanisms include hematogenous spread from distant infectious foci (e.g., infected catheter, urinary tract infection, dental caries, intravenous drug use, skin infection), direct extension from an adjacent infection (e.g., abdominal or retroperitoneal infection), or direct inoculation (e.g., following a spinal procedure). The patient's medical comorbidities predispose him to development of spinal infection. Known patient risk factors associated with spinal infection include advanced age (>60 years), diabetes, rheumatoid arthritis, chronic steroid use, and acquired immunodeficiency syndrome. In this patient, his chronic skin condition may be a potential source for the infection under discussion. However, all patients with spinal osteomyelitis without an obvious source should be evaluated for subacute bacterial endocarditis.

Physical examination reveals no posterior spinal tenderness. Sensory and motor functions are intact in both upper and lower extremities. The absence of spinal tenderness, fever, muscle spasm, and sciatic

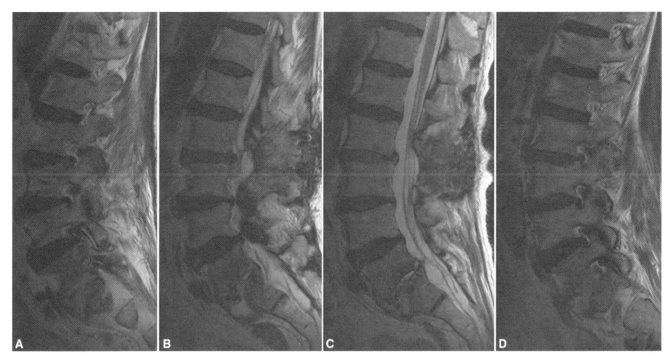

Figure 7.1.

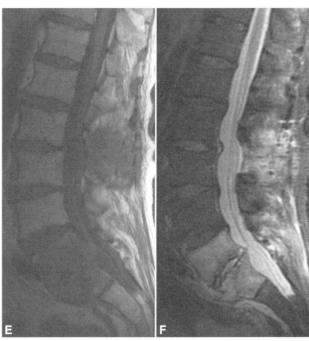

tension signs combined with a history of weight loss over 6 months support the diagnosis of chronic infection rather than acute or subacute infection.

Laboratory data include anemia as well as persistently elevated ESR and C-reactive protein levels. Anemia is not specifically correlated with infection but may represent a marker for underlying chronic disease. ESR is increased in over 90% of patients with infection but is a very nonspecific test and may be normal in low virulence infections. C-reactive protein levels are typically elevated in pyogenic infection and are considered more specific than ESR. However, increased ESR and C-reactive protein levels are not pathognomonic for infection. The white blood cell count is not reported. Studies document its elevation in less than half of cases of spinal infection. In this case, the laboratory tests may be falsely normal due to the patient's immunocompromised state. A prealbumin level is recommended in this case to assess baseline nutritional status and guide decision making. Poor preoperative nutritional status is associated with an increased rate of wound complications following surgical intervention.

A bacteriologic diagnosis is not documented in this case. Blood cultures should be obtained in patients with pyogenic infections although negative culture may occur in up to 75% of patients. Urine cultures should be obtained realizing that a patient with osteomyelitis may have a concurrent urinary infection with a different organism. Closed needle biopsy is necessary to provide a definite diagnosis in the absence of positive blood cultures. It is critical to obtain a bacteriologic diagnosis to guide subsequent antibiotic treatment. Therefore, antibiotics should be withheld until cultures are obtained.

Despite the fact that >50% of spinal infections are due to *Staphylococcus*, uncommon organisms are frequently encountered. For example, anaerobic infections are common in diabetics and in penetrating injuries. When the urinary tract is the source of infection, Proteus and *E. coli* species are common pathogens. *Pseudomonas aeruginosa* is associated with infections presenting in intravenous drug users and immunocompromised patients. The clinical scenario describes a 12-week course of antibiotic therapy but does not specify route of administration (intravenous vs. oral), antibiotic type, and whether antibiotics selection was guided by culture results.

Available diagnostic imaging studies in this case presentation are limited to lumbar MRI images with and without gadolinium contrast enhancement (Fig. 7.1A–F). Erect weight-bearing plain radiographs of the lumbar spine are important and should be performed concurrently with MRI. Plain radiographic findings associated with lumbar discitis/osteomyelitis include disc space narrowing, end-plate blurring or erosion, and bone destruction in adjacent vertebral bodies. MRI is the current gold standard for imaging pyogenic infection, and classic findings are demonstrated in this case. The infectious foci shows characteristic decreased intensity on the T1 weighted images (Fig. 7.1E) and increased signal intensity on T2 weighted images (Fig. 7.1A–C). Intravenous gadolinium contrast may be used as an adjunct in the MRI diagnosis of infection. The disc and involved regions of the adjacent vertebral bodies typically enhance in the presence of gadolinium (Fig. 7.1F). In addition, the gadolinium is helpful in identifying epidural abscess. An abscess will enhance along its periphery on T1 gadolinium images, while reactive granulation tissue will enhance in a more diffuse pattern. The diagnosis of epidural abscess is important to treatment decisions. This can be difficult with the only pathognomonic finding being a dark signal with rim enhancement on gadolinium images. Recently, administration of gadolinium has been shown to exacerbate renal failure in patients with

sepsis and elevated serum creatinine levels. Epidural phlegmon is commonly seen and does not necessarily indicate that surgery is required.

CT scanning complements the diagnostic information obtained from MRI as CT provides better depiction of bone detail than MRI. The enhancement noted on MRI in the vertebral bodies adjacent to an infected disc space represents edema. CT more reliably estimates the degree of bone destruction secondary to infection, which tends to be overestimated when MRI is the only available imaging study. Radionuclide studies (technetium, gallium, indium) may be useful in the early diagnosis and localization of spinal infection, but their sensitivity, specificity, accuracy, and spatial resolution are inferior to MRI and are not useful for surgical decision making.

DECLARATION OF SPECIFIC DIAGNOSIS

This patient has chronic discitis and osteomyelitis involving the L5-S1 disc and adjacent vertebral endplates. There is an epidural abscess ventral to the thecal sac at the level of the L5-S1 disc with extension distally behind the S1 vertebral body. In addition, there is an anterior paravertebral abscess at L5-S1.

BRAINSTORMING: WHAT ARE THE TREATMENT GOALS AND SURGICAL OPTIONS?

The treatment goals are

1. Eradicate the infection
2. Relieve axial pain
3. Prevent deterioration of neurologic status
4. Prevent development of spinal instability and spinal deformity
5. Avoid iatrogenic complications

The treatment options are classified into four broad categories: nonoperative, posterior surgery, anterior surgery, and combined approaches.

Nonoperative Treatment

Antibiotics can be temporarily discontinued and closed needle biopsy of the L5-S1 level performed. If a positive culture is obtained, culture-specific intravenous antibiotics can be administered for an additional 6 weeks. The patient may be immobilized in a lumbar orthosis during this period. Nutritional consultation can be obtained, and intervention to improve nutritional status can be implemented. Further treatment options can be reassessed at that time.

Posterior Surgical Procedures

A variety of posterior surgical procedures can be considered and include

1. Posterior lumbar decompression (bilateral laminotomies with preservation of facet joints and debridement of the L5-S1 disc space) and utilization of a lumbar orthosis and/or bed rest.
2. Posterior lumbar decompression, posterolateral L5-S1 fusion without posterior instrumentation
3. Posterior lumbar decompression, posterolateral L5-S1 fusion and posterior spinal instrumentation (pedicle screws and rods)
4. Posterior lumbar decompression, posterolateral L5-S1 fusion, posterior spinal instrumentation (pedicle screws and rods,) and transforaminal lumbar interbody fusion L5-S1. Options for interbody fusion include structural iliac autograft, structural allograft cages, titanium mesh cages, and carbon fiber or PEEK cages. RhBMP-2 and/or a bone graft extender (e.g., allograft) may be used in conjunction with any of the interbody fusion options.
5. Percutaneous suction/irrigation of the L5-S1 disc space followed by percutaneous external fixation L5 to ilium.

Anterior Surgical Procedures

Anterior surgical options include

1. Stand-alone anterior L5-S1 discectomy and fusion. Options for interbody fusion include structural iliac autograft, structural allograft cages, titanium mesh cages, and carbon fiber or PEEK cages. RhBMP-2 (Infuse) and/or a bone graft extender (e.g., allograft) may be used in conjunction with any of the interbody fusion options.
2. Anterior L5-S1 discectomy and fusion combined with anterior plate fixation.

Combined Anterior and Posterior Surgical Procedures

Combined anterior and posterior options include

1. Anterior L5-S1 discectomy and fusion combined with posterior lumbar decompression, posterolateral L5-S1 fusion, posterior spinal instrumentation (pedicle screws and rods). This may be performed on same day or in staged fashion on separate days.
2. Anterior L5-S1 discectomy and fusion combined with minimally invasive posterior lumbar decompression, minimally invasive posterior spinal instrumentation (pedicle screws and rods)

EVALUATION OF THE LITERATURE

To identify relevant publications on discitis and osteomyelitis of the lumbar spine, a Medline search was performed. Medline "in process" and non–indexed citations were searched as was EBM reviews-Cochrane database. Search strategies included the use of MeSH (medical subject headings) and key words. Key words included "osteomyelitis," "spondylitis," and "spine." A focused search of "osteomyelitis" and "spine" with subheadings of "surgical procedures" and "therapeutics" was performed. The search strategy identified 118 pertinent articles after limiting from 1950 to 2007. A similar search strategy was applied to Embase and revealed 40 articles. Search terms included the following: "osteomyelitis," "treatment," "surgery," "thoracic spine," "spine surgery," "thoracolumbar spine," "spine disease," "infection," "abscess," "bacterial infection," "bone and joint infection," "device infection." Google Scholar and PubMed were also searched with the following terms: "osteomyelitis," "spondylitis," and "spine" to capture all potentially relevant articles. Journals were hand searched as well including Spine, Journal of Spinal Disorders, and Journal of Bone and Joint Surgery (Am). There were 311 English language abstracts that were reviewed and 57 full text articles were read.

The literature review was synthesized to address the following pertinent questions with respect to pyogenic discitis and osteomyelitis in adult patients:

1. What are the results of nonoperative treatment including mortality?
2. What are the indications for surgical treatment?
3. How do results of various surgical approaches compare for treatment of lumbar pyogenic discitis and osteomyelitis?
4. Can posterior spinal instrumentation be utilized in the setting of an acute spinal infection without an increased rate of infection-related complications?
5. Are infection-related complications increased if combined anterior and posterior surgical procedures are performed under the same anesthetic versus performing the procedures in separate stages?
6. Are foreign bodies applied to the anterior spinal column such as structural allografts, cages, bone cement, and anterior spinal instrumentation safe and effective in the setting of acute infection?
7. Can bone morphogenic protein be used off label in the presence of infection?

DETAILED REVIEW OF PERTINENT ARTICLES

What are the Results of Nonoperative Treatment Including Mortality?

Prior to modern era of antibiotic treatment, mortality from pyogenic spinal infections exceeded 25%.[1] With the advent of effective antibiotic treatment, mortality rates declined to reach currently reported rates, which range from 2% to 17%.[2,3] Duration of infection and delay to diagnosis of infection have been demonstrated to play a role in determining the outcome of nonoperative treatment.[4,5] Nonoperative treatment is advised as initial treatment in the absence of neurologic deficit, extensive bony destruction, significant deformity, or clinically significant abscess formation. In some cases, nonoperative treatment may be indicated due to medical comorbidities, which preclude consideration of surgical intervention. Nonoperative treatment includes culture-directed antibiotic therapy and spinal immobilization with an orthosis and even temporary bed rest. In some cases of pyogenic infection, the combination of reactive bone formation, reactive osteophyte formation, and resultant disc space narrowing may lead to autofusion of the involved motion segment. The most consistent predictors of success for nonoperative treatment reported include age <60 years, competent immune status, infection with *S. aureus*, and decreasing value for ESR over the course of treatment.[6] Duration of intravenous antibiotic treatment has proved critical with administration of antibiotics for <4 weeks associated with treatment failure.[7,8] Antibiotic selection plays a critical role. It has been shown that antibiotics with a positive charge such as vancomycin, aminoglycosides, and clindamycin penetrate into the nucleus pulposus better than negatively charged antibiotics such as penicillin, oxacillin, and cephalosporins.[9] ESR and CRP are useful to monitor response to antibiotic treatment. MRI has been proposed as a means to predict failure of nonoperative treatment of pyogenic osteomyelitis.[10] Signal change on the T1-weighted sagittal image exceeding 90% involvement of an affected motion segment at the onset of treatment successfully predicted failure of medical management and the need for subsequent surgical treatment. Follow-up MRI studies may be used to monitor response to antibiotic treatment. Soft-tissue findings (i.e., paraspinal abscess, epidural abscess) rather than osseous findings should be the focus of attention on follow-up MRI scans.[11] Vertebral body enhancement and bone marrow edema may appear worse but may not correlate with the patient's clinical status.

Nonoperative treatment is reported as successful in up to 75% of appropriately treated patients.[2,12] However, criteria for success focus on infection cure, infection recurrence, kyphosis correction, and neurologic status following treatment. Few studies provide quality of life data following nonoperative treatment of pyogenic vertebral infection. Woertgen et al.[4] reported that quality of life measures derived from SF-36 scores were not restored in patients treated for pyogenic vertebral infection when compared to a normative population sample. Only 14% of patients were free of pain following treatment, and 31% of patients had an unfavorable outcome.

In summary, there is weak evidence based on multiple retrospective case series to support nonoperative treatment with culture-directed intravenous antibiotics (minimum duration 4 weeks) and spinal immobilization. The authors agree that the most appropriate candidate for nonoperative treatment is a neurologically intact patient with primarily disc space involvement, minimal involvement of adjacent vertebra, no kyphotic deformity, and who is not debilitated by systemic disease or immune suppression.[12] It is challenging to directly compare the outcomes of operative and nonoperative treatment as the indications for selecting each type of treatment are different and vary with the duration and extent of infection as well as individual patient factors.

What are the Indications for Surgical Treatment?

Current accepted indications for surgical intervention include

- To perform an open biopsy to identify a pathogen when closed biopsy negative or considered unsafe
- To treat a clinically significant abscess (e.g., associated with sepsis)
- To salvage a failed course of appropriate nonsurgical management (intravenous antibiotics) in a patient with persistently elevated ESR, CRP, or refractory severe back pain (e.g., preventing ambulation)
- To treat neurologic deficit due to spinal cord, cauda equina, or nerve root compression
- To treat significant progressive spinal deformity or extensive vertebral body destruction
- In cases where significant medical comorbidities make nonsurgical treatment unlikely to succeed (e.g., immune compromise, inability to comply with treatment recommendations), surgical intervention can also be considered.

In summary, the indications for surgical intervention for pyogenic spinal infections are consistent with the indications for surgical intervention for other types of spinal pathology, that is, to confirm a diagnosis through biopsy, prevent neurologic deficit by decompression of neural structures, and prevent and/or correct spinal deformity via spinal realignment and stabilization.

How Do Results of Various Surgical Approaches Compare for Treatment of Lumbar Pyogenic Discitis and Osteomyelitis?

Well-designed prospective trials comparing surgical options for spinal discitis/osteomyelitis of the spine do not exist. Current recommendations are based on observational cohort studies, retrospective studies, case series, and expert opinion.

Spinal discitis/osteomyelitis is a disease process, which predominantly affects the anterior spinal column. The principles of the anterior approach to the spinal column for treatment of infection were defined by Hodgson and Stock[13] for treatment of tuberculosis and subsequently applied to the treatment of pyogenic spinal infections. Laminectomy alone is rarely advocated for the treatment of pyogenic infection due to its destabilizing effect and association with deformity progression, worsening spinal instability, and neurologic deterioration. One series showed that 60% of patients with osteomyelitis treated with laminectomy without stabilization required additional surgery to treat recurrent infection, spinal instability, and secondary neurologic impairment.[14] Laminectomy without stabilization is advised only in the special circumstance of primary epidural abscess where anterior vertebral elements are uninvolved and when epidural abscess extends cranial and caudad at multiple levels.

The effectiveness of an anterior approach with debridement and autologous structural bone grafting of the resultant anterior column defect without the use of spinal instrumentation has been documented in many retrospective studies.[15–18] Disadvantages associated with this approach include the need for prolonged post-op immobilization, poor maintenance of deformity correction, risk of graft dislodgement, and donor site complications related to harvest of long structural autografts. However, in cases of discitis/osteomyelitis localized to a single disc space, without significant vertebral body destruction and located in an inherently stable spinal region (e.g., mid thoracic region), an isolated anterior approach with debridement and autologous structural bone grafting of the anterior column defect is sufficient treatment and spinal instrumentation is not necessary.

Although the use of anterior spinal instrumentation following anterior debridement and grafting has been described in the cervical spine,[19,20] few studies exist to evaluate efficacy of anterior instrumentation in treatment of thoracolumbar and lumbar discitis/osteomyelitis. The use of anterior spinal instrumentation is less accepted in the thoracolumbar and lumbar spinal regions due to concerns regarding poor screw purchase in osteoporotic bone, the need to include additional motion segments when compared to posterior procedures, and direct contact of instrumentation system with the formerly infected area. Hee et al.[21] reported major complications in two patients (10%) whose surgical procedure included anterior titanium screw-rod staple constructs. Patients in this series underwent anterior debridement and reconstruction followed by posterior spinal instrumentation and fusion. One patient died of sepsis, and one patient developed recurrent osteomyelitis. These negative experiences led the group to discontinue the use of anterior instrumentation in the management of spinal osteomyelitis. In contrast, Ruf et al.[22] reported use of anterior screw-rod fixation, titanium mesh, and posterior spinal instrumentation without any infection-related problems encountered with respect to the anterior metallic implants. In a study utilizing a variety of surgical approaches, O'Shaughnessy et al.[23] reported four cases of discitis/osteomyelitis treated through an anterior approach with a titanium mesh cage, rhBMP-2, and dual rod anterolateral screw-based instrumentation. All patients had disease restricted to the anterior spinal column at a single segment with an intact posterior tension band. No recurrent infections or wound problems were reported.

The combination of radical anterior debridement and bone grafting followed by posterior fusion and posterior instrumentation has been advocated to avoid the complications associated with isolated anterior approaches. Multiple case series support the use of posterior spinal instrumentation following anterior debridement and grafting in the treatment of spinal discitis/osteomyelitis.[24–28] Anterior decompression and fusion with autogenous graft followed by posterior instrumentation and fusion have been considered the procedure of choice for discitis/osteomyelitis complicated by deformity, neurologic deficit, or epidural abscess.[29] There has been debate whether the anterior and posterior procedures should be performed under the same anesthetic or in a staged manner due to concerns about dorsal spread of infection and bonding of bacteria to the posterior implants resulting in recurrent infection.

Comprehensive posterior approaches (posterior instrumentation combined with posterior decompression and debridement of the disc plus structural grafting of the anterior spinal column from a single posterior approach) have been proposed as an alternative to separate anterior and posterior procedures. In the thoracic region, posterior approaches (extracavitary, costotransversectomy, transpedicular) may avoid the morbidity associated with thoracotomy. In the lumbar region, posterior approaches avoid challenges associated with anterior exposure in the setting of anatomy distorted by inflammation and bony destruction. McGuire and Eismont[18] reported 13 patients treated for lumbar disc space infection with posterior debridement of the disc space and endplates followed by bilateral lateral iliac autograft without use of spinal instrumentation and noted that such cases were likely to heal with local kyphosis. Evidence to support comprehensive posterior approaches for vertebral osteomyelitis is limited to small retrospective case series. In the largest reported series,[14] 48% of patients underwent posterior debridement, posterior pedicle screw-rod fixation, and placement of gentamycin/PMMA chains. Two weeks later, autogenous iliac graft was placed in the anterior column via the posterior approach. Remaining patients underwent single-stage posterior debridement, posterior pedicle screw-rod fixation, and placement of autologous iliac graft from the posterior approach. The overall rate of recurrent infection was 5% in patients whose treatment included posterior spinal instrumentation. In a study utilizing a variety of surgical approaches, O'Shaughnessy et al.[23] reported eight patients treated with posterior instrumentation and fusion and structural grafting of the anterior spinal column from a posterior approach with use of rhBMP-2. No cases of recurrent or persistent infection were reported. Lumbar cases were treated with transforaminal lumbar interbody fusion with titanium mesh cages. Thoracic cases were treated with debridement and placement of titanium mesh cages via a posterolateral extracavitary approach. In three cases, a direct posterior approach was performed for patients with long-standing paraplegia in which the thecal sac was ligated and corpectomies performed through the spinal canal.

Minimally invasive posterior approaches have been advocated as an alternative to open spinal surgery in retrospective case series. However, proponents point out limitations of these techniques, which include their use only for early-stage single level infections limited to a single disc space in the lower thoracic or lumbar spine.[30] These techniques are contraindicated for cases of advanced infection, neural compression, kyphotic deformity, extensive bony destruction. Additional risks associated with these approaches include inadequate curettage of the posterior aspect of the disc space, recurrent or progressive deformity, and recurrence of infection.[29,31] Jeanneret and Magerl[32] proposed a procedure combining percutaneous suction and irrigation of disc space infection followed by posterior external fixation. Disadvantages of this technique included the need for additional procedures in half of patients and incomplete correction of kyphotic deformity. More recently, minimally invasive pedicle screw insertion has been proposed as a potential means to limit posterior dissection and blood loss in patients undergoing sequential anterior and posterior surgical procedures for thoracic and lumbar pyogenic infections.[33]

In summary, a strong recommendation (based on low quality evidence) is made to utilize an anterior surgical approach when possible for treatment of pyogenic discitis/osteomyelitis. The use of adjunctive posterior spinal instrumentation is supported in this setting. A posterior approach with laminectomy without stabilization is associated with significant complications and is not advised except in special circumstances. Evidence to support comprehensive posterior approaches for decompression, disc debridement, and stabilization is limited for treatment of pyogenic discitis/osteomyelitis. Minimally invasive posterior treatment approaches as an alternative to combined anterior and posterior surgical procedures are not supported based on current literature.

Can Posterior Spinal Instrumentation be Utilized in the Setting of an Acute Spinal Infection without an Increased Rate of Infection-related Complications?

Multiple studies over the past decade support the use of posterior spinal instrumentation in the setting of acute spinal infection following thorough and radical debridement.[34–37] Advantages associated with the use of posterior spinal instrumentation in this setting include the following: (a) preservation of spinal alignment and restoration of spinal stability following radical debridement; (b) increased fusion rates; (c) ability to correct kyphotic spinal deformities; (d) avoidance of graft collapse, graft dislodgement, and loss of deformity correction; (e) rapid patient mobilization and early rehabilitation; and (f) avoidance need for a spinal orthosis. Experimental and clinical evidence supports the concept that bone infections are better controlled with antibiotics and bone stabilization than with antibiotics alone in an unstable osseous environment.[38] Carragee and Lezza[26] reported long-term prospective follow-up of immune-suppressed patients with active thoracic and lumbar spinal infections treated with radical anterior debridement and posterior spinal instrumentation and fusion. The mean duration of parenteral antibiotic therapy following surgery was 11 weeks, and all patients had discontinuation of antibiotic treatment by 8 months after surgery. All patients were disease-free at final follow-up (8.1 years). There was only one case of recurrent infection, which was salvaged with debridement, retained instrumentation, and antibiotics. There was no evidence of gross, microscopic, culture, or PCR evidence of residual infection or occult colonization when the original surgical site was examined at autopsy or at the time of implant removal procedures. Stainless steel instrumentation was utilized in this study. Experimental studies have analyzed the interplay between infection and various metals. Such studies have shown that bacteria adhere and persist to a greater degree on stainless steel than titanium alloys.[39] This finding suggests that titanium alloys should be considered for use in patients with preexisting spinal infections.

In summary, a weak recommendation based on poor quality evidence (case series) supports the use of posterior spinal instrumentation in patients with acute spinal infection. Basic science studies suggest that titanium alloys may resist bacterial adherence and can be considered as an alternative to stainless steel implant constructs in this setting.

Are Infection-Related Complications Increased If Combined Anterior and Posterior Surgical Procedures be Performed Under the Same Anesthetic Versus Performing the Procedures in Separate Stages?

No randomized prospective studies directly compare two-stage versus single-stage (same day) anterior and posterior procedures in the treatment of pyogenic vertebral discitis/osteomyelitis. One successful protocol is to perform anterior surgical debridement with fusion, followed by a period of intravenous antibiotics and delayed (average of 14 days) instrumented posterior fusion. Dimar et al.[34] documented success using this protocol with resolution of infection in all patients without recurrence of infection in any case. Advantages of this staged approach include the opportunity for a period of intravenous antibiotics between surgical stages to provide better control of infection as well as the opportunity to stabilize the patient's overall medical condition. Disadvantages of this approach include the difficulty in rapidly mobilizing these elderly patients due to the need for external support or bed rest between stages as well as the risks of additional anesthesia and surgery.

Sequential (same day) anterior and posterior approaches have been advocated to avoid the risks associated with a staged approach. Potential advantages include lower blood loss, a shortened hospital stay, decreased perioperative complications, earlier mobilization of the patient, avoidance of risks/costs associated with a second anesthetic, and decreased patient/family anxiety as treatment occurs in a single operative session.[40] Many patients are at their lowest medical/surgical risk at the time of presentation and their overall medical condition may not be enhanced if surgical intervention is delayed. The benefits of sequential same day surgery with implantation of metallic spinal implants must be balanced against the theoretic risk of bacterial colonization of the fixation device with subsequent recurrence of infection when antibiotics are discontinued. Over the past decade, numerous studies support the sequential (same day) anterior and posterior approach. Carragee and Lezza[26] reported that

one patient out of 25 patients undergoing same day anterior and posterior surgery developed a postoperative wound infection. Successful eradication of infection without removal of implants was achieved following operative debridement in this patient. Kuklo et al.[41] reported 2 posterior wound infections in a series of 21 patients treated with same day anterior debridement and reconstruction combined with posterior instrumentation. Both patients were successfully treated with irrigation and debridement without infection reoccurrence. Korovessis et al.[42] reported no postoperative posterior wound infections in a series of 17 patients undergoing same day anterior and posterior procedures. One anterior wound infection was noted and was successfully treated with a single operative debridement.

In summary, evidence does not support the superiority of staged anterior and posterior surgery versus single-stage (same day) surgery for pyogenic discitis/osteomyelitis. The authors recommend that decision making be individualized on a case-by-case basis considering factors such as the patient's general medical condition, the presence/absence of systemic sepsis, patient response under anesthesia during the anterior procedure (e.g., hemodynamic stability), and inherent stability of the anterior spinal column construct following debridement.

Are Foreign Bodies Applied to the Anterior Spinal Column Such As Structural Allografts, Cages, Bone Cement, and Anterior Spinal Instrumentation Safe and Effective in the Setting of Acute Infection?

Options for anterior spinal column reconstruction following surgical debridement of discitis/osteomyelitis have evolved. Historically, autograft bone (ilium, rib, fibula) has been used most commonly.[43] Studies also report use of vascularized autografts (e.g., rib).[44] The use of alternative materials, including structural allograft and titanium mesh cages, has been reported. No studies specifically analyze use of carbon fiber or PEEK in the treatment of discitis/osteomyelitis.

The use of structural allografts for anterior spinal reconstruction has been reported as successful for a variety of spinal pathologies including spinal deformities, degenerative disorders, fractures, and spinal tumor reconstruction.[45–47] Few studies specifically analyze results of structural allografts for discitis/osteomyelitis. Schuster et al.[48] reported 39 patients treated with surgical stabilization including anterior reconstruction with fresh-frozen allografts. Two patients developed recurrent infection at a contiguous level. Both patients had a history of intravenous drug use. Allen et al.[49] reported on 11 patients treated with fresh-frozen allografts packed with BMP-2 (Infuse) and encountered no recurrent infections.

The success of titanium mesh cages for anterior spinal column reconstruction has been documented for tumor, trauma, deformity, and degenerative disorders.[50] Over the past decade, the utility and safety of titanium mesh cages have been extensively reported in the treatment of discitis/osteomyelitis. Ruf et al.[22] reviewed 88 consecutive cases of vertebral osteomyelitis treated with titanium mesh cages filled and surrounded with autograft iliac bone graft or bone cement and screw-rod constructs. Two postoperative wound infections were noted: one at the iliac crest donor site and one posterior wound infection. No adverse effects of titanium mesh cages in the presence of active infection were noted. Infection was eradicated in all patients. Fayazi et al.[51] reported 11 patients treated with staged anterior debridement and reconstruction with titanium mesh filled with cancellous allograft followed 1 week later by posterior instrumentation. No complications were attributed to the titanium mesh cages. No evidence of recurrent or residual infection was noted in any patient. Kuklo et al.[41] reported 21 patients treated with single-stage anterior debridement, reconstruction with a titanium mesh cage filled with allograft chips and demineralized bone matrix followed by posterior pedicle screw instrumentation. No cases of chronic infection or implant-related problems were noted. Korovessis et al.[42] described success with a similar protocol using titanium mesh cages in 14 patients. Liljenqvist et al.[52] reported 20 patients treated with one-stage posterior instrumentation and fusion followed by anterior debridement, decompression and anterior column reconstruction using an expandable titanium cage filled with morselized autologous bone graft. All cases were fused on follow-up radiographs, and all infections were eradicated.

No studies specifically analyze the use of polymethylmethacrylate bone cement (PMMA) in the thoracic or lumbar infections. Ruf et al.[22] describe filling titanium mesh cages with (PMMA) surrounded with autologous iliac bone graft in patients with extreme osteoporosis following anterior debridement of discitis/osteomyelitis and do not report any recurrence of infection with this technique. The use of an antibiotic-PMMA strut has been described for treatment of cervical pyogenic spondylitis,[53] but no reports specifically address the use of a PMMA construct for this indication in the thoracic or lumbar spine.

Conflicting results exist regarding use of anterior spinal instrumentation following anterior debridement of pyogenic discitis/osteomyelitis. One study reported recurrent osteomyelitis and sepsis following use of anterior titanium screw-rod constructs.[21] In contrast, another study reported no infections associated with use of anterolateral screw-rod constructs following debridement of osteomyelitis.[23]

In summary, there is weak evidence (small case series) that allograft and titanium cages when applied in osteomyletic vertebrae do not have an adverse effect on eradication of infection, are not associated with complications, and are associated with high fusion rates. The use of anterior spinal screw-rod instrumentation is not well supported and has been associated with persistence of infection and sepsis in small case series.

Can Bone Morphogenic Protein be Used Safely Off Label in the Presence of Infection?

The efficacy of rhBMP-2 (Infuse) in humans with active pyogenic vertebral infections is not yet defined, and its use in this setting is not FDA approved and considered "off-label use." An initial report by Allen et al.[49] described 14 patients who underwent circumferential fusion for pyogenic vertebral osteomyelitis. RhBMP-2 (Infuse) was inserted into anterior fresh-frozen allografts (11 patients) or titanium mesh cages (3 patients) and followed by posterior spinal instrumentation and fusion with autogenous iliac graft. The theoretical reason to apply rhBMP-2 was to improve tissue vascularity and osseous union in the challenging fusion environment of pyogenic vertebral osteomyelitis. At 2-year follow-up, there were no recurrences of infection. Osseous union was noted in all patients. No adverse effects were attributed to the use of rhBMP.

Aryan et al.[20] analyzed 15 patients with osteomyelitis treated with corpectomy, titanium cage-plate reconstruction, and placement of rhBMP-2. Supplemental posterior screw-rod instrumentation was used in ten patients. Measurement of CRP levels returned to normal over a 6-month period, and no recurrence of infection was noted. There were two postoperative posterior wound infections, which were treated with open packing and healing by secondary intention. Fusion was reported in all patients. O'Shaughnessy et al.[23] reported a series of 20 patients with osteomyelitis treated with rhBMP-2 as the primary bone graft material for anterior and posterior fusion. All patients were treated with posterior titanium implants. Anterior column defects were reconstructed with titanium mesh cages with rhBMP-2. Posterior fusion was performed with rhBMP-2 and milled allograft. Dosing of rhBMP-2 was uniform in all cases: discectomy (6 mg/level), corpectomy (24 mg/level), posterior fusion at infected level (12 mg/level), posterior fusion at levels not infected but included in posterior construct (4 mg/level). The standard concentration of rhBMP-2 (1.5 mg/mL) was used and applied to an absorbable collagen sponge carrier. One pseudarthrosis was noted and was treated successfully with revision surgery. CT scans were used to assess fusion following surgery in all cases. There was no documentation of intracanal bone growth, symptomatic soft-tissue swelling, or postoperative radiculitis. This study showed that rhB-MP-2 applied with a standard dosing regimen may provide an alternative for bone grafting in cases of vertebral osteomyelitis. However, as the previous studies consist of case series without control groups, they represent low-quality evidence regarding the benefits of rhBMP-2 in this setting.

In summary, there is weak evidence (small case series) that BMP-2 does not exert a negative effect on the eradication of spinal infection, is not associated with adverse events when used in the thoracic and lumbar spinal regions, and is associated with a consistently high fusion rate. Based on current literature, there is a weak recommendation regarding the use of BMP-2 in cages or allograft struts following anterior debridement of pyogenic discitis/osteomyelitis.

EVIDENTIARY TABLE AND SELECTION OF TREATMENT METHOD

The best available evidence dictates that the patient presented in the clinical scenario should be treated operatively. In order to evaluate the most appropriate surgical treatment, only articles pertaining to adult patients with thoracic and lumbar osteomyelitis treated with modern spinal reconstructive techniques were critically examined above and are summarized in Table 7.1. Issues central to decision making in this case include

- Choice of surgical approach: combined anterior and posterior approach versus comprehensive posterior approach (e.g., TLIF, PLIF)
- Single-stage (same day) anterior and posterior surgery versus staged anterior and posterior surgery:
- The use of posterior instrumentation
- Options for reconstruction of the anterior spinal column (e.g., autograft, allograft, titanium mesh)
- Whether or not to use rhBMP-2

DEFINITIVE TREATMENT PLAN

The patient in this clinical scenario should be managed with operative intervention as nonsurgical treatment with antibiotic therapy for 3 months has not led to resolution of infection. This patient would not be predicted to improve with additional nonoperative treatment due to advanced age, incompetent immune status, and persistent elevation of ESR over the course of treatment. In the 78-year-old patient under consideration, a 60 lb weight loss strongly suggests compromised nutritional and immune states. Associated medical comorbidities (diabetes, prostate cancer and the presence of an ileostomy), persistently elevated ESR and CRP, and the erosion of the anterior superior aspect of the S1 vertebral endplate noted on MRI are additional negative prognostic factors.

TABLE 7.1 Evidentiary Table.

Paper Author (Year)	Description	Summary of Results	Quality of Evidence
Operative Treatment Versus Nonoperative Treatment			
Woertgen et al. (2006)	Consecutive retrospective case series, measured quality of life data (SF-36)	62 patients, 45% nonoperative and 55% operative treatment. Surgically treated patients, especially those with placement of spinal instrumentation, experienced slightly better outcomes than patients treated nonoperatively. Overall complication rate is similar in both groups (32%). 31% of patients had unfavorable outcome. Three patients died during hospitalization	Low
O'Daly et al. (2008)	Consecutive retrospective case series, measured quality of life data (SF-36, ODI)	28 patients, 72% nonoperative and 28% operative treatment. No functional differences in outcome between patients treated operatively vs. nonoperatively. 17% death rate due to acute sepsis. 28% required readmission within 1 y. 66% had adverse outcomes. SF-36 scores do not return to level of normative population despite full recovery of neurologic deficit.	Low

(Continued)

TABLE 7.1 **Evidentiary Table.** (*Continued*)

Paper Author (Year)	Description	Summary of Results	Quality of Evidence
Anterior Approach for Surgical Treatment			
Fang et al. (1994)	Retrospective case series	39 patients. Anterior debridement, iliac or rib autograft and 3 wk of bed rest. 93% fusion rate.	Low
Matsui et al. (1998)	Retrospective case series	38 patients. Anterior debridement, iliac autograft and 1-mo bed rest. No recurrence of infection. One reoperation for pseudarthrosis.	Low
Posterior Approach for Surgical Treatment			
Rath et al. (1996)	Retrospective case series	43 patients. All treated with posterior approaches. 5 patients treated with decompression only, and 3 of these patients required additional surgery. Remaining patients treated with posterior debridement, pedicle fixation, and interbody fusion (18 patients were treated as single stage and 21 patients had second stage interbody fusion).	Low
Combined Anterior and Posterior Approaches, Miscellaneous Series			
Dimar et al. (2004)	Consecutive retrospective case series All infections resolved. No infection recurrence.	42 patients. Two-stage anterior debridement and strut graft (67% autograft, 16% allograft, 16% combination) followed by delayed PSF/PSI[a] (14 d).	Low
Caragee et al. (2008)	Prospective observational study, single cohort, consecutive series 1 anterior debridement + ASF/ASI 3 miscellaneous posterior approaches Disease-free survivorship was 96%. One recurrent infection. Antibiotic therapy discontinued within first 6 mo.	32 patients, mean follow-up 8 y. 25 single-stage anterior debridement/graft and PSF/PSI.	Strong
Ruf et al. (2007)	Consecutive retrospective case series	85 patients. 71% same day anterior/posterior and 29% staged procedures. Anterior debridement and titanium mesh with iliac autograft followed by PSF/PSI. Cage filled with antibiotic bone cement in cases with severe osteopenia. 15% complication rate. No recurrent infections	Low
Kuklo et al. (2006)	Consecutive retrospective case series	21 patients. Titanium mesh cages with allograft and demineralized bone matrix + PSF/PSI. Anterior and posterior procedures performed in single stage. All patients had resolution of infection. 2 wound infections.	Low
O'Shaughnessy et al. (2008)	Consecutive retrospective case series	20 patients. Titanium mesh cages with rhBMP-2 were utilized. A variety of approaches were used to debride the anterior column infection—anterior only, posterior only, and anterior/posterior. 4 patients were treated solely with anterior titanium spinal instrumentation. Posterior titanium instrumentation was utilized in 16 patients. No recurrent or persistent infection was noted.	Low

PSF/PSI: posterior spinal fusion/posterior spinal instrumentation
ASF/ASI: anterior spinal fusion/anterior spinal instrumentation

The preferred treatment based on strength of the literature would consist of surgical treatment utilizing a same day single-stage anterior and posterior approach. Antibiotics would be withheld until after tissue cultures for aerobic, anaerobic fungi and tuberculosis were obtained. Additional tissue would be sent for pathologic examination and special stains for possible pathogens. The choice of appropriate antibiotics would be made in consultation with an infectious disease specialist and would include vancomycin.

Initially, the patient would be placed supine on a Jackson table and an anterior retroperitoneal exposure of L5-S1 would be performed. The disc space and adjacent vertebra involved by osteomyelitis would be debrided. It most likely would be possible to adequately debride the epidural space by working through the disc space from the anterior approach. A titanium mesh cage filled with rhBMP-2 and morselized cancellous allograft would be placed. Alternatively, a structural allograft could be placed. If the patient's medical condition is not a contraindication, the patient would be turned prone using the Jackson turning frame. Posterior exposure of L5-S1 with placement of pedicle screws in L5 and bilateral iliac screws and rods would be performed. Addition of S1 alar screws could be considered based on whether bone in the sacral ala region was compromised by the infection based on review of preoperative CT studies. Partial laminectomies of L5 and S1 would be performed to permit additional decompression of the epidural abscess/granulation tissue, which is believed to be present on the preoperative MRI study. Posterior L5-S1 fusion would be performed using rh-BMP-2 and local bone graft from the laminectomy mixed with autograft obtained at the site of iliac screw insertion. Nutritional consultation would be obtained prior to and following surgery and a plan created to enhance perioperative nutritional status utilizing a feeding tube and/or total parenteral nutrition. Intravenous antibiotics would be continued postoperatively for a minimum of 6 weeks following surgery. Decision making regarding termination of antibiotics at that time would be based on the type of organism, ESR, and CRP when compared to preoperative levels.

In a 78-year-old patient with an ileostomy, some anterior spine access surgeons may be reluctant to perform an anterior surgical approach. As the infection is below the aortic bifurcation, anterior exposure is much less demanding than at the L4-5 level and the necessary surgical exposure can be achieved in most cases. However, if anterior surgery was not an option or if the L5-S1 level could not be accessed anteriorly due to scarring and inflammation, there is literature to support addressing this pathology from an entirely posterior approach.[14,23] Partial laminectomies of L5 and S1 and a transforaminal approach to the L5-S1 disc space with debridement of the disc and endplates would be

performed. Placement of titanium mesh cages with rhBMP-2 and iliac autograft would be performed. Insertion of pedicle screws in L5 and bilateral iliac screws and rods would be performed. Addition of S1 alar screws could be considered based on whether bone involvement or destruction by infection was evident on preoperative CT studies. Posterior L5-S1 fusion would be performed using rh-BMP-2 and local bone graft from the laminectomy mixed with autograft obtained at the site of iliac screw insertion.

In accordance with the method of grading recommendations set forth by Schunemann et al.[54] the proposed treatment would be considered a weak recommendation.

PREDICTING OUTCOMES

To adequately predict outcomes and counsel patients with discitis/osteomyelitis, it is necessary to rely on validated outcome measures. Studies that report only process measures (e.g., resolution of neurologic deficit, rate of infection recurrence, correction of preoperative kyphosis) tend to overestimate the success of treatment of patients with pyogenic discitis/osteomyelitis.

A long-term retrospective study of 253 patients with vertebral osteomyelitis showed that residual disability occurred in more than one third of survivors.[5] Neurologic compromise, time to diagnosis of infection, and hospital acquisition of infection were independent risk factors for adverse outcome in this study. Delay in diagnosis and neurologic impairment at diagnosis have been shown to be significant predictors of neurologic deficit at follow-up.[3] Appropriate surgical treatment with modern techniques can achieve disease-free survival in nearly all patients.[26] Woertgen et al.[4] reported that quality of life measures derived from SF-36 scores was not restored in patients treated for pyogenic vertebral infection when compared to a normative population sample. Only 14% of patients were free of pain following treatment, and 31% of patients had an unfavorable outcome. The study suggested that surgical management, particularly in conjunction with instrumentation, may be more beneficial than antibiotic therapy alone in patients with spinal infection. O'Daly et al.[3] analyzed long-term results following pyogenic infection using standardized outcome measures (Oswestry disability index, SF-36) and reached a similar conclusion noting that poor functional outcome following pyogenic spinal infection is common at long-term follow-up even in patients with apparent full neurologic recovery. In this study, SF-36 scores for patients with pyogenic spinal infection, even with apparent full neurologic recovery, did not return to levels of an age-matched normative population. Even in the modern era, permanent neurologic deficit and death are possible outcomes in cases of spinal osteomyelitis and the need for appropriate and timely management cannot be underestimated.

In counseling the patient in the current clinical scenario, appropriate surgery as outlined above would have a very high likelihood of eradicating his infection. However, spinal fusion in the seventh decade of life is associated with a very significant rate of perioperative complications and this is increased above age-adjusted normative data in this case due to the patient's multiple medical comorbidities. We would be especially concerned about the risk of postoperative wound infection in this patient with presumed poor nutritional status as evidenced by a recent 60 lb weight loss. Based on available outcome data,[4] we would estimate the patient's chance of an unfavorable outcome as at least one in three and his chance of a favorable outcome as less than two in three. If surgery is not performed, we would anticipate that bone destruction would increase and a deformity would develop at the lumbosacral junction, which would lead to increased pain and potential for progressive neurologic deficit. Although there is a chance that the L5-S1 disc space infection may progress to spontaneous ankylosis if surgery is not performed, this course would not be expected based on the patient's clinical profile.

SUMMARY

We are presented with a 78-year-old man who presents with a known history of discitis and osteomyelitis at L5-S1 being treated nonoperatively with antibiotic therapy for the past 12 weeks. The most appropriate treatment for this patient's problem at this time is anterior L5-S1 debridement and fusion combined with posterior fusion and posterior spinal instrumentation. Significant perioperative complications are possible. There is at least a one in three chance of an unfavorable outcome. Despite successful eradication of infection and successful spinal fusion, the patient's quality of life measures as determined by SF-36 scores is not likely to return to age-adjusted norms.

REFERENCES

1. Kulowski J. Pyogenic osteomyelitis of the spine: an analysis and discussion of 102 cases. *J Bone Joint Surg Am.* 1936;18(2):343–364.
2. Butler JS, Shelly MJ, Timlin M, et al. Nontuberculous pyogenic spinal infection in adults: a 12-year experience from a tertiary referral center. *Spine.* 2006;31(23):2695–2700.
3. O'Daly BJ, Morris SF, O'Rourke SK. Long-term functional outcome in pyogenic spinal infection. *Spine.* 33(8): E246–E253.
4. Woertgen C, Rothoerl RD, Englert C, et al. Pyogenic spinal infections and outcome according to the 36-item short form health survey. *J Neurosurg Spine.* 2006;4: 441–446.
5. McHenry MC, Easley KA, Locker GA. Vertebral osteomyelitis: long-term outcome for 253 patients from 7 Cleveland-area hospitals. *Clin Infect Dis.* 2002;34: 1342–1350.
6. Carragee, EJ. The clinical use of magnetic resonance imaging in pyogenic vertebral osteomyelitis. *Spine.* 1997;22(7):780–785.
7. Sapico FL, Montgomery JZ. Pyogenic vertebral osteomyelitis: report of nine cases and review of the literature. *Rev Infect Dis.* 1979;1754–1776.
8. Sapico FL. Microbiology and antimicrobial therapy of spinal infections. *Orthop Clin North Am.* 1996;27(1):9–13.
9. Riley LH, Banovac K, Maratinez OV, et al. Tissue distribution of antibiotics in the intervertebral disc. *Spine.* 19:2619–2625, 1994.
10. Hodges FS, McAtee S, Kirkpatrick JS, et al. The ability of MRI to predict failure of nonoperative treatment of pyogenic vertebral osteomyelitis. *J Spinal Disord Tech.* 2006;19(8):566–570.
11. Kowalski TJ, Layton KF, Berbari EF, et al. Follow-up MR imaging in patients with pyogenic spine infections: lack of correlation with clinical features. *Am J Neuroradiol.* 2007;28:693–699.
12. Rezai AR, Woo HH, Errico TJ, et al. Contemporary management of spinal osteomyelitis. *Neurosurgery.* 1999;44(5):1018–1025.
13. Hodgson AR, Stock FE. Anterior spinal fusion. A preliminary communication on the radical treatment of Pott's disease and Pott's paraplegia. 1956. *Clin Orthop* 1994; 300: 16–23.
14. Rath SA, Neff U, Schneider O, et al. Neurosurgical management of thoracic and lumbar vertebral osteomyelitis and discitis in adults: a review of 43 consecutive surgically treated patients. *Neurosurgery.* 1996;38(5):926–933.
15. Eismont FJ, Bohlman HH, Soni PL, et al. Pyogenic and fungal osteomyelitis with paralysis. *J Bone Joint Surg Am.* 1983;65:19–29.
16. Emery SE, Chan DP, Woodward HR. Treatment of hematogenous pyogenic vertebral osteomyelitis with anterior debridement and primary bone grafting. *Spine* 1989; 14: 284–291.
17. Fang D, Cheung KMC, Dos Remedios IDM, et al. Pyogenic vertebral osteomyelitis: treatment by anterior spinal debridement and fusion. *J Spinal Disord.* 1994;7(2):173–180.
18. McGuire RA, Eismont FJ. The fate of autogenous bone graft in surgically treated pyogenic vertebral osteomyelitis. *J Spinal Disord.* 1994;7(3):206–215.
19. Ames CP, Acosta FL Jr, Aryan HE. Infections of the spine. *Contemporary Spine Surgery.* 2008;9(10):1–5.
20. Aryan HE, Lu DC, Acosta FL, et al. Corpectomy followed by the placement of instrumentation with titanium cages and recombinant human bone morphogenetic protein-2 for vertebral osteomyelitis. *J Neurosurg Spine.* 2007;6: 23–30.
21. Hee HT, Majd ME, Holt RT, et al. Better treatment of vertebral osteomyelitis using posterior stabilization and titanium mesh cages. *J Spinal Disord.* 2002;15(2):149–156.

22. Ruf M, Stoltze D, Merk HR, et al. Treatment of vertebral osteomyelitis by radical debridement and stabilization using titanium mesh cages. *Spine.* 2007;32(9):E275–E280.

23. O'Shaughnessy BA, Kuklo TR, Ondra SL. Surgical treatment of vertebral osteomyelitis with recombinant human bone morphogenetic protein-2. *Spine.* 2008;33(5) E132–E139.

24. Cahill DW, Love LC, Rechtine GR. Pyogenic osteomyelitis of the spine in the elderly. *J Neurosurg.* 1992;74: 878–886.

25. Carragee EJ. Pyogenic vertebral osteomyelitis. *J Bone Joint Surg Am.* 1997;79(6): 874–880.

26. Carragee EJ, Lezza A. Does acute placement of instrumentation in the treatment of vertebral osteomyelitis predispose to recurrent infection: long-term follow-up in immune-suppressed patients. *Spine.* 2008;33(19):2089–2093.

27. Faraj AA, Webb JK. Spinal instrumentation for primary pyogenic infection report of 31 patients. *Acta Orthop Belg.* 2000;66(3):242–247.

28. Lee MC, Wang MY, Fessler RG, et al. Instrumentation in patients with spinal infection. *Neurosurg Focus.* 2004;17(6):1–6.

29. Hadjipavlou AG, Mader JT, Necessary JT, et al. Hematogenous pyogenic spinal infections and their surgical management. *Spine.* 2000;25(13):1668–1679.

30. Nagata, K, Ohashi T, Mamoru A, et al. Percutaneous suction aspiration and drainage for pyogenic spondylitis. *Spine.* 1998; 23(14):1600–1606.

31. Kensei N, Ohashi T, Mamoru A, et al. Percutaneous suction aspiration and drainage for pyogenic spondylitis. *Spine.* 1998. 23:1600–1606.

32. Jeanneret B, Magerl F. Treatment of osteomyelitis of the spine using percutaneous suction/irrigation and percutaneous external spinal fixation. *J Spinal Disord.* 1994;7:185–205.

33. Korovessis P, Repantis T, Iliopoulos P, et al. Beneficial influence of titanium mesh cage on infection healing and spinal reconstruction in hematogenous septic spondylitis. *Spine.* 2008;33:E759–E767.

34. Dimar JR, Carreon Ly, Glassman SD, et al. Treatment of pyogenic vertebral osteomyelitis with anterior debridement and fusion followed by delayed posterior spinal fusion. *Spine.* 2004;29(3):326–332.

35. Hsieh PC, Wienecke RJ, O'Shaughnessy BA, et al. Surgical strategies for vertebral osteomyelitis and epidural abscess. *Neurosurg Focus.* 2004;17(6):1–6.

36. Krodel A, Kruger A, Lohscheidt K, et al. Anterior debridement, fusion, and extrafocal stabilization in the treatment of osteomyelitis of the spine. *J Spinal Disord.* 1999;12(1):17–26.

37. Youssef JA, Vaughan SL, Denker MW, et al. Acute and chronic pyogenic vertebral osteomyelitis: is there a role for adjunctive internal fixation during surgical management. *Seminars Spine Surg.* 2004:162–173.

38. Arens S, Hansis M, Schlegel U, et al. Infection after open reduction and internal fixation with dynamic compression plates-clinical and experimental data. *Injury.* 1996;27:SC27–SC33.

39. Chang CC, Merritt K. Infection at the site of implanted materials with and without preadhered bacteria. *J Orthop Res.* 1994; 12:526–531.

40. Safran O, Rand N, Kaplan L, et al. Sequential or simultaneous, same-day anterior decompression and posterior stabilization in the management of vertebral osteomyelitis of the lumbar spine. *Spine.* 1998;23(17):1885–1890.

41. Kuklo TR, Potter BK, Bell RS, et al. Single-stage treatment of pyogenic spinal infection with titanium mesh cages. *J Spinal Disord Tech.* 2006; 19(5):376–382.

42. Korovessis P, Petsinis G, Koureas G, et al. Anterior surgery with insertion of titanium mesh cage and posterior instrumented fusion performed sequentially on the same day under one anesthesia for septic spondylitis of thoracolumbar spine: is the use of titanium mesh cages safe. *Spine.* 2006;31(9):1014–1019.

43. Matsui H, Hirano N, Sakaguchi Y. Vertebral osteomyelitis: an analysis of 38 surgically treated cases. *Eur Spine J.* 1998;7:50–54.

44. Bradford DS, Daher YH. Vascularized rib grafts and stabilization of kyphosis. *J Bone Joint Surg Br.* 68: 357–361,1986.

45. Vaccaro AR, Cirello J. The use of allograft bone and cages in fractures of the cervical, thoracic and lumbar spine. *Clin Orthop.* 2002;394:19–26.

46. Molinari RW, Bridwell KH, Klepps SJ, et al. Minimum 5-year follow-up of anterior column structural allografts in the thoracic and lumbar spine. *Spine.* 1999;24;10:967–972.

47. Lewandrowski K, Hecht AC, KeLaney TF, et al. Anterior spinal arthrodesis with structural cortical allografts and instrumentation for spine tumor surgery. *Spine.* 2004; 10:1150–1159.

48. Schuster JM, Avellino AM, Mann FA, et al. Use of structural allografts in spinal osteomyelitis: a review of 47 cases. *J Neurosurg.* 2000;93(1 Suppl):8–14.

49. Allen TR, Lee YP, Stimson E, et al. Bone morpphogenetic protein-2 (BMP) in the treatment of pyogenic vertebral osteomyelitis. *Spine.* 2007; 32(26):2996–3006.

50. Eck KR, Bridwell KH, Ungacta FF, et al. Analysis of titanium mesh cages in adults with minimum two-year follow-up. *Spine.* 2000;25:2407–2415.

51. Fayazi AH, Ludwig SC, Dabbah M, et al. Preliminary results of staged anterior debridement and reconstruction using titanium mesh cages in the treatment of thoracolumbar vertebral osteomyelitis. *Spine J.* 2004; 4:388–395.

52. Liljenqvist U, Lerner T, Bullmann V, et al. Titanium cages in the surgical treatment of severe vertebral osteomyelitis. *Eur Spine J.* 2003;12:606–612.

53. Chen JF, Lee ST. Antibiotic-polymethylmethacrylate strut: an option for treating cervical pyogenic spondylitis: case report. *J Neurosurg Spine.* 2006;5:90–95

54. Schunemann HJ, Jaeschke R, Cook DJ, et al. ATS Documents Development and Implementation Committee. An official ATS statement: grading the quality of evidence and strength of recommendations in ATS guidelines and recommendations. *Am J Respir Crit Care Med.* 2006; 174: 605–614.

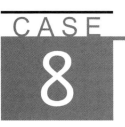

CASE 8

Rheumatoid Arthritis of the Cervical Spine

SEAN COMSTOCK, MD, FRCSC AND
MARCEL F. DVORAK, MD, FRCSC

EDITORS' CASE PRESENTATION

A 58-year-old woman with a 20-year history of rheumatoid arthritis presents with a complaint of neck pain and suboccipital headache for 7 years. For the past 6 months, she has had "clunking" with neck movement. She feels that her pain is worse with rotation and better while wearing a cervical orthosis. Besides having undergone bilateral wrist arthrodesis, she is in reasonably good medical condition. She has no bowel or bladder complaints and does not have upper extremity dexterity issues. She does not report imbalance while walking.

Her physical examination demonstrates stigmata of rheumatoid arthritis, including ulnar deviation of the digits at the metacarpophalangeal joints. At resting position, her head is held rotated 20 degrees to the right and slightly forward flexed. Upon palpation, the neck is nontender. Range of motion of the neck reveals 20 degrees of rotation to the right, 60 degrees to the left, flexion to one finger width to the chest, and extension to 20 degrees. She has pain at the extreme of flexion, which produces pain in the right shoulder. Motor, sensory, and reflex examinations are normal. Hoffman reflex is negative, and she has no Babinski sign.

Radiographic imaging studies are shown in Figures 8.1 to 8.3.

INTERPRETATION OF CLINICAL PRESENTATION

The clinical scenario describes a middle-aged woman with a long-standing history of rheumatoid arthritis. Her chief complaint is axial neck pain and suboccipital headache. This has been longstanding but lately has been associated with "clunking." These are common presenting symptoms related to rheumatoid involvement of the c-spine.[1-5] The suboccipital headache may be multifactorial and may very well be referred from the cervical spine. Rheumatoid involvement of the upper cervical spine may lead to suboccipital headache based simply on inflammatory degeneration of the upper cervical spine, compression of the posterior primary ramus of C2 or patterns of upper cervical instability including horizontal C1-2 instability or vertical atlantoaxial impaction (AAI),[6] which would need to be ruled out by imaging. The patient's pain is worse with rotation and alleviated with an orthosis in keeping with inflammatory degeneration and/or instability of the cervical spine.

Rheumatoid cervical spine involvement is more common in patients with more than a 10-year disease history of the disease and in whom peripheral fusions have been performed for erosive disease.[2,7-18] This patient has no issues with dexterity, gait, or voiding and thus has no symptoms of myelopathy.

The physical examination shows limited motion specifically in extension and in rotation to the right. Shoulder pain with flexion may indicate radicular irritation from subaxial or atlantoaxial subluxation (AAS) and must be ruled out with imaging. She has no weakness or sensory disturbance.

There are three commonly recognized patterns of cervical spine instability seen in rheumatoid arthritis and these include horizontal atlantoaxial subluxation (AAS); vertical atlantoaxial instability (AAI); and subaxial subluxation (SAS)

The plain radiographs included are flexion and extension lateral projections, an appropriate screening radiographic examination in the symptomatic rheumatoid population. Figure 8.1A and B are lateral cervical flexion and extension views that reveal an increase in the distance between the anterior arch of C1 and the odontoid in flexion, which reduces to normal alignment in extension. Although there are multiple levels of degeneration between C3 and C7,

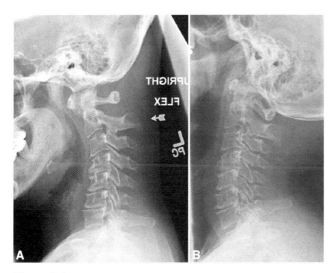

Figure 8.1.

there is no subluxation or instability. This is consistent with a finding of dynamic horizontal instability of the atlas (AAS) in which the atlas reduces completely on extension. The degree of this subluxation is difficult to interpret without absolute numbers. An anterior atlantodental interval (ADI) of >3 mm is consistent with AAS.[3,7,19–21] Boden et al. showed that if the posterior atlantodental interval (PADI) was <14 mm,

then there was an increased risk of spinal cord compression and myelopathy and stabilization was recommended.[9,22] In this case, the space available for the spinal cord is reduced in flexion, but the patient remains free of clinical signs and symptoms of spinal cord compression.[1,23,24] On the plain radiographs, vertical AAI does not appear to be present, although using measurement techniques such as Ranawat's criteria,[4,25] or the Redlund-Johnell method[26] are relatively imprecise. There is no appreciable SAS on these images.

The computerized tomography (CT) scan images (Fig. 8.2) provide further clinical information. The CT images confirm the horizontal AAS but, more importantly, demonstrate progression of the horizontal AAS toward vertical AAI. In Figure 8.2E, the right C1-2 articulation is severely degenerative and collapsed, leading to upward migration of the odontoid relative to the foramen magnum (seen on Figure 8.2B where the tip of the odontoid is at the level of McRae's line, which is the opening of the foramen magnum).

Note that on the paramedian sagittal and the coronal reformats, the atlanto-occipital joints are relatively uninvolved. The axial cut and the coronal reformat show the rotatory component to the AAS with C1 and the occiput rotated to the right. Another important

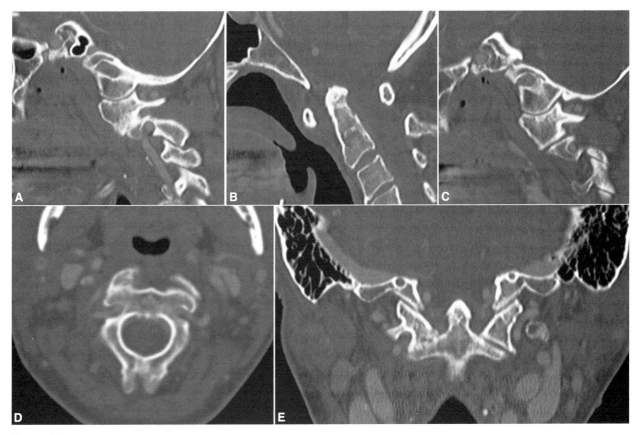

Figure 8.2.

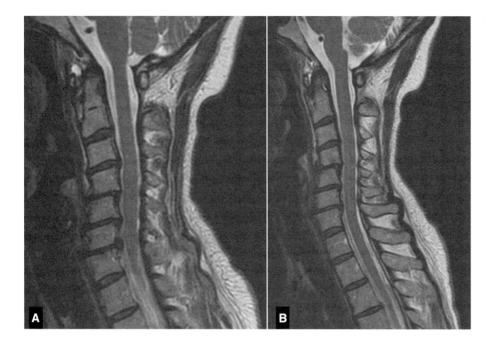

Figure 8.3.

observation is the course of the vertebral artery. It is very high in C2 and courses medially such that the pedicle isthmus of C2 appears very small in the sagittal and coronal diameters, although with a single image slice, it is difficult to assess completely.

Sagittal T2 midline MRI images are provided in Figure 8.3A and B, which at C1-2 show adequate space for cerebro-spinal fluid both anterior and posterior to the cord. There is no large pannus posterior to the dens and no Chiari malformation. The cervicomedullary angle is >135 degrees. There are areas of stenosis distally, most notably at C3-4, C4-5, and C5-6. The cord is indented, but there is no high signal, nor is there obliteration of the space for cerebro-spinal fluid.

DECLARATION OF SPECIFIC DIAGNOSIS

This patient has symptomatic, reducible atlantoaxial subluxation secondary to rheumatoid arthritis with very early vertical migration of the odontoid or vertical AAI.

BRAINSTORMING: WHAT ARE THE TREATMENT GOALS AND SURGICAL OPTIONS?

The treatment goals are

1. Alleviating pain
2. Avoiding complications, most significantly the development of myelopathy
3. Arresting the course of disease and progression of instability

4. Achieving stability
5. Rehabilitation without the need for rigid external immobilization

The treatment options are

1. Observation
2. Rigid cervical orthosis
3. Atlantoaxial fusion with sublaminar techniques
4. Atlantoaxial fusion with transarticular screws (TASs)
5. Atlantoaxial fusion with segmental screw and rod fixation
6. Occipitocervical arthrodesis

EVALUATION OF THE LITERATURE

To identify relevant publications on rheumatoid arthritis of the cervical spine, a Medline search was performed. Search strategies included the use of MeSH (medical subject headings) and key words. Key words included "cervical vertebrae," "arthritis, rheumatoid," and "instability." This produced 130 citations. Abstracts were reviewed for relevance, which excluded 64. The "related articles" function of PubMed was used and identified a further 169 citations. Reference sections were then hand searched to identify 66 further pertinent articles. Searching evidence based medicine reviews (EBMR) and the Cochrane database returned no results. Two-hundred thirty-five English language abstracts were reviewed, and 164 full-text articles were read.

DETAILED REVIEW OF PERTINENT ARTICLES

The overall quality of literature on the operative management of AAS in Rheumatoid Arthritis is moderate to low.[27,28]

Operative or Nonoperative Treatment

Rheumatoid involvement of the c-spine proceeds in a stepwise fashion: AAS untreated leads to AAI and, as the disease progresses, to SAS.[4,7,10–12,15,16,29–34] Atlantoaxial fusion can arrest the course of disease and prevent the development of AAI where the outcomes are less predictable.[35–39] Some authors disagree, thinking that the disease progresses regardless.[7,40] Surgery is indicated to prevent disease progression and neurologic injury,[9,29] with outcomes being related to preoperative neurologic function.[5,22,29,41] Even those with advanced myelopathy may have improvement as some authors recommend fusion even for those patients with high-grade myelopathy.[42]

Mortality rates of 10% to 40% have been reported in rheumatoid patients with cervical subluxation,[43,44,45] and, in AAS, have been reported to be eight times that of rheumatoid patients without AAS.[46] A significant reduction in mortality has been shown when instability is treated surgically,[39] as much as 38% in one study.[47]

Kauppi et al.[48–50] have looked at bracing as an alternative to fixation and have determined that a rigid orthosis can restrict AAS, but these patients were not followed over time. Others have concluded that nonoperative management does not change the natural history of disease.[5,51]

Chronic neck pain in the setting of radiographic instability that does not respond to nonnarcotic pain medication is an indication for surgery.[4,19,52–54] Pain itself is not always correlated to instability, nor instability to neurologic symptoms.[53,55]

There have been several prospective, controlled studies looking at operative vs. nonoperative management. Paus in a prospective cohort study concluded that since operative risk is small and the mortality high in rheumatoid subluxation, surgery is a reasonable option.[56] Krieg in a prospective cohort study looked at 7-year follow-up data of patients who had been fused and found that all patients were satisfied with their result.[57] Santavirta performed a prospective case-control study to look at fusion versus nonfusion and found that pain relief was 80% in operatively treated patients but only 12% in the nonoperative controls.[58] Matsunaga in 2003 in a case-control study showed that in rheumatoid patients with myelopathy, fusion increased the survival rate from 0% at 8 years to 84% at 5 and 37% at 10 years.[59]

In case presented, operative management is clearly indicated for a variety of reasons. First of all, this patient appears to have significantly disabling mechanical neck pain and referred suboccipital headache, both of which would likely be improved by arthrodesis. Similar to a wrist arthrodesis or subtalar arthrodesis in a patient with rheumatoid joint destruction, the surgical management of severe axial skeletal pain is an effective and reasonable treatment in these patients. Second of all, the AAS is dynamic and easily reducible by neck extension. While the instability is reducible, arthrodesis is technically easier and more likely to result in a stable fusion than if the patients' atlas was fixed in an anteriorly subluxed position. Once this instability leads to a fixed subluxation, then treatment may require either preoperative traction or intraoperative open reduction to realign C1 and C2 or possibly even direct decompression with a posterior C1 arch resection or anterior odontoidectomy, both of which increase the surgical morbidity and complexity. The final and most compelling reason to consider surgery in this patient is the early development of vertical migration of the odontoid or AAI. As the instability between the atlas and the axis progresses, the lateral masses of the atlas, particularly the inferior C1 articular processes, erode and the lateral masses collapse leading to AAI. It is important to note that this occurs with no degeneration of the occipitocervical joints but occurs through the atlantoaxial articulation. Performing a successful atlantoaxial arthrodesis while the instability is reducible will protect the patient against progression of the vertical migration of the odontoid and may very well allow the patient to avoid the morbidity of an occipitocervical fusion and possibly even an anterior odontoid resection in the future.[6,60]

There is an RCT underway to determine the timing of surgery in patients with AAS and no neurologic compromise;[61] however, results are as yet unavailable.

Sublaminar Techniques

There are a variety of posterior wiring techniques, most of which involve wiring the posterior arches of the atlas and the axis together with interposed structural bone graft.[62–64] Omura in 2002[65] published a prospective cohort study of 17 patients, 11 of whom underwent extensive Luque fusions. They showed better outcomes with regard to activities of daily living and neurologic improvement in the operative group.

Christensson in 2000 looked at a cross section of patients who had undergone posterior wiring techniques, reporting a 4% mortality and a 22% recurrent subluxation at 7 months.[66] Naderi et al.[67] in a biomechanical study showed that cable graft constructs were better than transarticular screws in resisting flexion and extension.

There are many low and very low quality studies demonstrating acceptable results ranging from 60% to 81% rates of successful outcomes[64,68–72] and 58%

to 100% fusion rates. However, all posterior wiring techniques rely on the postoperative use of a halo or rigid external orthosis.[25,62–64,71,73–86] Biomechanically, posterior wiring alone has been superseded by screw fixation techniques mainly due to the improved fusion rates that do not rely on external immobilization postoperatively.

Transarticular Screws

Biomechanical studies show that TAS, which are paired screws inserted in a caudal to cranial direction from the C2 lateral masses across the C1-2 articulation and into the lateral mass of the atlas, are known to provide improved fixation when compared to sublaminar techniques.[87–93] Cyr in 2008 showed that unicortical screws are biomechanically sufficient.[94] Although Tokuhashi suggested that a sublaminar clamp may offer increased stiffness over screws, failure of this implant has limited its use.[95]

Weidner, in a prospective case-control trial, demonstrated that using image guidance reduced but did not eliminate the risk of screw malposition.[96] Multiple retrospective analyses have shown the same.[97–100] Gebhard, in a cadaver study, observed no risk of vertebral artery injury and that the structure most at risk is the atlantooccipital joint.[101]

Yoshida showed that roughly 10% of C1-2 complexes were unsuitable for both TAS and C2 pedicle screws as they had either a superior or medially positioned vertebral artery that made safe passage of screws through the C2 isthmus impossible.[102] Others have shown the optimal end point to be 7 mm from the anterior tubercle of C1 on the lateral projection.[101,103] The screw length should be between 38 and 45 mm and should be measured preoperatively on the CT instead of the lateral radiograph.[101,104]

In a case-control study, Reilly showed a much higher union rate and lower complications in TAS versus posterior wiring.[105] Neo in a case-control study placed TAS in the most dorsal and medial aspect of the isthmus of C2. There were no complications despite a 12% incidence of high riding or medial vertebral artery. They concluded that one should aim for the dorsal cortex of the isthmus on the lateral.[106,107]

Dickman prospectively studied a series of 121 patients who underwent TAS, 16 unilaterally because of an anomalous vertebral artery. They achieved a 98% fusion rate. Five percent of screws were malpositioned, but none were associated with clinical sequelae.[108] Magerl's original description reported on 12 patients with TAS who had 100% fusion rate and 2 temporary neurologic injuries, as well as a malpositioned screw.[109]

Multiple retrospective studies have reported 82% to 100% fusion rates,[75,77,109–122] 80% to 100% pain relief,[111,116,119,122] 0% to 8% vertebral artery injury,[77,114,116,123–125]

0.5% mortality,[114] 0% to 17% complication rates,[113–116,119] and 0% to 14% malpositioned screws.[109,112,113,115,116,119,124] They have also shown that postoperative halo immobilization is not required.[122,126]

Segmental Screw-Rod Fixation

TASs may be contraindicated in 18% to 54% of cases because of anatomic variations.[90,124,127–130] Biomechanical studies have shown that segmental screw rod fixation between C1 and C2 is equivalent to TASs.[131–136] Laminar screws may be placed in C2 when safe placement of a C2 pedicle screw cannot be achieved. Some authors have shown that C2 laminar screws are equivalent to pedicle screws[137] while others that pedicle screws are stiffer.[133,138] Wright reported retrospectively on a series of ten patients treated with C2 laminar screws and reported no complications.[139] Eck has shown that unicortical screws are stronger in C1 than in the subaxial spine, but bicortical C1 screws are stronger than unicortical.[140]

Harms reported his initial series of 37 in 2001 with a 100% fusion rate and no complications at 6 to 24 months.[141] Aryan in 2008 reported a multicentre series of 102 patients treated with C1-2 segmental screw rod fixation. They showed a 98% fusion rate and a 4% rate of complications. Pars screws were used instead of C2 pedicle screws in 23 patients because of unfavorable vertebral artery anatomy.[142] Other retrospective studies have shown 100% fusion, 0% to 10% malposition, 0% vascular, and 0% neurological complications.[143–147]

Other Techniques

Some have shown that a transoral plate plus posterior wiring is as good as TAS.[148] Others have reported success with anterior TAS,[149] Olerud clamps,[150] TAS plus segmental screw-rod fixation,[147] and C2 pedicle screw and C1 cable.[151]

Literature Inconsistencies

This patient has a high-riding and medially located vertebral artery in C2. Despite a case-control trial and an observational study showing that TAS can be placed safely in these patients,[106,107] the preponderance of evidence would suggest otherwise and an up to 8% vertebral artery injury rate has been reported.[77,114,116,123–125] The observational studies by Yoshida et al.[102] and Resnick[130] would suggest that C2 pedicle screws are just as risky as transarticular screws.[143,145,146] Furthermore, if it did not prove possible to place pedicle screws in C2, pars screws or laminar screws would seem to be reasonable alternatives.[139,142]

The observational biomechanical studies are conflicting, but there are studies that generally suggest the superiority of screw fixation techniques over sublaminar wiring techniques.

EVIDENTIARY TABLE AND SELECTION OF TREATMENT METHOD

In this patient, polyaxial screw-rod fixation is best supported by the data. It is less risky than TASs to the vertebral artery and given her anatomy the best choice. The data supporting this treatment method are multiple biomechanical studies,[131,132,134–136] one large multicentre case series,[142] and six other retrospective studies.[141,143–147]

Posterior polyaxial screw-rod fixation will address the surgical goals in this patient. Fusion provides reliable pain relief,[2,5,29] has a low complication rate especially in neurologically intact patients,[29,33] and will arrest the course of disease.[35–39] The addition of instrumentation enables this to be achieved without the need for rigid external immobilization.[141–147] Although some authors would suggest instrumentation without bone graft, the majority of studies utilize autogenous iliac crest bone graft, either structural or morcellized (Table 8.1).

DEFINITIVE TREATMENT PLAN

Preoperative antibiotics would be given and the surgery would be conducted according to the original description by Harms:[141] Most of these patients should undergo awake fiberoptic intubation prior to being given a general anesthetic. Positioning is prone and is most safely accomplished with skull tong traction and rotation on a Stryker or Jackson table.

TABLE 8.1 Evidentiary Table: A Summary of the Quality of Evidence for Posterior Polyaxial Screw-Rod Fixation of Atlantoaxial Subluxation.

Paper Author (Year)	Description	Summary of Results	Quality of Evidence
Aryan et al. (2008)	Multicentre retrospective case series	102 patients 98% fusion rate 4% complications (wound infections) 16.4 mo follow-up	Very low
Gunnarsson et al. (2007)	Prospective case series	25 patients 100% fusion No complications 12 mo follow-up	Very low
Harms and Melcher (2001)	Retrospective case series	37 patients 100% fusion No complications 6–24 mo follow-up	Very low
Pham et al. (2000)	Retrospective case series	30 rheumatoid patients 100% fusion No complications 4.5 y follow-up	Very low
Stokes et al. (2002)	Retrospective case series	4 patients 100% fusion No complications Follow-up 12 mo	Very low
Stulik et al. (2007)	Retrospective case series	28 patients 100% fusion 3 malpositioned screws, no major sequelae Follow-up 17 mo	Very low
Vilela et al. (2006)	Retrospective case series	11 patients 100% fusion No complications Follow-up 6–24 mo	Very low

Lateral fluoroscopy confirms anatomical C1-2 alignment prior to prepping and draping. A posterior exposure of C1-2 includes exposure of the C1-2 lateral mass articulation over the superior surface of the C2 pars interarticularis. This joint is a key anatomic landmark for accurate placement of the C1 lateral mass screw.

The C1 lateral mass screw is inserted from an entry point in the middle of the junction of the C1 posterior arch and the midpoint of the posterior inferior part of the C1 lateral mass. The C1 screw is inserted in a straight or slightly convergent trajectory in an anterior-posterior direction and parallel to the plane of the C1 posterior arch in the sagittal direction, with the tip of the drill directed toward the anterior arch of C1. The C2 lamina or pars interarticularis screws are inserted by identifying the entry point with a high-speed burr. The pilot hole is prepared with a 2-mm drill bit while monitoring the alignment on fluoroscopy and direct observation. Integrity of the pilot hole is verified with a blunt probe. The hole is tapped, and a 3.5-mm polyaxial screw of the appropriate length is inserted.

If necessary, reduction of the C1 ring is performed by repositioning the patient's head and/or directly manipulating C1 and C2 using the screws, followed by fixation to the rods to maintain the alignment. If a definitive fusion is required, C1 and C2 are decorticated posteriorly, and cancellous bone taken from a small incision in the posterior iliac crest can be placed over the decorticated surfaces of C1 and C2.

Patients are mobilized on the 1st postoperative day and wear a soft cervical collar for 2 to 3 weeks. Care must be taken not to fix C1-2 in hyperlordosis as that may lead to subaxial kyphosis.[152,153]

Grading the Evidence for this Plan

The evidence to support the technical aspects of our treatment selection would be considered low as it is derived from observational studies of moderate quality. The treatment goals have been met in the six studies found in Table 8.1, but the quality of evidence showing effectiveness of this treatment is very low.

In accordance with the method of grading recommendations set forth by Schunemann et al.,[28] our proposed treatment would be considered a strong recommendation. This grading is based not only on the quality of evidence but on the risks and benefits of the proposed intervention. The benefits of atlantoaxial fusion in a symptomatic rheumatoid patient clearly outweigh the risks.

PREDICTING OUTCOMES

Kandziora in a prospective cohort study showed consistent pain relief and improvement in the Health Assessment Questionnaire after fusion.[154] Morbidity is low and outcome predictable in isolated AAS.[5,22,29,35,41,155]

Fusion has been shown to have a 62% to 92% chance of being successful at relieving pain.[47,156–161] With atlanto-axial fusion, there is a chance of developing SAS and neurologic deterioration in 5.5% to 21%,[37,162,163] and there will be decreased neck rotation postoperatively.[164] There is a 6% to 37% mortality[47,160,161] in fused patients at all stages of rheumatoid instability, but this may be up to 38% less than in non–operated patients.[47]

In our experience, this procedure has a predictable outcome and is indicated in symptomatic patients. In our center, patients with rheumatoid arthritis and symptomatic AAS are offered surgery if there are no contraindications. We would advise this patient of all the risks as above, especially the risk of infection, vertebral artery injury, and the general risks of surgery as well as medical risks. Many of these patients are on medications for their rheumatoid arthritis that complicate perioperative care, such as prednisone or methotrexate. We would further tell her that the intervention proposed would have a high likelihood of relieving her symptoms.

SUMMARY

We are presented with a 58-year-old woman with symptomatic AAS secondary to rheumatoid arthritis. The most appropriate treatment for this patient, considering the natural history of the condition, would consist of atlantoaxial fusion. Consideration of the anatomy of her vertebral arteries would make a polyaxial screw-rod construct the most logical choice and would give the most predictable result considering the evidence.

REFERENCES

1. Babic-Naglic D, Potocki K, Curkovic B. Clinical and radiological features of atlantoaxial joints in rheumatoid arthritis. *Z Rheumatol*. 1999;58(4):196–200.
2. Bouchaud-Chabot A, Liote F. Cervical spine involvement in rheumatoid arthritis: a review. *Joint Bone Spine*. 2002;69(2):141–154.
3. Cabot A, Becker A. The cervical spine in rheumatoid arthritis. *Clin Orthop Relat Res*. 1978;131:130–140.
4. Kim DH, Hilibrand AS. Rheumatoid arthritis in the cervical spine. *J Am Acad Orthop Surg*. 2005;13(7):463–474.
5. Monsey RD. Rheumatoid arthritis of the cervical spine. *J Am Acad Orthop Surg*. 1997;5(5):240–248.
6. Rana NA, Hancock DO, Taylor AR, et al. Upward translocation of the dens in rheumatoid arthritis. *J Bone Joint Surg Br*. 1973;55(3):471–477.
7. Agarwal AK, Peppelman WC Jr, Kraus DR, et al. The cervical spine in rheumatoid arthritis. *Br Med J*. 1993; 306(6870):79–80.
8. Conlon PW, Isdale IC, Rose BS. Rheumatoid arthritis of the cervical spine: an analysis of 333 cases. *Ann Rheum Dis*. 1966;25(2):120–126.

9. Dreyer SJ, Boden SD. Natural history of rheumatoid arthritis of the cervical spine. *Clin Orthop Relat Res*. 1999; 366:98–106.

10. Fujiwara K, Fujimoto M, Owaki H, et al. Cervical lesions related to the systemic progression in rheumatoid arthritis. *Spine*. 1998;23(19):2052–2056.

11. Fujiwara K, Owaki H, Fujimoto M, et al. A long-term follow-up study of cervical lesions in rheumatoid arthritis. *J Spinal Disord*. 2000;13(6):519–526.

12. Fujiwara K, Yonenobu K, Ochi T. Natural history of upper cervical lesions in rheumatoid arthritis. *J Spinal Disord*. 1997;10(4):275–281.

13. Mathews JA. Atlanto-axial subluxation in rheumatoid arthritis. A 5-year follow-up study. *Ann Rheum Dis*. 1974; 33(6):526–531.

14. Naranjo A, Carmona L, Gavrila D, et al. Prevalence and associated factors of anterior atlantoaxial luxation in a nation-wide sample of rheumatoid arthritis patients. *Clin Exp Rheumatol*. 2004;22(4):427–432.

15. Oda T, Fujiwara K, Yonenobu K, et al. Natural course of cervical spine lesions in rheumatoid arthritis. *Spine*. 1995;20(10):1128–1135.

16. Paimela L, Laasonen L, Kankaanpaa E, et al. Progression of cervical spine changes in patients with early rheumatoid arthritis. *J Rheumatol*. 1997;24(7):1280–1284.

17. Winfield J, Cooke D, Brook AS, et al. A prospective study of the radiological changes in the cervical spine in early rheumatoid disease. *Ann Rheum Dis*. 1981;40(2):109–114.

18. Wolfe BK, O'Keeffe D, Mitchell DM, et al. Rheumatoid arthritis of the cervical spine: early and progressive radiographic features. *Radiology*. 1987;165(1):145–148.

19. Lipson SJ. Rheumatoid arthritis in the cervical spine. *Clin Orthop Relat Res*. 1989;239:121–127.

20. Rana NA, Hancock DO, Taylor AR, et al. Atlanto-axial subluxation in rheumatoid arthritis. *J Bone Joint Surg Br*. 1973;55(3):458–470.

21. Taniguchi D, Tokunaga D, Hase H, et al. Evaluation of lateral instability of the atlanto-axial joint in rheumatoid arthritis using dynamic open-mouth view radiographs. *Clin Rheumatol*. 2008;27(7):851–857.

22. Boden SD, Dodge LD, Bohlman HH, et al. Rheumatoid arthritis of the cervical spine: a long-term analysis with predictors of paralysis and recovery. *J Bone Joint Surg Am*. 1993;75(9):1282–1297.

23. Ebraheim NA, Lu J, Yang H. The effect of translation of the C1-C2 on the spinal canal. *Clin Orthop Relat Res*. 1998; 351:222–229.

24. Grogono BJS. Injuries of the atlas and axis. *J Bone Joint Surg Br*. 1954;36-B(Aug):397–410.

25. Ranawat CS, O'Leary P, Pellicci P, et al. Cervical spine fusion in rheumatoid arthritis. *J Bone Joint Surg Am*. 1979;61(7):1003–1010.

26. Redlund-Johnell I, Pettersson H. Radiographic measurements of the cranio-vertebral region. Designed for evaluation of abnormalities in rheumatoid arthritis. *Acta Radiol Diagn (Stockh)*. 1984;25(1):23–28.

27. Fisher CG, Wood KB. Introduction to and techniques of evidence-based medicine. *Spine*. 2007;32(19 suppl): S66–S72.

28. Schunemann HJ, Jaeschke R, Cook DJ, et al. An official ATS statement: grading the quality of evidence and strength of recommendations in ATS guidelines and recommendations. *Am J Respir Crit Care Med*. 2006;174(5):605–614.

29. Boden SD. Rheumatoid arthritis of the cervical spine. Surgical decision making based on predictors of paralysis and recovery. *Spine*. 1994;19(20):2275–2280.

30. Castro S, Verstraete K, Mielants H, et al. Cervical spine involvement in rheumatoid arthritis: a clinical, neurological and radiological evaluation. *Clin Exp Rheumatol*. 1994;12(4):369–374.

31. Lipson SJ. Rheumatoid arthritis of the cervical spine. *Clin Orthop Relat Res*. 1984;182:143–149.

32. Neva MH, Kaarela K, Kauppi M. Prevalence of radiological changes in the cervical spine–a cross sectional study after 20 years from presentation of rheumatoid arthritis. *J Rheumatol*. 2000;27(1):90–93.

33. Shen FH, Samartzis D, Jenis LG, et al. Rheumatoid arthritis: evaluation and surgical management of the cervical spine. *Spine J*. 2004;4(6):689–700.

34. Weissman BN, Aliabadi P, Weinfeld MS, et al. Prognostic features of atlantoaxial subluxation in rheumatoid arthritis patients. *Radiology*. 1982;144(4):745–751.

35. Agarwal AK, Peppelman WC, Kraus DR, et al. Recurrence of cervical spine instability in rheumatoid arthritis following previous fusion: can disease progression be prevented by early surgery? *J Rheumatol*. 1992;19(9):1364–1370.

36. Casey AT, Crockard HA, Pringle J, et al. Rheumatoid arthritis of the cervical spine: current techniques for management. *Orthop Clin North Am*. 2002;33(2):291–309.

37. Kraus DR, Peppelman WC, Agarwal AK, et al. Incidence of subaxial subluxation in patients with generalized rheumatoid arthritis who have had previous occipital cervical fusions. *Spine*. 1991;16(10 suppl):S486–S489.

38. Papadopoulos SM, Dickman CA, Sonntag VK. Atlanto-axial stabilization in rheumatoid arthritis. *J Neurosurg*. 1991;74(1):1–7.

39. Tanaka N, Sakahashi H, Hirose K, et al. Results after 24 years of prophylactic surgery for rheumatoid atlantoaxial subluxation. *J Bone Joint Surg Br*. 2005;87(7): 955–958.

40. Pellicci PM, Ranawat CS, Tsairis P, et al. A prospective study of the progression of rheumatoid arthritis of the cervical spine. *J Bone Joint Surg Am*. 1981;63(3):342–350.

41. Lonner BS, Cammisa FP Jr, Ranawat CS. Rheumatoid arthritis of the cervical spine. *Semin Arthroplasty*. 1995; 6(3):193–201.

42. Casey AT, Crockard HA, Bland JM, et al. Surgery on the rheumatoid cervical spine for the non-ambulant myelopathic patient-too much, too late? *Lancet*. 1996; 347(9007):1004–1007.

43. Hamilton JD, Gordon MM, McInnes IB, et al. Improved medical and surgical management of cervical spine disease in patients with rheumatoid arthritis over 10 years. *Ann Rheum Dis*. 2000;59(6):434–438.

44. Mikulowski P, Wollheim FA, Rotmil P, et al. Sudden death in rheumatoid arthritis with atlanto-axial dislocation. *Acta Med Scand*. 1975;198(6):445–451.

45. Smith PH, Benn RT, Sharp J. Natural history of rheumatoid cervical luxations. *Ann Rheum Dis*. 1972;31(6): 431–439.

46. Riise T, Jacobsen BK, Gran JT. High mortality in patients with rheumatoid arthritis and atlantoaxial subluxation. *J Rheumatol*. 2001;28(11):2425–2429.

47. Falope ZF, Griffiths ID, Platt PN, et al. Cervical myelopathy and rheumatoid arthritis: a retrospective analysis of management. *Clin Rehabil.* 2002;16(6): 625–629.

48. Kauppi M, Anttila P. A stiff collar can restrict atlantoaxial instability in rheumatoid cervical spine in selected cases. *Ann Rheum Dis.* 1995;54(4):305–307.

49. Kauppi M, Anttila P. A stiff collar for the treatment of rheumatoid atlantoaxial subluxation. *Br J Rheumatol.* 1996;35(8):771–774.

50. Kauppi M, Neva MH, Kautiainen H. Headmaster collar restricts rheumatoid atlantoaxial subluxation. *Spine.* 1999;24(6):526–528.

51. Moncur C, Williams HJ. Cervical spine management in patients with rheumatoid arthritis: review of the literature. *Phys Ther.* 1988;68(4):509–515.

52. Ballard WT, Clark CR. Increased atlanto-axial instability secondary to an atraumatic fracture of the odontoid process in a patient who had rheumatoid arthritis. A case report. *J Bone Joint Surg Am.* 1995;77(8):1245–1248.

53. Floyd AS, Learmonth ID, Mody G, et al. Atlantoaxial instability and neurologic indicators in rheumatoid arthritis. *Clin Orthop Relat Res.* 1989;241:177–182.

54. Kankaanpaa U, Santavirta S. Cervical spine involvement in rheumatoid arthritis. *Ann Chir Gynaecol Suppl.* 1985;198:117–121.

55. Nguyen HV, Ludwig SC, Silber J, et al. Rheumatoid arthritis of the cervical spine. *Spine J.* 2004;4(3):329–334.

56. Paus AC, Steen H, Roislien J, et al. High mortality rate in rheumatoid arthritis with subluxation of the cervical spine: a cohort study of operated and nonoperated patients. *Spine.* 2008;33(21):2278–2283.

57. Krieg JC, Clark CR, Goetz DD. Cervical spine arthrodesis in rheumatoid arthritis: a long-term follow-up. *Yale J Biol Med.* 1993;66(3):257–262.

58. Santavirta S, Slatis P, Kankaanpaa U, et al. Treatment of the cervical spine in rheumatoid arthritis. *J Bone Joint Surg Am.* 1988;70(5):658–667.

59. Matsunaga S, Sakou T, Onishi T, et al. Prognosis of patients with upper cervical lesions caused by rheumatoid arthritis: comparison of occipitocervical fusion between c1 laminectomy and nonsurgical management. *Spine.* 2003;28(14):1581–1587; discussion 1587.

60. Morizono Y, Sakou T, Kawaida H. Upper cervical involvement in rheumatoid arthritis. *Spine.* 1987;12(8): 721–725.

61. Wolfs JF, Peul WC, Boers M, et al. Rationale and design of The Delphi Trial–I(RCT)2: international randomized clinical trial of rheumatoid craniocervical treatment, an intervention-prognostic trial comparing 'early' surgery with conservative treatment [ISRCTN65076841]. *BMC Musculoskelet Disord.* 2006;7:14.

62. Fielding JW, Hawkins RJ, Ratzan SA. Spine fusion for atlanto-axial instability. *J Bone Joint Surg Am.* 1976; 58(3):400–407.

63. Klimo P Jr, Binning M, Brockmeyer DL, et al. The lasso technique for posterior C1-C2 fusion. *Neurosurgery.* 2007;61(3 suppl):94–99; discussion 99.

64. McCarron RF, Robertson WW. Brooks fusion for atlantoaxial instability in rheumatoid arthritis. *South Med J.* 1988;81(4):474–476.

65. Omura K, Hukuda S, Katsuura A, et al. Evaluation of posterior long fusion versus conservative treatment for the progressive rheumatoid cervical spine. *Spine.* 2002; 27(12):1336–1345.

66. Christensson D, Saveland H, Rydholm U. Cervical spine surgery in rheumatoid arthritis: a Swedish nation-wide registration of 83 patients. *Scand J Rheumatol.* 2000; 29(5):314–319.

67. Naderi S, Crawford NR, Song GS, et al. Biomechanical comparison of C1-C2 posterior fixations. Cable, graft, and screw combinations. *Spine.* 1998;23(18):1946–1955; discussion 1955–1956.

68. Brattstrom H, Granholm L. Atlanto-axial fusion in rheumatoid arthritis. A new method of fixation with wire and bone cement. *Acta Orthop Scand.* 1976;47(6):619–628.

69. Coyne TJ, Fehlings MG, Wallace MC, et al. C1-C2 posterior cervical fusion: long-term evaluation of results and efficacy. *Neurosurgery.* 1995;37(4):688–692; discussion 692–693.

70. Maniker AH, Schulder M, Duran HL. Halifax clamps: efficacy and complications in posterior cervical stabilization. *Surg Neurol.* 1995;43(2):140–146.

71. Statham P, O'Sullivan M, Russell T. The Halifax Interlaminar Clamp for posterior cervical fusion: initial experience in the United Kingdom. *Neurosurgery.* 1993;32(3):396–398; discussion 398–399.

72. Zoma A, Sturrock RD, Fisher WD, et al. Surgical stabilisation of the rheumatoid cervical spine. A review of indications and results. *J Bone Joint Surg Br.* 1987; 69(1):8–12.

73. Agrillo U, Simonetti G, Hernandez R, et al. Halifax interlaminar clamps for posterior atlanto-axial arthrodesis with spinal fusion by "H" bone+graft. *J Neurosurg Sci.* 1994;38(2):105–110.

74. Chan DP, Ngian KS, Cohen L. Posterior upper cervical fusion in rheumatoid arthritis. *Spine.* 1992;17(3):268–272.

75. Coyne TJ, Fehlings MG, Martin RJ. C1-C2 transarticular screw fixation for treatment of C1-C2 instability. *J Clin Neurosci.* 1996;3(3):243–246.

76. Cybulski GR, Stone JL, Crowell RM, et al. Use of Halifax interlaminar clamps for posterior C1-C2 arthrodesis. *Neurosurgery.* 1988;22(2):429–431.

77. Farey ID, Nadkarni S, Smith N. Modified Gallie technique versus transarticular screw fixation in C1-C2 fusion. *Clin Orthop Relat Res.* 1999;359:126–135.

78. Fehring TK, Brooks AL. Upper cervical instability in rheumatoid arthritis. *Clin Orthop Relat Res.* 1987;221: 137–148.

79. Goldie I. A synopsis of surgery for rheumatoid arthritis (excluding the hand). *Clin Orthop Relat Res.* 1984;191: 185–192.

80. Griswold DM, Albright JA, Schiffman E, et al. Atlanto-axial fusion for instability. *J Bone Joint Surg Am.* 1978;60(3): 285–292.

81. Huang CI, Chen IH. Atlantoaxial arthrodesis using Halifax interlaminar clamps reinforced by halo vest immobilization: a long-term follow-up experience. *Neurosurgery,* 1996;38(6):1153–1156; discussion 1156–1157.

82. Moskovich R, Crockard HA. Atlantoaxial arthrodesis using interlaminar clamps: an improved technique. *Spine.* 1992;17(3):261–267.

83. Sheehan JM, Jane JA. Occipital bone graft for atlanto-axial fusion. *Acta Neurochir (Wien)*. 2000;142(6):661–666; discussion 667.

84. Sorensen KH, Husby J, Hein O. Interlaminar atlanto-axial fusion for instability. *Acta Orthop Scand*. 1978;49(4): 341–349.

85. Wilde GP, Hopkins JS. The use of acrylic bone cement for cervical fusion in patients with rheumatoid arthritis. *J R Soc Med*. 1988;81(9):523–525.

86. Yonezawa I, Arai Y, Tsuji T, et al. Atlantoaxial transar-ticular screw fixation and posterior fusion using ultra-high-molecular-weight polyethylene cable. *J Spinal Disord Tech*. 2005;18(5):392–395.

87. Hartl R, Chamberlain RH, Fifield MS, et al. Biomechani-cal comparison of two new atlantoaxial fixation tech-niques with C1–2 transarticular screw-graft fixation. *J Neurosurg Spine*. 2006;5(4):336–342.

88. Henriques T, Cunningham BW, Olerud C, et al. Biome-chanical comparison of five different atlantoaxial poste-rior fixation techniques. *Spine*. 2000;25(22):2877–2883.

89. Mitchell TC, Sadasivan KK, Ogden AL, et al. Biome-chanical study of atlantoaxial arthrodesis: transarticular screw fixation versus modified Brooks posterior wiring. *J Orthop Trauma*. 1999;13(7):483–489.

90. Nichols LA, Mukherjee DP, Ogden AL, et al. A biome-chanical study of unilateral posterior atlantoaxial tran-sarticular screw fixation. *J Long Term Eff Med Implants*. 2005;15(1):33–38.

91. Papagelopoulos PJ, Currier BL, Hokari Y, et al. Biome-chanical comparison of C1-C2 posterior arthrodesis techniques. *Spine*. 2007;32(13):E363–E370.

92. Richter M, Schmidt R, Claes L, et al. Posterior atlanto-axial fixation: biomechanical in vitro comparison of six different techniques. *Spine*. 2002;27(16):1724–1732.

93. Song GS, Theodore N, Dickman CA, et al. Unilateral posterior atlantoaxial transarticular screw fixation. *J Neurosurg*. 1997;87(6):851–855.

94. Cyr SJ, Currier BL, Eck JC, et al. Fixation strength of uni-cortical versus bicortical C1-C2 transarticular screws. *Spine J*. 2008;8(4):661–665.

95. Tokuhashi Y, Matsuzaki H, Shirasaki Y, et al. C1-C2 intra-articular screw fixation for atlantoaxial posterior stabilization. *Spine*. 2000;25(3):337–341.

96. Weidner A, Wahler M, Chiu ST, et al. Modification of C1-C2 transarticular screw fixation by image-guided surgery. *Spine*. 2000;25(20):2668–2673; discussion 2674.

97. Acosta FL Jr, Quinones-Hinojosa A, Gadkary CA, et al. Frameless stereotactic image-guided C1-C2 transartic-ular screw fixation for atlantoaxial instability: review of 20 patients. *J Spinal Disord Tech*. 2005;18(5):385–391.

98. Borm W, Konig RW, Albrecht A, et al. Percutaneous transarticular atlantoaxial screw fixation using a cannu-lated screw system and image guidance. *Minim Invasive Neurosurg*. 2004;47(2):111–114.

99. Kawaguchi Y, Ishihara H, Ohmori K, et al. Computer-assisted Magerl's transarticular screw fixation for atlan-toaxial subluxation. *J Orthop Sci*. 2002;7(1):131–136.

100. Kelleher MO, McEvoy L, Nagaria J, et al. Image-guided transarticular atlanto-axial screw fixation. *Int J Med Robot*. 2006;2(2):154–160.

101. Gebhard JS, Schimmer RC, Jeanneret B. Safety and accuracy of transarticular screw fixation C1-C2 using an aiming device. An anatomic study. *Spine*. 1998; 23(20):2185–2189.

102. Yoshida M, Neo M, Fujibayashi S, et al. Comparison of the anatomical risk for vertebral artery injury associated with the C2-pedicle screw and atlantoaxial transarticu-lar screw. *Spine*. 2006;31(15):E513–E517.

103. Nadim Y, Sabry F, Xu R, et al. Computed tomography in the determination of transarticular C1-C2 screw length. *Orthopedics*. 2000;23(4):373–375.

104. Ebraheim NA, Misson JR, Xu R, et al. The optimal transarticular c1–2 screw length and the location of the hypoglossal nerve. *Surg Neurol*. 2000;53(3): 208–210.

105. Reilly TM, Sasso RC, Hall PV. Atlantoaxial stabilization: clinical comparison of posterior cervical wiring tech-nique with transarticular screw fixation. *J Spinal Disord Tech*. 2003;16(3):248–253.

106. Neo M, Matsushita M, Iwashita Y, et al. Atlantoaxial transarticular screw fixation for a high-riding vertebral artery. *Spine*. 2003;28(7):666–670.

107. Neo M, Sakamoto T, Fujibayashi S, Nakamura T. A safe screw trajectory for atlantoaxial transarticular fixation achieved using an aiming device. *Spine*. 2005;30(9): E236–E242.

108. Dickman CA, Sonntag VK. Posterior C1-C2 transarticu-lar screw fixation for atlantoaxial arthrodesis. *Neurosur-gery*. 1998;43(2):275–280; discussion 280–281.

109. Jeanneret B, Magerl F. Primary posterior fusion C1/2 in odontoid fractures: indications, technique, and results of transarticular screw fixation. *J Spinal Disord*. 1992; 5(4):464–475.

110. Dickman CA, Sonntag VK. Surgical management of atlantoaxial nonunions. *J Neurosurg*. 1995;83(2): 248–253.

111. Eleraky MA, Masferrer R, Sonntag VK. Posterior atlan-toaxial facet screw fixation in rheumatoid arthritis. *J Neurosurg*. 1998;89(1):8–12.

112. ElSaghir H, Boehm H, Greiner-Perth R. Mini-open approach combined with percutaneous transarticu-lar screw fixation for C1-C2 fusion. *Neurosurg Rev*. 2005;28(1):59–63.

113. Fountas KN, Kapsalaki EZ, Karampelas I, et al. C1-C2 transarticular screw fixation for atlantoaxial instability. *South Med J*. 2004;97(11):1042–1048.

114. Gluf WM, Schmidt MH, Apfelbaum RI. Atlantoaxial transarticular screw fixation: a review of surgical indica-tions, fusion rate, complications, and lessons learned in 191 adult patients. *J Neurosurg Spine*. 2005;2(2):155–163.

115. Grob D, Jeanneret B, Aebi M, et al. Atlanto-axial fusion with transarticular screw fixation. *J Bone Joint Surg Br*. 1991;73(6):972–976.

116. Haid RW Jr. C1-C2 transarticular screw fixation: techni-cal aspects. *Neurosurgery*. 2001;49(1):71–74.

117. Haid RW Jr, Subach BR, McLaughlin MR, et al. C1-C2 transarticular screw fixation for atlantoaxial instabil-ity: a 6-year experience. *Neurosurgery*. 2001;49(1):65–68; discussion 69–70.

118. Ito H, Neo M, Fujibayashi S, et al. Atlantoaxial tran-sarticular screw fixation with posterior wiring using

polyethylene cable: facet fusion despite posterior graft resorption in rheumatoid patients. *Spine*. 2008; 33(15):1655–1661.

119. Liang ML, Huang MC, Cheng H, et al. Posterior transarticular screw fixation for chronic atlanto-axial instability. *J Clin Neurosci*. 2004;11(4):368–372.

120. Marcotte P, Dickman CA, Sonntag VK, et al. Posterior atlantoaxial facet screw fixation. *J Neurosurg*. 1993;79(2): 234–237.

121. Naseer R, Bailey SI. Atlantoaxial instability treated with transarticular screw fixation. *Int Orthop*. 2001;25(4): 268–271.

122. Stillerman CB, Wilson JA. Atlanto-axial stabilization with posterior transarticular screw fixation: technical description and report of 22 cases. *Neurosurgery*. 1993;32(6):948–954; discussion 954–955.

123. Coric D, Branch CL Jr, Wilson JA, et al. Arteriovenous fistula as a complication of C1-2 transarticular screw fixation. Case report and review of the literature. *J Neurosurg*. 1996;85(2):340–343.

124. Madawi AA, Casey AT, Solanki GA, et al. Radiological and anatomical evaluation of the atlantoaxial transarticular screw fixation technique. *J Neurosurg*. 1997;86(6):961–968.

125. Prabhu VC, France JC, Voelker JL, et al. Vertebral artery pseudoaneurysm complicating posterior C1–2 transarticular screw fixation: case report. *Surg Neurol*. 2001;55(1):29–33; discussion 33–34.

126. Wang C, Yan M, Zhou H, et al. Atlantoaxial transarticular screw fixation with morselized autograft and without additional internal fixation: technical description and report of 57 cases. *Spine*. 2007;32(6):643–646.

127. Chung SS, Lee CS, Chung HW, et al. CT analysis of the axis for transarticular screw fixation of rheumatoid atlantoaxial instability. *Skeletal Radiol*. 2006;35(9):679–683.

128. Nogueira-Barbosa MH, Defino HL. Multiplanar reconstructions of helical computed tomography in planning of atlanto-axial transarticular fixation. *Eur Spine J*. 2005;14(5):493–500.

129. Paramore CG, Dickman CA, Sonntag VK. The anatomical suitability of the C1-2 complex for transarticular screw fixation. *J Neurosurg*. 1996;85(2):221–224.

130. Resnick DK, Lapsiwala S, Trost GR. Anatomic suitability of the C1-C2 complex for pedicle screw fixation. *Spine*. 2002;27(14):1494–1498.

131. Hott JS, Lynch JJ, Chamberlain RH, et al. Biomechanical comparison of C1–2 posterior fixation techniques. *J Neurosurg Spine*. 2005;2(2):175–181.

132. Kuroki H, Rengachary SS, Goel VK, et al. Biomechanical comparison of two stabilization techniques of the atlantoaxial joints: transarticular screw fixation versus screw and rod fixation. *Neurosurgery*. 2005;56(1 suppl): 151–159; discussion 151–159.

133. Lapsiwala SB, Anderson PA, Oza A, et al. Biomechanical comparison of four C1 to C2 rigid fixative techniques: anterior transarticular, posterior transarticular, C1 to C2 pedicle, and C1 to C2 intralaminar screws. *Neurosurgery*. 2006;58(3):516–521; discussion 516–521.

134. Melcher RP, Puttlitz CM, Kleinstueck FS, et al. Biomechanical testing of posterior atlantoaxial fixation techniques. *Spine*. 2002;27(22):2435–2440.

135. Oda I, Abumi K, Sell LC, et al. Biomechanical evaluation of five different occipito-atlanto-axial fixation techniques. *Spine*. 1999;24(22):2377–2382.

136. Puttlitz CM, Goel VK, Traynelis VC, et al. A finite element investigation of upper cervical instrumentation. *Spine*. 2001;26(22):2449–2455.

137. Gorek J, Acaroglu E, Berven S, et al. Constructs incorporating intralaminar C2 screws provide rigid stability for atlantoaxial fixation. *Spine*. 2005;30(13):1513–1518.

138. Claybrooks R, Kayanja M, Milks R, et al. Atlantoaxial fusion: a biomechanical analysis of two C1-C2 fusion techniques. *Spine J*. 2007;7(6):682–688.

139. Wright NM. Posterior C2 fixation using bilateral, crossing C2 laminar screws: case series and technical note. *J Spinal Disord Tech*. 2004;17(2):158–162.

140. Eck JC, Walker MP, Currier BL, et al. Biomechanical comparison of unicortical versus bicortical C1 lateral mass screw fixation. *J Spinal Disord Tech*. 2007;20(7): 505–508.

141. Harms J, Melcher RP. Posterior C1-C2 fusion with polyaxial screw and rod fixation. *Spine*. 2001;26(22): 2467–2471.

142. Aryan HE, Newman CB, Nottmeier EW, et al. Stabilization of the atlantoaxial complex via C-1 lateral mass and C-2 pedicle screw fixation in a multicenter clinical experience in 102 patients: modification of the Harms and Goel techniques. *J Neurosurg Spine*. 2008;8(3): 222–229.

143. Gunnarsson T, Massicotte EM, Govender PV, et al. The use of C1 lateral mass screws in complex cervical spine surgery: indications, techniques, and outcome in a prospective consecutive series of 25 cases. *J Spinal Disord Tech*. 2007;20(4):308–316.

144. Pham XV, Bancel P, Menkes CJ, et al. Upper cervical spine surgery in rheumatoid arthritis: retrospective study of 30 patients followed for two years or more after Cotrel-Dubousset instrumentation. *Joint Bone Spine*. 2000;67(5):434–440.

145. Stokes JK, Villavicencio AT, Liu PC, et al. Posterior atlantoaxial stabilization: new alternative to C1–2 transarticular screws. *Neurosurg Focus*. 2002;12(1):E6.

146. Stulik J, Vyskocil T, Sebesta P, et al. Atlantoaxial fixation using the polyaxial screw-rod system. *Eur Spine J*. 2007;16(4):479–484.

147. Vilela MD, Jermani C, Braga BP. C1 lateral mass screws for posterior segmental stabilization of the upper cervical spine and a new method of three-point rigid fixation of the C1-C2 complex. *Arq Neuropsiquiatr*. 2006;64(3B):762–767.

148. Kandziora F, Kerschbaumer F, Starker M, et al. Biomechanical assessment of transoral plate fixation for atlantoaxial instability. *Spine*. 2000;25(12):1555–1561.

149. Lu J, Ebraheim NA, Yang H, et al. Anatomic considerations of anterior transarticular screw fixation for atlantoaxial instability. *Spine*. 1998;23(11):1229–1235; discussion 1236.

150. Cornefjord M, Henriques T, Alemany M, et al. Posterior atlanto-axial fusion with the Olerud Cervical Fixation System for odontoid fractures and C1-C2 instability in rheumatoid arthritis. *Eur Spine J*. 2003;12(1):91–96.

151. Xiao ZM, Zhan XL, Gong de F, et al. C2 pedicle screw and plate combined with C1 titanium cable fixation for the treatment of atlantoaxial instability not suitable for placement of C1 screw. *J Spinal Disord Tech.* 2008;21(7):514–517.

152. Kato Y, Itoh T, Kanaya K, et al. Relation between atlantoaxial (C1/2) and cervical alignment (C2-C7) angles with Magerl and Brooks techniques for atlantoaxial subluxation in rheumatoid arthritis. *J Orthop Sci.* 2006;11(4):347–352.

153. Yoshimoto H, Ito M, Abumi K, et al. A retrospective radiographic analysis of subaxial sagittal alignment after posterior C1-C2 fusion. *Spine.* 2004;29(2):175–181.

154. Kandziora F, Mittlmeier T, Kerschbaumer F. Stage-related surgery for cervical spine instability in rheumatoid arthritis. *Eur Spine J.* 1999;8(5):371–381.

155. Stirrat AN, Fyfe IS. Surgery of the rheumatoid cervical spine. Correlation of the pathology and prognosis. *Clin Orthop Relat Res.* 1993;293:135–143.

156. Clark CR, Goetz DD, Menezes AH. Arthrodesis of the cervical spine in rheumatoid arthritis. *J Bone Joint Surg Am.* 1989;71(3):381–392.

157. Conaty JP, Mongan ES. Cervical fusion in rheumatoid arthritis. *J Bone Joint Surg Am.* 1981;63(8):1218–1227.

158. Eyres KS, Gray DH, Robertson P. Posterior surgical treatment for the rheumatoid cervical spine. *Br J Rheumatol.* 1998;37(7):756–759.

159. McRorie ER, McLoughlin P, Russell T, et al. Cervical spine surgery in patients with rheumatoid arthritis: an appraisal. *Ann Rheum Dis.* 1996;55(2):99–104.

160. Ronkainen A, Niskanen M, Auvinen A, et al. Cervical spine surgery in patients with rheumatoid arthritis: longterm mortality and its determinants. *J Rheumatol.* 2006;33(3):517–522.

161. van Asselt KM, Lems WF, Bongartz EB, et al. Outcome of cervical spine surgery in patients with rheumatoid arthritis. *Ann Rheum Dis.* 2001;60(5):448–452.

162. Clarke MJ, Cohen-Gadol AA, Ebersold MJ, et al. Long-term incidence of subaxial cervical spine instability following cervical arthrodesis surgery in patients with rheumatoid arthritis. *Surg Neurol.* 2006;66(2):136–140; discussion 140.

163. Mukai Y, Hosono N, Sakaura H, et al. Sagittal alignment of the subaxial cervical spine after C1-C2 transarticular screw fixation in rheumatoid arthritis. *J Spinal Disord Tech.* 2007;20(6):436–441.

164. Sugimoto Y, Tanaka M, Nakanishi K, et al. Assessing the range of cervical rotation in patients with rheumatoid arthritis after atlantoaxial screw fixation using axial CT. *Spine.* 2007;32(21):2318–2321.

Cervical Epidural Abscess

YU-PO LEE, MD, HOSSEIN GHOFRANI, MD, AND STEVEN R. GARFIN, MD

▇ EDITORS' CASE PRESENTATION

A 48-year-old woman with a history of active intravenous drug abuse presents to the emergency department with a history of progressive inability to move her upper or lower extremities over the past 24 hours. She reports this at the end of a 1-week binge of drug use, after which she "woke up" and could not move her arms or legs. She also states that she had increasing neck pain for the past 4 days. Her medical history includes that she has hepatitis B, hepatitis C, smokes heavily but is HIV-negative.

Upon physical examination, she appears thin, malnourished, and cachexic. She is currently febrile and is ventilator dependent but is hemodynamically stable. White blood cell count, ESR, and C-reactive protein levels are elevated. Blood cultures, so far, are negative. She has 0/5 strength in her upper and lower extremities and decreased rectal tone. Sensory examination is limited as she cannot speak.

Radiographic imaging studies are shown in Figure 9.1A–E.

INTERPRETATION OF CLINICAL PRESENTATION

The clinical scenario describes a woman who has an active infection with a rapid decline in neurologic function. In the setting of rapid neurologic decline, the differential diagnosis for this patient would include vertebral osteomyelitis/discitis with subsequent spinal cord compression from the formation of an epidural abscess, disc herniation, transverse myelitis, Guillain-Barré syndrome, stroke, mycotic aneurysm, brain tumor, and vasculitis.

Once an initial inspection has been made and a differential diagnosis has been generated, a review of the patient's history and medical comorbidities should be performed to narrow the list of potential diagnoses. The risk factors for pyogenic vertebral osteomyelitis include intravenous drug use, diabetes, multiple medical comorbidities, morbid obesity, elderly patients, hepatic and renal failure, malnutrition, and tobacco use.[1,2] This patient has many of the risk factors for the development of pyogenic vertebral osteomyelitis, so this diagnosis remains high on our list.

Neck or back pain is the most common complaint in patients with pyogenic vertebral osteomyelitis and is noted in more than 90% of patients.[1,2] Elevated temperatures are also noted in 50% of patients. The cervical spine is affected approximately 10% of the time. Up to 18% of patients with a pyogenic spondylodiscitis will have spinal epidural abscesses and more than 50% of these patients will have neurologic deficits. Given this patient's 4-day history of neck pain prior to the onset of her neurologic symptoms, cervical spondylodiscitis is possible. The onset of her neurologic symptoms could also signal the formation of an epidural abscess.

The laboratory evaluation helps confirm or narrow the diagnosis of infection. Given the elevated white blood cell count, ESR, and C-reactive protein levels in conjunction with her rapid neurologic decline, vertebral osteomyelitis with spinal cord compression from the formation of an epidural abscess becomes the primary consideration. An elevated white blood cell count is found in approximately one third of pyogenic vertebral osteomyelitis cases.[1–3] An elevated ESR is noted over 95% of the time in these cases, and an elevated C-reactive protein level may be observed in virtually all cases. Positive blood cultures are recorded only 50% of the time, so negative blood cultures in this case by no means rule out a pyogenic infection.

The next step in the evaluation process is imaging to confirm the diagnosis. In this instance, MRI with gadolinium is the procedure of choice. The MRI

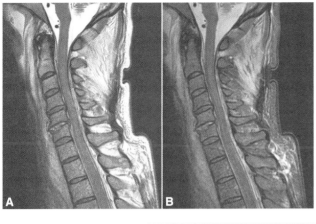 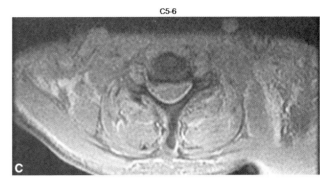

Figure 9.1.

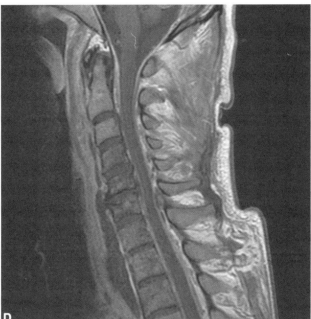 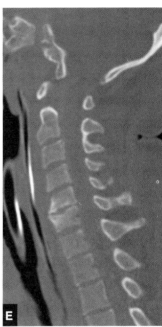

images (Figure 9.1A–D) provided show hyperintensity in the disc and endplates between C5 and C6. Endplate erosion and destruction are also noted between C5 and C6. The C5 and C6 vertebral bodies show characteristic inflammatory changes. The infected regions have decreased intensity on the T1-weighted sagittal image (Figure 9.1D) and increased intensity on T2-weighted images. This is certainly consistent with a pyogenic C5-6 spondylodiscitis. Also noted is a fluid collection behind the disc space and vertebral bodies of C5 and C6 (Figure 9.1D). This is suggestive of an epidural abscess behind C5 and C6. The abscess is indenting the spinal cord and causing cord compression at these levels (Figure 9.1C). This MRI finding could certainly explain her rapid neurologic decline in both her upper and lower extremities as well as the loss of her rectal tone. In addition, her dependence on the ventilator might also be related to the epidural abscess as it is high enough to disrupt the respiratory centers of her spinal cord.

The CT image provided shows endplate destruction between C5 and C6 (Figure 9.1E). These findings are consistent with a C5-6 spondylodiscitis and support the diagnosis of a cervical epidural abscess that originated from a pyogenic C5-6 spondylodiscitis.

DECLARATION OF SPECIFIC DIAGNOSIS

This patient has a pyogenic C5-6 spondylodiscitis with the formation of a ventral epidural abscess.

BRAINSTORMING: WHAT ARE THE TREATMENT GOALS AND SURGICAL OPTIONS?

The treatment goals are

1. Eradication of the infection
2. Maximize recovery of neurologic function
3. Maintain spinal alignment and ensuring continued stability
4. Early mobilization
5. Rehabilitation and healing

The treatment options are

1. Antibiotics and medical management
2. Anterior decompression with anterior instrumentation only
3. Anterior decompression and instrumentation with supplemental posterior instrumentation

EVALUATION OF THE LITERATURE

A Medline search was performed to find articles concerned about different aspects of cervical epidural abscess. Search strategies included the use of MeSH (medical subject headings) and key words. Key words included "cervical epidural abscess," "spinal epidural abscess," and "spinal infection." Subheadings of classification, etiology, symptoms, complications, treatment, radiography, and mortality were also searched. This search resulted in 649 articles including 89 review articles. After limiting our search to articles in English language and to those published after 1960, 329 articles including 51 review articles were found. Most of the publications were case reports or case series (230 of 329). About 60 abstracts were read, and 35 articles were reviewed.

DETAILED REVIEW OF PERTINENT ARTICLES

Operative or Nonoperative Treatment

Overall, the quality of evidence guiding treatment in patients with cervical epidural abscesses is fair to poor. The literature review revealed no randomized prospective studies. The literature consists primarily of case reports or retrospective reviews of patients with epidural abscesses. There was, however, a meta-analysis performed on spinal epidural abscesses.[4] The meta-analysis pooled together all the case reports, case series, and retrospective reviews from 1954 to

1997. This generated a pool of 915 patients. Of these 915 patients, treatment details were available for 639 patients. Only 72 (11%) of the 639 patients were treated exclusively with antibiotic treatment alone.

While these case reports and case series indicate that some patients may be successfully treated with antibiotics alone, the authors of the majority of these papers noted that this should only be done in patients who are not septic and do not have significant neurologic symptoms.[4] Furthermore, despite the successful medical management of epidural abscesses in some of the cases, sudden neurological deterioration of patients receiving appropriate antibiotic therapy has been noted.[2-7] Unfortunately, the true success rate of nonoperative treatment for cervical epidural abscesses is difficult to discern from the literature. Many cases were most likely selectively reported, and unsuccessful attempts at medical management were not reported once the patient had surgery.

In patients who are septic or who have significant neurologic deficits, the literature supports surgical intervention. In one of the first comprehensive reviews on spinal epidural abscesses, Dandy reported on 32 patients who were all treated nonoperatively.[8] Of these 32 patients, 26 died (81%). Since then, the literature has indicated a reduction in the mortality rate from 34% to 16% from 1954 to 1980. The overall mortality rate seems to be fairly constant at 15% since 1980.[8] It is believed that increased awareness and early intervention, along with improved antibiotic treatments and surgical intervention, have played a significant role in mortality reduction. In a recent retrospective review by Boström et al. published in 2008, the authors noted a 6.5% mortality rate.[9] Also noteworthy was the fact that many of the patients who had surgery experienced partial or complete neurologic recovery. The retrospective reviews evaluated in the literature search support the hypothesis that patients with sepsis or neurologic deficits will have improved outcomes with surgery compared to nonoperative care.[2-15] In patients who are not septic and do not have any neurologic deficits, nonoperative management is an option. However, these patients need to be followed very closely as neurologic decline, despite appropriate antibiotic treatment, has been noted in multiple studies.[4,6-15]

Hence, we would recommend surgical treatment for this patient. While she is hemodynamically stable and thus probably not septic, she has severe neurologic deficits. While the quality of the available literature on cervical epidural abscesses is fair to poor, it is consistent in recommending surgical intervention in patients who have severe neurologic deficits. In fact, there were no studies found reporting good outcomes in patients who had cervical epidural abscesses with neurologic deficits who were treated with antibiotics alone. Thus, we can confidently recommend surgical intervention in this case. The number of retrospective reviews supporting surgery combined with the absence of any articles supporting nonoperative treatment in this case gives considerable support to this argument.

Timing of Surgery

Once the decision to operate has been made, the surgeon must decide when to operate. In the clinical scenario provided, the literature argues for immediate surgical decompression. In the retrospective reviews of cervical epidural abscesses, it was noted that patients with neurologic deficits may recover neurologic function with surgical decompression.[2–7,9–15] It was also noted that patients with neurologic deficits had improved recovery if they were operated on sooner.[4,6,7,9–15] In a study by Rigamonti et al.[2] the authors noted that patients who presented with severe neurologic deficits had a worse outcome if they were treated more than 24 hours later. Poor outcome occurred in 9 of 19 patients (47%) treated after 24 hours, whereas it occurred in only 1 of 10 patients (10%) treated promptly. This hypothesis is supported by multiple other retrospective reviews.[4,6,7,9–15] Thus, we would recommend early surgical decompression for this patient. While the optimal time period before surgery still remains in doubt, the literature supports earlier surgical intervention when the patient has a neurologic deficit. The quality of the literature upon which this hypothesis is based is fair to poor because the literature consists primarily of case reports and retrospective reviews. However, it is consistent in recommending earlier versus later intervention.[2–7,9–15]

EVIDENTIARY TABLE AND SELECTION OF TREATMENT METHOD

The best available evidence dictates that the patient presented in the clinical scenario should be treated operatively. The following questions would then be whether surgery should be performed from an anterior or combined anterior and posterior approach and also whether or not fusion with instrumentation is appropriate in the setting of infection. In order to evaluate the most appropriate surgical treatment, only articles pertaining to adult patients with cervical epidural abscesses treated with modern spinal instrumentation were critically examined. These results are summarized in Table 9.1.

Anterior Versus Posterior Decompression and Fusion

Selection of the appropriate surgical technique for this patient comes from an analysis of five studies that utilized modern spinal instrumentation. In a retrospective review by Ruf et al.[16] 88 patients with vertebral osteomyelitis were treated with anterior debridement and fusion with titanium cages and anterior plating. Thirteen patients with cervical epidural abscesses were also included in this study. The authors noted a solid bony fusion in all the patients without any recurrence of infection at the last follow-up despite the use of titanium cages and titanium plates. Furthermore, they observed significant clinical improvement in pain score, Frankel's classification, and blood parameters in all patients. In another study by McGuire and Eismont,[17] 27 patients with vertebral osteomyelitis were treated with anterior debridement and fusion.[17] The authors noted that they were able to eradicate the infection in all of the patients. Furthermore, the authors found that placement of autogenous bone graft at the time of primary debridement did not hinder eradication of the infection. Critical review of the remaining four studies also showed that anterior decompression was an effective method of eradicating infection and that concurrent fusion with anterior plating at the time of debridement did not result in recurrent infection.[5,18–20] Therefore, anterior debridement and fusion with instrumentation are appropriate.

Autogenous Strut Grafting Versus Titanium Cages

The use of titanium cages has become more popular in the setting of infection. The various sizes of footplates and lengths available with titanium cages make them attractive in the setting of infection in which corpectomies must be performed. In the study by Ruf et al.[16] all 13 patients successfully fused with the use of titanium cages. Thus, there is some evidence that titanium cages are effective in forming a solid fusion.

However, the majority of the literature currently advocates the use of autograft in the setting of infection. In the study by McGuire and Eismont,[17] the authors used strut autograft and achieved a 96% fusion rate. Also, they reported no recurrence of infection. Based upon this and multiple other retrospective reviews, autogenous bone is still the graft of choice in the setting of infection, though bone packed in a titanium mesh cage is a viable option.[4–15,18–20]

Supplemental Posterior Instrumentation

We would also advocate supplemental posterior fixation in this setting. In a study by Dimar et al.[20] 42 patients with vertebral osteomyelitis underwent anterior debridement and fusion with delayed posterior fixation. This study included five patients with cervical osteomyelitis. All patients had resolution of their infections with no recurrence. In the patient

TABLE 9.1 **Evidentiary Table.**

Paper Author (Year)	Description	Summary of Results	Quality of Evidence
Ruf et al. (2007)	Retrospective case series	88 patients with vertebral osteomyelitis treated operatively. Titanium mesh cages were used to reconstruct the anterior vertebral column in all cases. All patients showed a solid bony fusion without any recurrence of infection at last follow-up. Changes in pain score, Frankel's classification, and blood parameters demonstrated a significant clinical improvement in all patients.	Very low
McGuire and Eismont (1994)	Retrospective case series	27 patients with vertebral osteomyelitis were treated with autogenous bone grafting. Infection resolution occurred equally well in all cases. Arthrodesis occurred in 96% of the cases (26 of 27 patients).	Very low
Osenbach et al. (1990)	Retrospective case series	40 patients with vertebral osteomyelitis were reviewed. 27 patients were treated surgically. 8 of 19 patients who had neurologic deficits regained full function while 9 improved, 1 remained unchanged, and 1 died.	Very low
Nakase et al. (2006)	Retrospective case series	9 patients with vertebral osteomyelitis and epidural abscesses were treated operatively in two stages. No evidence of recurrence or residual infection was observed in any patient.	Very low
Dimar et al. (2004)	Retrospective case series	42 patients with vertebral osteomyelitis were treated with anterior debridement and fusion followed by delayed posterior stabilization and fusion. All patients had resolution of their infections with no recurrence. There were two deaths. Neurologic deficits resolved in all patients.	Very low

described in this scenario, we would be concerned about osteoporosis and poor bone quality. Hence, posterior fixation would reduce the risk of subsidence or migration of the anterior graft. However, we would advocate waiting until the patient's medical condition improved before subjecting her to another procedure. In addition, waiting a week would allow better control of the infection before more instrumentation and bone graft are placed in her posterior cervical spine. Lastly, it must be remembered that she has sustained a severe neurologic injury. Delayed posterior instrumentation would also give here spinal cord a chance to recover before she must be flipped over and placed prone for a prolonged period of time.

DEFINITIVE TREATMENT PLAN

In the clinical scenario provided, our patient has a pyogenic spondylodiscitis at C5 and C6 with an epidural abscess extending behind the bodies of C5 and C6. Since the compression is occurring anteriorly, the recommendation in this patient would be to do an anterior decompression and fusion with delayed supplemental posterior instrumentation. In order to completely evacuate the epidural abscess, a corpectomy of both the C5 and C6 vertebral bodies would need to be performed. A review of the literature shows that many patients with a cervical epidural abscess may present with either frank pus or with a phlegmon.[4,6–15] A corpectomy of the C5 and C6 vertebral bodies would completely evacuate any residual pus and decompress the spinal cord if a phlegmon had developed behind the C5 or C6 vertebral bodies. Furthermore, removal of the C5 and C6 vertebral bodies would help to eradicate the infection by removing any residual sources of infection.

Once the corpectomies of C5 and C6 have been performed, we would recommend strut grafting with autogenous bone. While Ruf et al., have shown success with titanium cages in the setting of infection, the vast majority of the literature published to date supports the use of autogenous bone in the setting of infection.[4–16,18–20] There is sufficient evidence supporting the use of an anterior plate to prevent dislodgment of the graft to warrant its use.[18–20] In addition, we would recommend supplemental posterior instrumentation at a later date to decrease the risk of infection and to improve the fusion rate, particularly if C4 and C7 appear osteopenic/osteoporotic.

Grading the Evidence for This Plan

The evidence to support the technical aspects of our treatment selection would be considered low as it is derived from retrospective reviews of moderate quality. The treatment goals have been met in the six studies found in Table 9.1. Anterior debridement and fusion with instrumentation resulted in complete resolution of the infection in all of the cases. Also, fusion rates were >90% in all of the studies.

In accordance with the method of grading recommendations set forth by Schunemann et al.[21] our proposed treatment would be considered a **strong recommendation**. The grading paradigm utilized is necessary because it not only considers the quality of evidence but also addresses the benefits, harms, and burdens of the proposed interventions.

PREDICTING OUTCOMES

In the clinical scenario provided, the outcome will most likely be poor. Hlavin et al. reported no improvement for any of their seven patients with paralysis, despite surgical treatment between 6 and 12 hours after the onset of paralysis.[7] This observation has been consistently noted in multiple other studies.[10–12] Hence, once paralysis has set in, the chance of significant neurologic recovery is not high. However, surgery is still indicated in this patient because it gives her the best

chance of possible neurologic recovery. In addition, cultures obtained during surgery will be important to guide antibiotic treatment since her blood cultures were initially negative.

SUMMARY

We are presented with a 48-year-old woman who has developed a cervical epidural abscess. The most appropriate treatment for this patient would be a C5 and C6 corpectomy with thorough debridement of any pus or phlegmon ventral to the spinal cord with a C4-7 anterior instrumented fusion with iliac crest bone graft strut from C4-7. Posterior instrumentation from C4-7 may be performed at a later day to improve fusion rates. This procedure gives her the best chance of eradication of her infection and also yields high fusion rates. Unfortunately, the outcome will most likely be poor because she has already developed complete paralysis in both her upper and lower extremities. However, this plan gives her the best chance for neurologic recovery and eradication of her infection.

REFERENCES

1. Sampath P, Rigamonti D. Spinal epidural abscess: a review of epidemiology, diagnosis, and treatment. *J Spinal Disord*. 1999;12(2):89–93.
2. Rigamonti D, Liem L, Sampath P, et al. Spinal epidural abscess: contemporary trends in etiology, evaluation, and management. *Surg Neurol*. 1999;52(2):189–196.
3. Carragee EJ. Pyogenic vertebral osteomyelitis. *J Bone Joint Surg Am*. 1997;79(6):874–880.
4. Reihsaus E, Waldbaur H, Seeling W. Spinal epidural abscess: a meta-analysis of 915 patients. *Neurosurg Rev*. 2000;23(4):175–204.
5. Hadjipavlou AG, Mader JT, Necessary JT, et al. Hematogenous pyogenic spinal infections and their surgical management. *Spine*. 2000;25(13):1668–1679.
6. Khanna RK, Malik GM, Rock JP, et al. Spinal epidural abscess: evaluation of factors influencing outcome. *Neurosurgery*. 1996;39:958–964.
7. Hlavin ML, Kaminski HJ, Ross JS. Spinal epidural abscess: a ten-year perspective. *Neurosurgery*. 1990;27:177–184.
8. Dandy WE. Abscesses and inflammatory tumors in the spinal epidural space (so called pachymeningitis externa). *Arch Surg*. 13:477–494.
9. Boström A, Oertel M, Ryang Y, et al. Treatment strategies and outcome in patients with non-tuberculous spinal epidural abscess–a review of 46 cases. *Minim Invasive Neurosurg*. 2008;51(1):36–42.
10. Nakase H, Matsuda R, Tamaki R, et al. Two-stage management for vertebral osteomyelitis and epidural abscess: technical note. *Neurosurgery*. 2006;58(6):E1219.
11. Pereira CE, Lynch JC. Spinal epidural abscess: an analysis of 24 cases. *Surg Neurol*. 2005;63(suppl 1):S26–S29.

12. Tang HJ, Lin HJ, Liu YC, et al. Spinal epidural abscess–experience with 46 patients and evaluation of prognostic factors. *J Infect.* 2002;45(2):76–81.

13. Akalan N, Ozgen T. Infection as a cause of spinal cord compression: a review of 36 spinal epidural abscess cases. *Acta Neurochir (Wien).* 2000;142(1):17–23.

14. Darouiche RO, Hamill RJ, Greenberg SB, et al. Bacterial spinal epidural abscess. Review of 43 cases and literature survey. *Medicine (Baltimore).* 1992;71(6):369–385.

15. Nussbaum ES, Rigamonti D, StandifordH. Spinal epidural abscess: a report of 40 cases and review. *Surg Neurol.* 1992;38:225–231.

16. Ruf M, Stoltze D, Merk HR, et al. Treatment of vertebral osteomyelitis by radical debridement and stabilization using titanium mesh cages. *Spine.* 2007;32(9):275–280.

17. McGuire RA, Eismont FJ. The fate of autogenous bone graft in surgically treated pyogenic vertebral osteomyelitis. *J Spinal Disord.* 1994;7(3):206–215.

18. Osenbach RK, Hitchon PW, Menezes AH. Diagnosis and management of pyogenic vertebral osteomyelitis in adults. *Surg Neurol.* 1990;33(4):266–275.

19. Nakase H, Matsuda R, Tamaki R, et al. Two-stage management for vertebral osteomyelitis and epidural abscess: technical note. *Neurosurgery.* 2006;58(6):1219.

20. Dimar JR, Carreon LY, Glassman SD, et al. Treatment of pyogenic vertebral osteomyelitis with anterior debridement and fusion followed by delayed posterior spinal fusion. *Spine.* 2004;29(3):326–332.

21. Schunemann HJ, Jaeschke R, Cook DJ, et al. ATS Documents Development and Implementation Committee. An official ATS statement: grading the quality of evidence and strength of recommendations in ATS guidelines and recommendations. *Am J Respir Crit Care Med.* 2006;174:605–614.

22. Torda AJ, Gottlieb T, Bradbury R. Pyogenic vertebral osteomyelitis: analysis of 20 cases and review. *Clin Infect Dis.* 1995;20(2):320–328.

SPINAL TUMORS AND FRACTURES

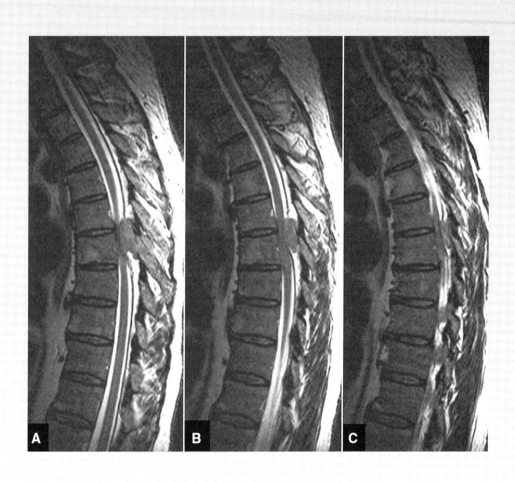

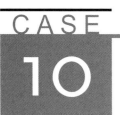

Metastatic Prostate Tumor with Fracture at L3

ILYA LAUFER, MD, ERIC LIS, MD, AND MARK H. BILSKY, MD

EDITORS' CASE PRESENTATION

A 61-year-old man with a history of prostate cancer presents with low back pain and right lower extremity pain. Prostate cancer was initially diagnosed in 2002, for which he underwent a prostatectomy and radiation; he is currently receiving chemotherapy. He also has a complaint of generalized fatigue. He feels back fatigue with ambulation but, in addition, feels a substantial amount of back pain when he tries to lie supine. The patient expresses the feeling of being hunched over, particularly with ambulation. He has no bowel or bladder complaints.

Physical examination demonstrates a noticeable kyphotic posture of the low back with some prominence of the L3 spinous process. However, he is grossly neurologically intact to motor, sensory, and reflex testing. He has some mild tenderness to palpation of the low back. Magnetic resonance (MR) images and plain radiographs are shown in Figures 10.1 to 10.3.

INTERPRETATION OF CLINICAL PRESENTATION

The clinical scenario reveals a man with a known history of prostate carcinoma who presents with low back and right lower extremity pain. The patient is presumably 6 years from his initial diagnosis. Based on the fact that he is currently receiving chemotherapy, we can assume that he is castrate insensitive and has failed prior hormonal androgen deprivation therapy, suggesting that he has advanced disease. Relevant information for restaging him at this point would include a prostate-specific antigen level and recent 18-FDG-PET or CT of the chest, pelvis, and abdomen.

His history suggests two important clinical components that need to be assessed to make proper treatment recommendations:

1. Low back pain in combination with a kyphotic posture and prominent L3 spinous process suggests the presence of a lumbar fracture with deformity. In terms of decision making, the question is whether this deformity is stable. A large number of cancer patients present with burst fractures and deformity in the lumbar spine but have no significant movement-related pain and are considered stable. However, this patient does, in fact, have mechanical back pain symptoms relevant to lying flat. This may represent pressure on the kyphotic spinous process but more likely represents straightening of unstable kyphosis and, thus, mechanical pain.
2. The patient has right leg pain. If this pain is worse with axial load, the pain would be consistent with a mechanical radiculopathy. This represents a mechanical symptom caused by narrowing of the neural foramen when sitting or standing, as opposed to soft-tissue compression from tumor. Additional studies should be undertaken to ensure that the lower extremity pain is, in fact, radicular. This workup includes plain radiographs of the pelvis, hips, and lower extremities and/or bone scan, and possible right lower extremity MR. His legs should be examined for swelling and pain on palpation with consideration given to lower extremity Doppler ultrasound; 18-FDG-PET may be a useful screen for systemic disease and the presence of lower extremity pathology.

Most commonly, patients with adenocarcinoma of prostate origin present with sclerotic, osteoblastic bone metastases: Burst or compression fractures in prostate

Figure 10.1.

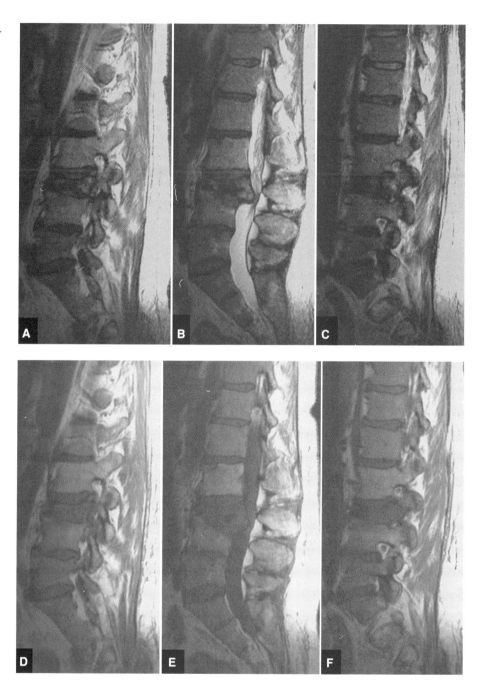

Figure 10.2.

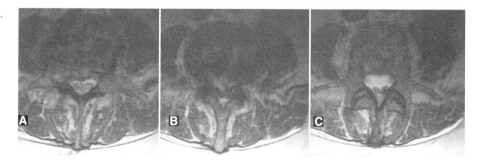

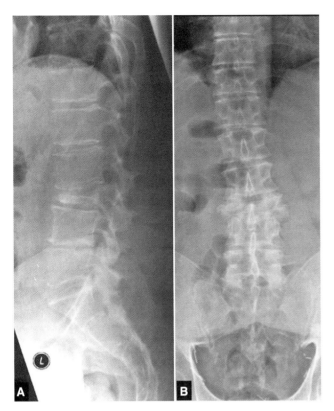

Figure 10.3.

carcinoma are most commonly osteoporotic resulting from androgen deprivation. Although certainly not definitive on plain radiographs, this patient's spinal segments adjacent to the fracture do not appear to be osteoporotic. Findings on the MR scan suggest that the fractures are from lytic tumor destruction and not osteoporosis. This determination is based on the presence of vertebral body (VB) and bilateral pedicle involvement. Epidural and neuroforaminal soft-tissue tumor extension are also suggestive of tumor. If concerned, 18-FDG-PET may be helpful in differentiating osteoporotic from tumor—fracture in this patient. In a recent study examining 18-FDG-PET in patients undergoing percutaneous needle biopsy, all patients with a lytic tumor and an standard uptake value greater than two were confirmed to have tumor on needle biopsy. While late-stage prostate carcinoma may develop fractures, a needle biopsy is warranted to confirm the diagnosis of prostatic adenocarcinoma, establish whether there has been transformation to a small cell variant, or detect the unlikely presence of a second primary.

The MR does explain the symptoms present in this patient. The L3 burst fracture is consistent with the observed deformity and back pain (Figs 10.1A–F, 10.2A–C and 10.3A,B). The films are also consistent with mechanical radiculopathy, which is most commonly seen with a burst fracture resulting in foraminal compression. This compression is best appreciated on the sagittal T1-weighted images.

DECLARATION OF SPECIFIC DIAGNOSIS

This patients has an L3 pathologic burst fracture and kyphosis with bilateral neuroforaminal involvement resulting in a right L3 mechanical radiculopathy.

BRAINSTORMING: WHAT ARE THE TREATMENT GOALS AND SURGICAL OPTIONS?

As with all spinal metastases, the goals of therapy are palliative with the intention of achieving pain and local tumor control, maintenance or improvement of neurologic function, and mechanical stability. The treatment goals follow the NOMS assessment, which includes Neurologic, Oncologic, Mechanical instability, and Systemic and medical comorbidities.[1,2] All four assessments should be considered in this patient. The principal considerations are neurologic and mechanical instability as the patient is unstable and has a kyphotic deformity resulting in axial-load-induced right L3 radiculopathy. The oncologic issue relates to the radiosensitivity of prostate carcinoma in an attempt to achieve durable tumor control. The systemic disease assessment reflects the patient's ability to withstand the proposed procedure, expected survival, and consideration of chemotherapy to treat systemic disease if present.

The treatment options fall into four general categories:

1. Radiation alone, either conventional external beam radiation therapy (cEBRT), for example, 30 Gy in 300 cGy per fraction, or stereotactic radiosurgery (SRS), for example, 24 Gy single fraction
2. Brace treatment
3. Minimally invasive procedures using percutaneous VB cement augmentation, either vertebroplasty or kyphoplasty with or without the addition of percutaneous pedicle screws
4. Open surgery in the form of posterolateral decompression/posterior or circumferential instrumentation, retroperitoneal decompression/anterior instrumentation, or combined retroperitoneal and posterolateral decompression/circumferential instrumentation

EVALUATION OF THE LITERATURE

In order to identify relevant publications on the treatment of mechanical radiculopathy in solid tumor metastases, specifically prostate carcinoma, a literature search was performed. Search strategies included the use of MESH headings and key words. These words included the following: prostate carcinoma, metastasis, solid tumor, pathologic spine fracture, vertebroplasty, kyphoplasty, percutaneous cement augmentation, radiation therapy (RT) and spine metastasis, and SRS and spine metastasis. All relevant abstracts were reviewed and pertinent articles were perused.

DETAILED REVIEW OF PERTINENT LITERATURE

The quality of literature relevant to mechanical instability and radiculopathy resulting from pathologic burst fractures is low to very low. Treatment decisions are based on literature review and expert opinion.

Radiation Therapy

Effective treatment of this patient is principally dictated by the need to palliate and resolve the mechanical radiculopathy. RT is a very effective treatment modality for achieving local tumor control of metastatic prostate carcinoma[3,4] but will not effectively treat mechanical radiculopathy. This follows the dictum that no amount of radiation will stabilize an unstable spine. Prostate carcinoma is an exception to the rule that solid tumors are radioresistant to cEBRT. A small number of retrospective studies have demonstrated the marked radiosensitivity of prostate carcinoma in terms of reduction of soft-tissue tumor and durable tumor control. Maranzano and Latini[5] reported a series of patients with high-grade epidural spinal cord compression. In that series, patients with prostate carcinoma maintained ambulation in 8/9 (89%) and recovered ambulation in 6/11 (55%) cases. Due to the favorable response in most patients using cEBRT, limited data exist regarding the use of SRS for the treatment of prostate carcinoma. However, responses to SRS are histology independent and thus should also be effective therapy for local tumor control.[6,7] Despite the marked radiosensitivity of prostate carcinoma, RT is contraindicated as initial therapy in this patient because it will not address the mechanical instability.

RT should be used as an adjunct following a stabilizing procedure to achieve local tumor control. Castrate-insensitive prostate carcinoma tends to be locally aggressive with early recurrences following resection. SRS can be safely administered in the early postoperative period[8] which may be an argument to use this modality instead of cEBRT. The beams used to deliver SRS are administered from multiple directions reducing the soft-tissue side effects and therefore wound issues compared to cEBRT. If the patient requires an open procedure, our preference would be the use of SRS as a postoperative adjuvant within 2 to 4 weeks of the surgery. If the decision is percutaneous cement augmentation, cEBRT can effectively be delivered with little morbidity.

Brace

A paucity of data exists to support brace treatment in the presence of gross spinal instability resulting from a pathologic fracture. Mechanical radiculopathy is worse in axial load, which limits the usefulness of brace application for mechanical radiculopathy. Cancer patients tend to tolerate braces poorly given multiple other medical issues and often previous procedure. If the patient cannot tolerate any surgical procedure, it may be worth a brace trial.

Minimally Invasive Procedures

Minimally invasive procedures, particularly percutaneous VB cement augmentation, often provide effective palliation for mechanical pain. Multiple series have demonstrated excellent pain palliation resulting from pathologic fractures in the metastatic population.[9–13]

Hentschel et al.,[13] reported a series of pathologic fractures treated with either vertebroplasty or kyphoplasty. Of the 53 patients treated, 17 patients presented with 18 fractures that had contraindications to cement augmentation procedures as described in previous reports.[10,14–17] These contraindications included VB collapse >75%, epidural extension of disease >20% of the spinal canal diameter, radiculopathy, or posterior VB fracture with cortical disruption. VAS scores were reduced from 8 to 2 with the only complication being transient radiculopathy and extravasation of cement anterior to the VB. Unfortunately, the L3 burst fracture under review had all of the contraindications with the addition of bilateral pedicle and neuroforaminal involvement. The risk of extravasation of PMMA into the spinal canal is extremely high in this case. In an unpublished series from Memorial Sloan-Kettering Cancer Center, mechanical radiculopathy responded poorly to VB cement augmentation and routinely required salvage with open surgery.

Percutaneous pedicle screws, as an adjunct to vertebroplasty or kyphoplasty, offer a potential solution to the treatment of mechanical radiculopathy by preventing axial load–induced compression of the neural foramen. Currently, there are no data in the literature to support percutaneous screw augmentation in this scenario.

Open Surgery

Open surgery has been used effectively to treat mechanical radiculopathy and kyphosis in cancer patients followed by RT to achieve local tumor control. Three open surgical options exist for the treatment of this patient: (1) right-sided retroperitoneal resection of L3 VB with anterior strut and plate, (2) single-stage posterolateral resection with posterior or circumferential fixation, and (3) two-stage combined anterior-posterolateral resection with circumferential fixation. All of these modalities are supported in the literature for the treatment of epidural disease, but none have specifically addressed mechanical radiculopathy. Considering the mechanism of mechanical radiculopathy, the primary focus of the operation is decompression of the right neural foramen and achieving spinal stability. The other principal consideration is that the median survival of patients with castrate insensitive prostate carcinoma with metastatic spine disease is 12 months and all patients in one series died of systemic disease at 2 years. Our preference is for a single-stage posterolateral approach.[1,18–21] This provides access to perform a unilateral or bilateral facetectomy, neuroforaminal and epidural decompression, and VB resection and reconstruction. In principle, this procedure is better tolerated than a two-staged combined approach. An anterior stand-alone approach is reasonable as well, however; metastatic cancer patients are at risk for osteoporosis and adjacent segment progression.[22–29] Cancer patients benefit often from posterior supplementation of anterior reconstruction.[30]

Hardware considerations in metastatic spine tumors must take into account the deformity, the probability of osteoporotic bone, and adjacent segment progression. Posterior segmental fixation is principally performed using pedicle screw-rod techniques as opposed to sublaminar hooks or wires.[1] Pedicle screws provide for three-column fixation and obviate the need for encroachment into the spinal canal. Typically posterior fixation should be extended two levels superior and inferior to the diseased level in order to prepare for adjacent segment progression. Although few data exist, supplemental PMMA may improve pedicle screw fixation in osteoporotic bone.[31] In this patient, posterior fixation can be extended superiorly to T12 to prevent a junctional kyphosis if that patient has extended survival, otherwise L1 may be adequate. Inferiorly, pedicle screws are placed at L4 and L5.

A large number of anterior constructs have been used in cancer reconstruction. PMMA with or without Steinman pins or chest tubes is durable in compression. PMMA is excellent for reconstruction in osteoporotic bone following veretebrectomy.[20,25,27] Additionally, this construct can effectively be terminated in the midvertebral body without regard for an intact endplate. Other anterior reconstruction techniques that can be placed anteriorly or posteriorly are allograft bone,[32] PEEK carbon fiber,[33] or titanium cages.[34] Expandable cages have often been used for anterior reconstruction in tumor patients.[35]

All of the referenced publications are based on retrospective review of patient records or prospective observation of patient outcomes without control groups. Therefore, all of the literature on this subject falls into the very low quality of evidence category. Furthermore, most of publications include an array of radiation and chemotherapeutic treatments delivered at various times in reference to the surgical decompression, which further complicates literature analysis.

EVIDENTIARY TABLE AND SELECTION OF TREATMENT METHOD

As mentioned above, the main consideration in this patient is restoration of spinal stability in order to treat his mechanical radiculopathy. While none of the surgical or biomechanical studies directly evaluate mechanical radiculopathy in the setting of metastatic disease, all of the surgical series where modern instrumentation techniques were employed report excellent pain relief outcomes. While in most publications, it may be difficult to separate outcomes of back pain and radicular pain, radicular pain must have been included in some of the series.

None of the publications report the results of a direct comparison of anterior and posterior approaches to the VB. Therefore, the decision must be based on the preference of the surgeon and the ability of the patient to undergo anterior or combined approaches. *For this reason, an evidentiary table was not formulated.* Anterior approach in the lumbar spine generally carries the risk of damage of major organs or vascular structures. Many of the patients with metastatic disease already had abdominal surgery or radiation, further complicating the operation. Therefore, our preference has been to avoid the anterior approach and to use the posterolateral approach whenever possible. In our hands, the posterolateral approach has allowed excellent ventral decompression and reconstruction in all patients with vertebral metastases. Furthermore, we generally do not attempt to perform a gross-total resection of the tumor. Our goal is adequate cord or nerve root decompression with mechanical stabilization of the spine. Once these two goals are achieved, patients can be effectively treated with radiation in order to achieve local tumor control. The quality of the data supporting treatment of prostate metastases to the spine with radiation falls in categories that range from very low to moderate.[5,36–38]

DEFINITIVE TREATMENT PLAN

Based on the presence of mechanical radiculopathy, the literature supports open surgery followed by RT. This patient should undergo an L2-4 posterolateral laminectomy, complete right L3 and superior L4 facetectomy, and posterior resection of the L3 VB, L2-3, L3-4 laminectomy. Reconstruction includes T12-L5 pedicle screw fixation and L2-4 anterior reconstruction using PMMA and Steinman pins or cage. Follow-up SRS or cEBRT should be used for local tumor control 2 to 4 weeks postoperatively.

PREDICTING OUTCOMES

Surgery followed by radiation should provide meaningful palliation in terms of local durable tumor control and relief of mechanical radiculopathy. Based on the published experience with surgical decompression and stabilization of vertebral metastases, in conjunction with postoperative RT, we expect more than 90%[1,39] probability of pain relief with 95% probability of durable local tumor control.[7] This is congruent with our experience in treating these patients. The patients must be informed of the potential complications such as wound infection or dehiscence, along with the possible requirement of postdischarge rehabilitation. Furthermore, this operation must always be placed in the context of the patient's systemic disease and further treatment.

SUMMARY

We are presented with a male patient with L3 radiculopathy related to an L3 pathologic fracture from metastatic prostate cancer. Surgery would give this patient the best possible chance at symptom relief. It is our preference to perform this through an all-posterior approach that includes posterolateral decompression, PMMA reconstruction of the resected portions of the VB, and posterior instrumentation. Good outcomes can be expected in terms of local tumor control and pain relief.

REFERENCES

1. Wang JC, Boland P, Mitra N, et al. Single-stage posterolateral transpedicular approach for resection of epidural metastatic spine tumors involving the vertebral body with circumferential reconstruction: results in 140 patients. Invited submission from the Joint Section Meeting on Disorders of the Spine and Peripheral Nerves, March 2004. *J Neurosurg.* 2004;1:287–298.

2. Bilsky M, Smith M. Surgical approach to epidural spinal cord compression. *Hematol Oncol Clin North Am.* 2006;20:1307–1317.

3. Cereceda LE, Flechon A, Droz JP. Management of vertebral metastases in prostate cancer: a retrospective analysis in 119 patients. *Clin Prostate Cancer.* 2003;2:34–40.

4. Katagiri H, Takahashi M, Inagaki J, et al. Clinical results of nonsurgical treatment for spinal metastases. *Int J Radiat Oncol Biol Phys.* 1998;42:1127–1132.

5. Maranzano E, Latini P. Effectiveness of radiation therapy without surgery in metastatic spinal cord compression: final results from a prospective trial. *Int J Radiat Oncol Biol Phys.* 1995;32:959–967.

6. Gerszten PC, Burton SA, Ozhasoglu C, et al. Radiosurgery for spinal metastases: clinical experience in 500 cases from a single institution. *Spine.* 2007;32:193–199.

7. Yamada Y, Bilsky MH, Lovelock DM, et al. High-dose, single-fraction image-guided intensity-modulated radiotherapy for metastatic spinal lesions. *Int J Radiat Oncol Biol Phys.* 2008;71:484–490.

8. Rock JP, Ryu S, Shukairy MS, et al. Postoperative radiosurgery for malignant spinal tumors. *Neurosurgery.* 2006;58:891–898; discussion 891–898.

9. Fourney DR, Schomer DF, Nader R, et al. Percutaneous vertebroplasty and kyphoplasty for painful vertebral body fractures in cancer patients. *J Neurosurg.* 2003;98: 21–30.

10. Weill A, Chiras J, Simon JM, et al. Spinal metastases: indications for and results of percutaneous injection of acrylic surgical cement. *Radiology.* 1996;199:241–247.

11. Cotten A, Dewatre F, Cortet B, et al. Percutaneous vertebroplasty for osteolytic metastases and myeloma: effects of the percentage of lesion filling and the leakage of methyl methacrylate at clinical follow-up. *Radiology.* 1996;200:525–530.

12. Tseng YY, Yang ST, Tu PH, et al. Minimally invasive vertebroplasty in the treatment of pain induced by spinal metastatic tumor. *Minim Invasive Neurosurg.* 2008;51: 280–284.

13. Hentschel SJ, Burton AW, Fourney DR, et al. Percutaneous vertebroplasty and kyphoplasty performed at a cancer center: refuting proposed contraindications. *J Neurosurg Spine.* 2005;2:436–440.

14. Amar AP, Larsen DW, Esnaashari N, et al. Percutaneous transpedicular polymethylmethacrylate vertebroplasty for the treatment of spinal compression fractures. *Neurosurgery.* 2001;49:1105–1114; discussion 1114–1105.

15. Barr JD, Barr MS, Lemley TJ, et al. Percutaneous vertebroplasty for pain relief and spinal stabilization. *Spine.* 2000;25:923–928.

16. Cotten A, Boutry N, Cortet B, et al. Percutaneous vertebroplasty: state of the art. *Radiographics.* 1998;18:311–320; discussion 320–313.

17. Peters KR, Guiot BH, Martin PA, et al. Vertebroplasty for osteoporotic compression fractures: current practice and evolving techniques. *Neurosurgery.* 2002;51:S96–S103.

18. Street J, Fisher C, Sparkes J, et al. Single-stage posterolateral vertebrectomy for the management of metastatic disease of the thoracic and lumbar spine: a prospective study of an evolving surgical technique. *J Spinal Disorder Tech.* 2007;20:509–520.

19. Bilsky MH, Boland P, Lis E, et al. Single-stage posterolateral transpedicle approach for spondylectomy, epidural decompression, and circumferential fusion of spinal metastases. *Spine.* 2000;25:2240–2249, discussion 2250.

20. Klekamp J, Samii H. Surgical results for spinal metastases. *Acta Neurochirurgica.* 1998;140:957–967.

21. Jansson KA, Bauer HC. Survival, complications and outcome in 282 patients operated for neurological deficit due to thoracic or lumbar spinal metastases. *Eur Spine J.* 2006;15:196–202.

22. Ernstberger T, Bruning T, Konig F. Vertebrectomy and anterior reconstruction for the treatment of spinal metastases. *Acta Orthop Belg.* 2005;71:459–466.

23. Gokaslan ZL, York JE, Walsh GL, et al. Transthoracic vertebrectomy for metastatic spinal tumors. *J Neurosurg.* 1998;89:599–609.

24. Seifert V, van Krieken FM, Bao SD, et al. Microsurgery of the cervical spine in elderly patients. Part 2: Surgery of malignant tumourous disease. *Acta Neurochirurgica.* 1994;131:241–246.

25. Harrington KD. Anterior cord decompression and spinal stabilization for patients with metastatic lesions of the spine. *J Neurosurg.* 1984;61:107–117.

26. Siegal T. Surgical decompression of anterior and posterior malignant epidural tumors compressing the spinal cord: a prospective study. *Neurosurgery.* 1985;17:424–432.

27. Sundaresan N, Galicich JH, Lane JM, et al. Treatment of neoplastic epidural cord compression by vertebral body resection and stabilization. *J Neurosurg.* 1985;63:676–684.

28. Onimus M, Schraub S, Bertin D, et al. Surgical treatment of vertebral metastasis. *Spine.* 1986;11:883–891.

29. Atanasiu JP, Badatcheff F, Pidhorz L. Metastatic lesions of the cervical spine. A retrospective analysis of 20 cases. *Spine.* 1993;18:1279–1284.

30. Manabe S, Tateishi A, Abe M, et al. Surgical treatment of metastatic tumors of the spine. *Spine.* 1989;14:41–47.

31. Frankel BM, Jones T, Wang C. Segmental polymethylmethacrylate-augmented pedicle screw fixation in patients with bone softening caused by osteoporosis and metastatic tumor involvement: a clinical evaluation. *Neurosurgery.* 2007;61:531–537; discussion 537–538.

32. Lewandrowski KU, Hecht AC, DeLaney TF, et al. Anterior spinal arthrodesis with structural cortical allografts and instrumentation for spine tumor surgery. *Spine.* 2004;29:1150–1158; discussion 1159.

33. Schulte M, Schultheiss M, Hartwig E, et al. Vertebral body replacement with a bioglass-polyurethane composite in spine metastases—clinical, radiological and biomechanical results. *Eur Spine J.* 2000;9:437–444.

34. Akamaru T, Kawahara N, Tsuchiya H, et al. Healing of autologous bone in a titanium mesh cage used in anterior column reconstruction after total spondylectomy. *Spine.* 2002;27:E329–E333.

35. Crocker M, James G, Ibrahim A, et al. Posterior approach vertebrectomy in the thoracolumbar spine with expandable cage reconstruction: indications and techniques based on eight cases. *Br J Neurosurg.* 2008;22:235–240.

36. Zelefsky MJ, Scher HI, Krol G, et al. Spinal epidural tumor in patients with prostate cancer. Clinical and radiographic predictors of response to radiation therapy. *Cancer.* 1992;70:2319–2325.

37. Greenberg HS, Kim JH, Posner JB. Epidural spinal cord compression from metastatic tumor: results with a new treatment protocol. *Ann Neurol.* 1980;8:361–366.

38. Turner S, Marosszeky B, Timms I, et al. Malignant spinal cord compression: a prospective evaluation. *Int J Radiat Oncol Biol Phys.* 1993;26:141–146.

39. Sundaresan N, Rothman A, Manhart K, et al. Surgery for solitary metastases of the spine: rationale and results of treatment. *Spine.* 2002;27:1802–1806.

Thoracic Epidural Tumor

JOHN CHI, MD, MPH AND NING LIN, MD

EDITORS' CASE PRESENTATION

A 62-year-old man with a history of non-Hodgkin lymphoma was referred to the emergency department by his oncologist for a 1-week history of progressive band-like back pain radiating to his chest and increasing difficulty with ambulation. Currently, he is unable to stand without assistance. He has no bowel or bladder complaints and has no history of any other substantial medical comorbidities. He has recently finished a course of chemotherapy.

Physical examination reveals a normal appearing male and no cachexic. He has lower extremity hyperreflexia (3+) and five beats of clonus on the right side. Sensation is grossly intact. Strength testing shows 2/5 hip flexion, 2/5 knee extension, 4/5 plantar and dorsiflexion, with the right side being slightly stronger than the left. He has intact rectal tone and perianal sensation. Laboratories are relatively normal with no signs of coagulopathy.

Radiographic imaging studies are shown in Figures 11.1 to 11.3.

INTERPRETATION OF CLINICAL PRESENTATION

This case describes an upper middle-aged man with known oncological history who presents with radiating back and chest pain and difficulty ambulating. The onset of symptoms is fairly rapid and has occurred in the absence of any injury or trauma, and there is significant motor dysfunction, thus indicating that this is an urgent problem. Physical examination reveals myelopathy as evidenced by hyperreflexia and clonus in the lower extremities, localizing the problem to the thoracic spine with involvement of the spinal cord above the conus medullaris. Further localization can be

specified based on the dermatomal level of radiating back and chest pain. Given the history of non-Hodgkin lymphoma, the time course of symptoms, and the absence of trauma, secondary malignancy with epidural spread and possible pathologic fracture in the thoracic spine should be strongly considered. Other differential diagnoses include herniated thoracic disc, spinal cord tumor, spinal infection/abscess, spinal hemorrhage, primary malignancy of the spine, spinal fracture, and spinal inflammatory processes.

The spinal column is one of the most frequent sites of secondary disease in metastatic cancer.[1,2] The percentage of patients with symptomatic spinal metastases is estimated to be 5% to 10% of all cancer patients[3,4] and, in certain autopsy series, up to 90% of cancer patients had vertebral lesions.[5,6] The vast majority of spinal metastases are extradural involving the bony elements and epidural space, with intradural or intramedullary spinal cord metastases occurring infrequently. Pain is the most common symptom in spinal metastases occurring in up to 90% of patients, which can be axial, mechanical, and/or radicular in nature. Axial and mechanical pain suggest bony destruction and pathologic fracture, while radicular pain suggests epidural compression and nerve root impingement. This patient presents with back pain and radicular pain, which is consistent with an epidural tumor that involves the bony spine and is causing compression on thoracic nerve roots.

Neurologic symptoms are the second most common symptom in spinal metastases occurring in about 70% to 80% of patients and can include weakness, loss of sensation, and/or bowel/bladder dysfunction. Neurologic symptoms indicate compression of the spinal cord from epidural tumor mass and/or bony compression secondary to a pathologic fracture or deformity. Motor deficit frequently lags behind the onset of back pain by days to weeks for patients with epidural spinal compression, and up to two thirds of patients are nonambulatory when diagnosed.[5,7,8] Later manifestations of epidural spinal compression include sensory deficits, such as a spinal sensory level or Lhermitte sign, and sphincter dysfunction.

Figure 11.1.

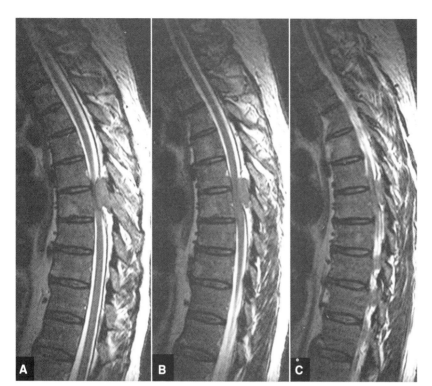

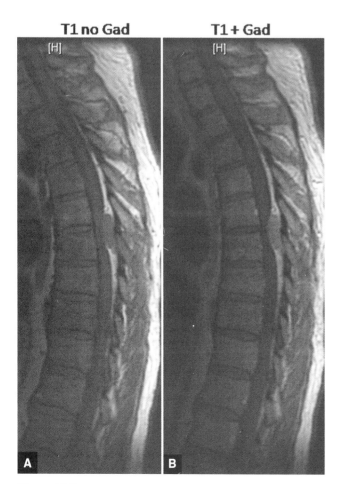

Figure 11.2.

This patient's motor symptoms include bilateral leg weakness, hyperreflexia, and clonus in the right leg, which all indicate significant spinal cord compression. There is proximal greater than distal leg weakness and suggestion of right greater than left weakness as well, which would indicate a lateralized compression. Multiple studies suggest that pretreatment neurological status is a reliable predictor of posttreatment functional outcome. Thus, prompt recognition and diagnosis of spinal metastases causing significant epidural compression, as in this case, are of vital importance to the prognosis of these patients.

MRI is the most sensitive diagnostic test for metastases to the spine, and gadolinium should be administered whenever cancer is suspected or a compressive mass lesion detected. The axial and sagittal MRI images of the thoracic spine are available for review. Imaging reveals a posterolateral compressive epidural mass with involvement of the left lateral bony elements (lamina, spinous process, pedicle, and transverse process) (Fig. 11.3A–H). The mass occupies more than 50% of the spinal canal and enhances after gadolinium administration (Fig. 11.2A and B). There is T2 signal change within the cord (Figs. 11.1A–C and 11.3A), indicating significant and rapid compression and swelling. Precise localization can be performed by counting from C2 or L5 levels if available on sagittal views, or based on the thoracolumbar junction as visualized by the last level of fully formed floating ribs. This lesion appears to be at the apex of normal thoracic kyphosis (generally T6-7). There is no indication of a pathologic fracture given the preserved

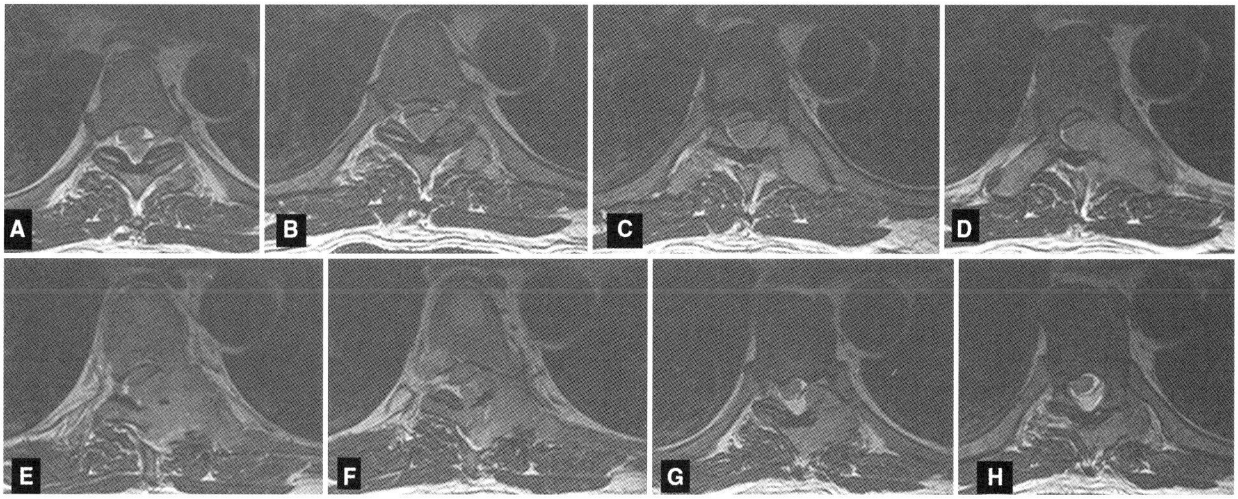

Figure 11.3.

height and shape of the vertebral bodies and lack of contrast enhancement in the bodies. Nevertheless, there is extensive involvement of the posterolateral bony elements, which correlates with the patients back pain and suggests impending or pathologic instability. Further imaging could include CT, to aid in treatment planning and to evaluate bone integrity and assessment of stability, but is not considered mandatory.

As with any patient with an oncologic history and likely metastatic disease, cancer staging is important for global understanding of disease burden. Given the urgency of this patient's presentation, staging with a PET CT or other modalities can be deferred if urgent treatment is required. Additionally, as with any patient who had received prior chemotherapy or radiation therapy, blood lab values should be carefully reviewed to assess coagulopathy, thrombocytopenia, anemia, and leukopenia, which could affect treatment options.

DECLARATION OF SPECIFIC DIAGNOSIS

This patient has a thoracic epidural spinal mass causing spinal cord compression with bony involvement likely from secondary non-Hodgkin lymphoma.

BRAINSTORMING: WHAT ARE THE TREATMENT GOALS AND SURGICAL OPTIONS?

The treatment goals are

1. Direct decompression of the spinal cord via resection of the mass lesion
2. Preservation of neural elements
3. Maintaining spinal alignment and ensuring continued stability

4. Obtain tissue for histopathologic diagnosis
5. Rehabilitation and healing

The treatment options are

1. Percutaneous tissue biopsy for diagnosis confirmation
2. High-dose steroids
3. Adjuvant chemotherapy/radiation therapy alone
4. Surgical decompression alone, with follow-up adjuvant therapy
5. Surgical decompression with stabilization and follow-up adjuvant therapy

EVALUATION OF THE LITERATURE

A thorough literature search was performed on PubMed with "spinal epidural metastasis" included in the subject/abstract sections. A total of 226 articles were retrieved and when qualified with "surgery" or "surgical management," 103 articles were found. Earlier publications tended to be focused on different radiation dosages, fractionation, and other outcome studies after radiotherapy. The role of surgery has been better defined recently for the treatment of spinal epidural metastases. Emphasis was placed on the quality of the studies, with prospective, randomized, controlled trials having more weight than other designs.

DETAILED REVIEW OF PERTINENT ARTICLES

Surgery with Radiation Versus Radiation Alone

Radiotherapy traditionally has been used to prevent further tumor growth, ameliorate pain, and maintain ambulation for patients with epidural metastases.

Prognostic factors for radiotherapy include pretreatment neurological status, type of tumor, radiation sensitivity of tissue type, and extent of subarachnoid block seen on MRI.[5] A number of series demonstrate that 80% to 100% of patients who are ambulatory when treatment begins will maintain ambulation, and about one third of those who are not mobile will regain mobility.[5,7,9] Radiotherapy is noninvasive and is preferred in patients with overall poor performance and limited life expectancy. Complications are generally low but do include bone marrow suppression, spinal cord necrosis, and skin irritation.

Harrington[10,11] created a staging system for patients with epidural metastasis based mainly on neurologic deficits and instability. Nonsurgical management was recommended for stage 1 (no significant neurological involvement) to stage 3 (neurological involvement without bony invasion) disease, which he considered to be milder. The patient in this case presented with an epidural mass invading through the posterior column of the thoracic spine and causing cord compression and significant neurological deficit. The patient is nonambulatory at the time of presentation. According to the above classification, the patient is categorized stage 5, for which radiation therapy alone may not be enough to achieve adequate disease control.

The role of surgery was traditionally limited in the treatment of spinal epidural metastases. Earlier studies compared simple laminectomies, laminectomies plus radiation, and radiation alone and failed to show any benefits for patients who underwent laminectomies.[12,13] Recent advancements in surgical techniques introduced direct circumferential decompression of the spinal cord and multilevel spinal fusion to achieve immediate mechanical stability. A number of surgical series[3,14–16] and a recent multicenter, prospective, randomized trial[17] indicate that radical surgical decompression followed by radiotherapy is superior compared with radiation alone. Subgroup analysis of the same study indicates that age is an important factor to determine postoperative benefits for patients with epidural cord compression. There was no difference in outcome between treatments for patients >65 years of age.[18]

EVIDENTIARY TABLE AND SELECTION OF TREATMENT METHOD

Based on the current literature, the patient should undergo surgical decompression followed by radiation therapy (Table 11.1). One caveat for this recommendation comes from the type of tumor involved in this case. Lymphoma is highly radiosensitive and patients with lymphomas (as well as those with leukemia, multiple myeloma, and germ-cell tumors) were excluded from the multicenter randomized study discussed above.[17] Therefore, there is no direct evidence to support the recommendation of surgery. However, inference from multiple studies and severity of this patient's neurological symptoms suggest that direct surgical decompression offers the best chance to regain ambulatory ability and achieve long-term durable results. For a patient with rapid symptom development, surgery offers the most immediate method of decompression. Radiation treatment can take days to weeks to be effective.

Nevertheless, confirmation of histologic pathology with radiation therapy and chemotherapy is a viable option for a patient with non-Hodgkin lymphoma and should be discussed.[19–23] In patients with significant comorbidities and/or frail overall conditions, surgery may not be the best option. Additionally, in patients with less acute and less dramatic presenting symptoms with a very radiosensitive tumor-like lymphoma, radiation alone can be an excellent treatment option.

High-dose steroids have a role in any patient with spinal cord compression secondary to tumor and neurologic symptoms, especially weakness. Decadron (10–100 mg) has been used and should be started as soon as possible after presentation.[24] In the event that there is no previous oncologic history, steroid use can interfere with pathologic diagnosis; therefore, the decision to use them should be tailored to the clinical urgency of the situation.

Anterior Versus Posterior Surgical Approaches

Anterior and anterolateral spinal decompression have been described in several surgical series for spinal metastases that involve mainly the vertebral body.[3,14,16,25] These approaches spare the posterior elements of the spinal cord, which are often intact and thus afford better stability. The patient in this case, however, has cancer metastasized to the spinous process, lamina, pedicle, invading epidural space and paraspinal soft tissues. The majority of the disease is located posteriorly and posterolaterally. Therefore, a posterior approach will offer better exposure for the surgical resection of the metastatic tumor.

Direct Posterior Versus Posterolateral Transpedicular Decompression

For this patient, direct laminectomy can provide access for adequate decompression of the posterior compression. To address the posterolateral involvement, additional exposure is needed to access tumor in the pars, pedicle, neuroforamen, and lateral epidural space. Transpedicular approaches, including costotransversectomy and lateral extracavitary exposure, are especially well suited to provide excellent visualization of the neural elements and working room for

TABLE 11.1	Evidentiary Table: A Summary of the Quality of Evidence for Direct Surgical Resection with Instrumented Fusion Followed by Radiation to Treat Spinal Epidural Metastases.		
Paper Author (Year)	**Description**	**Summary of Results**	**Quality of Evidence**
Patchell et al. (2005)	Multicenter, randomized, prospective trial comparing surgery followed by radiation and radiation alone.	A total of 50 patients were randomized to surgery and radiotherapy and 51 to radiotherapy alone. Overall, 84% of patients were ambulatory after surgery and 57% after radiotherapy. Patients treated with surgery retained the ability to walk for a median of 122 d, whereas those treated with radiotherapy alone, 13 d. Of 32 patients who entered the study nonambulatory, 62% regained ambulation after surgery and 19% after radiation. The study was stopped after an interim analysis.	High
Klimo et al. (2005)	Meta-analysis of 24 surgical series and 4 radiation series, mostly uncontrolled cohort studies. Ambulatory ability and rescue rates were primary outcome measures.	A total of 999 surgical patients and 543 radiation patients were included. Surgical patients were 1.3 times more likely to be ambulatory after treatment and twice as likely to regain ambulatory function. Overall ambulatory rate is 85% after surgery and 64% after radiation. Primary pathology was the principal factor determining survival.	Medium
North (2005)[30]	Retrospective case series	Of 61 patients included in the study, 52 (85%) were ambulatory preoperatively and 59 (97%) postoperatively. 81% of those who survived 6 mo remained ambulatory, and 66% of those alive at 1.6 y. The median postoperative survival was 10 mo.	Low

decompression. For ventral epidural spread, sacrifice of the exiting nerve root is necessary and usually of little consequence if carefully performed. CSF leak is rare but could lead to pseudomeningocele formation.

Considerations on Instrumentation and Arthrodesis

Patients with metastatic disease of the spine usually require stabilization after posterior decompressive surgery because of interruption of the posterior elements and likely wide spread bony involvement of cancer.[26,27] Vertebrectomy and transpedicular approaches would require instrumented reconstruction. For posterolateral approaches, at least two levels above and below the level of decompression are included in the reconstruction. In cases where laminectomy alone is adequate, instrumented arthrodesis is not required unless the decompression is at the apex of the thoracic kyphosis (T6-7) or thoracolumbar junction (T11-L1). Wound complications have been shown to be higher for surgery performed after external radiation; therefore, if surgery and radiation are recommended, surgery

should be performed first with at least 2 to 4 weeks allowed for wound healing prior to radiation doses.[28]

DEFINITIVE TREATMENT PLAN

The patient in this clinical scenario should be managed with operative decompression and stabilization primarily because of the significant neurologic dysfunction observed over a short period of time. Intravenous steroids should be administered if there is a delay in surgery. Decompression should be achieved via a posterior approach with posterolateral exposure for maximal decompression. Complete laminectomy (bilateral) with left-sided removal of the pars, transverse process, and pedicle would allow for a transpedicular decompression of the lateral spinal canal. Stabilization would include pedicle screw at two to three levels above and below the decompressed level, given that the spine is partially destabilized by involvement of the left-sided pedicle and facet complex and that the lesion is at the apex of the thoracic kyphosis. Tissue should be sent for permanent pathologic examination. Adjuvant chemotherapy and radiation therapy should also follow surgery once appropriate wound healing has occurred.

Grading the Evidence for this Plan

The evidence to support the technical aspects of our treatment selection would be considered medium to high. There is one class I study supporting the role of surgery in malignant epidural spinal cord compression from secondary solid tumors. Similar class I evidence does not exist specifically for hematologic tumors but can be inferred from existing evidence. If surgery is performed in the way recommended, then instrumentation is strongly advised, though there is little class I or class II evidence for this. Radiotherapy is also an option for treatment in this patient and has medium class II level evidence in the literature.[19,20,22]

PREDICTING OUTCOMES

The outcome for this patient can be assessed in severaldifferent ways. Ambulation status is a good dichotomous outcome measure that is easy to assess. Ambulation can be graded as nonambulatory, ambulatory with assist (cane or walker), or independently ambulatory. Based on class I data for solid tumor metastases to the spine, the chance of remaining ambulatory or regaining ambulation is higher after surgery than radiation alone.[17] One caveat is that patient age does interact with this benefit; thus, older patients may not enjoy as much of a benefit from surgery compared to radiation.[18]

Quality of life is another outcome that can be measured by surveys such as SF-36. Though there are no large studies indicating the benefit of quality of life after surgery or radiation, there is a general consensus that if pain and/or neurologic function is improved or maintained after treatment, quality of life is also improved. The main confounder of quality of life measures in cancer is that medical treatments and the natural course of the disease can have major alterations on quality of life, independent of those attributable to surgical treatment. Improvement of pain is another outcome to be measured, and in several retrospective studies, there seems to be substantial improvement in pain after surgery in which unstable lesions are stabilized. It is important to note that for pathologic fractures without epidural compression, minimally invasive vertebroplasty/kyphoplasty can be effective.[29] Surgical outcomes are generally good in appropriately selected patients. Patients with >6 months life expectancy, well-controlled systemic disease, and good functional status can expect to have low rates of complications. Complications from surgery for spinal cancer do include

nerve injury, CSF fistula, pneumothorax, chylothorax, instrumentation failure, surgical hematoma, and surgical site infection. Combined rates of complications range from 5% to 25%.[28]

SUMMARY

We are presented with a 62-year-old man with a history of non-Hodgkin lymphoma with pain and neurologic dysfunction from epidural compression of the spinal cord. The most appropriate treatment, considering the timing of symptoms and severity of dysfunction, would be a surgical decompression and stabilization at the affected level. Preservation of ambulation, improvement in quality of life, and relief of pain can all be expected with a fairly low surgical complication rate.

REFERENCES

1. Aaron AD. The management of cancer metastatic to bone. *JAMA*. 1994;272:1206–1209.
2. Ryken TC, Eichholz KM, Gerszten PC, et al. Evidence-based review of the surgical management of vertebral column metastatic disease. *Neurosurg Focus*. 2003;15:E11.
3. Sundaresan N, Galicich JH, Bains MS, et al. Vertebral body resection in the treatment of cancer involving the spine. *Cancer*. 1984;53:1393–1396.
4. Winn HR, ed. *Youmans Neurological Surgery*. Vol 4, 5th ed. WB Saunders Company, Philadelphia, 2004.
5. Prasad D, Schiff D. Malignant spinal-cord compression. *Lancet Oncol*. 2005;6:15–24.
6. Wong DA, Fornasier VL, MacNab I. Spinal metastases: the obvious, the occult, and the impostors. *Spine*. 1990;15:1–4.
7. Bach F, Larsen BH, Rohde K, et al. Metastatic spinal cord compression. Occurrence, symptoms, clinical presentations and prognosis in 398 patients with spinal cord compression. *Acta Neurochir (Wien)*. 1990;107:37–43.
8. Husband DJ. Malignant spinal cord compression: prospective study of delays in referral and treatment. *BMJ*. 1998;317:18–21.
9. Martenson JA Jr, Evans RG, Lie MR, et al. Treatment outcome and complications in patients treated for malignant epidural spinal cord compression (SCC). *J Neurooncol*. 1985;3:77–84.
10. Harrington KD. Metastatic disease of the spine. *J Bone Joint Surg Am*. 1986;68:1110–1115.
11. Harrington KD. Orthopedic surgical management of skeletal complications of malignancy. *Cancer* 1997;80:1614–1627.
12. Sorensen S, Borgesen SE, Rohde K, et al. Metastatic epidural spinal cord compression. Results of treatment and survival. *Cancer*. 1990;65:1502–1508.
13. Young RF, Post EM, King GA. Treatment of spinal epidural metastases. Randomized prospective comparison of laminectomy and radiotherapy. *J Neurosurg*. 1980;53:741–748.

14. Harrington KD. Anterior cord decompression and spinal stabilization for patients with metastatic lesions of the spine. *J Neurosurg*. 1984;61:107–117.

15. Klimo P Jr. Thompson CJ, Kestle JR, et al. A meta-analysis of surgery versus conventional radiotherapy for the treatment of metastatic spinal epidural disease. *Neuro Oncol*. 2005;7:64–76.

16. Overby MC, Rothman AS. Anterolateral decompression for metastatic epidural spinal cord tumors. Results of a modified costotransversectomy approach. *J Neurosurg*. 1985;62:344–348.

17. Patchell RA, Tibbs PA, Regine WF, et al. Direct decompressive surgical resection in the treatment of spinal cord compression caused by metastatic cancer: a randomised trial. *Lancet*. 2005;366:643–648.

18. Chi JH, Gokaslan ZL, McCormick P, et al. Selecting treatment for patients with malignant epidural spine cord compression—does age matter? Results from a randomized clinical trial. *Spine*. 2008;34:431–435.

19. Maranzano E, Bellavita R, Rossi R, et al. Short-course versus split-course radiotherapy in metastatic spinal cord compression: results of a phase III, randomized, multicenter trial. *J Clin Oncol* 2005;23:3358–3365.

20. Maranzano E, Latini P. Effectiveness of radiation therapy without surgery in metastatic spinal cord compression: final results from a prospective trial. *Int J Radiat Oncol Biol Phys*. 1995;32:959–967.

21. Maranzano E, Latini P, Beneventi S, et al. Comparison of two different radiotherapy schedules for spinal cord compression in prostate cancer. *Tumori*. 1998;84:472–477.

22. Maranzano E, Latini P, Perrucci E, et al. Short-course radiotherapy (8 Gy × 2) in metastatic spinal cord compression: an effective and feasible treatment. *Int J Radiat Oncol Biol Phys*. 1997;38:1037–1044.

23. Maranzano E, Trippa F, Chirico L, et al. Management of metastatic spinal cord compression. *Tumori*. 2003;89:469–475.

24. Loblaw DA, Laperriere NJ. Emergency treatment of malignant extradural spinal cord compression: an evidence-based guideline. *J Clin Oncol*. 1998;16:1613–1624.

25. Tomita K, Kawahara N, Kobayashi T, et al. Surgical strategy for spinal metastases. *Spine*. 2001;26:298–306.

26. Heary RF, Bono CM. Metastatic spinal tumors. *Neurosurg Focus*. 2001;11:e1.

27. Rompe JD, Eysel P, Hopf C, et al. Decompression/stabilization of the metastatic spine. Cotrel-Dubousset-Instrumentation in 50 patients. *Acta Orthop Scand*. 1993;64:3–8.

28. Bilsky MH, Fraser JF. Complication avoidance in vertebral column spine tumors. *Neurosurg Clin N Am*. 2006;17:317–329.

29. Chi JH, Gokaslan ZL. Vertebroplasty and kyphoplasty for spinal metastases. *Curr Opin Support Palliat Care*. 2008;2:9–13.

30. North RB, LaRocca VR, Schwartz J, et al. Surgical management of spinal metastases: analysis of prognostic factors during a 10-year experience. *J Neurosurg Spine*. 2005;2:564–573.

12 L1 Fracture with Paraplegia

TODD D. MCCALL, MD, DANIEL R. FASSETT, MO, MBA, HARSH PARIKH, BA, AND ALEXANDER VACCARO, MD

■ EDITORS' CASE PRESENTATION

A 41-year-old man was ejected from the front windshield of his car after a motor vehicle collision. He presented to the trauma department intubated and unconscious. At the scene, he was reported to be moving his arms but not his legs. The patient's non–spine injuries include bilateral pulmonary contusions and a closed head injury. He is now hemodynamically stable five hours after the injury.

Physical examination is limited because the patient is not awake and is not moving spontaneously. He has no rectal tone and has an absent bulbocavernosus reflex. He has no appreciable reflexes in his lower extremities. In addition to his thoracolumbar injury, he has nondisplaced lamina fractures of C5 and C6 but no evidence of ligamentous injury, translation, kyphosis, or misalignment.

Radiographic imaging studies are shown in Figures 12.1 and 12.2.

INTERPRETATION OF THE CLINICAL PRESENTATION

This case involves a middle-aged man with a high-energy mechanism of injury. Individuals ejected from a motor vehicle have, on average, a higher ISS (Injury Severity Score), length of hospital stay, and mortality rate compared with those not ejected.[1] Strict adherence to ATLS (Advanced Trauma Life Support) protocols is critical to maximize the patient's chance of survival.[2] This patient has two injuries (brain and pulmonary) that are potentially life threatening and therefore take precedence over a spine or spinal cord injury. First, pulmonary contusions can contribute

to increased mortality by leading to acute respiratory distress syndrome, pneumonia, or sepsis.[3,4] In this case, the patient's respiratory status has presumably been stabilized with intubation and mechanical ventilation. Second, the closed head injury may represent a serious threat to the patient. The description of the patient's neurological status suggests a GCS (Glasgow Coma Score) of 8 or less, which in the context of the mechanism of injury is very worrisome for a traumatic brain injury. Prior to any thoughts of surgical intervention for a spine injury, the patient's neurological exam must improve or intracranial pressures must be measured and determined to be stable in a tolerable range.

The description of the patient's neurological examination is suggestive of a severe spinal cord injury. The bulbocavernosus reflex is a spinal cord reflex arc mediated by sacral nerve roots 1 to 3 in which the anal sphincter contracts after a controlled pull on the glans penis or Foley catheter. This reflex can be lost because of spinal shock or direct injury to the conus medullaris. The loss of lower extremity reflexes suggests a lower motor neuron injury, which can also occur at the conus medullaris where the central nervous system transitions to the peripheral nervous system. Thus, the examination is most consistent with an injury at the level of the conus medullaris, which would imply a spine injury in an adult between T12 and L2.[5] A spinal cord injury at a higher level would be expected to cause brisk or pathological reflexes. The spinal cord injury should not be at the level of the cervical spine because the function of the upper extremities appears to be intact.

The Frankel or American Spinal Injury Association (ASIA) grading system is the most commonly used classification of spinal cord injuries. Based on the information provided, the patient most likely has a Frankel grade A spinal cord injury, although a grade B injury cannot be excluded. A Frankel grade A injury is defined by a complete loss of motor and sensory functions, while a grade B injury has a complete loss of

Figure 12.1.

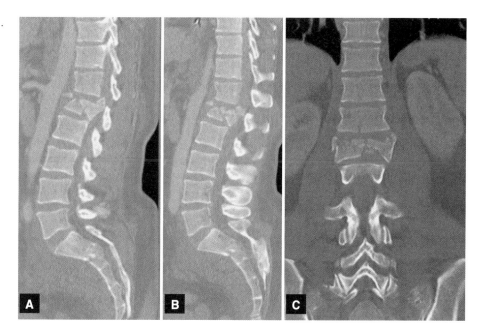

motor function but not sensory function. Since we do not explicitly know the status of the patient's sensory function, a grade B injury cannot be excluded, although a complete spinal cord injury is assumed because there is no documented neurological function in the lower extremities.

The computed tomography scans include axial images of T12 and L1, as well as sagittal views of the thoracolumbar spine. The axial images of T12 (Fig. 12.2A and B) demonstrate a sagittal split fracture that involves the vertebral body and right lamina. The axial images of L1 (Fig. 12.2C and D) show a burst fracture with 100% canal compromise, which correlates well with a complete neurological injury of the conus medullaris. There is also a fracture of the right lamina. There is no appreciable widening of the T12/L1 facet joints. The sagittal views (Fig. 12.1A and B) clearly demonstrate an L1 burst fracture. There is 22 degrees of kyphosis from the superior endplate of T12 to the inferior endplate of L2, with 40% loss of L1 vertebral body height. Furthermore, there appears to be a mild

increase in the distance of the posterior elements from T12 to L1 on Figure 12.1A.

DECLARATION OF SPECIFIC DIAGNOSIS

This patient has an L1 axial burst fracture (Magerl A3.3.3 injury) and T12 sagittal split fracture (Magerl A2.1 injury) with associated complete conus medullaris spinal cord injury.[6]

BRAINSTORMING: WHAT ARE THE TREATMENT GOALS AND THE SURGICAL OUTCOMES?

The treatment goals are

1. Primum non nocere (first, do no harm)
2. Stabilization of the spine

T11   **T12**

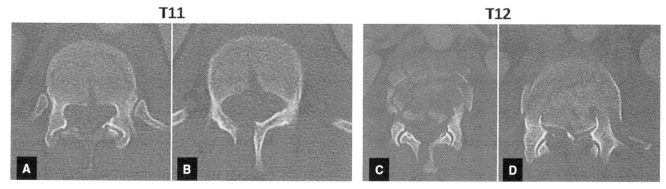

Figure 12.2.

3. Maximize functional recovery
4. Decompression of neural elements
5. Restoration and long-term maintenance of radiographic measures

The treatment options are

1. Bracing or casting
2. Posterior fixation with pedicle screws (short or long segment construct)
3. Anterolateral corpectomy, strut graft, and instrumentation
4. Combined anterior and posterior approach, using a short segment construct

EVALUATION OF THE LITERATURE

To identify relevant publications on burst fractures of the thoracolumbar spine, a PubMed search was performed with the phrases "thoracolumbar" and "burst fracture," which produced a total of 322 citations in the English language. All abstracts were reviewed and articles were excluded if they included fewer than 10 patients or specifically pertained to patients who were osteoporotic or adolescent, had no neurological deficits, had lower lumbar burst fractures, or were treated with antiquated instrumentation constructs. The remaining 81 articles were carefully reviewed, and any additional references that were identified in the articles were also reviewed.

DETAILED REVIEW OF PERTINENT ARTICLES AND EVIDENTIARY TABLE

This patient has two specific issues that must be addressed: the L1 burst fracture and the complete spinal cord injury. The burst fracture itself is a controversial topic with regard to the optimal treatment. However, the spinal cord injury raises additional controversies including the timing of surgery and role of decompressing the central spinal canal. This review of pertinent articles first focuses on the topics of operative or nonoperative treatment, the timing of surgery, and decompression of the central canal. The evidentiary table and accompanying discussion focus on the selection of a surgical plan. It should be noted that other important but contentious issues, such as the medical management of spinal cord injuries with blood pressure maintenance and corticosteroid therapy, are excluded because they are beyond the scope of this chapter.

A complete spinal cord injury is a significant clinical consideration. Acutely, a patient unable to walk has a higher risk of hospital complications such as pneumonia and deep venous thrombosis.[7] Over a longer term, functional outcomes are hindered and other complications, such as Charcot spine, can arise.[8] Thus, an optimal study in the context of this case would specifically only include patients with thoracolumbar burst fractures and complete spinal cord injuries. There were no articles that specifically met these criteria. Some studies only included burst fractures without neurological deficits, which are not included in this discussion. The remaining articles have a mixed patient population of neurologically intact, incomplete spinal cord injuries, and complete spinal cord injuries. Patients with complete spinal cord injuries are generally a small minority.

Operative or Nonoperative Treatment

Several studies have either retrospectively or prospectively directly compared operative and nonoperative treatments for the management of thoracolumbar burst fractures.[9–13] Several of these studies specifically excluded patients with neurological deficits[10,12,13] and are therefore not applicable to this case. Two studies comparing operative and nonoperative treatment of thoracolumbar burst fractures included patients with neurological deficits[9,11]; however, neither study was randomized, and patients with severe neurological injuries (Frankel grade A or B) were treated only operatively. Thus, we could not identify any contemporary studies comparing operative and nonoperative treatment in a patient population similar to this case. In their prospective comparison of operative and nonoperative treatments, Hitchon et al.[11] concluded that patients should undergo surgery if they have neurological deficits, >20 degrees of angular deformity, >50% canal compromise, or >50% loss of anterior vertebral body height. Other authors have made similar recommendations.[9,14,15] There appears to be a general consensus that the degree of angular kyphosis, percent canal compromise, and presence of significant canal compromise in this case are all reasonable indications for surgical intervention in the absence of strong evidence to guide treatment.

In recent years, the Spine Trauma Study Group has developed the Thoraco-Lumbar Injury Classification and Severity (TLICS) scale to guide both the classification and the treatment of thoracolumbar injuries.[16] The TLICS scale is based on three distinct variables of the injury: (1) injury morphology, (2) integrity of the posterior ligamentous complex, and (3) neurological status. The grading system is not complicated, which contributes to good interobserver and intraobserver reliability.[17] In this case, the patient receives a morphology score of 2 for a compression burst fracture. The integrity of the posterior ligamentous complex receives a score of 2 because it is indeterminate whether there is injury. Finally, a complete neurological injury receives a score of 2, for a total score of 6. Because a score of 5 or higher indicates a surgical injury, the TLICS scale recommends operative treatment for this case.

Timing of Surgery

The question of whether early surgical decompression of the spinal cord results in better neurological recovery in cases of spinal cord injury has received considerable attention with no definitive answers. Fehlings and Perrin[18] performed a systematic literature review to assess the timing of surgical intervention for acute spinal cord injury, which included 67 articles. Nineteen animal studies consistently demonstrated that neurological recovery was improved with early decompression. The same results were not been borne out in human studies. One prospective randomized trial published by Vaccaro et al.[19] did not find a difference between early (<72 hours) and late (>5 days) decompression for cervical spinal cord injuries. This study was considered class II (moderate quality) evidence because a large portion of patients were lost to follow-up. Other class II and III (poor quality) studies have had mixed results, with some studies concluding that early surgical decompression confers no benefit,[20,21] while others found that early surgical decompression was advantageous.[22–24] For patients with complete spinal cord injuries, the possibility of neurological improvement with decompression is even more doubtful than with incomplete injuries.[21,25,26] Overall, there is no clear evidence at this time that early decompression improves neurological recovery in cases of spinal cord injury.

Central Canal Decompression

The potential of canal clearance contributing to neurological recovery has also been the topic of many publications. In a review by Boerger and Dickson[27] addressing the issue of surgical canal clearance, they included 60 articles in their analysis. Only three of the articles were prospective, and no articles included a control group or randomization. When data were pooled, the average Frankel score improvement in patients with spinal cord injuries due to burst fractures was 0.83 for patients treated with surgery and 0.97 for those treated nonoperatively. The authors concluded that there is currently no convincing evidence that surgical decompression influences neurological outcome. The role of central canal decompression in cases of complete spinal cord injury is even more questionable because of the poor rate of neurological improvement. For example, in a study of 105 cases treated with anterior decompression for thoracic or lumbar spine fractures, none of 34 patients with complete spinal cord injuries recovered any function below the level of injury.

Surgical Approach

The literature search identified 17 clinical studies that met our inclusion criteria. The three studies by Been and Bouma,[28] Hitchon et al.[29] and Sasso et al. were cohort studies with control groups but were graded as poor quality since there was no randomization and the studies were retrospective. The remaining studies were all graded as very poor quality because they were cohort studies without control groups. Most studies evaluated posterior and/or anterolateral constructs, but three studies by Been and Bouma,[28] Payer,[30] and Tezer et al.[31] specifically looked at combined anterior plus posterior constructs. The results of all 17 clinical studies are summarized in Table 12.1.

TABLE 12.1   Evidentiary Table.

Authors (Year)	Description	Summary of Results	Quality Rating
Been and Bouma (1999)	Retrospective cohort study Comparison of combined anterior plus posterior instrumentation and short segment pedicle screw fixation	Retrospective cohort of 46 patients with thoracolumbar burst fractures and at least 50% canal compromise treated with either combined anterior and posterior stabilization (Group 1) or short segment posterior pedicle fixation alone with the AO internal fixator (Group 2). 39% of patients had neurological injury. Mean follow-up of 6 y. Bony fusion occurred in all patients. Loss of reduction of −5 degrees occurred significantly more often in Group 2 (68%) than in Group 1 (7%), but the kyphotic angle at last follow-up examination did not significantly differ between groups. Mean loss of correction was 2.1 degrees in Group 1 and 8.2 degrees in Group 2. Clinical outcome was also similar between groups with regard to pain.	Low

(Continued)

TABLE 12.1 **Evidentiary Table.** *(Continued)*

Authors (Year)	Description	Summary of Results	Quality Rating
Hitchon et al. (2006)	Retrospective cohort study Comparison of anterolateral and posterior constructs	Retrospective review of 63 thoracolumbar fractures (T11-L2) treated with decompression and either an anterolateral ($N = 38$) or posterior ($N = 25$) construct. The anterolateral group had either dual rods and screws ($N = 31$) or plate and screws ($N = 7$) placed, while the posterior group had pedicle screws ($N = 18$), pedicle screws and hooks ($N = 6$), or hooks alone ($N = 1$). Mean preoperative Frankel score was 3.7 in the anterolateral group and 3.5 in the posterior group. Mean clinical follow-up period of 1.8 y except SF-36 scores were obtained a mean of 5.8 y after surgery. The mean angular deformities in the anterolateral and posterior groups preoperatively were 11.9 and 4.1 degrees, postoperatively 2.0 and 3.4 degrees, and at last follow-up examination 4.5 and 9.8 degrees, respectively. The difference in angular deformity between groups at last follow-up examination was statistically significant. No significant difference in SF-36 score, Frankel scores, or complication rates postoperatively between groups.	Low
Sasso et al. (2006)	Retrospective cohort study Comparison of anterior strut graft or posterior short segment fixation	Retrospective review of 53 patients with unstable burst fractures treated by either an anterior strut graft and plate ($N = 40$) or posterior short segment fixation ($N = 23$). Posterior construct included pedicle screws 1 level above and below fracture as well as laminar hooks 1 level below and 2 levels above. 47 patients with neurological deficits, including 9 with complete injuries. Mean follow-up of 53 mo in posterior group and 31 mo in anterior group. Mean postoperative correction of kyphosis was 15.3 degrees in the anterior group and 14.1 degrees in the posterior group, which was not a significant difference. At last follow-up examination, the anterior group had a mean loss of correction of 1.8 degrees, which was significantly less than the 8.1 degrees loss in the posterior group. 5/9 (56%) had some neurological improvement after surgery.	Low
Akalm et al. (1994)	Cohort study No control group	Cohort of 44 patients with thoracolumbar burst fractures treated with short segment pedicle fixation using the AO spinal internal fixator. 59% of patients had a neurological deficit, including 18% with a Frankel grade A injury. Mean follow-up period of 28.8 months. Significant improvement was noted for spinal canal compromise, local kyphotic deformity, and anterior vertebral body height. The local kyphotic angle improved from 20.2 degrees preoperatively to 4.3 degrees postoperatively and 6.5 degrees at last follow-up. Half of grade A patients neurologically improved.	Very low

(Continued)

TABLE 12.1 **Evidentiary Table.** *(Continued)*

Authors (Year)	Description	Summary of Results	Quality Rating
Alvine et al. (2004)	Retrospective cohort study No control group	Retrospective cohort of 40 patients with thoracolumbar burst fractures treated with pedicle screw fixation, of which 36 constructs were short segment. Mean follow-up period of 52 mo. For thoracolumbar junction fractures, the preoperative, postoperative, and follow-up mean angular measurements were 15, 4, and 9 degrees, respectively. The mean anterior vertebral body collapse was 37%, 15%, and 16%. 7 of 14 patients with neurological injury had improvement. Pseudarthrosis rate of 8% and reoperation rate of 23%.	Very low
Benson et al. (1992)	Prospective cohort study No control group	Prospective cohort of 25 patients who underwent short segment pedicle screw fixation with the AO internal fixator for unstable thoracolumbar burst fractures. 14 patients with neurological deficits, including 2 patients with Frankel grade A injuries. Mean follow-up period of 22 mo. Mean sagittal kyphosis improved from + 16 degrees preoperatively to −4 degrees postoperatively. A mean of 9 degrees of correction was lost at last follow-up examination. Canal compromise improved from a mean of 42%–28%. Neither of the patients with grade A injuries improved neurologically. No instances of pseudarthrosis, and no reoperations were required. 33% of patients had intermittent back pain.	Very low
Bernucci et al. (1994)	Cohort study No control group	Cohort of 41 patients with thoracolumbar burst fractures treated by short segment pedicle screw fixation. Mean follow-up period of 19.9 mo. Kyphotic deformity significantly improved from 13.4 degrees preoperatively to −1 degrees postoperatively. A significant loss of correction occurred to a final kyphosis of 5.4 degrees at last follow-up examination. Vertebral body height followed a similar pattern.	Very low
Boucher et al. (2001)	Cohort study No control group	Cohort of 24 patients treated for lumbar burst fractures with short segment pedicle screw fixation. Mean follow-up period of 3.2 ys. 6 patients had a neurological deficit. Mean kyphosis was 16.9 degrees preoperatively, 6.3 degrees postoperatively, and 12.4 at last follow-up examination. Canal compromise improved from 54.4% to 29.6%. SF-36 and Oswestry questionnaires found a high level of functional outcome, with no correlation to radiographic findings.	Very low
Esses et al. (1991)	Prospective cohort study No control group	Prospective multicenter trial evaluating the use of the AO internal fixator for the treatment of unstable thoracolumbar injuries, including 61 burst fractures. 19 patients with neurological deficits, including 5 with Frankel grade A injuries. All but 3 patients had short segment pedicle screw constructs. Mean kyphosis improved from 18 degrees preoperatively	Very low

(Continued)

TABLE 12.1	Evidentiary Table. (Continued)		
Authors (Year)	**Description**	**Summary of Results**	**Quality Rating**
		to 3 degrees postoperatively, with no long-term follow-up monitoring. Mean improvement in canal clearance was 30%. One patient with a grade A injury improved to grade C. No instances of pseudarthrosis at 6 mo.	
Inamasu et al. (2008)[32]	Retrospective cohort study No control group	Retrospective cohort of 32 patients with unstable injuries from T11-L2 and neurological deficits treated with pedicle screw fixation 2 vertebrae above and below the level of injury. Patients treated within 7 d of injury. Excluded 4 patients treated anteriorly who had progressively worsening neurological examination. 17 of the patients had burst fractures. ASIA classifications included 15 grade A, 8 grade B, 7 grade C, and 2 grade D. Mean follow-up period of 18 mo. No ASIA grade A and 6/8 grade B patients remained nonambulatory. All other patients became ambulatory. One case of hardware failure, but bony fusions still occurred.	Very low
Kaneda et al. (1997)[33]	Cohort study No control group	Cohort of 150 patients with a thoracolumbar burst fracture and neurological deficit treated with anterior corpectomy and placement of a Kaneda device. Mean follow-up period of 8 years. Average kyphosis of 19 degrees preoperatively improved to 7 degrees at discharge and 8 degrees at last follow-up examination. 95% had improvement of at least 1 Frankel grade. 93% fusion rate, with 10 patients requiring posterior instrumentation.	Very low
McDonough et al. (2004)	Retrospective cohort study No control group	Retrospective cohort of 30 patients with thoracolumbar burst fractures treated with anterior corpectomy and Z-plate fixation. 46% of the patients had an incomplete neurological deficit. Mean follow-up period of 27 mo. Mean preoperative kyphosis of 18 degrees improved to 6 degrees at first follow-up examination and 8 degrees at last follow-up examination. No statistical analysis performed. All patients with neurological deficits improved at least one Frankel grade. One patient required supplemental posterior fixation.	Very low
Payer (2006)	Prospective cohort study No control group	Prospective cohort of 20 patients with unstable thoracolumbar junction burst fractures treated with a posterior bisegmental fixation followed by anterior corpectomy and titanium cage placement. 14 of the patients had neurological deficits. Follow-up period of 24 mo. Mean preoperative regional kyphosis of 16 degrees was improved to 2 degrees of lordosis postoperatively. Mean loss of kyphosis correction was 3 degrees at 24 mo. No cases of hardware failure. 12/14 patients with neurological deficits had average improvement of 1.5 grades on the ASIA scale. This included 3/6 patients with initial complete paraplegia (ASIA A) who improved 3 grades. Mean VAS of 1.6 at follow-up examination.	Very low

(Continued)

TABLE 12.1   **Evidentiary Table.** *(Continued)*

Authors (Year)	Description	Summary of Results	Quality Rating
Tezer et al. (2005)	Retrospective cohort study No control group.	Retrospective cohort of 48 patients with thoracolumbar burst fracture and associated with flexion-distraction injury. All patients treated with combined posterior pedicles screws and anterior corpectomy, strut graft, and anterior rod. Mean follow-up period of 70 mo. Mean correction of kyphosis was 98%. No loss of correction at follow-up examination. 8/11 patients with neurological injury had some improvement.	Very low
Viale et al. (1993)	Cohort study No control group	Cohort of 27 patients who underwent transpedicular decompression and short segment pedicle screw fixation for the treatment of lumbar burst fractures. All patients had a neurological deficit, with 4 patients initially being a Frankel grade A. Median follow-up period of 18.7 mo. Both kyphosis and vertebral body height significantly improved postoperatively, but no long-term radiographic results were reported. 17 patients exhibited complete neurological recovery, and 75% of Frankel grade A patients showed improvement.	Very low
Wang et al. (2008)	Retrospective cohort study No control group	Retrospective cohort of 27 patients with thoracolumbar burst fractures treated with short segment pedicle screw fixation. 6 of the patients had incomplete neurological deficits. Mean follow-up period of 2.7 ys. Mean anterior vertebral body height ratio significantly improved from 44% preoperatively to 90% postoperatively. A mean 3.8% loss of height at last follow-up examination was not significant. Significant improvement in mean Cobb angle (16.3–3.1 degrees) and sagittal index (19.3–2.9 degrees) noted postoperatively. Significant loss of correction at final follow-up examination was noted with both the Cobb angle (11.5 degrees) and sagittal index (8.4 degrees). Authors concluded the collapse of the disc contributes to 94% of the loss of correction. All patients with neurological deficits improved at least one Frankel grade.	Very low
Wiggins et al. (1999)	Retrospective cohort study No control group	Retrospective cohort of 21 patients with an unstable thoracolumbar burst fracture treated with anterior corpectomy, titanium mesh cage, and Kaneda device. 11 patients had a neurological deficit but no complete injuries. Mean 15-mo follow-up period. Preoperative kyphosis of 18.8 degrees improved to 0.1 degrees at last follow-up examination. Compared with a previously published cohort of burst fractures treated with posterior constructs, anterior group had better results for correction of kyphosis and pain. However, posterior surgical group treated with a variety of instrumentation systems including Harrington distraction rods and Luque rings.	Very low

SF-36, Short Form 36.

The success of a surgical approach can be measured by many parameters. Historically, radiographic measures such as canal decompression and kyphotic angulation have received the most attention. However, pain and functional scores are more important from the perspective of the patient. Quantifying radiographic differences between surgical approaches should be qualified with the question of whether these differences are clinically significant. Thus, the following discussion attempts not only to compare the various radiographic outcome measures between surgical treatments but also to place them in a clinical context.

Central Canal Decompression

In 1990, Esses et al.[34] published a prospective randomized-control trial comparing anterior decompression and Kostuik-Harrington instrumentation with pedicle screw fixation using the AO internal fixator in the treatment of unstable burst fractures. This study was not included in the evidentiary table because the anterior instrumentation was outdated and potentially contributed to an unusually high loss of correction of kyphosis in the anterior group. However, the anterior instrumentation should not affect the canal decompression, which was significantly better in the anterior (57.1%) group than in the posterior (29.9%) group. This study provides good quality evidence that anterior surgery is superior to posterior surgery for improving canal clearance. Several studies have provided very poor quality evidence that canal decompression with a posterior approach ranges from 15% to 39%.[14,35–37] As discussed, the benefit of canal decompression in cases of incomplete and complete spinal cord injury remains unproven.

Kyphotic Deformity

Sasso et al.[38] retrospectively reviewed 53 patients with unstable burst fractures treated with either anterior strut graft and plating or short segment pedicle screw fixation. The mean postoperative kyphosis correction for the anterior (15.3 degrees) and posterior (14.1 degrees) groups was not significantly different. At a mean follow-up of 53 months, there was significantly less loss of kyphosis correction with the anterior (1.8 degrees) group than with the posterior (8.1 degrees) group, providing poor quality evidence that an anterior approach is superior to a posterior approach for maintaining kyphosis correction. In a similar study providing poor quality evidence, Hitchon et al.[29] found that posterior surgery resulted in significantly more kyphosis at last follow-up examination than an anterior approach. This result is difficult to generalize because the posterior group had an average initial kyphosis correction of only 0.7 degrees, which is an order of magnitude smaller than any other study. The final study offering poor quality evidence by Been and

Bouma[28] found that a loss of more than 5% kyphosis correction occurred significantly less often in a combined approach (7%) than with short segment pedicle fixation (68%). However, the final kyphosis angle was not different between groups because the posterior group was overcorrected initially.

Numerous studies provide very poor quality evidence that posterior short segment pedicle screw fixation initially improves kyphotic deformity between and 10.3 and 20 degrees.[14,35–40] Long-term loss of correction ranges from 2.2 to 9 degrees, resulting in a net final correction of 4.5 to 13.7 degrees. In comparison, very poor quality evidence has shown that anterior surgery corrects kyphosis between 12 and 18.7 degrees, which is similar to posterior results.[41–43] However, the anterior approach loses only 1 to 2 degrees of correction, with a net gain of 10 to 11 degrees. A combined approach has similar results to an anterior approach.[30,31]

Taken together, poor and very poor quality evidence suggests that anterior and posterior approaches can gain a similar amount of correction of kyphosis but that more loss of correction over time occurs with a posterior construct. A recent article by Wang et al.[44] found that 94% of the loss of correction with posterior surgery occurs because of collapse of the disk spaces. If loss of correction occurs at the disk spaces, then less loss would be expected with an anterior approach because the disks are removed and replaced with the strut graft.

Functional Status and Pain

Despite the better maintenance of kyphosis correction than anterior surgery offers, there is a notable lack of evidence supporting a clinical benefit of an anterior versus posterior approach. In the study by Hitchon et al.[29] anterior and posterior groups did not have significant differences in mean Short Form-36 scores, Frankel scores, and complication rates despite the significantly worse kyphosis in the posterior group at last follow-up examination. Likewise, Been and Bouma[28] found no difference in pain between posterior and combined surgery. Finally, in a cohort of 24 patients treated with short segment pedicle screw instrumentation, Boucher et al.[36] found no correlation between radiographic outcomes and Short Form-36 or Oswestry Disability Index scores. Wiggins et al.[43] did report that anterior corpectomy and fusion resulted in a better pain outcome than posterior surgery. However, the posterior group was a historical control group of which a large portion of patients were treated with outdated instrumentation constructs such as Harrington distraction rods and Luque rings.

Complications and Surgical Morbidity

The evidence suggests that anterior and posterior approaches have similar pseudarthrosis rates.[28] Very poor quality evidence has found a pseudarthrosis rate between 0% and 8% for posterior surgery[14,37,39] and 7% for anterior surgery.[41] Very poor quality evidence has found that a posterior approach incurs significantly less blood loss during surgery and consumes less time.[34,45]

EVIDENTIARY TABLE AND SELECTION OF TREATMENT METHOD

Available evidence does not provide any strong evidence to guide treatment decisions in this case of an L1 burst fracture with a concurrent T12 sagittal split fracture and complete conus medullaris spinal cord injury. On the basis of the recommendations of multiple authors and the TLICS scale, this patient should be managed with operative treatment. It is doubtful that early surgical decompression is a viable option, given the patient's closed head injury. Since there is no clear benefit of early surgical decompression, it would be reasonable to wait until the patient's other injuries have stabilized and the risks of surgery minimized.

The mild widening of the posterior elements suggestive of posterior ligamentous disruption favors posterior stabilization. Although a posterior approach will likely result in mildly more kyphosis long-term, current evidence suggests that functional and pain outcomes will not be adversely affected with a posterior approach. Because of the adjacent level fracture at T12, pedicle screws would be placed two levels below and above the level of the burst fracture, although this determination is admittedly based on clinical experience and not data. We are unaware of any clinical studies addressing the issue of adjacent burst and sagittal split fractures, so there is no available evidence to guide this decision. However, a biomechanical study did show that a construct with pedicle screws at four levels is superior to an anterior construct and equivalent to a combined anterior plus posterior.[46]

There is no convincing evidence that decompression of the canal would improve the neurological outcome in this patient. On the other hand, there is no good quality evidence showing that decompression does *not* improve neurological recovery. Until canal decompression has been convincingly demonstrated to be ineffective, we believe that it is reasonable to attempt canal decompression to maximize a patient's chance of recovery. In this case, the posterior longitudinal ligament is likely disrupted, and therefore canal decompression would be performed with a laminectomy and transpedicular approach instead of by ligamentotaxis. The laminectomy would also provide autograft for a formal fusion, which could be supplemented with a graft extender. There are data demonstrating that short segment pedicle fixation for burst fractures does not require fusion, but those studies did not

involve laminectomies with disruption of the posterior elements and are therefore not applicable to this case.[47,48]

Our surgical plan emphasizes those goals we believe are most important. The first goal of treatment is to not harm the patient, which is why we do not emphasize early surgery in this case. The second goal is stabilization of the spine, and our proposed construct with pedicle screws two levels above and below the burst fracture has been demonstrated to be similar to a combined anterior plus posterior construct biomechanically. The third goal of functional recovery is not affected by the choice of surgical approach. The final goals of neural decompression and maintaining correction of radiographic measurements are better obtained with an anterior approach but are of uncertain clinical significance and therefore considered less important.

DEFINITIVE TREATMENT PLAN

The patient in this clinical scenario should be managed with surgical stabilization because of the degree of kyphotic deformity, neurological injury, and likely injury to the posterior ligamentous complex. A posterior approach is favored to address any injury to the posterior tension band. After exposure from the level of the pedicles of T10 to L3, neural decompression would be achieved with a L1 laminectomy. Transpedicular removal of vertebral body fragments would allow for further decompression. Pedicle screws would be placed bilaterally at T10, T11, L2, and L3. Pedicle screws and rods could then be used to introduce distraction and lordosis across L1. The combination of distraction and previous removal of vertebral body fragments would then allow bony fragments retropulsed into the central canal to be pushed back into the vertebral body. Finally, autograft and graft extender as needed could be placed for a posterolateral arthrodesis.

Grading the Evidence for this Plan

In accordance with the method of grading recommendations set forth by Schunemann et al.,[49] our proposed treatment would be considered a strong recommendation. Although there is only low and very low quality of evidence for outcome measures, the benefits of spine stabilization are deemed to clearly outweigh the risks and morbidity of surgery.

PREDICTING OUTCOMES

The most important outcome from the patient's perspective is recovery of the spinal cord injury. Unfortunately, large studies have found that the chance of a functionally meaningful recovery from a complete spinal cord injury is not good. Benzel and Larson[50] reported that all 34 patients with complete spinal cord injuries after thoracic or lumbar spine injuries achieved no neurological improvement. Another large study of 154 patients with spinal cord injuries secondary to motor vehicle accidents found that 93% of patients with complete injuries had no improvement.[51] There is reason to give patients some small measure of hope, however, as reports of grade A injuries improving 2 or 3 grades have sporadically been published.[30,37]

The literature suggests at least a 90% chance of solid bony fusion.[14,37,39] Over time, approximately 5 degrees of kyphosis would recur, which would be clinically insignificant.[14,35-40]

We would counsel the patient that the goal of surgery is to stabilize the spine to allow for mobilization. Although we would decompress the spinal cord and, in theory, maximize the chance of neurological recovery, it would be performed with the understanding that significant recovery is doubtful. In our experience, functional impairment from a surgical fusion is minimal compared with the disability of a complete spinal cord injury. As such, the risks and morbidity of a thoracolumbar surgery are acceptable in this case, given the severity of the injury.

SUMMARY

We are presented with a 41-year-old man who has incurred both an L1 complete burst fracture and a T12 sagittal split fracture with an associated complete spinal cord injury. A posterior surgical approach for decompression and stabilization is warranted given the degree of kyphosis, neurological injury, and likelihood of posterior ligamentous injury. The patient's functional outcome will be limited by recovery of the spinal cord injury. Radiographically, some mild kyphosis will likely occur over time without clinical consequence.

REFERENCES

1. Gongora E, Acosta JA, Wang DS, et al. Analysis of motor vehicle ejection victims admitted to a level I trauma center. *J Trauma.* 2001;51:854–859.
2. Harris MB, Sethi RK. The initial assessment and management of the multiple-trauma patient with an associated spine injury. *Spine.* 2006;31:S9–S15; discussion S36.
3. Perl M, Gebhard F, Bruckner UB, et al. Pulmonary contusion causes impairment of macrophage and lymphocyte immune functions and increases mortality associated with a subsequent septic challenge. *Crit Care Med.* 2005;33:1351–1358.
4. Wu J, Sheng L, Ma Y, et al. The analysis of risk factors of impacting mortality rate in severe multiple trauma patients with posttraumatic acute respiratory distress syndrome. *Am J Emerg Med.* 2008;26:419–424.
5. Malas MA, Salbacak A, Buyukmumcu M, et al. An investigation of the conus medullaris termination level during the period of fetal development to adulthood. *Kaibogaku Zasshi.* 2001;76:453–459.
6. Magerl F, Aebi M, Gertzbein SD, et al. A comprehensive classification of thoracic and lumbar injuries. *Eur Spine J.* 1994;3:184–201.
7. Aito S. Complications during the acute phase of traumatic spinal cord lesions. *Spinal Cord.* 2003;41:629–635.
8. Staloch MA, Hatem SF. Charcot spine. *Emerg Radiol.* 2007;14:265–269.
9. Dai LY. Remodeling of the spinal canal after thoracolumbar burst fractures. *Clin Orthop Relat Res.* 2001;382:119–123.
10. Denis F, Armstrong GW, Searls K, et al. Acute thoracolumbar burst fractures in the absence of neurologic deficit. A comparison between operative and nonoperative treatment. *Clin Orthop Relat Res.* 1984;189:142–149.
11. Hitchon PW, Torner JC, Haddad SF, et al. Management options in thoracolumbar burst fractures. *Surg Neurol.* 1998;49:619–626; discussion 626–617.
12. Shen WJ, Liu TJ, Shen YS. Nonoperative treatment versus posterior fixation for thoracolumbar junction burst fractures without neurologic deficit. *Spine.* 2001;26:1038–1045.
13. Wood K, Buttermann G, Mehbod A, et al. Operative compared with nonoperative treatment of a thoracolumbar burst fracture without neurological deficit. A prospective, randomized study. *J Bone Joint Surg Am.* 2003;85-A:773–781.
14. Benson DR, Burkus JK, Montesano PX, et al. Unstable thoracolumbar and lumbar burst fractures treated with the AO fixateur interne. *J Spinal Disord.* 1992;5:335–343.
15. Willen J, Anderson J, Toomoka K, et al. The natural history of burst fractures at the thoracolumbar junction. *J Spinal Disord.* 1990;3:39–46.
16. Vaccaro AR, Lehman RA Jr, Hurlbert RJ, et al. A new classification of thoracolumbar injuries: the importance of injury morphology, the integrity of the posterior ligamentous complex, and neurologic status. *Spine.* 2005;30:2325–2333.
17. Rihn JA, Anderson DT, Harris E, et al. A review of the TLICS system: a novel, user-friendly thoracolumbar trauma classification system. *Acta Orthop.* 2008;79:461–466.
18. Fehlings MG, Perrin RG. The timing of surgical intervention in the treatment of spinal cord injury: a systematic review of recent clinical evidence. *Spine.* 2006;31:S28–S35; discussion S36.
19. Vaccaro AR, Daugherty RJ, Sheehan TP, et al. Neurologic outcome of early versus late surgery for cervical spinal cord injury. *Spine.* 1997;22:2609–2613.
20. McKinley W, Meade MA, Kirshblum S, et al. Outcomes of early surgical management versus late or no surgical intervention after acute spinal cord injury. *Arch Phys Med Rehabil.* 2004;85:1818–1825.
21. Pollard ME, Apple DF. Factors associated with improved neurologic outcomes in patients with incomplete tetraplegia. *Spine.* 2003;28:33–39.

22. Chen TY, Dickman CA, Eleraky M, et al. The role of decompression for acute incomplete cervical spinal cord injury in cervical spondylosis. *Spine.* 1998;23:2398–2403.

23. La Rosa G, Conti A, Cardali S, et al. Does early decompression improve neurological outcome of spinal cord injured patients? Appraisal of the literature using a meta-analytical approach. *Spinal Cord.* 2004;42:503–512.

24. Mirza SK, Krengel WF III, Chapman JR, et al. Early versus delayed surgery for acute cervical spinal cord injury. *Clin Orthop Relat Res.* 1999;359:104–114.

25. Botel U, Glaser E, Niedeggen A. The surgical treatment of acute spinal paralysed patients. *Spinal Cord.* 1997;35:420–428.

26. Petitjean ME, Mousselard H, Pointillart V, et al. Thoracic spinal trauma and associated injuries: should early spinal decompression be considered? *J Trauma.* 1995;39:368–372.

27. Boerger To, Limb D, Dickson RA. Does 'Canal clearance' affect neurological outcome after thoraculumbar burst fractures? *Bone Joint Surg Br.* 2000;82:629–635.

28. Been HD, Bouma GJ. Comparison of two types of surgery for thoraco-lumbar burst fractures: combined anterior and posterior stabilisation vs. posterior instrumentation only. *Acta Neurochir (Wien).* 1999;141:349–357.

29. Hitchon PW, Torner J, Eichholz KM, et al. Comparison of anterolateral and posterior approaches in the management of thoracolumbar burst fractures. *J Neurosurg Spine.* 2006;5:117–125.

30. Payer M. Unstable burst fractures of the thoraco-lumbar junction: treatment by posterior bisegmental correction/fixation and staged anterior corpectomy and titanium cage implantation. *Acta Neurochir (Wien).* 2006;148:299–306; discussion 306.

31. Tezer M, Ozturk C, Aydogan M, et al. Surgical outcome of thoracolumbar burst fractures with flexion-distraction injury of the posterior elements. *Int Orthop.* 2005;29:347–350.

32. Inamasu J, Guiot BH, Nakatsukasa M. Posterior instrumentation surgery for thoracolumbar junction injury causing neurologic deficit. *Neurol Med Chir (Tokyo).* 2008;48:15–21; discussion 21.

33. Viale GL, Silvestro C, Francaviglia N, et al. Transpedicular decompression and stabilization of burst fractures of the lumbar spine. *Surg Neurol.* 1993;40:104–111.

34. Esses SI, Botsford DJ, Kostuik JP. Evaluation of surgical treatment for burst fractures. *Spine.* 1990;15:667–673.

35. Akalm S, Kis M, Benli IT, et al. Results of the AO spinal internal fixator in the surgical treatment of thoracolumbar burst fractures. *Eur Spine J.* 1994;3:102–106.

36. Boucher M, Bhandari M, Kwok D. Health-related quality of life after short segment instrumentation of lumbar burst fractures. *J Spinal Disord.* 2001;14:417–426.

37. Esses SI, Botsford DJ, Wright T, et al. Operative treatment of spinal fractures with the AO internal fixator. *Spine.* 1991;16:S146–150.

38. Sasso RC, Renkens K, Hanson D, et al. Unstable thoracolumbar burst fractures: anterior-only versus short-segment posterior fixation. *J Spinal Disord Tech.* 2006;19:242–248.

39. Alvine GF, Swain JM, Asher MA, et al. Treatment of thoracolumbar burst fractures with variable screw placement or Isola instrumentation and arthrodesis: case series and literature review. *J Spinal Disord Tech.* 2004;17:251–264.

40. Bernucci C, Maiello M, Silvestro C, et al. Delayed worsening of the surgical correction of angular and axial deformity consequent to burst fractures of the thoracolumbar or lumbar spine. *Surg Neurol.* 1994;42:23–25.

41. Kaneda K, Taneichi H, Abumi K, et al. Anterior decompression and stabilization with the Kaneda device for thoracolumbar burst fractures associated with neurological deficits. *J Bone Joint Surg Am.* 1997;79:69–83.

42. McDonough PW, Davis R, Tribus C, et al. The management of acute thoracolumbar burst fractures with anterior corpectomy and Z-plate fixation. *Spine.* 2004;29:1901–1908; discussion 1909.

43. Wiggins GC, Rauzzino MJ, Shaffrey CI, et al. A new technique for the surgical management of unstable thoracolumbar burst fractures: a modification of the anterior approach and an outcome comparison to traditional methods. *Neurosurg Focus.* 1999;7:e3.

44. Wang XY, Dai LY, Xu HZ, et al. Kyphosis recurrence after posterior short-segment fixation in thoracolumbar burst fractures. *J Neurosurg Spine.* 2008;8:246–254.

45. Danisa OA, Shaffrey CI, Jane JA, et al. Surgical approaches for the correction of unstable thoracolumbar burst fractures: a retrospective analysis of treatment outcomes. *J Neurosurg.* 1995;83:977–983.

46. Eichholz KM, Hitchon PW, From A, et al. Biomechanical testing of anterior and posterior thoracolumbar instrumentation in the cadaveric spine. Invited submission from the Joint Section Meeting on Disorders of the Spine and Peripheral Nerves, March 2004. *J Neurosurg Spine.* 2004;1:116–121.

47. Sanderson PL, Fraser RD, Hall DJ, et al. Short segment fixation of thoracolumbar burst fractures without fusion. *Eur Spine J.* 1999;8:495–500.

48. Wang ST, Ma HL, Liu CL, et al. Is fusion necessary for surgically treated burst fractures of the thoracolumbar and lumbar spine? A prospective, randomized study. *Spine.* 2006;31:2646–2652; discussion 2653.

49. Schunemann HJ, Jaeschke R, Cook DJ, et al. An official ATS statement: grading the quality of evidence and strength of recommendations in ATS guidelines and recommendations. *Am J Respir Crit Care Med.* 2006;174:605–614.

50. Benzel EC, Larson SJ. Functional recovery after decompressive operation for thoracic and lumbar spine fractures. *Neurosurgery.* 1986;19:772–778.

51. Moslavac S, Dzidic I, Kejla Z. Neurological outcome in road traffic accidents with spinal cord injury. *Coll Antropol.* 2008;32:583–586.

C4 Fracture

JOHN C. FRANCE, MD

A 52-year-old woman presents to the emergency department after being rear-ended in her car. She presented in a cervical collar with a complaint of neck pain and left shoulder pain. She had no other associated injuries. She works as a real-estate agent and relies on her voice for her livelihood.

Physical examination demonstrates that she is neurologically intact to motor, strength, and reflex testing of the upper and lower extremities. She has pain to palpation in the upper cervical spine but no palpable deformities or step-off. Rectal tone is normal and perianal sensation is intact.

Radiographic images are shown in Figure 13.1A–F.

INTERPRETATION OF CLINICAL PRESENTATION

Because this is a low-energy motor vehicle accident, it is likely that the initial patient evaluation will be made by the emergency room physician. Although low energy, it does represent a trauma and the patient should be evaluated with a primary and secondary survey according to ATLS (Advanced Trauma Life Support) protocols. Based on the history given, we know that her only complaint and relevant finding is neck pain radiating to her shoulder. Because the radiating pain does not extend beyond her shoulder and her motor and sensory exam are intact, the pain likely represents musculoskeletal pain rather than neurological pain.

Given that no associated injuries are identified, a decision must be made regarding cervical clearance or the need for further radiographic assessment. Because she has neck pain, this patient would not meet the NEXUS or Canadian C-spine rules for clearance

without imaging. The traditional means of imaging would have included an anteroposterior (AP), odontoid, and lateral cervical plain radiographs. If such films revealed evidence of an injury, then a CT would be indicated to characterize that injury, but if no evidence of injury was identified, then, given the history of pain and trauma, a CT scan would still be indicated to look for more occult pathology. With this thought process in mind and given the literature on helical CT scanning as a screening tool in trauma, this patient would proceed directly to a helical CT scan as the primary means of evaluating her for a cervical fracture, subluxation, or dislocation.

Figure 13.1A–F shows images from her CT evaluation. Figure 13.1A is a sagittal cut through the left facets and demonstrates a minimally displaced fracture of the superior facet of C4, but it involves almost the entire facet, which is nicely shown in the magnified view of Figure 13.1E. The joint itself is not dislocated, but the inferior facet of C3 is following the fractured superior facet of C4 as it shifts forward. In Figure 13.1B, we see a midsagittal image slightly to the left and there appears to be a minimal anterolisthesis of C3 on C4, but in Figure 13.1C, there is a midsagittal image slightly to the right without an anterolisthesis, implying that there is a rotational component. The axial view in Figure 13.1F confirms the rotation with forward subluxation on the left since the posterolateral corner of the C3 body is shifted anterior to the C4 uncinate process. Also, the facet fracture on the left is again seen with a normal right facet joint in this view. Figure 13.1D is a sagittal cut through the right facet and is normal.

These radiographic findings clearly explain the neck pain. This pattern of injury could potentially be associated with a spinal cord injury but more commonly would include a root injury (C4 in this case) if there was a neurological injury. In this specific case, it might be difficult to fully rule out a root injury because the C4 root is cephalad to the roots that make up the brachial plexus making a specific sensory-motor exam unreliable. At this level, a subtle root injury would be unlikely to alter the decision making; thus, it is unnecessary to consider it further.

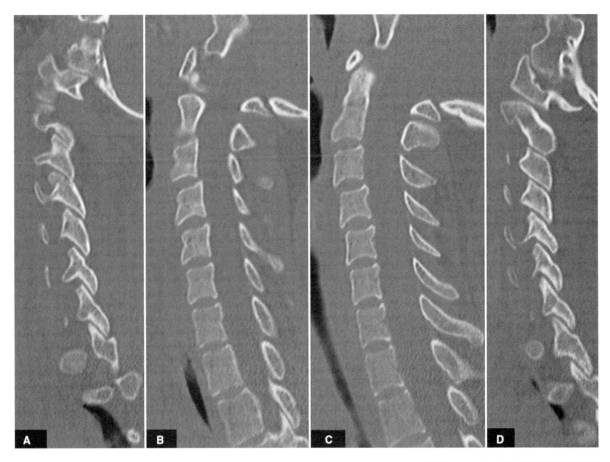

Figure 13.1.

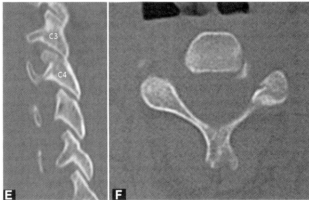

Additional imaging may be justified. If one is considering nonoperative treatment as an option, which is a possibility in this patient, then an AP and lateral plain films should be done as a baseline that could be used in comparison to future films to rule out interval increase in subluxation. An MRI would give additional information regarding the discoligamentous status that may alter the decision between nonoperative and operative management and may alter the direction of surgical intervention (posterior vs. anterior). It could reveal disruption of the posterior ligamentous complex greater than expected from the subtle subluxation on the CT images. Such a finding would confirm the need for surgical stabilization. Also a significant disc herniation could make the anterior approach favorable.

If an MRI is ordered, then it should be a trauma protocol with sagittal short T1 inversion recovery (STIR) or other T2 fat-suppressed series to highlight edema or ligamentous disruption. If based on the CT images one has decided to pursue surgical treatment and the surgeon's preferred direction of surgical stabilization for this fracture is anterior, then the information to be gained from an MRI would be superfluous. Because the subluxation is minimal and little reduction will be required, the concerns about creating a neurological deficit from an unrecognized disc herniation during a posterior stabilization are not prominent in this case. Therefore, even if one had decided that this patient required surgical stabilization and the surgeon preferred a posterior approach, then the MRI may also be unnecessary.

DECLARATION OF SPECIFIC DIAGNOSIS

The diagnosis is a left unilateral superior facet fracture with mild rotary subluxation of C3 on C4 without neurological deficit.

BRAINSTORMING: WHAT ARE THE TREATMENT GOALS AND THE SURGICAL OPTIONS?

The treatment goals for this patient can be divided into early and long-term goals. The initial goal is to impart enough stability to avoid further subluxation and neurological injury. The amount of subluxation is minimal and restoration of alignment may not be critical, but one would want to avoid further subluxation. The method chosen to establish enough stability to allow bony healing of the superior facet to create long-term stability should allow early and full mobility of the patient.

In the long-term, the goal of treatment is to maximize function. The greatest factor determining this will be the amount of pain that the patient is experiencing so minimizing late pain is probably the dominant long-term goal. Secondarily, it would be good to preserve motion across the C3-4 segment but not at the cost of pain that limits function.

The options for treatment are as follows:

1. Immobilization in a rigid collar
2. Immobilization in cervicothoracic orthosis or a halo-vest
3. Anterior discectomy and fusion at C3-4
4. Posterior fusion at C3-4, potentially C3-5
5. Anterior-posterior fusion C3-4.

EVALUATION OF THE LITERATURE

A literature search was performed using PubMed as the data base search engine. A variety of search terms/phrases were used to identify articles pertaining to facet fractures. We used cervical facet fractures, facet fractures, and facet fracture-dislocation, which identified

137, 446, and 123 articles, respectively, with much overlap between searches. The titles were reviewed, and abstracts potentially pertaining to or possibly including treatment of unilateral cervical facet fractures were read. From these abstracts, 40 articles were selected that dealt specifically with unilateral facet fractures or the broader topic of unilateral facet dislocations that could potentially be pertinent to or include some discussion of facet fractures without dislocation. These articles were read and their references searched for any additional relevant articles.

DETAILED REVIEW OF PERTINENT ARTICLES

Most articles reviewed dealt primarily with unilateral facet-dislocations or fracture-dislocations. The literature available to guide treatment of unilateral facet fractures without dislocation is much more limited. With the current practice of using helical CT scans as the means of radiographically screening trauma patients for injury, the identification of unilateral facet fractures with minimal to no displacement seems to have increased.[1]

Predicting Early Instability

Because the most important early goal is to prevent loss of alignment and potential new onset of neurological deficit, one must attempt to predict which injuries are most likely to be unstable. There are three articles that look at CT and one using MRI parameters to define which facet fractures are the most unstable.

The only article using MRI is from 1997 and was a retrospective review of 24 unilateral facet/lateral mass fractures, most of which were initially nondisplaced or minimally displaced.[2] Twelve patients were treated operatively and 12 nonoperatively. The anterior longitudinal ligament (ALL), posterior longitudinal ligament (PLL), the interspinous ligament, and the facet capsules were assessed for injury. The operative group included seven patients considered to be minimally or nondisplaced (<1–2 mm) on the initial CT that subsequently displaced in either a Minerva brace or Miami-J collar. They did not report any late development of neurological deficit, but six of the seven had evidence of injury to at least three of the ligamentous structures evaluated on MRI. In the nonoperative group, there were three patients who also had injury to at least three structures but were lost to follow-up. The other nonoperative patients had less ligamentous injury.

Three studies looked at CT alone as a predictor of instability. In 1994, Shanmuganathan et al.[3] used CT scans of 40 patients to look at the incidence and role of facet fractures in unilateral facet dislocations. They found the incidence to be 73% and that injury occurred at a greater rate at the more caudal segments. Interestingly, they asserted that the facet fractures created greater instability, but noted that when a facet fracture was present, there was a statistically significantly lower incidence of neurological injury ($p = 0.006$). More recently, Ebraheim et al.[4] studied facet morphology in cadavers and on patient CT scans and found that dislocation was more common at C5-6 and C6-7. The superior articular facets at C6 and C7 had significantly less slope relative to the horizontal, less height, and smaller AP diameter relative to the more cephalad facets. They felt this variation in anatomy made dislocation easier in the event of injury to the caudal levels.

The best attempt to use radiographic findings to predict which patients will fail nonoperative treatment comes from Spector et al.[5] who looked retrospectively at 24 patients with unilateral facet fractures who were all initially treated nonoperatively. Five of these patients failed nonoperative treatment (four subluxated, one increased radiculopathy). The presence of radiculopathy and the location of superior or inferior facet did not correlate with failure. The two factors that were most predictive of failure were the absolute height of the fracture as measured on a sagittal CT reconstruction ($p = 0.0002$) and the fracture height as a percent of the intact contralateral lateral mass ($p = 0.026$). In fact, no patient with <1 cm actual height or <40% relative height failed nonoperative treatment. Although there was no significant progression in neurological deficit in the above studies with external immobilization, there is a case report of transient tetraparesis from an unrecognized superior facet fracture.[6]

Compliance with immobilization devices was considered by Kalayci et al.[7] They reported two patient cases, one of which failed nonoperative management (defined as increased subluxation requiring surgery) who was noncompliant and another who successfully completing nonoperative treatment who was compliant.

Predicting Late Pain and Outcomes

Comparisons between nonoperative and operative management of unilateral facet dislocations have been retrospectively studied in larger case series,[8–10] and operative treatment has been demonstrated to be superior for maintenance of anatomic alignment, avoidance of late surgery, and minimizing late pain. Only one study is available that compares operative and nonoperative Health Related Quality of Life (HRQoL) outcomes for cervical facet fractures.[11] Dvorak et al. retrospectively looked at 90 patients with cervical facet fracture that included displaced and nondisplaced fractures. They used the SF-36 with focus on the bodily pain (BP) and physical component score (PCS), and the American Academy of Orthopaedic Surgeons (AAOS)/ North American Spine Society (NASS) cervical spine questionnaire (NASS PD) as their primary outcome measures. Of the 18 patients treated nonoperatively, 17 were nondisplaced superior facet fractures. There were a total of 40 nondisplaced facet fractures (32 superior and 8 inferior); the remainder of these patients were treated surgically. The surgical group was divided into early (<18 months) and late (>18 months) follow-up. The later operative follow-up group had the best outcomes. The SF36-PCS was statistically better for the surgical group as compared to the nonsurgical group ($p = 0.017$). In addition, the SF36-BP and NASS PD scores trended to favor the surgical group ($p = 0.22$ and $p = 0.074$ respectively). Scores for both the operative and nonoperative groups were below normative data.

One study found no effect of preinjury canal diameters on neurological or pain outcomes.[12] Only initial neurological injury and fracture severity appeared to influence the end result.

Approach for Surgery (Anterior or Posterior)

There are no studies that directly compare surgical approaches for this specific injury pattern (nondisplaced facet fracture) and no studies that prospectively compare anterior versus posterior surgery for facet dislocations. Traditionally, facet injuries have been handled posteriorly due to favorable biomechanics, but anterior procedures may be able to achieve enough clinical stability to provide good end results.[13] There are only retrospective case series that look at anterior and posterior stabilization procedures. Dvorak et al.[11] could not reach any conclusions that favored one approach over the other due to sample size. Renaudin et al.[14] found that four patients with facet chip fractures with subluxation who also had radiculopathy benefited from the posterior approach that afforded more direct access for foraminal decompression of the offending bony fragment. Rabb et al.[15] demonstrated satisfactory results from anterior discectomy and fusion for unilateral facet fractures with at least 2 mm subluxation. Johnson et al.[16] were also able to obtain good results in 87% of patients with traumatic cervical flexion distraction injuries using anterior cervical plating, but they raised concern for failure of fixation in those patients who had vertebral endplate fractures and facet fractures (13% loss of reduction).

EVIDENTIARY TABLE AND SELECTION OF TREATMENT METHOD

From the above articles, we have selected those that are most pertinent to this case study of a nondisplaced or minimally displaced cervical facet fracture in a neurologically intact patient and included them in an evidentiary table (Table 13.1). From this data, we can offer a treatment plan to address both the goal of early stabilization and late satisfactory functional outcomes.

TABLE 13.1	Evidentiary Table.			
Paper Author (Year)	**Description**	**Summary of Results**		**Quality of Evidence**
Spector et al. (2006)	Retrospective cohort study No control group	24 patients with unilateral minimally displaced facet fractures All nonoperatively treated, five fail due to subluxation or increased radicular complaints Height of facet fracture (1 cm) and percent height of facet fracture relative to contralateral intact lateral mass (40%) correlate with loss of reduction and late surgery		Low
Dvorak et al. (2007)	Retrospective cohort study compares nonoperative and operative HRQoL outcomes Outcomes compared with normative data	90 patients unilateral facet injuries Includes 32 superior facet fractures without displacement Compare late outcomes for function and pain between operative and nonoperative groups All patients scored lower than normative data, but the operative patients appear to be statistically better on SF 36-PCS and trend better on SF 36-BP and NASS PD		Moderate
Johnson et al. (2004)	Retrospective case series	107 patients with cervical flexion distraction injuries treated operatively via anterior approach 13% loss of reduction Patients with facet fractures and vertebral endplate fractures at greatest risk		Very low

It appears that *early stability* can be inferred from the CT evaluation. Although MRI scans are playing a larger role in assessment of this type of injury, there have been no studies since Halliday[2] in 1997 that have looked at the role of MRI in predicting stability of nondisplaced facet fractures. Halliday looked at four ligamentous components, namely, the facet region, interspinous ligament, ALL, and PLL and concluded that injury to at least three of the four constituted instability. Our case does not provide an MRI so these data are not included in our treatment decision. But, an MRI as part of the decision process for this type of patient may be worthwhile. The best data about CT come from the Spector study.[5] It would support an initial course of nonoperative treatment and would predict that spinal alignment could be maintained with hard collar immobilization to definitive healing. The height of our fracture is <1 cm and <40% of the intact contralateral lateral mass. In their study, no patient suffered loss of alignment when those criteria were met so this would favor a **nonoperative** approach.

Since we can assume that nonoperative treatment has a good probability of maintaining alignment, the next issue is one of late functional and pain-related outcomes. The only study available to aid us

in our treatment decision is the one by Dvorak et al.[11] Because 17 of the 18 patients treated nonoperatively had minimally displaced superior facet fractures, we can gain significant insight since this matches our case example. The pain and disability outcome measures in this study statistically significantly favored the operative treatment group in those followed >18 months. The actual scores were only 8% to 10% improved making it difficult to determine whether or not they are clinically significant. On the other hand, the operative patients as a whole had more severe injuries. Because that group included the dislocations, one would expect any bias to favor the nonoperative group. Perhaps this strengthens their conclusions that operative treatment should be considered for all facet fractures. Based on this data, one would have to favor an **operative** approach even if the alignment could be maintained in a collar.

Lastly, if operative treatment is selected, the next step is to determine whether the fusion should be done *anteriorly or posteriorly*. The current literature fails to definitively dictate in favor of either approach so this remains entirely up to the surgeon. We can offer some guidance from what is available. The posterior approach remains an excellent option, has been used for a long time, and is sound biomechanically. It does involve turning the patient prone, which carries some displacement risk, and it is more destructive to soft tissues, namely the paraspinal muscles. The posterior approach offers a more direct means of foraminal decompression that may have resulted from the fracture fragment, which would be unnecessary in this case of a neurologically intact patient. The anterior approach, although not as strong biomechanically, can provide clinically adequate stability for this purpose. If used in the face of facet fracture, one has to be careful since the facets may not provide enough translational stability, particularly if the motion segment is overdistracted during graft insertion. Thus, either an **anterior or posterior** approach can be chosen based on our evidence.

DEFINITIVE TREATMENT PLAN

For our patient, I would recommend **operative** stabilization and would perform it through a **posterior** approach. The patient is neurologically intact, so no decompression is necessary. Even in the face of radiculopathy, the evidence does not require decompression or even surgery for a reasonable rate of resolution. The density of any radiculopathy would have to be factored in the decision but is not required for our patient.

Given the size of the superior facet fracture in this patient, one could be confident that further displacement is unlikely even with nonoperative treatment. The concern that I have for this individual patient is that there is already some mild rotary subluxation. This is clearly not a dislocation or even a perched facet, but the amount of rotary subluxation or fracture displacement that would be considered "nondisplaced" is not well elucidated in any of the literature reviewed. There is some reference to 2 to 3 mm and 11 degrees of angulation (no angulation present in our patient), but this is clearly not a nondisplaced fracture. The amount of displacement and the knowledge that functional and pain outcomes tend to be better with surgical management would push me over the edge toward surgical treatment. One would not be faulted for choosing nonoperative treatment because even in the unlikely event of increased subluxation in the collar, the risk of significant neurological deterioration is unexpected and not reported in the literature reviewed. Additionally, it could be argued that the improvement in functional outcome measures is minimal and late pain could be addressed with a fusion procedure at that time. In my practice, it is rare for a patient to return with enough complaints of pain or dysfunction to warrant a late fusion.

I have traditionally stabilized these injuries with a posterior approach since that is the region of injury. If the superior facet fracture was a little larger and I thought the lateral mass would not hold a screw to allow a two-level posterior fusion, then I would approach this anteriorlym, taking great care to not overdistract and achieve good extension to minimize the risk of loss of reduction. In this case, the approach should be chosen based on the procedure with which the individual surgeon is most comfortable and familiar.

Grading the Evidence for this Plan

The grade of recommendation is being determined in accordance with the guidelines set forth by Schunemann et al.[17] The quality of studies forming the basis for a decision to recommend surgery is low to moderate and for the direction of approach is low. The studies are all retrospective and either cohort or case series with no prospective or randomized clinical trials. The studies used in the review and evidentiary table make up only part of the final strength of the recommendation for treatment. The final strength of recommendation must include a consideration of the benefits, harms, and burdens of the proposed interventions. Also, surgeon expert opinion and experience as well as patient factors such as comorbidities and preferences should be taken into account.

In accordance with the method of grading recommendations set forth by Schunemann et al., our proposed treatment would be considered a **weak recommendation**. The potential harm to the patient by selecting nonoperative treatment appears to be subtle in the way of mild pain or functional deficit and the nonoperative approach would be less costly initially. However, the patient numbers in all studies are relatively low, and thus care must be taken when determining the final treatment recommendation. This is a case where a clear discussion with the patient to determine their concerns and desires will play a large role in the final treatment decision.

PREDICTING OUTCOMES

The only literature available to assess HRQoL outcomes for this group of patients is that of Dvorak et al., which would indicate that no matter which treatment is selected, the patient's pain and function measures will remain less than normative data even after 18 months postinjury. With operative treatment, the outcome measures can be slightly improved. If one chooses nonoperative treatment but remains vigilant on follow-up (i.e., upright x-rays are taken prior to discharge and after 1–2 weeks), then any subsequent displacement can be detected early and treatment can be changed to operative care. The risk of neurological deterioration while immobilized in a collar appears to be unlikely.

I frequently begin nonoperative treatment for those facet fractures that are nondisplaced and only on occasion need to switch to surgical care. Similar to the literature, I have not experienced neurological deterioration with additional subluxation in these patients. I follow these patients 1 to 2 years postinjury, although many trauma patients are lost to follow-up. It is rare that they have enough pain or dysfunction to consider late fusion procedures. The persistence of radiculopathy with persistent root compression is the exception, but this is not the case in our case example. This is definitely a patient whom I would directly involve in the treatment decision process since the literature-derived treatment recommendations are weak.

SUMMARY

Our patient has a minimally rotationally subluxated unilateral superior facet fracture and is neurologically intact. How much of this rotary subluxation is acceptable is very unclear in the literature. Based on the size of the fragment, it is unlikely to displace further with nonoperative treatment. However, the late pain and functional status of the patient can perhaps be improved with operative treatment. Although this is a patient and injury I would treat operatively, this recommendation is weak and a choice for nonoperative treatment could not be faulted as long as the follow-up was vigilant. The approach to surgical treatment is based on surgeon's preference.

REFERENCES

1. Lin JT, Lee JL, Lee ST. Evaluation of occult cervical spine fractures on radiographs and CT. *Emerg Radiol*. 2003;10(3):128–134.
2. Halliday AL, Henderson BR, Hart BL, et al. The management of unilateral lateral mass/facet fractures of the subaxial cervical spine: the use of magnetic resonance imaging to predict instability. *Spine*. 1997;22(22):2614–2621.
3. Shanmuganathan K, Mirvis SE, Levine AM. Rotational injury of cervical facets: CT analysis of fracture patterns with implications for management and neurologic outcome. *Am J Roentgenol*. 1994;163(5):1165–1169.
4. Ebraheim NA, Patil V, Liu J, et al. Morphometric analyses of the cervical superior facets and implications for facet dislocation. *Int Orthop*. 2008;32(1):97–101.
5. Spector LR, Kim DH, Affonso J, et al. Use of computed tomography to predict failure of nonoperative treatment of unilateral facet fractures of the cervical spine. *Spine*. 2006;31(24):2827–2835.
6. Nyunt BA. Unrecognized fracture through the base of superior articular facet of cervical spine presenting with transient tetraparesis. *Injury*. 1995;26(8):563–564.
7. Kalayci M, Cagavi F, Acikgoz B. Unilateral cervical facet fracture: presentation of two cases and literature review. *Spinal Cord*. 2004;42(8):466–472.
8. Beyer CA, Cabanela ME. Unilateral facet dislocations and fracture-dislocations of the cervical spine: a review. *Orthopedics*. 1992;15(3):311–315.
9. Beyer CA, Cabanela ME, Berquist TH. Unilateral facet dislocations and fracture-dislocations of the cervical spine. *J Bone Joint Surg Br*. 1991;73(6):977–981.
10. Koivikko MP, Myllynen P, Santavirta S. Fracture dislocations of the cervical spine: a review of 106 conservatively and operatively treated patients. *Eur Spine J*. 2004;13(7):610–616.
11. Dvorak MF, Fisher CG, Aarabi B, et al. Clinical outcomes of 90 isolated unilateral facet fractures, subluxations, and dislocations treated surgically and nonoperatively. *Spine*. 2007;32(26):3007–3013.
12. Lintner DM, Knight RQ, Cullen JP. The neurologic sequelae of cervical spine facet injuries: the role of canal diameter. *Spine*. 1993;18(6):725–729.
13. Duggal N, Chamberlain RH, Park SC, et al. Unilateral cervical facet dislocation: biomechanics of fixation. *Spine*. 2005;30(7):E164–E168.
14. Renaudin J, Snyder M. Chip fracture through the superior articular facet with compressive cervical radiculopathy. *J Trauma*. 1978;18(1):66–67.
15. Rabb CH, Lopez J, Beauchamp K, et al. Unilateral cervical facet fractures with subluxation: injury patterns and treatment. *J Spinal Disord Tech*. 2007;20(6):416–422.
16. Johnson MG, Fisher CG, Boyd M, et al. The radiographic failure of single segment anterior cervical plate fixation in traumatic cervical flexion distraction injuries. *Spine*. 2004;29(24):2815–2820.
17. Schunemann HJ, Jaeschke R, Cook DJ, et al. An official ATS statement: grading the quality of evidence and strength of recommendations in ATS guidelines and recommendations. *Am J Respir Crit Care Med*. 2006;174(5):605–614.

Metastatic Renal Tumor of L4 After Failed Kyphoplasty

GREGORY S. MCLOUGHLIN, MD
AND DARYL R. FOURNEY, MD, FRCSC, FACS

EDITORS' CASE PRESENTATION

A 68-year-old woman with a history of known metastatic renal cell carcinoma presents with a history of a destructive lesion of L4. She has a primary complaint of left leg pain, with a lesser complaint of back pain. She underwent a kyphoplasty about a month and a half ago that did not improve her pain. Lower extremity pain is described as radiating into her thigh, down to the knee, and intermittently into the lower leg. She has no bowel or bladder complaints.

Physical exam demonstrates that her gait is normal. She has decreased sensation in the left L4 distribution. Strength is 5/5 in the upper and lower extremities. Her reflexes are 2+ in the upper and lower extremities. She has negative straight leg raises. Alignment of the cervical spine is grossly normal.

Radiographic imaging studies are demonstrated in Figures 14.1 to 14.3.

INTERPRETATION OF CLINICAL PRESENTATION

The clinical scenario describes a woman with spinal metastasis secondary to known renal cell carcinoma. Her chief complaint is that of pain, primarily localized to the left leg, but involves her back to a lesser extent. The right leg is not affected. The fact that her pain periodically radiates below the knee suggests that there is a radicular component to her symptoms.[1] It is important to note that her bowel and bladder are unaffected, which is crucial when contemplating involvement of the conus medullaris or cauda equina. Her physical examination is remarkable for mild symmetric hyperreflexia. Her gait and motor exam are reassuring, in the sense that there is no evidence of an upper or lower motor neuron lesion. A lower motor neuron deficit would suggest significant nerve root dysfunction, while an upper motor neuron deficit would indicate compression of the spinal cord or cerebral involvement. It is important to remember that renal cell carcinoma has a propensity for intracerebral metastasis, which could manifest solely as unilateral leg weakness in this setting.

The patient had recently undergone an L4 kyphoplasty. The procedure involves the injection of polymethylmethacrylate (PMMA) into the vertebral body using a percutaneous transpedicular approach.[2] In contradistinction to vertebroplasty, kyphoplasty utilizes a balloon to locally dilate the vertebral body prior to injection of the cement. Kyphoplasty has been purported to offer greater vertebral body height restoration with less risk of cement extravasation; however, the relative merits of the two techniques are controversial.[3] In the setting of spinal malignancy, vertebral augmentation has been used to provide relief of mechanical back pain by stabilizing the pathological collapse of the vertebral body.[4]

The available images demonstrate the metastatic tumor of L4 and confirm that a kyphoplasty had been performed at this level. Figure 14.1A–D shows T2-weighted images in the sagittal and paramedian planes. The sagittal alignment of the spine is preserved, and normal lumbar lordosis is present. There is no evidence of vertebral body collapse at any of the lumbar levels. In the midsagittal plane, there is no significant central stenosis. However, on the parasagittal images, it becomes apparent that there is attenuation of the thecal sac by epidural tumor along the posterolateral

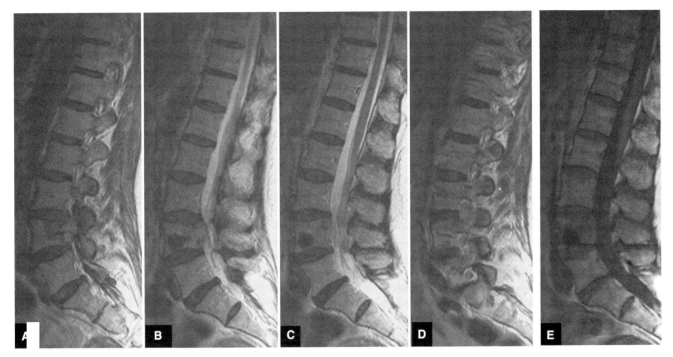

Figure 14.1.

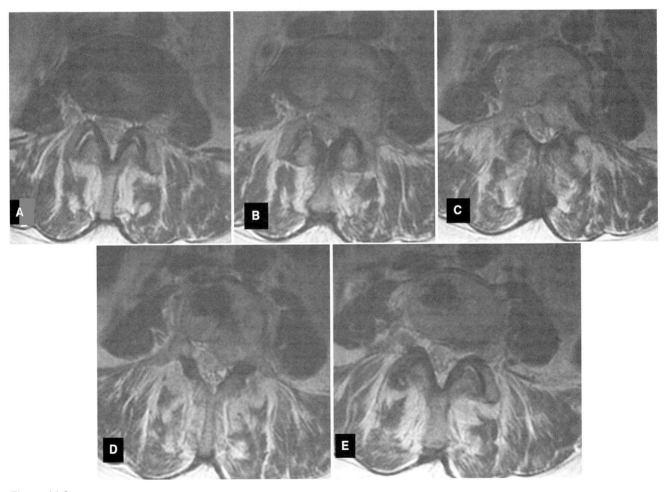

Figure 14.2.

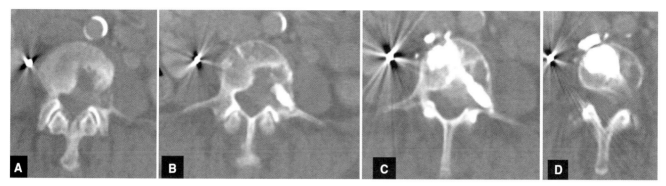

Figure 14.3.

aspect of the vertebral body. The left L4 pedicle is also expanded by tumor. The overall effect is compression of the left L4 nerve root within the lateral recess and L4/5 neural foramen. Note the area of hypointensity within the vertebral body; this is the PMMA that had been injected previously during the kyphoplasty.

Figure 14.1E is a T1-weighted sagittal MRI that again demonstrates the adequate sagittal alignment of the spine. This image is without gadolinium contrast, so the pathology of L4 is represented by areas of hypointensity within the posterior vertebral body. The intensely hypointense region is the PMMA.

The T2-weighted axial MR images provided in Figure 14.2 are most helpful in defining the radiologic pathology. Figure 14.2A represents a slice through the L3-4 disc space, and the remaining cuts continue caudally. Of particular importance is the T2-isotense tumor involving the left L4 posterior vertebral body and pedicle. This results in severe stenosis of the left L4 lateral recess, undoubtedly contacting and compressing the exiting left L4 nerve root. Further caudally (Fig. 14.2E), both nerve roots are seen exiting their respective foramina, indicating that the left L4 nerve root remains intact. This likely explains part of the patient's symptomatology, namely the left radicular pain. There is some displacement of the thecal sac medially due to the mass, although this does not result in severe central canal stenosis. Note that the left superior facet of L4 is partially involved with tumor but sparing the remaining facet joints above and below the tumor.

Figure 14.3A–D shows axial CT images (bone-window algorithm) and is best at illustrating the PMMA from the kyphoplasty procedure and the extent of bone destruction by tumor. Note the local destruction of bone involving the posterior aspect of the vertebral body. The injected PMMA is evident as the intensely hyperdense material within the vertebral body. The PMMA was injected unilaterally along the left pedicle, and PMMA is visible along the cannulation path. A small amount of PMMA is evident anterior to the vertebral body, which represents extravasation of cement (Fig. 14.3C). On CT, the tumor is barely visible as a slightly hyperdense mass coinciding with the tumor's location on the MR images.

DECLARATION OF SPECIFIC DIAGNOSIS

This patient is experiencing left radicular lower extremity pain and axial back pain secondary to metastatic involvement of the left L4 vertebral body, pedicle, foramen, and facet. Her main complaint is left L4 radiculopathy due to metastatic epidural tumor involving the L4/5 neural foramen and lateral recess. The previous kyphoplasty was not successful because this procedure is indicated for painful vertebral body fracture. In the present case, the tumor only involves the posterolateral aspect of the vertebral body, and therefore there is no vertebral collapse. Although some kyphoplasty cement is located in the left L4 pedicle, the cement does not appear to be compressing the nerve root.

BRAINSTORMING: WHAT ARE THE TREATMENT GOALS AND SURGICAL OPTIONS?

The treatment goals are

1. Preservation of neurological status
2. Decompression of compressed neural elements
3. Restoration of segmental stability
4. Provision of symptomatic relief

The treatment options are

1. Radiation therapy
2. Posterior decompression
3. Posterior decompression and stabilization
4. Anterior decompression and stabilization
5. Combined anterior/posterior decompression and stabilization

EVALUATION OF THE LITERATURE

To provide an evidence-based treatment plan, a comprehensive literature search was carried out on metastatic tumors of the spine. Embase, Medline, and the Cochrane Review databases were interrogated with the following key words: "spine," "metastasis," "instability," "decompression," "radiculopathy," "fusion," "vertebroplasty," and "kyphoplasty." The key words "spine and metastasis" were sequentially combined with the other key words during the literature search process. All searches were limited to English articles published between 1974 and 2009. Articles specifically limited to regions of the mobile spine aside from the lumbar spine were excluded. The search strategy revealed a total of 3,218 publications among the databases. Of these, 294 articles were relevant to the clinical question. These abstracts were reviewed, and of these, 26 papers were selected for in-depth analysis.

DETAILED REVIEW OF PERTINENT ARTICLES

When contemplating surgery, consideration is given to the neurological status of the patient, the type of tumor the patient has, the stage of the spinal tumor, the radiosensitivity of the tumor, the chemosensitivity of the tumor, and the presence of medical comorbidities.[5,6] An expected survival >3 months is suggested in the literature before surgery is offered.[7] These parameters are built on experience and observational studies, so the evidence supporting these algorithms is poor.

The vast majority of articles published regarding the surgical management of epidural spinal disease were of low-quality evidence. Of the literature available to the search parameters, only one randomized, nonblinded trial is published.[8]

The landmark study by Patchell et al.[8] randomized patients with metastatic epidural spinal cord compression into two arms: those treated with radiotherapy alone and those treated with decompressive surgery and radiotherapy. We should point out that all patients in this trial had *spinal cord* compression by metastatic tumor. Patients with radiculopathy alone were not candidates for the trial; however, it is still the best evidence we have comparing surgical and nonsurgical treatment.

A clear benefit to the surgical arm was noted, with respect to preserving ongoing mobility (122 vs. 13 days, $p = 0.003$) or recovery of mobility (62% vs. 19%, $p = 0.01$). According to this data, patients who retained some degree of lower extremity motor function (i.e., were not completely paraplegic beyond 48 hours), who had limited medical comorbidities, and had a life expectancy beyond 3 months benefited from surgery and radiotherapy more so than radiotherapy alone. These data are helpful in designing treatment algorithms for patients with spinal metastatic disease and emphasize the importance of acting quickly before paraplegia occurs. An important exception to this strategy is the presence of radiosensitive tumors, for which radiation may be given up front.

The study by Patchell et al.[8] provides good clinical evidence regarding the efficacy of surgery and radiotherapy to functional outcome. A recent prospective, multicenter study by Ibrahim et al.[9] focused on these patients' quality of life. Several clinical parameters were analyzed, including the type of surgery performed (i.e., en bloc vs. debulking procedure or palliative decompression) and overall survival. Quality of life parameters included preoperative and postoperative mobility status, neurological impairment, continence, and daily activity performance. A total of 223 patients were included in the study. Postoperatively, 71% of patients reported improved pain control. During the follow-up period, 53% of patients regained or retained their ability to mobilize independently, and 39% regained urinary continence.

Although the literature suggests that a more extensive surgical excision is associated with prolonged survival,[7,10,11] there is no randomized data dictating which procedure should be performed for any given patient. Recent advancements in technical and hardware technology have made aggressive anterior-poster tumor resection and reconstruction feasible.[12–14] Prior to this, surgery consisted of laminectomy alone. This was often associated with a poor outcome since the procedure led to significant iatrogenic instability if the anterior column was weakened by tumor.[15]

One of the features of the clinical case included in this discussion is the kyphoplasty that was performed on our patient. This procedure does have merit in the management of metastatic spine disease, provided the appropriate indications are followed. A prospective study by Pflugmacher et al.[16] reports a 2-year evaluation regarding the efficacy of kyphoplasty for vertebral body collapse secondary to metastasis. A pain visual analogue scale (VAS) and the Oswestry Disability Index (OSD) were recorded from 65 patients preoperatively and at 3, 6, 12, and 24 months postoperatively. The mean outcome of these scales improved postoperatively ($p < 0.0001$) and remained stable during the 24-month follow-up period. The authors concluded that kyphoplasty provides long-term pain relief and improved functional status for appropriately selected patients. Patients who may benefit from kyphoplasty include those experiencing refractory pain due to pathological compression fractures. Contraindications for the procedure include epidural compression of the neural elements and pain that is primarily radicular in nature.[17,18]

Renal cell carcinoma is poorly responsive to radiation therapy, and therefore, this would be a poor choice for the palliation of symptomatic epidural compression. It would be most appropriately administered as an adjuvant to surgery.[19] Stereotactic radiosurgery and intensity-modulated radiotherapy are potential options, but most reported series employed these modalities when surgery was not feasible and radiation therapy had failed.[20,21]

EVIDENTIARY TABLE AND SELECTION OF TREATMENT METHOD

The best available evidence suggests that our patient should be treated with tumor resection, internal stabilization, and postoperative radiation therapy. This will provide the patient with the best chance of preserving her current functional status. It is very likely that she will experience significant pain relief postoperatively. Her pattern of pain is primarily radicular, which is a contraindication for kyphoplasty (Table 14.1).

Although no guidelines exist regarding the selection of a surgical approach, an argument is made for en bloc resection. Renal cell carcinoma is radioresistant, and Biorini et al.[14] have reported long-term survival following en bloc resection of isolated renal cell spinal metastasis. The status of the primary tumor is important when making this decision; solitary spinal metastasis in the setting of a well-controlled primary tumor provides a strong incentive to achieve local control. If the primary tumor is not controlled, then a less aggressive surgical

excision may be warranted. Either way, it is imperative that the epidural tumor be removed to decompress the neural elements. This will likely destabilize an already compromised motion segment, and it will be necessary to internally fixate the spine. Depending on the degree of resection, this will take the form of a short- or long-segment fixation. Because radiotherapy is often given postoperatively, a fusion is not likely to occur and a formal fusion procedure is not necessary.

Based on the available data, our patient would undergo a simultaneous combined anterior-posterior approach with the goal of en bloc spondylectomy. The thecal sac and nerve roots will be completely decompressed. The anterior column will be stabilized with an expandable anterior cage or the chest-tube/PMMA technique introduced by Errico et al.[22] A posterior short-segment fixation (L3-5) is performed. A formal fusion procedure is not necessary. Postoperatively, once the wound has sufficiently healed, the patient will undergo adjuvant radiotherapy.

En bloc resection is an aggressive choice but is most appropriate in the setting of radioresistant solitary vertebral metastasis. A second choice, with a lower chance for early morbidity but less chance for long-term disease control, is an intralesional resection.

DEFINITIVE TREATMENT PLAN

Prior to surgery, the patient is placed on steroids and preoperative embolization is performed.[19] The technique for this procedure would be that described

TABLE 14.1	Evidentiary Table: A Selected Summary of the Quality of Evidence for Surgery and Kyphoplasty for the Treatment of Metastatic Epidural Spinal Disease.		
Paper Author (Year)	**Description**	**Summary of Results**	**Quality of Evidence**
Patchell et al. (2005)	Prospective, randomized, nonblinded study	101 patients to receive radiotherapy alone, or surgery and radiotherapy Patients treated with surgery were more likely to retain or regain the ability to walk Study stopped prematurely due to the significant benefit incurred by the surgery arm	High
Ibrahim et al. (2008)	Prospective observational study	223 patients underwent surgery 71% improvement in pain, 53% regained independent mobility 39% regained urinary continence en bloc associated with longer survival	Low
Pflugmacher et al. (2008)	Prospective observational study	65 patients treated with kyphoplasty Significantly improved VAS and OSD postoperatively Results sustained during 24 mo follow-up	Low

by Fourney et al.,[23] consisting of a simultaneous anterior-posterior approach. This technique offers adequate exposure anteriorly to remove the involved vertebral body en bloc and reconstruct the anterior column. The patient can be turned 90 degrees (without the need for redraping) to the fully prone position for resection of the posterior columns and placement of stabilization devices.

The patient is placed in the right lateral decubitus position upon a Wide Lateral Access Table (Jackson OSI Table, Union City, California). Antibiotics are given upon induction. A retroperitoneal incision is connected to the posterior midline incision over the index level. This is confirmed by intraoperative fluoroscopy. Skin flaps are reflected and the paraspinal muscles are mobilized and retracted with a Penrose drain. Simultaneously, a midline posterior incision is made by a second surgical team. Pedicle screws are placed at L3 and L5. The laminae and facets of L4 are removed, with careful attention not to enter tumor along the left pedicle. The right pedicle is cut across its base with a thread-wire saw.[13] A single rod is placed on the right side, to maintain vertebral alignment while the spondylectomy is completed.

The L4 vertebral body followed anteriorly on the left side and the segmental vessels are identified and divided along the midposition of the vertebral body. The vertebral body is dissected free from the peritoneum, and radical discectomies are performed at the L3-4 and L4-5 levels. Along its right side, the vertebral body has to be dissected free of the psoas muscle from the posterior approach, as described by Tomita et al.[13] The thecal sac is mobilized and gently retracted to expose the vertebral body and pedicle contralateral to the tumor. This is drilled until the contralateral retroperitoneum is encountered and the vertebral body circumferentially dissected free of the adjoining tissues. The tumor is then delivered en bloc with care to protect the thecal sac. A marginal resection is expected along the dura and nerve root sleeve. Great care is taken not to enter the tumor, but given the location of disease within the neural foramen, it is not unlikely to have a small area of intralesional resection.

The left-sided rod can now be fixed to the pedicle screws and then cross-links are applied. Reconstruction of the anterior column utilizes a cage or chesttube technique with PMMA.[22] An anterior plate is not necessary if the cage is expandable or alternatively placed under compression by the pedicle screws. The wound is irrigated. Subfascial drains are placed and the wound closed in layers. Postoperatively, the patient is managed in the ICU and early mobilization is encouraged.

In accordance with the method of grading recommendations set forth by Schunemann et al.[24] our proposed treatment would be considered a **strong recommendation (low-quality evidence)**.

PREDICTING OUTCOMES

According to the available data, our patient should expect to experience significant reduction in her preoperative pain following decompression of the left L4 nerve root and stabilization of the motion segment. Her functional status should be preserved.

It is our experience that timely decompression for radiculopathy can result in remarkable recovery of function with time. Radicular pain is often relieved immediately postoperatively, and the patient's narcotic requirement is drastically reduced over time. If the bladder or bowel function is affected prior to surgery, it is not likely that significant recovery will take place (although this does happen on the rare occasion).

Prior to surgery, it is crucial for the patient to understand the rationale behind the procedure. It should be emphasized that the goal of surgery is the relief of pain and prevention of a neurological deficit. A blood transfusion is to be expected.[23] Renal cell carcinoma metastasis can be very vascular, and consideration should be given to preoperative embolization.[19] The morbidity and mortality of the procedure need to be clearly explained, along with the expected postoperative course. For the above-mentioned surgery, a morbidity of 27% and a 30-day mortality of 0% are reported.[23] The possibility of recurrent tumor in the future should be discussed as well. Alternative treatments (such as radiotherapy alone, intralesional surgery, stereotactic radiosurgery, or ongoing conservative management) must be discussed along with the potential risks and benefits of each approach.

SUMMARY

The case presented is a 68-year-old woman with persistent radicular and back pain following a kyphoplasty for metastatic renal cell carcinoma of L4. The kyphoplasty was not successful most likely because the main complaint was radiculopathy due to epidural metastasis within the lateral recess and neural foramen and there was no pathologic fracture. Following an extensive literature search, the available data were assessed to assist in the selection of the most appropriate treatment regimen. Based on the current data, the patient would best be served by undergoing an en bloc resection of the tumor. This would provide her with the best chance of long-term local disease control while preserving her functional status and providing her with significant symptomatic relief.

REFERENCES

1. Bilsky M, Lis E, Raizer R, et al. The diagnosis and treatment of metastatic spinal tumor. *Oncology.* 1999;4:459–469.

2. Chi J, Gokaslan Z. Vertebroplasty and kyphoplasty for spinal metastases. *Curr Opin Support Palliat Care.* 2008;2:9–13.

3. Fourney D, Schomer D, Nader R, et al. Percutaneous vertebroplasty and kyphoplasty for painful vertebral body fractures in cancer patients. *J Neurosurg Spine.* 2003;98:21–30.

4. Humle P, Krebs J, Ferguson J, et al. Vertebroplasty and kyphoplasty: a systematic review of 69 clinical studies. *Spine.* 2006;31(17):1963–2001.

5. George R, Jeba J, Ramkumar G, et al. Intervention for the treatment of metastatic extradural spinal cord compression in adults. *Cochrane Database Syst Rev.* 2008;8(4).

6. Cole J, Patchell R. Metastatic epidural spinal cord compression. *Lancet.* 2008;7(5):459–466.

7. Sciubba D, Nguyen T, Gokaslan Z. Solitary vertebral metastasis. *Orthop Clin N Am.* 2009;40:145–154.

8. Patchell R, Tibbs P, Regine W, et al. Direct decompressive surgical resection in the treatment of spinal cord compression caused by metastatic cancer: a randomized trial. *Lancet.* 2005;366:643–648.

9. Ibrahim A, Crockard A, Antonietti P, et al. Does spinal surgery improve the quality of life for those with extradural (spinal) osseous metastases? An international multicenter prospective observational study of 223 patients. *J Neurosurg Spine.* 2008;8:271–278.

10. Witham T, Khavkin Y, Gallia G, et al. Surgery insight: current management of epidural spinal cord compression from metastatic spine disease. *Nat Clin Pract Neurol.* 2006;2(2):87–94.

11. Sundaresan N, Rothman A, Manhart K, et al. Surgery for solitary metastases of the spine: rational and results of treatment. *Spine.* 2002;27(16):1802–1806.

12. Yao K, Boriani S, Gokaslan Z, et al. En bloc spondylectomy for spinal metastases: a review of techniques. *Neurosurg Focus.* 2003;15(5):E6.

13. Tomita K, Kawahara N, Baba H, et al. Total en bloc spondylectomy for solitary spinal metastases. *Int Orthop.* 1994;18:291–298.

14. Boriani S, Biagini R, De Lure F, et al. En bloc resections of bone tumors of the thoracolumbar spine: a preliminary report of 29 patients. *Spine.* 1996;21(16):1927–1931.

15. Siegal T, Siegal T. Surgical decompression of anterior and posterior malignant epidural tumor compressing the spinal cord: a prospective study. *Neurosurgery.* 1985;17(3):424–432.

16. Pflugmacher R, Taylor R, Agarwal A, et al. Balloon kyphoplasty in the treatment of metastatic disease of the spine: a 2-year prospective evaluation. *Eur Spine J.* 2008;17:1042–1048.

17. Wenger M, Markwalder TM. Vertebroplasty combined with pedicular instrumentation. *J Clin Neurosci.* 2008;15:257–262.

18. Pflughmacher R, Beth P, Schroeder RJ, et al. Balloon kyphoplasty for the treatment of pathological fractures in the thoracic and lumbar spine caused by metastasis: one-year follow-up. *Acta Radiologica.* 2007;1:89–95.

19. Jackson R, Gokaslan Z, Loh SG. Metastatic renal cell carcinoma of the spine: surgical treatment and results. *J Neurosurg Spine.* 2001;94:18–24.

20. Sheehan J, Jagannathan J. Review of spinal radiosurgery: a minimally invasive approach for the treatment of spinal and paraspinal metastases. *Neurosurg Focus.* 2008;25(2):E18.

21. Gong Y, Wang J, Bai S, et al. Conventially-fractionated image-guided intensity modulated radiotherapy (IG-IMRT): a safe and effective treatment for cancer spinal metastasis. *Radiat Oncol.* 2008;22:3–11.

22. Errico T, Cooper P. A new method of thoracic and lumbar body replacement for spinal tumors: technical note. *Neurosurgery.* 1993;32(4):678–680.

23. Fourney D, Abi-Said D, Rhines L, et al. Simultaneous anterior-posterior approach to the thoracic and lumbar spine for the radical resection of tumors followed by reconstruction and stabilization. *J Neurosurg Spine.* 2001;94:232–244.

24. Schunemann H, Jaeschke R, Cook D, et al. ATS documents development and implementation committee. An official ATS statement: grading the quality of evidence and strength of recommendations in the ATS guidelines and recommendations. *Am J Respir Crit Care Med.* 2006;174:605–614.

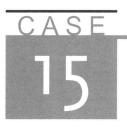

CASE 15

Thoracolumbar Flexion-Distraction Injury

STEPHEN P. KINGWELL, MD, FRCSC AND
CHARLES G. FISHER, MD, MHSC(EPI), FRCSC

■ EDITORS' CASE PRESENTATION

A 38-year-old woman presents to the emergency department with a complaint of pain at the thoracolumbar junction following a ski injury in which she ran into a gate. Immediately following the injury, she experienced pain in the abdomen and thoracolumbar region of the spine. She does not report any lower extremity numbness or weakness. She has no other associated injuries and has no other relevant medical history.

Physical examination reveals a healthy, fit-appearing woman. Her abdomen is tender and has a transverse bruise across its lower aspect. She has active bowel sounds. Upon examination of her back, she has intact skin, though there is some swelling about the thoracolumbar junction. She has a palpable interspinous process gap in this region, as well as tenderness. Her neurological examination reveals intact motor, sensory, and reflex functions. She has intact perianal sensation and normal rectal tone.

Radiographic imaging studies are shown in Figures 15.1 to 15.3.

INTERPRETATION OF CLINICAL PRESENTATION

The clinical scenario describes a woman of childbearing age who was involved in a recreational accident of moderate energy. The chief complaint of thoracolumbar pain would suggest a spinal injury; however, the initial approach to this patient must adhere to ATLS protocols.[1,2] Striking a gate while skiing could potentially lead to a compressive or distractive force to the spinal column, depending on the body area of contact. The concomitant abdominal and thoracolumbar pain would raise the possibility of a flexion-distraction injury (FDI). Furthermore, a lack of neurological deficit is consistent with an FDI as the incidence of neurological injury is lower for this thoracolumbar trauma subgroup than patients with burst fractures or fracture-dislocations.[3] The incidence of neurological deficits in patients with FDIs is reported to be between 11% to 32%.[4–8] Importantly, the diagnostic priority must be adherence to the primary survey with the abdominal pain being assessed by the trauma team leader or general surgeon.

The transverse bruising on the abdomen represents the likely contact area of the gate. This finding is analogous to the so-called seatbelt sign classically found on victims of motor vehicle collisions wearing lap belts.[7–11] In this case, the gate acts as a fulcrum and the thoracolumbar spine is flexed and subjected to a distractive force starting posteriorly.[4,6,12] The spinal injury that is most likely to occur in a neurologically intact patient subjected to this mechanism is a thoracolumbar FDI. There is a 44% to 67% incidence of concomitant abdominal trauma in patients with FDIs.[4,7–9,13,14] The clinician must recognize this relationship because the abdominal trauma may be life threatening and the diagnosis can be unnecessarily delayed. Classically, hollow viscus structures, such as the intestines, are most at risk.[8,15]

The presence of swelling, tenderness, and an interspinous gap at the thoracolumbar junction is consistent with an FDI. Still, the absence of these signs would not exclude an FDI as the sensitivity of these findings is poor. Lee et al.[16] found that the diagnostic accuracy for detecting posterior ligamentous complex (PLC) injury by palpation was 54% compared to 97% for fat-suppressed T2 sequence magnetic resonance imaging (MRI). Both techniques were compared to operative findings. Though sensitivity and specificity were generally low, it is valuable to appreciate that a palpable gap had a 93% positive predictive value of intraoperative PLC disruption.[16]

The computerized tomography (CT) scan images available include two paramedian reformatted images,

Figure 15.1.

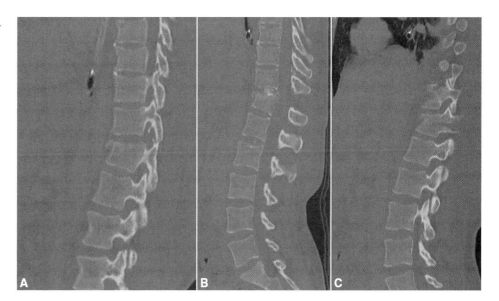

a midline sagittal reformat, and a representative axial cut through the facets at the injury level. Figure 15.1A demonstrates failure of the anterior column in compression, distraction through the posterior disc space, and a unilateral facet subluxation on the left at T12. Mild anterior compression fractures are noted at T8 and T9. In the midline, there is a similar degree of anterior compression, a focal kyphosis at the injury level, and a widened interspinous space (Fig. 15.1B). Figure 15.1C shows a transverse fracture through the right pedicle and thus, the injury pattern involves both bony and soft-tissue structures. The axial CT cut through the

T11-12 disc space demonstrates an absence of the T12 superior articular process on the left, which is in keeping with the unilateral facet subluxation (Fig. 15.2).

Representative fat-suppressed T2-weighted images in the sagittal and paramedian planes are shown in Figure 15.3. Figure 15.3A shows increased signal in the interspinous and supraspinous ligaments at T11-12 with widening of the interspace. There is evidence of a hematoma in the disc space. A line of increased signal is visualized in the vertebral body, which represents the compression fracture. Of note, there is no evidence of ongoing neural compression at the level of the conus medullaris; nor is there evidence of an epidural hematoma or intramedullary hematoma at this level. No signal change is seen within the conus on the available images. Figure 15.3B clearly shows the pedicle fracture on the right with resultant widening. The T11-12 facet joint appears to be intact on the right. On the left, the facet joint is subluxated and there is increased signal, which suggests disruption of the facet capsule (Fig. 15.3C).

DECLARATION OF SPECIFIC DIAGNOSIS

This patient has a T11-12 FDI with bony and disco-ligamentous disruption.

BRAINSTORMING: WHAT ARE THE TREATMENT GOALS AND SURGICAL OPTIONS?

The treatment goals are

1. Obtaining a reduction and normal spinal alignment
2. Preservation of neural elements

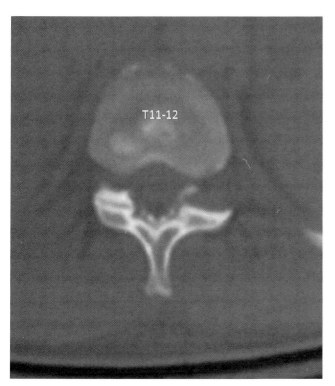

T11-12

Figure 15.2.

Figure 15.3.

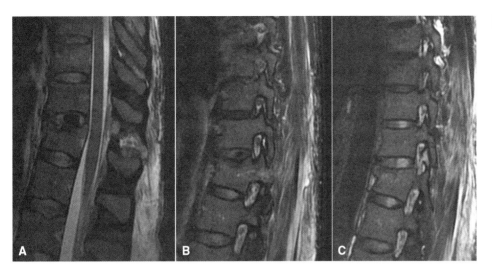

3. Maintaining spinal alignment and ensuring continued stability

4. Early mobilization

5. Rehabilitation and healing

The treatment options are

1. Brace/Casting with or without closed reduction

2. Percutaneous/minimally invasive reduction and instrumentation

3. Open reduction and short-segment or multilevel fixation

4. Fusion or no formal fusion

EVALUATION OF THE LITERATURE

To identify relevant publications on flexion-distraction injuries of the thoracolumbar spine, a Medline search was performed. Search strategies included the use of MeSH (medical subject headings) and key words. Key words included "flexion distraction," "chance" within three words of "fractures," and "seatbelt or seat belt" within three words of "fractures." A focused search of "spinal fractures" with subheadings of mortality, classification, complications, radiography, rehabilitation, surgery, and therapy was performed. The results for "spinal fractures" were then combined with thoracic vertebrae or lumbar vertebrae to identify patients with flexion-distraction injuries within larger heterogeneous studies on spinal fractures. Journals were hand searched and references were reviewed to identify pertinent articles. The search strategy revealed 1,410 potential publications after limiting from 1950 to 2007. The same search strategy was applied to Embase and revealed 268 results. Medline "in process" and nonindexed citations were searched as was EBM reviews-Cochrane database. There were 131 English language abstracts that were reviewed and 35 full text articles read.

DETAILED REVIEW OF PERTINENT ARTICLES

Operative or Nonoperative Treatment

Overall, the quality of evidence pertaining to FDIs in the thoracolumbar spine is poor. The literature review revealed only one prospective cohort study and one retrospective cohort study with a cross-sectional outcome analysis.[14,17] Nevertheless, these studies in addition to numerous case series represent the best available evidence.

Although most thoracolumbar trauma classification systems adequately categorize an injury, they usually fall short in specifying or directing management based on important clinical radiographic parameters. This consistent limitation amongst classifications led to a new scoring system devised by a panel of experts that utilized the injury morphology, integrity of the PLC, and the neurologic status of the patient.[18] According to the Thoracolumbar Injury Classification and Severity Score (TLICS), our patient would receive a total score of four. The compression injury morphology receives a score of one, no points for intact neurology, and a score of three for an injured PLC. A score of four can be considered for nonoperative or operative intervention. Although this classification has been found to be reliable, and has face validity and content validity, its ultimate acceptance will depend on the results of the criterion validity studies currently being conducted.

As such, for the purpose of this chapter, the decisions concerning how to manage this patient will be based on a thoughtful analysis of three factors: patient factors, literature evidence, and clinical expertise, specifically related to stability and healing issues.

Patient Factors

This patient has an FDI at T11-12 with a suspected intra-abdominal injury. Although there is uncertainty regarding the precise abdominal pathology, an orthosis is likely contraindicated and would probably not be well tolerated in this patient.

NEUROLOGIC STATUS

In this case, there is no neurologic deficit and therefore no requirement for operative decompression.

Spinal Stability

In the setting of an FDI, analyzing the degree of soft-tissue disruption is an essential component of the decision-making process. When the injury pattern involves primarily ligamentous structures, there is concern that healing will be incomplete and resultant instability and delayed neurologic deterioration could occur. Expert opinion and pathophysiological rationale would suggest that an FDI with a substantial discoligamentous injury is unlikely to heal with nonoperative methods.[7,13,14,17,19–25] In this case, the patient's injury is primarily bony on the right and soft tissue on the left. The fact that this patient has a facet subluxation is important based on the study by LeGay et al.[7] Eighteen patients with flexion-distraction injuries were reviewed and nonoperative treatment resulted in fair or poor results in 60% of patients with "facet involvement." However, this study was retrospective and the duration of bed rest (average 4.1 weeks) would not be considered acceptable by today's standards.

Thus, the ultimate question is what distribution and degree of soft tissue and bony injury will lead to adequate healing with nonoperative treatment? The answer is elusive as a selection bias is present in the studies available for review. Demonstrably, our patient, with an abdominal injury and ligamentous spine injury, is typically treated surgically. A useful guideline to assist with this dilemma is from the work of Schunemann et al.[26]

In order to offer clinical recommendations, it is suggested that the clinician consider the quality of the evidence in addition to the perceived benefits, harms, and burdens of the interventions. On an individual level, patient preference will influence the variables considered above. However, without specific knowledge of the weight of various outcomes or risks from their perspective, the clinician must be the patient's surrogate. The results of the three studies in Table 15.1, which utilized modern spinal instrumentation and are more representative of our patient, demonstrate that surgical treatment results in acceptable disease-specific outcome scores and health-related quality of life (HrQoL) outcome scores. Furthermore, surgical complications and radiographic failure are uncommon. From retrospective case series, nonoperative treatment has a more unpredictable outcome with respect to nonunion and radiographic deterioration.[5,7,13] For this particular patient, **operative treatment is selected** because of

TABLE 15.1	Evidentiary Table: A Summary of the Quality of Evidence for Posterior, Single-Level Fixation of Thoracolumbar Flexion-Distraction Injuries.		
Paper Author (Year)	**Description**	**Summary of Results**	**Quality of Evidence**
Finkelstein et al. (2003)	Prospective cohort study No control group	21 patients with bony and ligamentous FDIs were treated with a standard technique of single-level fixation. Significant radiographic correction, no loss of correction Mean Oswestry score of 11.5 and 88% reporting minimal disability at 20 mo	Low
Miyanji et al. (2006)	Retrospective cohort study with cross-sectional outcome analysis Outcomes compared with normative data and patient recall	40 patients (25 operative, 15 nonoperative) with thoracolumbar FDIs treated with single-level instrumentation and fusion. HrQoL was significantly worse for surgically treated FDIs at 3 y compared to recall baseline/normative data No difference in HrQoL between nonoperative and recall/normative data No relationship between kyphosis and functional outcome	Low
Liu et al. (2003)	Retrospective case series	23 patients with thoracolumbar FDIs treated surgically if ligamentous or initial kyphosis >15 degrees Average radiologic correction was 9.5 degrees No validated outcome score	Very low

proven benefit, low risk, and fewer treatment-related burdens, such as brace wear in the setting of an abdominal injury, potentially slower mobilization, and closer radiographic follow-up due to the greater potential for deformity progression.

Other reported indications for surgical intervention include initial kyphosis >10 to 17 degrees; however, there is little evidence to support such one-dimensional indications.[13,17,20,27]

Literature Inconsistencies

The study by Miyanji et al.[14] would suggest that non-operatively treated patients have superior HrQOL outcomes as compared to operatively treated patients with FDIs. The type of treatment had an influence on the SF-36 mental component score (MCS) and the North American Spine Society (NASS) pain and disability score as lower scores were more likely in the surgically treated group. These findings can be attributed to the fact that nonoperatively treated patients were preselected because of a bony injury, reducible kyphosis, and lack of concomitant abdominal injuries that would have precluded the use of a brace. Furthermore, their regression analysis demonstrated that only an "associated other system injury" independently influenced the SF-36 physical component score (PCS). The patient in our clinical scenario would still have been treated operatively according to the surgical indications set forth by Miyanji et al.

EVIDENTIARY TABLE AND SELECTION OF TREATMENT METHOD

The best available evidence dictates that the patient presented in the clinical scenario should be treated operatively. In order to evaluate the most *appropriate* surgical treatment, only articles pertaining to adult patients with thoracolumbar FDIs treated with modern spinal instrumentation were critically examined. These results are summarized in Table 15.1.

Open or Percutaneous (Minimally Invasive) Reduction and Stabilization

The concept of minimally invasive or percutaneous stabilization of FDIs is appealing, given that short-segment instrumentation has been shown to be clinically sound for this particular injury. Two case reports of temporary percutaneous stabilization of bony FDIs followed by implant removal have been described, the rationale for which was preserving segmental motion long-term.[28,29] Presently, there is not enough evidence to support this technique for this patient and **open reduction** is favored.

Short-Segment or Multilevel Fixation

Selection of the appropriate surgical technique for this patient comes from an analysis of two studies that utilized modern spinal instrumentation.[17,20] In a prospective cohort study by Finkelstein et al.[17] 21 patients with FDIs were treated with single-level fixation. Significant improvements in kyphosis were noted at 29 months, the mean Oswestry score was 11.5, and 88% of patients reported only minimal disability. This represents the only series of a standardized surgical technique for FDIs. The components of this technique were the following: positional reduction, neural monitoring, midline posterior approach, posterior decompression, further gentle compression reduction using interspinous wiring, single-level screws or hooks (depending on pedicle fractures) to form a neutralization construct, and iliac crest autograft over the adjacent transverse processes. Liu et al.[20] also utilized short-segment instrumentation at one level above and below the injury. Although radiographic kyphosis improved, no validated outcome score was utilized to judge clinical outcomes. Only one mechanical failure occurred in thirty patients at 85 months. Therefore, **short-segment fixation** is appropriate.

Fusion or No Formal Fusion

The fact that surgically treated burst fractures have been adequately managed without a formal fusion suggests that bony FDIs could be treated in a similar manner.[30,31] In our clinical scenario, we have elected to treat the patient operatively because of concerns that there is not enough bony surface to heal and as such a **formal fusion** should be carried out.

DEFINITIVE TREATMENT PLAN

The patient in this clinical scenario should be managed with operative stabilization primarily because of the soft-tissue injury and the associated abdominal injury. Initial reduction is obtained through positioning on bolsters on a radiolucent table. Instrumentation would include pedicle screws at T11 and L1 and a formal fusion between T11 and T12. Final reduction can be achieved through a compression maneuver under direct visualization once the ligamentum flavum is removed over the injured interspace. The flavum is removed to prevent any infolding and subsequent narrowing of the canal with reduction. Implant removal can be considered at 9 to 12 months, although the goal of preserving motion at the thoracolumbar junction is questionable. Alternatively, a laminar hook could be used at T12 on the right and a pedicle screw on the left at T12 to preserve the integrity of T12-L1. This would be consistent with **single-level fixation**. Both constructs are safe in the hands of fellowship-trained spine surgeons and have been shown to maintain spinal alignment in patients with FDIs while allowing early mobilization. The role for postoperative bracing is unclear as it was a component of the protocol in only two of the relevant studies reviewed.[17,20]

Grading the Evidence for this Plan

The evidence to support the technical aspects of our treatment selection would be considered low as it is derived from observational studies of moderate quality. The treatment goals have been met in the three studies found in Table 15.1. Single-level fixation has clearly been shown to result in immediate and sustained correction of kyphosis, no neurologic deterioration, and the postoperative protocols have all allowed for early mobilization.

In accordance with the method of grading recommendations set forth by Schunemann et al.[26] our proposed treatment would be considered a **strong recommendation**. The grading paradigm utilized is necessary because it not only considers the quality of evidence but also addresses the benefits, harms, and burdens of the proposed interventions. Furthermore, the benefits of short-segment fixation in a patient with a bony/ligamentous FDI, in whom a brace is likely contraindicated, clearly outweigh the harms and burdens of such an intervention.

PREDICTING OUTCOMES

To adequately predict outcomes and counsel patients with this injury, one has to rely on validated outcome measures, since radiographic outcomes rarely correlate with patient satisfaction.[14,17,32] Previously cited studies using modern instrumentation would suggest that a lasting improvement of 10 degrees in overall kyphosis can be expected.[17,20] Miyanji et al.[14] found a 14-point decrease on the SF-36 PCS for surgically treated patients with FDIs compared to normative data. Over 90% of individuals with such a score report that they are restricted during vigorous activities; a PCS score of 39 is worse than chronic conditions such as rheumatoid arthritis and congestive heart failure.[33] A predictor of poor outcome on the SF-36 PCS was associated "other system injury" and surgical treatment negatively influenced SF-36 MCS and NASS pain/disability scores independently.[14] Our patient would have both of these negative predictors of outcome.

The results of Finkelstein et al.[17] would suggest that the outcome of surgical treatment in patients with FDIs is somewhat better. The disease-specific instrument utilized was the Oswestry Functional Assessment Questionnaire, and the average score of 11.5 is similar to the population mean of 10.14.[34] Eighty-eight percent of their study patients reported minimal disability. Again, substantial abdominal injury was related to greater disability on the Oswestry index. Overall, our patient can expect a good radiographic outcome and

some degree of physical impairment at 2 to 3 years. The severity of the abdominal injury will have a significant influence on the patient's functional outcome.

Patient preference is an important component of evidence-based medicine.[35] Preoperative counseling requires a frank discussion of the treatment options and their inherent risks, benefits, potential outcomes, and associated burdens. The information conveyed must contain the best available evidence and expert opinion. Importantly, the delivery must consider the fact that the patient has sustained a significant injury and their ability to understand this information may be impaired.

These results are in keeping with my experience as a spine surgeon and should drive the clinician to be selective with surgical treatment and offer nonoperative treatment when factors such as patient preference, an absence of abdominal trauma, and a bony injury pattern are present. Less invasive surgical techniques and attempts to preserve segmental motion are important considerations that require further investigation.

SUMMARY

We are presented with a 38-year-old woman who sustained a T11-12 FDI and suspected intra-abdominal trauma. The most appropriate treatment for this patient's spinal injury, considering the combined bony and ligamentous injury, would consist of operative reduction and stabilization from T11-L1 with a formal fusion from T11-12. A sustained radiological correction with some degree of persistent physical impairment can be expected. Her functional outcome will be somewhat dependent on the severity of her concomitant injuries.

REFERENCES

1. American College of Surgeons Committee on Trauma. *Advanced Trauma Life Support Program for Doctors*. 7th ed. Chicago, IL: American College of Surgeons, 2004.
2. Harris MB, Sethi RK. The initial assessment and management of the multiple-trauma patient with an associated spine injury. *Spine*. 2006;31(suppl):9–15.
3. Gertzbein SD. Scoliosis Research Society: multicenter spine fracture study. *Spine*. 1992;17:528–540.
4. Gertzbein SD, Court-Brown CM. Flexion-distraction injuries of the lumbar spine: mechanisms of injury and classification. *Clin Orthop*. 1988;227:52–60.
5. Gumley G, Taylor TK, Ryan MD. Distraction fractures of the lumbar spine. *J Bone Joint Surg Br*. 1982;64:520–525.
6. Magerl F, Aebi M, Gertzbein SD, et al. A comprehensive classification of thoracic and lumbar injuries. *Eur Spine J*. 1994;3:184–201.
7. LeGay DA, Petrie DP, Alexander DI. Flexion-distraction injuries of the lumbar spine and associated abdominal trauma. *J Trauma*. 1990;30:436–444.

8. Green DA, Green NE, Spengler DM, et al. Flexion-distraction injuries to the lumbar spine associated with abdominal injuries. *J Spinal Disord*. 1991;4:312–318.

9. Smith WS, Kaufer H. Patterns and mechanisms of lumbar injuries associated with lap seat belts. *J Bone Joint Surg Am*. 1969;51:239–254.

10. Howland WJ, Curry JL, Buffington CB. Fulcrum fracture of the lumbar spine. *JAMA*. 1965;193:240–241.

11. Garrett JW, Braunstein PW. Seat belt syndrome. *J Trauma*. 1962;2:220–238.

12. Rennie W, Mitchell N. Flexion distraction fractures of the thoracolumbar spine. *J Bone Joint Surg Am*. 1973;55:386–390.

13. Anderson PA, Henley MB, Rivara FP, et al. Flexion distraction and chance injuries to the thoracolumbar spine. *J Orthop Trauma*. 1991;5:153–160.

14. Miyanji F, Fisher CG, Keynan O, et al. Flexion-distraction injuries of the thoracolumbar spine: health-related quality of life and radiographic outcomes. *Top Spinal Cord Inj Rehabil*. 2006;12:58–69.

15. Vaccaro AR, Kim DH, Brodke DS, et al. Diagnosis and management of thoracolumbar spine fractures. *J Bone Joint Surg Am*. 2003;12:2456–2470.

16. Lee HM, Kim HS, Kim DJ, et al. Reliability of magnetic resonance imaging in detecting posterior ligamentous complex injury in thoracolumbar spinal fractures. *Spine*. 2000;25:2079–2084.

17. Finkelstein JA, Wai EK, Jackson SS, et al. Single-level fixation of flexion distraction injuries. *J Spinal Disord Tech*. 2003;16:236–242.

18. Vaccaro AR, Lehman RA, Hurlbert RJ, et al. A new classification of thoracolumbar injuries: the importance of injury morphology, the integrity of the posterior ligamentous complex, and neurologic status. *Spine*. 2005;30:2325–2333.

19. Denis F. The three column spine and its significance in the classification of acute thoracolumbar spinal injuries. *Spine*. 1983;8:817–831.

20. Liu YJ, Chang MC, Wang ST, et al. Flexion-distraction injury of the thoracolumbar spine. *Injury*. 2003;34:920–923.

21. Gertzbein SD, Court-Brown CM. Rationale for the management of flexion-distraction injuries of the thoracolumbar spine based on a new classification. *J Spinal Disord*. 1989;2:176–183.

22. McGuire RA, Freeland AE. Flexion-distraction injury of the thoracolumbar spine. *Orthopedics*. 1992;15:379–381.

23. Triantafyllou SJ, Gertzbein SD. Flexion distraction injuries of the thoracolumbar spine: a review. *Orthopedics*. 1992;15(3):357–364.

24. Vanichkachorn JS, Vaccaro AR. Nonoperative treatment of thoracolumbar fractures. *Orthopedics*. 1997;20:948–953.

25. Yu WY, Siu CM. Seat belt injuries of the lumbar spine—stable or unstable? *Paraplegia*. 1989;27:450–456.

26. Schunemann HJ, Jaeschke R, Cook DJ, et al. ATS Documents Development and Implementation Committee. An official ATS statement: grading the quality of evidence and strength of recommendations in ATS guidelines and recommendations. *Am J Respir Crit Care Med*. 2006;174:605–614.

27. Neumann P, Nordwall A, Osvalder AL. Traumatic instability of the lumbar spine: a dynamic in vitro study of flexion-distraction injury. *Spine*. 1995;20:1111–1121.

28. Beringer W, Potts E, Khairi S, et al. Percutaneous pedicle screw instrumentation for temporary internal bracing of nondisplaced bony Chance fractures. *J Spinal Disord Tech*. 2007;20:242–247.

29. Eichinger JK, Arrington ED, Kerr GJ, et al. Bony flexion-distraction injury of the lower lumbar spine treated with instrumentation without fusion and early implant removal: a method of treatment to preserve lumbar motion: two-year follow-up of a teenage patient. *J Spinal Disord Tech*. 2007;20:93–96.

30. Sanderson PL, Fraser RD, Hall DJ, et al. Short segment fixation of thoracolumbar burst fractures without fusion. *Eur Spine J*. 1999;8:495–500.

31. Wang ST, Ma HL, Liu CL, et al. Is fusion necessary for surgically treated burst fractures of the thoracolumbar and lumbar spine?: a prospective, randomized study. *Spine*. 2006;31:2646–2652.

32. Weinstein JN, Collalto P, Lehmann TR. Thoracolumbar "burst" fractures treated conservatively: a long-term follow-up. *Spine*. 1988;13:33–38.

33. Ware JE, Snow KK, Kosinski M, et al. *SF-36 Health Survey: Manual and Interpretation Guide*. Boston, MA: The Health Institute, 1993.

34. Fairbank JCT, Pynsent PB. The Oswestry Disability Index. *Spine*. 2000;25:2940–2953.

35. Fisher CG, Wood KB. Introduction to and techniques of evidence-based medicine. *Spine*. 2007;32(suppl):66–72.

Metastatic Tumor of the Cervical Spine

JOSEPH H. SCHWAB, MD

EDITORS' CASE PRESENTATION

A 61-year-old woman with a history of renal cell carcinoma detected and treated 4 years ago with nephrectomy has a complaint of neck pain. She reports that her pain is aggravated by activity, particularly with neck rotation. She does not have any subjective weakness, numbness, or tingling in the upper or lower extremities. She has been using high-dose narcotic medication for her "cancer pain," though this has become increasingly less effective. She is currently receiving chemotherapy for oncological management and has not had radiation to the neck. She reports no other relevant comorbidities and is otherwise medically fit.

Examination reveals a fit, healthy woman. Overall, her neck range of motion is decreased by about 60% and she prefers to hold her neck in a neutral position. She has pain with the extremes of motion. She has tenderness to palpation of the upper cervical spine. She is neurologically intact to motor, sensory, and reflex testing. She has no other pertinent positives on examination.

Complete oncological workup reveals no other metastatic lesions.

Plain radiographic, magnetic resonance, CT, and arteriographic images are shown in Figures 16.1 to 16.4.

INTERPRETATION OF CLINICAL PRESENTATION

This 61-year-old female presents with a history of renal cell carcinoma as well as neck pain that is not being well controlled with narcotic pain medicine. Her pain

is worse with activity, and she does not have neurologic signs or symptoms. If I were encountering this patient for the first time in my clinic, I would feel the need to rule out metastatic renal cell carcinoma as the cause of her pain. I would be concerned that she has an unstable cervical spine based on her history of activity-related pain not responding to narcotics. Without looking at the images, her pain pattern seems more like that of instability rather than "cancer pain" per se. The instability may be due to the cancer; however, I think of "cancer pain" when the patient's symptoms are present even at rest or while in bed. The distinction is important because "cancer pain" may respond to chemotherapy or radiation, while "instability" pain will not respond to either.

Her physical examination is helpful in particular because it does not reveal myelopathy. However, her tendency to hold her head in a neutral position and the pain at extremes of motion further my concern for instability.

Figure 16.1 demonstrates a destructive lesion in the body of C3. There is focal collapse at this level seen on the lateral view. This image is quite helpful and it correlates well with her history and physical examination. The fact that she is tender in her upper cervical spine is not surprising based on these images. The anterior/posterior view does not demonstrate the destructive lesion as well due to the overlying mandible.

The CT scans demonstrate the lytic nature of this tumor the best. It also reveals the destruction of C2, which I did not appreciate on the plain x-rays. Nearly half of the body is destroyed on the left side. The vertebral artery on the left is embedded within the tumor; however, it does appear patent.

The T1- and T2-weighted MRIs demonstrate a large soft-tissue mass particularly posteriorly on the left side. The spinal cord is displaced by the mass. Her angiogram reveals a very vascular tumor, which correlates well with the patient's history of renal cell carcinoma as these tumors can be quite vascular.

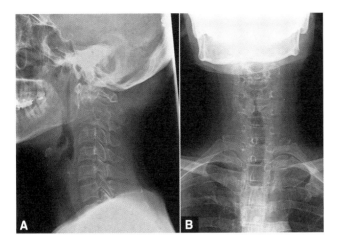

Figure 16.1.

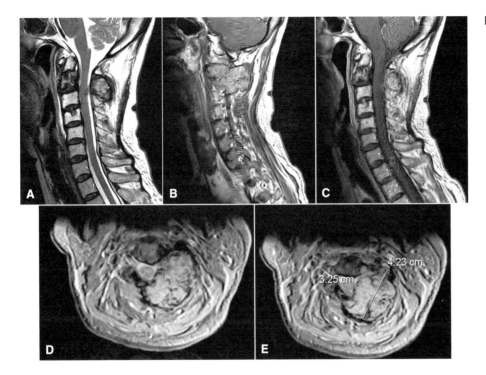

Figure 16.2.

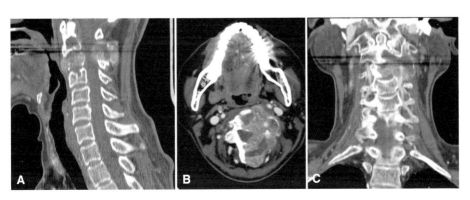

Figure 16.3.

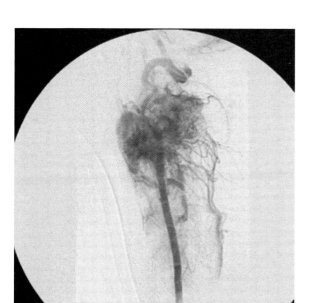

Figure 16.4.

DECLARATION OF SPECIFIC DIAGNOSIS

This 61-year-old woman with neck pain and a lytic lesion with large soft-tissue mass likely has metastatic renal cell carcinoma in the cervical spine.

BRAINSTORMING: WHAT ARE THE TREATMENT GOALS AND THE SURGICAL OPTIONS?

The treatment goals are to

1. Stabilize the spine
2. Prevent spinal cord compromise
3. Improve her pain
4. Improve/maintain quality of life

The treatment options are

1. Radiation alone
2. Surgical decompression with spinal stabilization
3. Surgical excision with spinal stabilization
4. Posterior stabilization
5. Anterior and posterior stabilization

EVALUATION OF THE LITERATURE

A search of the literature was carried out using the Pubmed search engine. I searched with the intent of reviewing articles specifically dealing with renal metastasis to the spine or skeleton. The first search used the key words *renal cell metastasis* and *bone metastasis*, which delivered 640 papers. A second search utilized *spine metastasis* instead of bone metastasis. Fifty-two articles were discovered. The titles of these articles were read and those that seemed relevant were further explored by reading the abstract. If the abstract seemed pertinent, then the entire article was reviewed.

Subsequent searches utilizing PubMed were performed using the key words *embolization, renal cell,* and/or *balloon occlusion*. Abstracts were scanned and pertinent articles were read. Subsequently, a search was performed using the key words *cervical spine, corpectomy,* and *biomechanics*. Abstracts were scanned and relevant articles were reviewed. Additionally, the bibliographies or particularly well-written articles were scanned for relevant articles, which were subsequently reviewed.

DETAILED REVIEW OF PERTINENT ARTICLES

Surgery and Radiation Versus Radiation Alone

There has been a prospective, randomized, non-blinded trial comparing surgery plus radiation therapy versus radiation alone for spinal cord compression from metastatic disease published by Patchell et al.[1] The patient in our example falls within most of the inclusion criteria of the study with some notable exceptions. She is over 18 years old and has metastatic disease with spinal cord compression. She has at least one sign or symptom (in this case pain) that is referable to her disease. Her lesion has not been confirmed as a metastatic lesion. A biopsy would have been necessary for her to be included in the randomized trial; it is necessary prior to begin treating this patient.

Our patient has a fracture at C3, which is noted on the lateral plain radiograph. This would have excluded her from the Patchell et al.[1] study as they would have classified her as unstable. All patients in the study were treated with high-dose corticosteroids including a bolus of 100-mg dexamethasone followed by 24 mg every 6 hours until the onset of radiation or surgery. Once randomized, patients underwent surgery or started radiation within 24 hours. Radiation included a total dose of 30 Gy in ten fractions.[1] Surgery was tailored to each patients needs.

The primary endpoint was the ability to walk after treatment. They defined walking as the ability to take a total of four steps with or without a gait aid. The study found that those patients who underwent surgical decompression followed by radiation maintained the ability to walk longer than those patients who underwent radiation alone. Furthermore, those patients who were unable to walk regained the ability to walk more frequently than those patients who underwent radiation alone. Finally, they found that those patients who underwent surgery survived longer than those who did not. These data have been used in support of surgical decompression for patients with symptomatic spinal cord compression.[1] The patient in this study would not have been randomized in their trial as she would have been classified as unstable. Radiation therapy will not render her spine stable, and randomizing her to the radiation arm of the study would have biased the data against radiation.

A follow-up study has been performed using the data from the prospective, randomized study mentioned above. Post hoc analysis of the data revealed that age <65 is an important predictor of ambulatory status and survival.[2]

Although there are no data proving that surgery is better for those patients with an unstable spine due to pathologic fracture, most physicians would not be comfortable treating such conditions nonoperatively. It is unlikely that contrary data will ever be collected in a randomized trial. Harrington classified spinal metastasis into five categories based on neurologic compromise and bone destruction: (1) no neurologic involvement, (2) bony involvement without collapse, (3) major neurologic involvement without bony involvement, (4) vertebral collapse with pain resulting from instability, and (5) vertebral collapse with instability and neurologic involvement. He recommended surgical intervention for those patients in category 4 or 5, both of which have instability.[3]

Oncologic Considerations

Assuming the pathologic diagnosis is metastatic renal cell carcinoma and that oncologic staging has not revealed any other site of disease in the setting of an unstable cervical fracture, the primary question becomes what type of surgery to perform rather than whether or not to operate.

There are two main points to consider with regard to surgery. The first issue pertains to the oncologic management of the tumor, and the second pertains to the stability of the spine. The first issue to consider is how aggressive to be with regard to tumor excision. The surgical approach must be guided by survival expectations. The three options that exist are palliative (laminectomy alone) decompression, aggressive debulking, and en bloc excision. There are no randomized trials comparing the three options. However, there have been several proposed mechanisms by which one can make this decision.

The classification by Tomita et al.[4] is based on the growth pattern of the tumor as well as the extent of metastasis. Our patient has a solitary renal cell metastasis. Her tumor would be given a score of 2 out of a possible 3 for renal cell metastasis. She has no visceral metastasis, and so she would be given a score of 1 out of 3. A score of 2 in this category represents a patient with treatable visceral metastasis, whereas a score of 3 is a patient with untreatable visceral metastasis. She has an isolated bony metastasis and so would also receive a score of 1 out of 2. A score of 2 represents multiple metastases. Her total score would be a 4 out of a possible 10. Tomita states that a patient with this clinical scenario ought to be approached with a goal of "middle term local control." They recommend a marginal or intralesional excision. They report a correlation coefficient of 0.690 using their prognostic system.[4]

A second classification system by Tokuhashi et al.[5] uses several more parameters in its decision tree: the patient's performance status, number of extra spinal bony metastases, the number of metastases in vertebrae, whether visceral metastases were present and whether they were resectable, the primary tumor type, and the Frankel grade. The primary tumor type is weighed more heavily than other parameters with a maximum score of 5 as opposed to the others that have a maximum score of 2. The highest score a patient could be given would be a 15. Our patient would be given a score of 13 out of 15. The scoring system would predict that she would live longer than 1 year, and they would recommend excisional surgery. They subgrouped their patients into three groups based on their prognosis. Group 1 survived <6 months, group 2 survived between 6 months and a year, and group 3 survived more than a year. They report that their prognostic scheme is correct in over 87% of cases.[5] They did not provide a correlation coefficient, which would give us an idea of how often their predictions were correct above that which you would expect from chance alone.

In a separate study analyzing only those patients with solitary spinal metastases, Sundaresan et al.[6] found that those patients with solitary renal metastases survived a median of 36 months. He recommended considering complete surgical excision for these patients.[6]

A more recent study concluded that surgery improved the quality of life of patients with spinal metastases by providing pain relief, maintaining mobility, and maintaining bowel and bladder function.[7] Nearly half of their patients had been treated with aggressive debulking, and 28% had been treated with en bloc excision. Renal cell carcinoma was one of the three most common histological subtypes in their groups treated with en bloc or aggressive debulking surgery.[7] Patients from these two groups had a median Tomita score of 5, which places them in the same Tomita group as our patient with a score of 4.

Based on the studies described above, we should perform either an aggressive debulking procedure or an en bloc resection for our patient. The implied advantage of en bloc excision would be increased survival. This would have to be weighed against the complications encountered with en bloc excision surgery. First, we should examine whether there are any data supporting en bloc excision for renal cell carcinoma in terms of survival advantage. There have been several retrospective reviews of the surgical management of renal cell metastases in the bones of the extremity.

In a retrospective review of bony metastases from renal cell carcinoma, which included 26 cases of solitary metastasis, the authors found that three parameters were found to influence survival in a positive way. The presence of only one osseous metastasis, wide resection of the metastasis, and a history of nephrectomy all correlated with survival. This study included four patients with solitary metastasis from the spine.[8] A second study from the Mayo Clinic, which analyzed 60 patients, did not find that a wide resection improved survival.[9] A large study from M.D. Anderson of 295 patients also failed to show a benefit to wide excision. While there is some evidence that wide excision is useful, there are larger series that contradict this finding.[10] It is not possible to make firm recommendations for or against wide excision based on these data, which are taken from cases of the extremity in most instances.

As mentioned previously, the merits of en bloc excision must be weighed against the possible complications of en bloc excision. Bandiera et al.[11] reported 43 major and 29 minor complications in 28 patients demonstrating the morbidity associated with en bloc excision in the spine. Some of these complications are severe and include death.

En bloc removal of the tumor is not the same as wide excision of the tumor. Based on the Enneking classification, a wide margin includes the entire tumor with a cuff of normal tissue around it.[12] A wide excision is not possible in this setting without removing the dura, which has been described for primary malignant disease.[13] It has not been described in the metastatic setting. In light of this, the surgical margin will be at best marginal and most likely intralesional.

It is important to remember that our goal of local control need not be carried solely by the surgeon. The role of radiation therapy in the management of tumors is evolving. The increased use of radiosurgery, intensity-modulated radiation therapy, as well as proton and carbon ion therapy offers significant promise. One prospective study reported local control rates over 90% using stereotactic radiation without surgery.[14] Furthermore, proton and carbon ion radiation have shown promise in treating "radioresistant" sarcomas, and they may play a larger role in the treatment of metastases in the future.[15]

Finally, the role of systemic therapy for renal cell metastasis is also evolving. There have been no prospective trials evaluating the benefit of systemic therapy in the local management of spinal metastasis. However, there have been prospective, randomized trials evaluating the efficacy of newer targeted agents including sunitinib (Sutent, Pfizer) and bevacizumab (Avastin, Genentech/Roche) in the management of metastatic renal cell carcinoma. Sunitinib targets VEGF-2, PDGF-Beta, c-kit, and Flt -3 tyrosine kinases, while bevacizumab targets VEGF. Sunitinib delayed progression of the tumor by 6 months when compared with interferon alone in patients with metastatic disease.[16] Similarly, bevacizumab delayed tumor progression by 3 to 5 months when given with interferon versus to interferon alone.[17,18] There are additional studies comparing the use of other targeted agents in the management of renal cell metastasis. Predicting survival in metastatic renal cell metastasis is a moving target. It is important for surgeons treating these conditions to be aware of the advances so they can alter their treatment algorithm accordingly.

Reconstructive Considerations

The patient has tumor compressing her spinal cord from the posterior and lateral margins. In addition, much of her C3 vertebral body and part of the C2 body have been destroyed. We must now weigh whether to proceed from posterior or anterior or both.

Posterior stabilization alone is an option and has been advocated by some.[19,20,21] This usually involves instrumenting more levels above and below the level of vertebral body involvement than would be performed if an anterior construct were added. In our case, it would likely involve fusion to the occiput down to the lower cervical spine. If an anterior reconstruction is entertained, then the posterior fixation need not encompass the occiput. In this case, screws placed in the lateral masses of C1 and the remaining pedicle of C2 are necessary.[22,23]

In our case, the C3 body is fractured and the C2 body is partially destroyed. A second stage using the anterolateral approach would allow these two vertebrae to be debulked from tumor as well as reconstructed. An anterior approach alone could be considered; however, this would not address the tumor burden posteriorly, which is displacing the spinal cord. In addition, there are good biomechanical data indicating that the addition of posterior stabilization provides a significant advantage after multilevel corpectomy in the cervical spine.[24] Furthermore, good long-term clinical results have been reported with anterior/posterior reconstruction after multilevel cervical corpectomy.[25]

Options for C2 and C3 reconstruction include static or expandable cages as well as methylmethacrylate. The odontoid and much of the C2 body are not involved with tumor. The transverse ligament and its attachments are intact. However, the superior facet of C2 is destroyed on one side and it will need to be reinforced. Reconstruction of the defect left after tumor excision can be readily performed with methylmethacrylate. Several retrospective studies have documented its safety as a means of corpectomy reconstruction in the cervical spine when combined with anterior plating.[26,27] A recent biomechanical model in the thoracic spine revealed that the combination of posterior instrumentation with anterior methylmethacrylate more than reconstitutes the rigidity of the spine.[28] A provocative approach for C2 corpectomy reconstruction utilizes a C2 prosthesis.[29] In our case, the remaining C2 body and the odontoid process will not be removed obviating the need for a prosthesis. In addition, this will allow us to expose the spine via a high cervical/retropharyngeal approach as opposed to a transoral approach.

Embolization

An important thing to consider is embolization. This is particular true in cases in which intralesional excision is expected. There have not been any prospective randomized studies evaluating the benefits of embolization for bony metastasis. However, there have been several retrospective reviews supporting its use as a means to reduce intra-operative blood loss.[30–33] Tomita et al. report embolizing not only the level of the tumor but the level above and below. They have found that this method significantly reduced blood loss without causing an increase in neurologic decline. This study was also retrospective.[34]

Balloon Occlusion of the Vertebral Artery

The vertebral artery is encased by the mass in this patient, and it is important to understand the potential neurologic consequences of its ligation. Evaluation of the relative importance of the vertebral artery to cerebral blood flow can be accomplished via balloon occlusion of the involved artery. There are retrospective studies regarding this technique in the management of head and neck aneurysms as well as the management of vertebral artery injuries.[35–37] While the technique has also been described in the treatment of primary and metastatic tumors of the spine, there have been no prospective trials.[38,39]

EVIDENTIARY TABLE AND SELECTION OF TREATMENT METHOD

The best available evidence leads us toward pursuing surgery in this case. The only randomized controlled study evaluating whether surgery plus radiation versus radiation alone would not have included our patient. She would have been excluded since she met their criteria for instability. I have included the article in my summary table as well as a subsequent post hoc analysis and a prospective study on the subject. They are the best studies to date on the problem of spinal cord compression from metastatic disease. All three indicate that surgery has a significant positive influence on outcome in patients with metastatic spine disease. While the issue of spine instability secondary to metastatic disease has not been specifically addressed in the literature, the risks of attempting nonoperative management are clearly outweighed by the known risks of surgery. In making my final recommendations regarding surgery, I am using the criteria outlined by Schunemann et al.[40] The criteria utilize the available evidence from the literature but mandate that the surgeon and patient balance the benefits, harms, and burdens of said intervention with the quality of the clinical evidence from the literature. In this case, the patient is in pain and she has a fracture. Her spine is unstable, and a potential consequence of further instability is damage to her spinal cord. This must be balanced with known but more predictable risks inherent in surgery. A surgical approach to this patient's problem is **strongly recommended** (Table 16.1).

Determining the type of surgery and the aggressiveness with which to pursue surgery can be aided with the literature available. In addition, and more importantly, the personal goals of the patient should be considered. The data available support surgery, but the type of surgery is not clear. Available retrospective studies evaluating the effect of wide resection for metastatic renal cell carcinoma are conflicting. In addition, the decision regarding surgery should be made in conjunction with the medical and radiation oncologists. The extent to which they can help control local disease as well as the patients' willingness to undergo such treatments is telling.

Both of the available prognostic surgical algorithms advise removing the tumor. A gross total resection would be the goal in this case.[41,42] While it is not possible to obtain a wide margin, this does not mean that aggressive surgery is not warranted. In some ways, the difficulty of intralesional resection in renal cell carcinoma is equal to en bloc excision due to its vascularity. A gross total resection will require both an anterior and a posterior approach. Again, it is important to think of the oncologic goals of surgery first and then meshing them with the stability goals. For instance, it is possible to perform a posterior decompression and occipital cervical fusion for this patient without attempting a gross total resection. Her spine can be decompressed and rendered stable in this manner; however, it would

TABLE 16.1 Evidentiary Table: A Summary of the Quality of Evidence for Comparison of Primarily Anterior Corpectomy Versus Laminoplasty for Multilevel Cervical Spondylotic Myelopathy.

Paper Author (Year)	Description	Summary of Results	Quality of Evidence
Patchell et al. (2005)	RCT comparing surgery plus XRT vs. XRT alone for high-grade spinal cord compression	Surgery plus XRT was superior to XRT alone regarding overall survival, function, and ambulation. Note: Patients with instability were excluded	Low
Tokuhashi et al. (2005)	Retrospective data used to develop a prognostic scoring system designed to help physicians decide when surgery is advisable	This scoring system proved useful with a correlation coefficient of 0.69 Note: Surgery is recommended based on this system, but the specific type of surgery is not clear	Low
Tomita et al. (1997)	Retrospective data used to develop a prognostic scoring system designed to help physicians decide when surgery is advisable	This system has been modified over time and it has been shown to be a useful tool when surgery is being considered Note: Surgery is recommended based on this system, but the specific type of surgery is not clear	Low
Shannon et al. (2004)	This biomechanical study was designed to evaluate anterior vertebral body reconstruction with methylmethacrylate combined with posterior fixation after corpectomy	Anterior reconstruction with methylmethacrylate combined with posterior fixation was equivalent to structural allograft in this model. Note: This was not a cervical spine model	Low
Singh et al. (2004)	Biomechanical study comparing different methods of cervical spine fixation following corpectomy	This study supports anterior and posterior reconstruction after multilevel corpectomy	Low

provide a less than optimal oncologic outcome. My recommendation would be for an anterior and a posterior approach to this tumor. Based on the grading recommendations set forth by Schunemann et al., my proposed treatment would be considered a **weak recommendation**.

Once the decision has been made to pursue anterior and posterior surgery, then the reconstruction options must be considered. An anterior construct utilizing methylmethacrylate with or without a titanium cage has the support of several retrospective studies. Additionally, there are good biomechanical data supporting the use of methylmethacrylate in anterior constructs particularly when they are used in conjunction with posterior instrumentation. Posterior lateral mass screws in C1 and pedicle screws into C2 have been shown to provide the most stability of all C1-2 reconstructive options. A combination of anterior structural support combined with posterior instrumentation including C1 lateral mass and C2 pedicle screws is **strongly recommended.**

DEFINITIVE TREATMENT PLAN

The treatment of this patient will include 3 major points that include surgery, radiation, and systemic therapy. The surgical portion will include preoperative embolization as well as a balloon occlusion study of the left vertebral artery. Assuming the embolization was successful and that collateral flow existed after occluding the left vertebral artery, I would begin with a posterior approach. The posterior approach would involve laminectomy at C2 and C3. The proximal and distal extent of the vertebral artery, above and below the tumor, would be identified and ligated. The left C2 and C3 nerve roots would be identified and protected. Aggressive removal of the left sided mass would be performed. The anterior aspect of the spine would be accessible due to the excision of the artery and roots as well as the fact that the tumor had destroyed the pedicle of C2. All gross tumor would be removed. Lateral mass screws would be placed into C1, and a pedicle screw would be placed into C2 on the right side. Lateral mass screws would be placed from C3 through C5. An anterior retropharyngeal approach would then allow the remaining tumor to be removed from C2 and C3. A titanium cage would be fitted into the defect left after removing the tumor. The cage would be filled with methylmethacrylate. The bone cement would be used to replace the superior facet of C2 on the left. An anterior plate placed would be inserted into what remained of the C2 body and also into the C4 body.

PREDICTING OUTCOMES

The patient has metastatic renal cell carcinoma. There is evidence that metastasectomy can improve survival; long-term survival has been noted in a subset of patients.[8,43] However, that seems to be the exception. A large series of surgically treated, metastatic renal cell carcinoma to bone indicated that over 50% of patients had died by 12 months. Thirty percent of patients were alive at 2 years and 10% at 5 years.[10] Still, there is cause for hope as targeted therapies have demonstrated increased disease-free survival up to 6 months. Our patient does fall into a more favorable category in that she has had a nephrectomy, her first metastasis occurred several years after her primary tumor was removed, she has no visceral metastasis, and she is <65 years of age.[2,8,44] Furthermore, she has not been treated with any systemic therapy so that there is hope that she will be a responder. Her reconstruction is sound, and it is likely that her quality of life will be improved with my plan.[7]

Treatments are evolving and the survival patterns of these patients are likely to change over time. Patients with metastatic disease pose a very difficult problem and all decisions should be made in collaboration with the patient's wishes as well as the recommendations of the medical and radiation oncologists.

SUMMARY

A 61-year-old woman with a pathologic cervical fracture along with spinal cord compression from metastatic renal cell carcinoma was presented. Surgical stabilization is indicated for the fracture alone; however, her prognosis is relatively good and so a sound oncologic procedure must also be considered. We have recommended a circumferential decompression and reconstruction of her cervical spine. The construct recommended is based on sound biomechanical data. She has several prognostic factors in her favor and it is hopeful that she will respond to targeted therapy. With good luck, she could be alive in 5 years.

REFERENCES

1. Patchell RA, et al. Direct decompressive surgical resection in the treatment of spinal cord compression caused by metastatic cancer: a randomised trial. *Lancet.* 2005;366(9486):643–648.
2. Chi JH, et al. Selecting treatment for patients with malignant epidural spinal cord compression-does age matter? Results from a randomized clinical trial. *Spine.* 2009;34(5):431–435.
3. Harrington KD. Metastatic disease of the spine. *J Bone Joint Surg Am.* 1986;68(7):1110–1115.
4. Tomita K, et al. Surgical strategy for spinal metastases. *Spine.* 2001;26(3):298–306.
5. Tokuhashi Y, Ajiro Y, Umezawa N. Outcome of treatment for spinal metastases using scoring system for preoperative evaluation of prognosis. *Spine.* 2009;34(1):69–73.
6. Sundaresan N, et al. Surgery for solitary metastases of the spine: rationale and results of treatment. *Spine.* 2002;27(16):1802–1806.
7. Ibrahim A, et al. Does spinal surgery improve the quality of life for those with extradural (spinal) osseous metastases? An international multicenter prospective observational study of 223 patients. Invited submission from the Joint Section Meeting on Disorders of the Spine and Peripheral Nerves, March 2007. *J Neurosurg Spine.* 2008;8(3):271–278.
8. Jung ST, et al. Treatment of osseous metastases in patients with renal cell carcinoma. *Clin Orthop Relat Res.* 2003(409):223–231.
9. Fuchs B, Trousdale RT, Rock MG. Solitary bony metastasis from renal cell carcinoma: significance of surgical treatment. *Clin Orthop Relat Res.* 2005(431):187–192.
10. Lin PP, et al. Patient survival after surgery for osseous metastases from renal cell carcinoma. *J Bone Joint Surg Am.* 2007;89(8):1794–1801.
11. Bandiera S, et al. Complications of en bloc resections in the spine. *Orthop Clin North Am.* 2009;40(1):125–131, vii.
12. Enneking WF. A system of staging musculoskeletal neoplasms. *Clin Orthop Relat Res.* 1986(204):9–24.
13. Biagini R, et al. En bloc vertebrectomy and dural resection for chordoma: a case report. *Spine.* 2003;28(18): E368–E372.
14. Svedman C, et al. A prospective Phase II trial of using extracranial stereotactic radiotherapy in primary and metastatic renal cell carcinoma. *Acta Oncol.* 2006;45(7): 870–875.
15. DeLaney TF, et al. Phase II study of high-dose photon/ proton radiotherapy in the management of spine sarcomas. *Int J Radiat Oncol Biol Phys,* 2009;74(3):732–739.
16. Motzer RJ, et al. Sunitinib versus interferon alfa in metastatic renal-cell carcinoma. *N Engl J Med.* 2007;356(2): 115–124.
17. Escudier B, et al. Bevacizumab plus interferon alfa-2a for treatment of metastatic renal cell carcinoma: a randomised, double-blind phase III trial. *Lancet.* 2007;370 (9605):2103–2111.
18. Rini BI, et al. Bevacizumab plus interferon alfa compared with interferon alfa monotherapy in patients with metastatic renal cell carcinoma: CALGB 90206. *J Clin Oncol.* 2008;26(33):5422–5428.

19. Bilsky MH, et al. Diagnosis and management of a metastatic tumor in the atlantoaxial spine. *Spine.* 2002;27(10):1062–1069.

20. Fourney DR, et al. Management of atlantoaxial metastases with posterior occipitocervical stabilization. *J Neurosurg.* 2003;98(2 suppl):165–170.

21. Shin H, et al. Occipitocervical fusion after resection of cranioverterbral junction tumors. *J Neurosurg Spine.* 2006;4(2):137–144.

22. Puttlitz CM, et al. Stability analysis of cranioverterbral junction fixation techniques. *J Bone Joint Surg Am.* 2004;86-A(3):561–568.

23. Harms J, Melcher RP. Posterior C1-C2 fusion with polyaxial screw and rod fixation. *Spine.* 2001;26(22):2467–2471.

24. Singh K, et al. Biomechanical comparison of cervical spine reconstructive techniques after a multilevel corpectomy of the cervical spine. *Spine.* 2003;28(20):2352–2358; discussion 2358.

25. Acosta FL Jr, et al. Long-term biomechanical stability and clinical improvement after extended multilevel corpectomy and circumferential reconstruction of the cervical spine using titanium mesh cages. *J Spinal Disord Tech.* 2008;21(3):165–174.

26. Timlin M, et al. Management of metastatic tumors to the spine using simple plate fixation. *Am Surg.* 1995;61(8):704–708.

27. Miller DJ, et al. Coaxial double-lumen methylmethacrylate reconstruction in the anterior cervical and upper thoracic spine after tumor resection. *J Neurosurg.* 2000;92(2 suppl):181–190.

28. Shannon FJ, et al. Biomechanical analysis of anterior poly-methyl-methacrylate reconstruction following total spondylectomy for metastatic disease. *Spine.* 2004;29(19):2096–2012.

29. Jeszenszky D, et al. C2 prosthesis: anterior upper cervical fixation device to reconstruct the second cervical vertebra. *Eur Spine J.* 2007;16(10):1695–1700.

30. Wallace S, et al. Embolization of renal carcinoma. *Radiology,* 1981;138(3):563–570.

31. Chatziioannou AN, et al. Preoperative embolization of bone metastases from renal cell carcinoma. *Eur Radiol.* 2000;10(4):593–596.

32. Layalle I, et al. Arterial embolization of bone metastases: is it worthwhile? *J Belge Radiol.* 1998;81(5):223–225.

33. Rehak S, et al. The role of embolization in radical surgery of renal cell carcinoma spinal metastases. *Acta Neurochir (Wien).* 2008;150(11):1177–1181; discussion 1181.

34. Tomita K, et al. Total en bloc spondylectomy for spinal tumors: improvement of the technique and its associated basic background. *J Orthop Sci.* 2006;11(1):3–12.

35. Sorteberg A, et al. Angiographic balloon test occlusion and therapeutic sacrifice of major arteries to the brain. *Neurosurgery.* 2008;63(4):651–660.

36. Anxionnat R, et al. Treatment of hemorrhagic intracranial dissections. *Neurosurgery.* 2008;62(6 suppl 3):1525–1531.

37. Herrera DA, Vargas SA, Dublin AB. Endovascular treatment of traumatic injuries of the vertebral artery. *Am J Neuroradiol.* 2008;29(8):1585–1589.

38. Bilsky MH, et al. Operative management of metastatic and malignant primary subaxial cervical tumors. *J Neurosurg Spine.* 2005;2(3):256–264.

39. Khalil IM, et al. Aneurysmal bone cyst of the cervical spine in a child: case report and review of the surgical role. *Surg Neurol.* 2006;65(3):298–303; discussion 303.

40. Schunemann HJ, et al. An official ATS statement: grading the quality of evidence and strength of recommendations in ATS guidelines and recommendations. *Am J Respir Crit Care Med.* 2006;174(5):605–614.

41. Tokuhashi Y, et al. A revised scoring system for preoperative evaluation of metastatic spine tumor prognosis. *Spine.* 2005;30(19):2186–2191.

42. Tomita K, et al. Total en bloc spondylectomy. A new surgical technique for primary malignant vertebral tumors. *Spine.* 1997;22(3):324–333.

43. Eggener SE, et al. Risk score and metastasectomy independently impact prognosis of patients with recurrent renal cell carcinoma. *J Urol.* 2008;180(3):873–878; discussion 878.

44. Toyoda Y, et al. Survival and prognostic classification of patients with metastatic renal cell carcinoma of bone. *Eur Urol.* 2007;52(1):163–168.

Thoracolumbar Burst Fracture

CHRISTOPHER S. BAILEY, MD, FRCSC, MSC

EDITORS' CASE PRESENTATION

A 46-year-old man presents with a chief complaint of back pain at the thoracolumbar junction following a ski injury in which he fell forcefully upon his buttocks. He has no complaints of numbness, tingling, or weakness. He is otherwise healthy and has no other injuries. Physical examination demonstrates minimal tenderness at the thoracolumbar junction. There is no swelling or palpable gap in the area. He is fit otherwise and is neurologically intact.

Radiographic imaging studies are shown in Figure 17.1A–E.

INTERPRETATION OF CLINICAL PRESENTATION

This case describes a 46-year-old man who has sustained a significant axial load to his spine while skiing and is now complaining of pain at the thoracolumbar region. It will be assumed that a complete assessment was performed identifying only this isolated spinal injury.[1] The mechanism of injury suggests that the patient most likely has sustained a burst fracture. Therefore, two important factors must be determined from the history, physical examination, and imaging studies: (1) whether an associated neurological injury has occurred (e.g., conus medullaris, cauda equina, or nerve root) and (2) the integrity of the posterior column. The posterior column was described by Denis to include the osseous posterior elements dorsal to and including the pedicles, as well as the facet and associated soft tissues including the capsules, ligamentum flavum, interspinous ligament, and supraspinous ligament.[2,3]

Both the history and physical examination exclude the possibility of an associated neurological injury.

With respect to thoracolumbar burst fractures, it is rare that a delayed significant neurological deficit will develop if it did not occur initially at the time of fracture.[4] However, it should be remembered that if nonoperative treatment is ultimately chosen, ambulation can produce lumbar radiculopathy, which is otherwise not detectable when the patient is recumbent.[5] In this case, it is unknown whether the patient was able to ambulate or ski following the injury, but this information would provide some insight into the "stability" of the fracture from both neurological and mechanical perspectives.

Determining whether the posterior column is competent is critical to assessing mechanical stability of this fracture.[6,7] Based on the AO classification, a burst fracture is produced by an axial load compression force, which does not disrupt the integrity of the posterior column.[8] This needs to be differentiated from a flexion-distraction or shear force, which will disrupt the posterior column, rendering the fracture unstable. History is important in identifying the injury mechanism. In this case, a direct load to the buttocks suggests a compression force. The physical exam of this patient identified minimal posterior tenderness in the location of the fracture with no palpable gap or swelling in the area. However, physical exam, specifically palpation for a gap, has a low negative predictive value and sensitivity (i.e., large possibility of a false negative), so it should not be relied upon to exclude posterior column injury in this patient.[9]

The axial CT cut (Fig. 17.1D) demonstrates a vertebral body fracture with associated retropulsion of bone into the spinal canal, producing an approximate 20% compromise. This confirms that at least a two column burst fracture has occurred. The facet joints at the level of this axial cut show no evidence of subluxation or widening. The sagittal CT cut (Fig. 17.1E) reveals an L2 burst fracture, which involves only the superior endplate, which is the most common pattern of fracture.[10] The kyphotic deformity approximates 10 degrees measured using the Cobb technique.[11] This represents a total deformity of approximately 20 degrees beyond

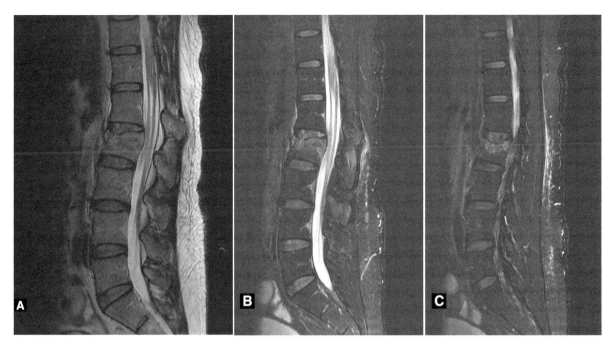

Figure 17.1.

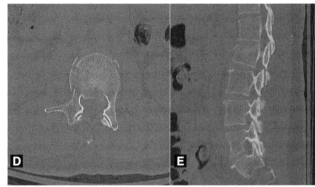

the 10 degrees of normal lordosis expected at this level.[12,13] This image confirms that the L1-2 and L2-3 facet joints are not subluxated, and there is no evidence of a distraction or shear fracture involving the posterior elements.

Three sagittal images are available from the MRI, which are T2 weighted with and without fat suppression (Fig. 17.1A–C). These images confirm the diagnosis of an L2 superior endplate burst fracture with an associated high signal in the superior aspects of the vertebral body and L1-2 disc. The ligamentum flavum and supraspinous ligaments appear to be in continuity. Some increased signal is seen within the interspinous ligaments and dorsal to the supraspinous ligament at the L2 level, which is suggestive of some degree of injury but not indicative of posterior column instability in light of the intact supraspinous ligament and ligament flavum. It has been demonstrated that MRI is highly accurate in detecting injury to the posterior ligamentous complex,[9,14] but the accuracy of determining the severity of the injury has not been determined.

DECLARATION OF SPECIFIC DIAGNOSIS

This patient has a so-called stable L2 burst fracture. It is described as stable because it is not associated with a neurological deficit or a mechanically destabilizing injury to the posterior elements such as a flexion-distraction injury or fracture-dislocation.

BRAINSTORMING: WHAT ARE THE TREATMENT GOALS AND THE TREATMENT OPTIONS?

Treatment goals:

1. Provide spinal stability to ensure early mobilization with adequate pain control
2. Prevent significant progression of deformity
3. Minimize the risk of neurological deterioration

4. Minimize the risk of treatment related complications

5. To ensure the best long-term functional outcome

Treatment options:

1. Prolonged recumbency followed by a thoracolumbosacral immobilization

2. Thoracolumbosacral orthosis (TLSO) and early mobilization

3. Postural kyphosis correction and percutaneous instrumentation

4. Open posterior realignment and stabilization ± fusion

5. Anterior corpectomy, instrumentation, and fusion

6. Combined anterior and posterior procedure

EVALUATION OF THE LITERATURE

A comprehensive literature search was undertaken utilizing the electronic databases of Medline (1966–2007), Embase (1980–2007), CINAHL (1982–2007), and Cochrane–EBM Reviews and controlled trials using the following MeSh and text word headings: fracture, and burst, and thoracolumbar or thoracic or lumbar, and intact neurolog$ or without neurolog$. Studies meeting the following criteria were included: thoracolumbar burst fracture (T10-L2); age 16 years or older; no neurological deficit; operative or nonoperative treatment; an outcome measure including radiographic, pain, function, disability, or health related quality of life assessment; and published in English. Bibliographies of selected articles were reviewed to detect other pertinent citations. One hundred and sixty two

abstracts were reviewed. Of these, 23 met all inclusion criteria.[4,15–36] The most common reasons for exclusion of articles were heterogeneous nature of the patient cohort (e.g., the inclusion of patients with neurological deficit, differing types of fractures) or report of only lower lumbar fractures. Moreover, studies in which the subgroup data from patients meeting the inclusion criteria could be extracted from the heterogeneous cohort were included in the review.

DETAILED REVIEW OF PERTINENT ARTICLES AND EVIDENTIARY TABLE

Operative or Nonoperative Treatment

To help decide whether to operate or to treat non-operatively, the literature search provides four original studies and one review: two retrospective case series by Kraemer et al. and Butler et al.[22,27] a randomized controlled trial (RCT) by Wood et al.[36] a quasi-RCT by Shen et al.,[34] and a systematic review by Thomas et al.[4] (Table 17.1). Also, one prospective study applied the Load Sharing Classification (LSC) to a cohort of nonoperatively treated patients so as to predict final outcomes.[18] It should be noted that a Cochrane Systematic review comparing operative versus nonoperative treatment was published in 2008 and was therefore not identified by the current literature review.[37] However, the Cochrane review included only the RCT by Wood et al. and therefore would not have contributed additional data to this analysis.

The RCT by Wood et al.[36] provides the best evidence by which to direct treatment. However, it should be considered moderate-quality evidence due to a number of methodological issues, which were well outlined in

| TABLE 17.1 | Operative Versus Nonoperative Treatment. |

Paper Author (Year)	Description	Summary of Results	Level of Evidence
Wood et al. (2003)	RCT	Anterior or posterior surgery; cast/custom TLSO for 12–16 wk, AAT with orthosis, Nonop group superior in SF-36 function, RMD, Oswestry (NSD); no difference in kyphosis or VAS pain	Moderate
Shen et al. (2001)	Quasi-RCT	Short-segment posterior instrumentation + fusion; custom TLSO for 3 mo, AAT with orthosis, op group superior VAS pain and Greenough LBOS early; op group less final kyphotic deformity	Moderate
Kraemer et al. (1996)	Case series	Anterior or posterior surgery; nonspecified nonoperative, no difference final RMD, SF-36, SF-36 pain, kyphosis	Very low
Butler et al. (2005)	Case series	Short-segment posterior instrumentation + fusion; custom TLSO for 3 mo followed by 6–12 wk TLSO, immediate AAT with cast, less pain in non-op group, improved kyphosis correction in surgical group	Very low

the systematic review by Thomas et al.[4] Fifty-three of fifty-five consecutive subjects were randomized to either nonoperative treatment (postural reduction plus 12–16 weeks cast or TLSO) or surgical treatment (posterior or anterior construct based on surgeon's preference). At a mean follow-up of 44 months, there were no differences in Visual Analogue Scale (VAS) pain or Oswestry Disability Index scores, but the nonoperative group was superior in the Roland Morris Disability (RMD) and SF-36 physical role and function scores. Although average kyphosis was significantly improved in the operative group compared to the nonoperative group at discharge, at final follow-up, there was no significant difference. The mean hospital stay was almost three days shorter for the nonoperative group. The operative cohort endured a combined nineteen complications in comparison to two in the nonoperative group. Initial hospital cost was significantly greater for the operative group.

Shen et al. compared 47 patients treated with a custom TLSO worn for 3 months with immediate ambulation as tolerated to 33 patients treated by reduction followed by short-segment instrumentation and posterior autograft fusion. At the time of enrollment, seven patients initially randomized to operative treatment immediately crossed over to the nonoperative arm, breaking the randomization process. Thus, the study must be downgraded from high-quality evidence to moderate-quality evidence. The mean hospital stay was not significantly different, but the cost was four times greater for the surgical cohort. The surgical group had significantly less pain as measured by VAS at 1 and 3 months, which equalized afterward. The surgical group had a significantly higher Greenough low back outcome score (LBOS) at 1, 3, and 6 months, with no difference later. The mean kyphosis at 2 years was 24 degrees in the nonoperative arm and 12 degrees in the surgical arm. Five patients required a second surgery for hardware removal.

To help predict prognosis, Aligizakis et al.[18] prospectively assessed the functional outcome of 60 consecutive patients treated with 6 months of a TLSO. They found that 55 of 60 patients had a satisfactory outcome and a LSC score of 3 or 4. The remaining five patients had a LSC score of 5 or 6, and all had unsatisfactory outcomes. This observational study represents low-quality evidence. A significant drawback of the study is that even though the Denis Pain and work scales were used to assess outcome, the definition of "satisfactory" was not clearly defined and apparently arbitrary. Despite this drawback and low-quality evidence, the assertion that a LSC score of 5 or 6 prognosticates a poor outcome compels one to more strongly consider surgery for such a patient.

However, this result can be refuted by both the studies of Shen et al.[34] and Wood et al.[36] Shen et al. did not directly report the LSC score in their study; however,

they did report two of the three components of the LSC as a combined score called the load share score. They also reported the kyphosis angle, which is the third component of the LSC. For the nonoperative group, the average load share score was 4.1 and the mean presenting kyphosis was 21 degrees.[34] Because a kyphosis of 21 degrees is awarded three points in the LSC,[38] the average LSC for the nonoperative group must be 5 or greater. Given that there is no significant difference in load share score, kyphosis, and final outcome between treatment groups would refute the suggestion that an LSC score of 5 or more necessitates surgery to improve outcome. Similarly, Wood et al.[36] reported individual data for each subject allowing a minimal LCS score of 5 to be assigned for 13 of the patients treated conservatively (kyphosis >9 degrees receives a score of 3 and the minimal score for the remaining two components of the LSC must each equal 1). Eleven of these 13 patients are reported to have minimal to no pain and a RMD of <3/24 at final outcome. Therefore, an LCS score should not help direct the decision to operate or treat conservatively due to the contradicting studies' results.

In summary, the RCTs of Shen et al.[34] and Wood et al.[36] represent moderate-quality evidence that for long-term outcome there is no difference between surgical treatment and a TLSO for a neurologically intact patient with a thoracolumbar burst fracture. Shen et al. demonstrated that a superior improvement existed in pain for 3 months and in functional outcome for 6 months in the surgically treated group. However, my post hoc analysis of the presented data reveals that, although statistically significant, the minimum clinically important difference for pain[39,40] was detected until only 1 month and for functional outcome at only 3 months.[41] Shen et al. also demonstrated a smaller residual posttraumatic kyphosis in the operative group. However, the systematic review by Thomas et al.[4] found no correlation between subjective outcome and kyphosis. Both the Shen and Wood articles describe a higher complication rate and repeat surgery rate for the operative treatment cohorts. Finally, the pertinent articles detailed above are well generalized to the patient described in the case presentation. Therefore, there is moderate-quality evidence to suggest the additional risk of surgery in the current patient is not justified.[4]

Nonoperative Treatment

The literature search identified seven case series providing low-quality to very low-quality evidence regarding the outcome of conservatively treated patients with neurologically intact thoracolumbar burst fractures (Table 17.2). The results, however, are very similar in that they show high success rates as measured by pain and work status.[18,19,24–26,30] These findings are consistent with those of the studies comparing operative and nonoperative treatment. Wood et al. demonstrated an

TABLE 17.2	Nonoperative Treatment.		
Paper Author (Year)	**Description**	**Summary of Results**	**Level of Evidence**
Cantor et al. (1993)	Prospective cohort	Total contact TLSO 14–24 wk, AAT with orthosis, 15/18 very little/no pain on pain scale of Denis; 95% satisfactory score on Work scale of Denis, <5 degrees kyphosis progression, 15/18 very little/no pain on pain scale of Denis; 95% satisfactory score on Work scale of Denis, <5 degrees kyphosis progression	Low
Aligizakis et al. (2002)	Prospective cohort	Custom TLSO for 6 mo, AAT, 50/60 no or minimal pain (Denis), 55 returned to work, average 2 degrees kyphotic deformity progression, 50/60 no or minimal pain (Denis), 55 returned to work, average 2 degrees kyphotic deformity progression	Low
Mumford et al. (1993)	Case series	Bed rest for average 31 d (range: 7–61 d), bracing for average 12 wk (range: 2–24), 66% good or excellent outcome based on Denis work status and VAS pain, 66% good or excellent outcome based on Denis work status and VAS pain	Very low
Shen and Shen (1999)	Case series	Jewitt brace or no orthosis, AAT, 32/38 very little/no pain (Denis); 3 unable to work; 6 degrees maximum kyphosis progression	Very low
Chan et al. (1993)	Case series	Cast, 8/8 no or minimal pain, preinjury work capacity, 6 degrees maximum deformity progression, 8/8 no or minimal pain, preinjury work capacity, 6 degrees maximum deformity progression	Very low
Chow et al. (1996)	Case series	Cast or Jewitt brace for 12–24 mo, AAT with orthosis, 19/24 no or minimal pain, slight progression (average 2.3 degrees) of kyphosis, 19/24 no or minimal pain, slight progression (average 2.3 degrees) of kyphosis	Very low
Aligizakis et al. (2002)	Case series	4-wk strict recumbency followed by 6 mo TLSO, 25/30 no, or minimal pain (Denis), some kyphotic deformity progression	Very low

RMD, Roland Morris Disability Questionnaire.

average VAS pain of 1.9, RMD of 3.9 (low disability), and Oswestry score of 10.7 (0–20 indicates minimal disability).[36] Shen et al.[34] found an average 2-year VAS pain of 1.5 and Greenough LBOS of 65, which corresponds to excellent patient status.

A variety of nonoperative treatment methods have been used in these studies including body cast, custom TLSO, hyperextension Jewett brace, and no brace in association with variable mobilization protocols ranging from 4 weeks of strict recumbency to immediate activity as tolerated (AAT). Although none of the studies were designed to determine the ideal conservative treatment protocol, it is clear that early mobilization and less restrictive orthosis are not required to achieve a successful outcome. The extreme example of this was described in the study by Shen

and Shen.[33] While only 9 of the 38 patients who were prescribed a Jewett brace actually wore it, more than 80% of patients reported little to no pain and only three patients were precluded from work because of pain. The ideal duration of treatment in a brace is also unknown, but based on the findings of this review, it appears that extended wear longer than 12 weeks is not necessary. In my experience, this is in keeping with current standards of practice.

SELECTION OF TREATMENT METHOD

Based on the evidence identified by the literature search, I would recommend the patient be treated conservatively with an off-the-shelf orthosis such as a Jewett extension brace and immediate ambulation as tolerated. There is moderate-quality evidence to support treating the patient nonoperatively using a brace with immediate ambulation.

All original treatment goals would be satisfied with the recommended treatment plan.

1. Brace treatment provides adequate spinal stability to allow for early mobilization. Both the studies by Wood et al.[36] and Shen et al.[34] comparing operative to nonoperative treatment found a shorter mean hospital stay for those patients treated nonoperatively.

2. Some progression of kyphotic deformity will occur with brace treatment but a number of studies demonstrated that it is <7 degrees from initial deformity. Importantly, the degree of posttraumatic kyphosis was not found to correlate with clinical outcome.[4,16,21,22,25,26,30,31,33,34] Certainly, the average residual kyphosis will likely be less if the patient is treated with surgery. Apart from cosmesis, there is no detrimental implication to outcome.

3. Treatment with a brace poses minimal risk of neurological deterioration.[4] Furthermore, the severity of spinal canal compromise cannot be considered an indication for surgery in the neurologically intact patient as at least some resorption of retropulsed fragments over time with gradual reconstitution of the spinal canal diameter is expected.[18,24,25,33,34,42–45] However, as cautioned previously, with initial mobilization, a radiculopathy can occur that may require surgical intervention to facilitate mobilization, although this is unlikely.[5]

4. Treatment-related complications are unlikely with conservative treatment and much less in frequency and severity compared to those demonstrated with operative treatment (Tables 17.1 and 17.2). The most common complication reported with nonoperative treatment is a urinary tract infection, which most likely is related to catheterization secondary to transient urinary retention.

5. Brace treatment has a high likelihood of achieving successful functional outcome as described in the evidentiary Tables 17.1 and 17.2. There is moderate-quality evidence that nonoperative treatment is at least equal to operative treatment for this patient.

DEFINITIVE TREATMENT PLAN

At the time of initial hospitalization, both physiotherapy and occupational therapy would clear the patient for discharge. The patient would be required to wear the brace for 10 to 12 weeks. A 90-degree hip flexion precaution would be implemented. The patient would be discharged with adequate oral analgesia. Weekly follow-up with upright x-rays would be required for the first 3 weeks to ensure that an unexpected progressive kyphotic deformity did not occur. I would expect no more that 7 to 10 degrees of further kyphosis from the initial (recumbent) measurement. Isometric core stability exercise would be started as soon as the patient could tolerate and continued during the duration of the brace treatment. When the brace was discontinued, the patient would initially wean from the brace and then begin an extensive rehabilitation directed by physiotherapy.

In accordance with the method of grading recommendations set forth by Schunemann et al., the proposed treatment would be considered a strong recommendation based on moderate-quality of evidence.[46] To be considered a strong recommendation, the benefits of the treatment must clearly outweigh the harms and burdens. This has been demonstrated by the evidence outlined above, would be in keeping with the preference of the patient (if surgery does not provide a superior outcome then why have it!), and is consistent with my experience as a spine surgeon.[5]

PREDICTING OUTCOMES

According to the literature, it is most likely that this patient will have an excellent outcome. As illustrated in Tables 17.1 and 17.2, the evidence suggests that over 80% of patients who sustain a thoracolumbar burst fracture without neurological deficit and no posterior column instability will have little to no pain at final follow-up and return back to their preinjury level of activity and work status.[18,19,22,24–26,33,34,36] In the context of health-related quality of life, Wood et al.[36] reported that the average score for the eight dimensions of health assessed by the SF-36 was similar to the general population norms. A residual kyphotic deformity of <30 degrees will be present in this patient's case, and it will likely not produce significant pain or dysfunction.[4,16,21,22,25,26,30,31,33,34]

My experience as an orthopaedic spine surgeon is similar to what the evidence demonstrates. The interim analysis of an ongoing multicentered RCT comparing brace treatment to no orthosis for the treatment of thoracolumbar burst fractures has shown very similar results: mean VAS pain <3 by 3 months, mean RMD score of 3 by 6 months, mean SF-36 physical component summary score to be 90% of normal at 1 year, and an average kyphotic deformity of 16 degrees (SD = 6 degrees).[5]

Therefore, taking into account the evidence and my personal experience, I would counsel this patient that surgery is not superior to brace treatment for his injury.

In addition, there is an 80% chance if treated with a TLSO that he will have little to no pain and return to near normal function within 3 to 6 months. I would also inform him that there is a small chance that this fracture will require surgical intervention and the risks and complications associated with brace treatment are small. Furthermore, the patient would be advised that he will have a residual gibbus at the thoracolumbar junction but that it is unlikely to cause significant symptoms or dysfunction.

SUMMARY

A 46-year-old man complaining of back pain at the thoracolumbar junction following a ski injury in which he fell forcefully upon his buttocks is presented. The history and physical examination are consistent with a burst fracture. Investigations confirm an L2 burst fracture without a significant posterior column injury, thus ruling out an associated flexion-distraction injury. As this fracture is stable from a mechanical and neurological perspective, and there are no patient factors excluding nonoperative treatment, I would make a strong recommendation to treat him with a Jewett brace and early mobilization.

REFERENCES

1. Harris MB, Sethi RK. The initial assessment and management of the multiple-trauma patient with an associated spine injury. *Spine*. 2006 May 15;31(11 suppl):S9–S15.

2. Denis F. The three column spine and its significance in the classification of acute thoracolumbar spinal injuries. *Spine*. 1983 Nov;8(8):817–831.

3. Denis F. Spinal instability as defined by the three-column spine concept in acute spinal trauma. *Clin Orthop*. 1984 Oct;(189):65–76.

4. Thomas KC, Bailey CS, Dvorak MF, et al. Comparison of operative and nonoperative treatment for thoracolumbar burst fractures in patients without neurological deficit: a systematic review. *J Neurosurg Spine*. 2006 May;4(5):351–358.

5. Bailey CS, Dvorak MF, Thomas KC, et al. TLSO versus No orthosis for the treatment of thoracolumbar burst fractures: Interim analysis of a multi-centred randomized clinical equivalence trial. *J Neurosurg Spine*. 2009 Sep;11:295–303.

6. James KS, Wenger KH, Schlegel JD, et al. Biomechanical evaluation of the stability of thoracolumbar burst fractures. *Spine*. 1994 Aug 1;19(15):1731–1740.

7. Oxland TR, Panjabi MM, Southern EP, et al. An anatomic basis for spinal instability: a porcine trauma model. *J Orthop Res*. 1991 May;9(3):452–462.

8. Magerl F, Aebi M. A comprehensive classification of thoracic and lumbar injuries. In: Aebi M, ed. *AO ASIF Principles in Spine Surgery*. Germany: Springer, 1998:20–41.

9. Lee HM, Kim HS, Kim DJ, et al. Reliability of magnetic resonance imaging in detecting posterior ligament complex injury in thoracolumbar spinal fractures. *Spine*. 2000 Aug 15;25(16):2079–2084.

10. Denis F, Armstrong GW, Searls K, et al. Acute thoracolumbar burst fractures in the absence of neurologic deficit. A comparison between operative and nonoperative treatment. *Clin Orthop Relat Res* 1984 Oct;(189):142–149.

11. Cobb JR. Outline for the study of scoliosis. Instructional course lectures, the American Academy of Orthopaedic surgeons 5:261–275, 1948.

12. Bernhardt M, Bridwell KH. Segmental analysis of the sagittal plane alignment of the normal thoracic and lumbar spines and thoracolumbar junction. *Spine*. 1989 Jul;14(7):717–721.

13. Jackson RP, McManus AC. Radiographic analysis of sagittal plane alignment and balance in standing volunteers and patients with low back pain matched for age, sex, and size. A prospective controlled clinical study. *Spine*. 1994 Jul 15;1914):1611–1618.

14. Haba H, Taneichi H, Kotani Y, et al. Diagnostic accuracy of magnetic resonance imaging for detecting posterior ligamentous complex injury associated with thoracic and lumbar fractures. *J Neurosurg*. 2003 Jul;99 (1 suppl):20–26.

15. Akbarnia BA, Crandall DG, Burkus K, et al. Use of long rods and a short arthrodesis for burst fractures of the thoracolumbar spine. A long-term follow-up study. *J Bone Joint Surg Am*. 1994 Nov;76(11):1629–1635.

16. Alanay A, Acaroglu E, Yazici M, et al. Short-segment pedicle instrumentation of thoracolumbar burst fractures: does transpedicular intracorporeal grafting prevent early failure? *Spine*. 2001 Jan 15;26(2):213–217.

17. Alanay A, Acaroglu E, Yazici M, et al. The effect of transpedicular intracorporeal grafting in the treatment of thoracolumbar burst fractures on canal remodeling. *Eur Spine J*. 2001 Dec;10(6):512–516.

18. Aligizakis A, Katonis P, Stergiopoulos K, et al. Functional outcome of burst fractures of the thoracolumbar spine managed non-operatively, with early ambulation, evaluated using the load sharing classification. *Acta Orthop Belg*. 2002 Jun;68(3):279–287.

19. Aligizakis A, Katonis P, Stergiopoulos K, et al. Conservative management of thoracolumbar burst spine fractures using gertzbein and load shearing classification. *Eur J Orthop Surg Traumatol*. 2002 Apr 20;12:36–41.

20. Andress HJ, Braun H, Helmberger T, et al. Long-term results after posterior fixation of thoraco-lumbar burst fractures. *Injury*. 2002 May;33(4):357–365.

21. Briem D, Lehmann W, Ruecker AH, et al. Factors influencing the quality of life after burst fractures of the thoracolumbar transition. *Arch Orthop Trauma Surg*. 2004 Sep;124(7):461–468.

22. Butler JS, Walsh A, O'Byrne J. Functional outcome of burst fractures of the first lumbar vertebra managed surgically and conservatively. *Int Orthop*. 2005 Feb;29(1):51–54.

23. Butt MF, Farooq M, Mir B, et al. Management of unstable thoracolumbar spinal injuries by posterior short segment spinal fixation. *Int Orthop*. 2007 Apr;31(2):259–264.

24. Cantor JB, Lebwohl NH, Garvey T, et al. Nonoperative management of stable thoracolumbar burst fractures with early ambulation and bracing. *Spine.* 1993 Jun 15;18(8):971–976.

25. Chan DP, Seng NK, Kaan KT. Nonoperative treatment in burst fractures of the lumbar spine (L2-L5) without neurologic deficits. *Spine.* 1993 Mar 1;18(3):320–325.

26. Chow GH, Nelson BJ, Gebhard JS, et al. Functional outcome of thoracolumbar burst fractures managed with hyperextension casting or bracing and early mobilization. *Spine.* 1996 Sep 15;21(18):2170–2175.

27. Kraemer WJ, Schemitsch EH, Lever J, et al. Functional outcome of thoracolumbar burst fractures without neurological deficit. *J Orthop Trauma.* 1996;10(8):541–544.

28. Kramer DL, Rodgers WB, Mansfield FL. Transpedicular instrumentation and short-segment fusion of thoracolumbar fractures: a prospective study using a single instrumentation system. *J Orthop Trauma.* 1995;9(6):499–506.

29. Laursen M, Hoy K, Hansen ES, et al. Recombinant bone morphogenetic protein-7 as an intracorporal bone growth stimulator in unstable thoracolumbar burst fractures in humans: preliminary results. *Eur Spine J.* 1999;8(6):485–490.

30. Mumford J, Weinstein JN, Spratt KF, et al. Thoracolumbar burst fractures. The clinical efficacy and outcome of nonoperative management. *Spine.* 1993 Jun 15;18(8):955–970.

31. Sanderson PL, Fraser RD, Hall DJ, et al. Short segment fixation of thoracolumbar burst fractures without fusion. *Eur Spine J.* 1999;8(6):495–500.

32. Sasso RC, Cotler HB. Posterior instrumentation and fusion for unstable fractures and fracture-dislocations of the thoracic and lumbar spine. A comparative study of three fixation devices in 70 patients. *Spine.* 1993 Mar 15;18(4):450–460.

33. Shen WJ, Shen YS. Nonsurgical treatment of three-column thoracolumbar junction burst fractures without neurologic deficit. *Spine.* 1999 Feb 15;24(4):412–415.

34. Shen WJ, Liu TJ, Shen YS. Nonoperative treatment versus posterior fixation for thoracolumbar junction burst fractures without neurologic deficit. *Spine.* 2001 May 1; 26(9):1038–1045.

35. Sochacki MA, Brantigan JW. Surgical treatment of L1 burst fracture: a case report. *Nebr Med J.* 1995 Dec;80(12): 354–356.

36. Wood K, Butterman G, Mehbod A, et al. Operative compared with nonoperative treatment of a thoracolumbar burst fracture without neurological deficit: a prospective, randomized study. *J Bone Joint Surg Am.* 2003 May; 85-A(5):773–781.

37. Yi L, Jingping B, Gele J, et al. Operative versus nonoperative treatment for thoracolumbar burst fractures without neurological deficit. *Cochrane Database Syst Rev.* 2006;(4):CD005079.

38. McCormack T, Karaikovic E, Gaines RW. The load sharing classification of spine fractures. Spine 1994 Aug 1; 19(15):1741–1744.

39. Kovacs FM, Abraira V, Royuela A, et al. Minimal clinically important change for pain intensity and disability in patients with nonspecific low back pain. *Spine.* 2007 Dec 1;32(25):2915–2920.

40. Ostelo RW, Deyo RA, Stratford P, et al. Interpreting change scores for pain and functional status in low back pain: towards international consensus regarding minimal important change. *Spine.* 2008 Jan 1;33(1):90–94.

41. Khatri M, Murray M, Greenough CG. Minimal clinically important difference in low back outcome score in individuals with low back pain. *J Bone Joint Surg Br.* 2004;86-B(suppl II 115).

42. de Klerk LW, Fontijne WP, Stijnen T, et al. Spontaneous remodeling of the spinal canal after conservative management of thoracolumbar burst fractures. *Spine.* 1998 May 1;23(9):1057–1060.

43. Fidler MW. Remodelling of the spinal canal after burst fracture. A prospective study of two cases. *J Bone Joint Surg Br.* 1988 Nov;70(5):730–732.

44. Scapinelli R, Candiotto S. Spontaneous remodeling of the spinal canal after burst fractures of the low thoracic and lumbar region. *J Spinal Disord.* 1995 Dec;8(6):486–493.

45. Yazici M, Atilla B, Tepe S, et al. Spinal canal remodeling in burst fractures of the thoracolumbar spine: a computerized tomographic comparison between operative and nonoperative treatment. *J Spinal Disord.* 1996 Oct;9(5):409–413.

46. Schunemann HJ, Jaeschke R, Cook DJ, et al. An official ATS statement: grading the quality of evidence and strength of recommendations in ATS guidelines and recommendations. *Am J Respir Crit Care Med.* 2006 Sep 1; 174(5):605–614.

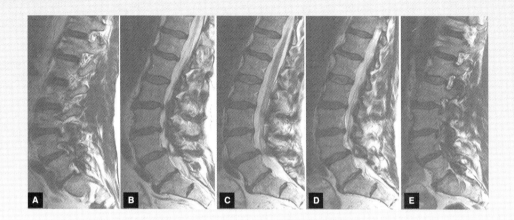

Single-Level Lumbar Degenerative Spondylolisthesis with Stenosis I

MANISH K. SETHI, MD AND MITCHEL B. HARRIS, MD

■ EDITORS' CASE PRESENTATION

A 63-year-old woman presents with a complaint of low back pain and right leg pain for the past year and a half. Pain radiates from her low back to her right calf and foot. She has no subjective complaint of weakness but feels that she has some "good days" and "bad days." She has undergone a course of physical therapy. The patient has had a number of selective nerve root blocks and other epidural injections but has not had long-standing pain relief. Despite these treatments, she feels she has become worse over time. Though her primary complaint in the right lower extremity, she does have some fatigue of her bilateral lower extremities with ambulation. Pain is worse with extension and a bit better with flexion. Additionally, she has a history of infrequent occurrences of loss of bladder control over the past several months.

Physical examination reveals 4/5 dorsiflexion weakness on the right compared to the left. Reflexes and sensation are normal. She has a somewhat positive straight-leg raise on the right side, negative on the left. She has minimal tenderness to palpation of the back, has normal gait, and has normal posture and alignment. Range of motion of the low back is limited in both flexion and extension by pain.

Radiographic imaging studies are shown in Figure 18.1A–D.

INTERPRETATION OF CLINICAL PRESENTATION

The patient's symptoms are consistent with lumbar spinal stenosis (LSS). She describes both radicular symptoms and axial pain, and her overall presentation is consistent with neurogenic claudication. Coupled with her age, this clinical presentation and history are classic for LSS.[1,2] Furthermore, these symptoms are alleviated with bending forward, which again is most suggestive of spinal stenosis. In a study of 93 adults with back pain by Katz et al.,[3] the finding of pain radiating into the buttocks or more distally had a sensitivity for the diagnosis of lumbar stenosis of 88% and a specificity of 34%.

The clinical examination identified weakness of the tibialis anterior muscle, innervated by the exiting L4 root. The presence of a positive straight-leg raise is not specific for LSS. Similarly, the presence of activity related to low back pain is consistent with but certainly not specific for LSS. Amundsen et al.[2] demonstrated the close relationship between these physical findings and LSS. Katz et al.[3] demonstrated that patients with abnormal gait demonstrated >90% sensitivity for LSS.

The patient presents with flexion and extension films of the lumbar spine, which demonstrate a Grade 1 spondylolisthesis at L4-5. L4-5 disc space narrowing along with end plate sclerosis and facet hypertrophy is also appreciated. The spondylolisthesis appears relatively stable as there is no obvious angular or translational motion in either flexion or extension. However, as Nizard et al.[4] point out, the use of flexion and extension lumbar radiographs to assess stability is neither highly sensitive nor specific.

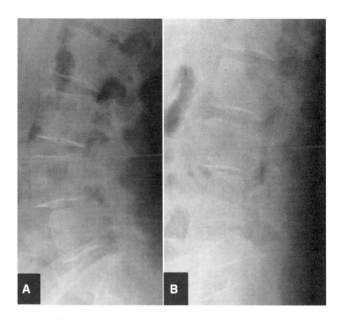

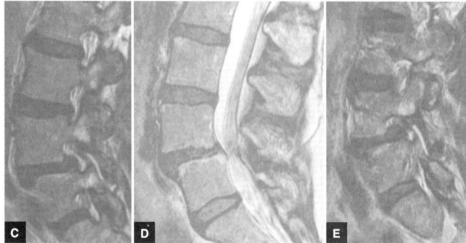

Figure 18.1.

On review of the MRI, with specific attention to the T2 sagittal images, one finds a disc herniation at L4-5 superimposed upon a grade 1 spondylolisthesis leading to evidence of single-level stenosis. One also notes a vacuum disc phenomenon at this level. There is clear evidence of Modic changes at the endplates of both the L4 and L5 vertebral bodies. The discs above and below L4-5 appear well hydrated with a very minimal disc protrusion at L3-4. On review of the paramedian imaging, one finds severe foraminal stenosis affecting the right L4 root secondary to the disc pathology and facet arthropathy. The traversing L5 nerve root is compressed by the disc at this level. The left parasagittal image reveals minimal foraminal stenosis in the left L4-5 foramen.

One must be cautious in interpreting MRI evidence and correlate with physical findings. Boden et al. have demonstrated that 21% of asymptomatic individuals aged 60 to 80 years had MRI evidence of lumbar stenosis.[5] Other studies have corroborated these findings.[6] However, with regard to diagnosing lumbar stenosis, MRI remains the gold standard study with high interobserver and intraobserver reliability.[7]

The imaging is consistent with both the physical examination findings and the patient's complaints. Her right-sided radicular symptoms together with weakness of ankle dorsiflexion are consistent with the significant foraminal stenosis on the right side at L4-5. The patient's report of lower back pain, neurogenic claudication, and occasional urinary incontinence coupled with the report that these symptoms improve on bending forward is consistent with the single-level lumbar stenosis demonstrated at L4-5 on MRI.

DECLARATION OF SPECIFIC DIAGNOSIS

In considering the patient's complaints, physical exam findings, and radiographic imaging, her diagnosis is that of single-level degenerative spondylolisthesis with spinal stenosis at L4-5. She has severe right-sided L4 root compromise originating from foraminal stenosis.

BRAINSTORMING: WHAT ARE THE TREATMENT GOALS AND SURGICAL OPTIONS

The treatment goals are

1. Relief of radicular pain and back pain
2. Improvement of neurogenic claudication
3. Improvement of urinary incontinence
4. Improvement in quality of life

The treatment options are

Conservative

1. A supervised course of physical therapy
2. Selective nerve root blocks and other epidural injections

Surgical

3. Decompression without fusion
4. L4-5 decompression with posterolateral instrumented fusion
5. L4-5 decompression with posterolateral fusion without instrumentation
6. L4-5 decompression and instrumented transforaminal lumbar interbody fusion (TLIF)
7. L4-5 decompression and instrumented posterior lumbar interbody fusion (PLIF) with posterolateral fusion

EVALUATION OF THE LITERATURE

In order to identify relevant publications on single-level lumbar degenerative spondylolisthesis with stenosis, Medline and PubMed searches were performed. Key words included the following: "lumbar stenosis," "spondylolisthesis," and "single level." Subheadings included "conservative treatment" and "surgical treatment." This search identified 1,200 abstracts that were reviewed. From this search, 150 articles were read and reference lists were reviewed. The search was limited from 1970 until the present.

DETAILED REVIEW OF PERTINENT ARTICLES

As mentioned previously, there are multiple treatment options for a patient with single-level lumbar degenerative spondylolisthesis with stenosis.

The following discussion will review the literature surrounding each of these treatments.

CONSERVATIVE TREATMENT

Katz and Harris[1] point out the lack of high-quality prospective controlled trials in evaluating conservative treatment (including physical therapy) of patients with lumbar stenosis. However, the two recent major prospective cohort studies of patients with lumbar stenosis both advocate an extended period of conservative treatment including physical therapy prior to surgery.[8,9] As noted in the illustrative case history, our patient continued to have symptoms in a progressive fashion despite a trial of physical therapy.

She also received epidural steroid injections, which provided transient improvement. The benefits of epidural steroid injections in the treatment of spinal stenosis are not consistent. In patients with lumbar stenosis, studies have demonstrated the utility of epidural steroids for periods from 1 to 2 years.[10,11] However, other studies have demonstrated minimal effect and have called for randomized controlled trials.[12–14]

With respect to conservative treatment, the patient had attempted both of the above-mentioned modalities without sustained relief of her symptoms prior to presentation. As such, we would move to offer her surgery for pain relief as well as to avoid further progression of her leg weakness.

Recent randomized trials lend evidence to the decision to move forward with surgical treatment. They demonstrate the benefits of surgery as compared to conservative treatment, after failure of the two major modalities of conservative treatment (physical therapy and injections). In two studies, one involving 94 patients and the other 289 patients, patients demonstrated significant improvement of symptoms after surgical management of lumbar stenosis compared to those patients managed conservatively.[15,16] However, a single observational cohort study following lumbar stenosis patients over a decade has demonstrated no major difference between the two modalities at the 10-year mark.[17]

Decompression Without Fusion

Pursuing surgery in this patient would begin with a thorough decompression at L4-5 with particular attention placed on the foraminal compression of the fourth nerve root on the right side. Decompression alone, however, would not be sufficient given the patient's accompanying spondylolisthesis. While patients with only lumbar stenosis benefit from decompression alone, those with associated spondylolisthesis often demonstrate further instability leading to an exacerbation of symptoms, particularly noted in association with activity.[18] Lombardi et al.[19] demonstrated significant improvement in 90% of patients with lumbar degenerative spondylolisthesis with stenosis treated with decompression and fusion as compared to 33% of similar patients treated with decompression alone. Ghogawala et al.[20] demonstrated significant improvement in both the Owestry Disability Index and Short Form 36 (SF-36) responses in similar patients treated with decompression and fusion as compared to those treated with decompression alone. However, a recent study has argued that similar patients do as well with laminoplasty decompression alone as compared to laminectomy and fusion.[21]

Given the literature described above and its demonstration of less favorable outcomes of patients with degenerative lumbar stenosis with grade I spondylolisthesis treated with decompression alone, we would recommend both a decompression and fusion. However, there remains a debate on the role of instrumentation in these patients.

Decompression and Posterolateral Fusion with and Without Instrumentation

In one of the few prospective controlled trials in the area, Fischgrund et al. compared the results of patients with degenerative lumbar stenosis with spondylolisthesis treated with decompression and fusion with or without instrumentation. In the 67 patients involved, the study demonstrated an 82% successful fusion rate in those with instrumentation as opposed to a 45% successful fusion rate in patients decompressed and fused without instrumentation.[22] However, while pedicle screws improved the fusion rate, there was no significant difference in clinical outcomes between the two groups at 2-year follow-up. In a prospective study conducted with 71 patients, France et al. also demonstrated no benefit in clinical outcomes with instrumentation in a similar patient population over 2 years. His study also demonstrated similar fusion rates with and without instrumentation.[23] Another recent randomized prospective study with 129 patients has suggested that LSS patients without instability fair better without instrumentation, whereas those who are unstable are more likely to achieve long-term improvement with instrumented fusion.[25]

To add to this debate, we consider a study by Kornblum et al.,[23] which was a follow-up study of 47 patients who underwent single-level decompression and uninstrumented fusion for degenerative lumbar stenosis with spondylolisthesis from the Fischgrund et al.'s study. This group demonstrated a significant difference in clinical outcomes between patients who achieved fusion as opposed to those with pseudoarthrosis with an average follow-up of 7.8 years. This

study demonstrated that while short-term clinical results perhaps are not influenced by the rates of fusion, longer-term results are.[23] In long-term follow-up ranging from 5 to 10 years of 49 patients similar to the case scenario presented here treated with decompression and instrumented posterolateral fusion, more than 80% of patients demonstrated significant improvement in symptoms and satisfaction with the procedure.[24]

Therefore, given the better long-term outcomes of patients with instrumented fusions as compared to those without, we would argue for the use of instrumentation given the demonstrated relationship between successful arthrodesis and long-term patient satisfaction in this patient group. Importantly, the literature has also demonstrated an increased complication rate with instrumentation as compared to noninstrumented fusion. For example, Bjarke et al. demonstrated a higher reoperation rate in patients with instrumentation in a prospective randomized trial involving 129 patients with 5-year follow up.[25] The instrumented group had a 25% reoperation rate, most commonly entailing removal of instrumentation with and without second fusion, compared with a 14% reoperation rate in the noninstrumented group.

TRANSFORAMINAL-LUMBAR INTERBODY FUSION AND POSTERIOR LUMBAR INTERBODY FUSION

Both TLIF and PLIF procedures have been advocated as a means to an increased fusion rate in patients compared to posterolateral fusion alone.[26] No randomized studies have demonstrated the purported advantage in patients with stenosis and degenerative spondylolisthesis. Studies comparing PLIF and TLIF have demonstrated similar rates of fusion with higher complication rates (dural tears) among PLIF patients.[27,28] As such, recent trends of interbody fusion have moved away from PLIF toward TLIF.[29]

Given the patient's unilateral facet hypertrophy in this clinical scenario, along with the significant foraminal stenosis, a TLIF with its requisite unilateral facetectomy could be implemented in either an open or mini-open TLIF procedure.[30] This decision would be based more on personal experience than available high-quality evidence.

LITERATURE INCONSISTENCIES

As noted throughout the discussion so far, there is a lack of randomized controlled trials in treating patients like the one presented in this case. The literature is in need of more studies like that of Fischgrund et al.[23] The majority of literature guiding surgical options is limited to retrospective cohort models. Furthermore, it seems that the findings of these prospective controlled trials are occasionally at odds with the retrospective data. For example, Fischgrund's study demonstrated no improvement in clinical outcomes in patients similar to the one presented here with instrumented fusion while retrospective studies did demonstrate a benefit.

EVIDENTIARY TABLE AND SELECTION OF TREATMENT METHOD

Table 18.1 summarizes the key studies noted above in guiding treatment. As mentioned in the discussion above, the patient in this case has failed conservative treatment and as such would benefit from surgical intervention. Given the literature and long-term outcomes demonstrated (see Table 18.1), we would move

forward with single-level L4-5 wide decompression and instrumented posterolateral fusion. While TLIF is an interesting option and offers great potential, the literature does not offer enough guidance with respect to long-term outcomes in the patient presented here.

DEFINITIVE TREATMENT PLAN

The patient in this scenario would best be treated with single-level L4-5 decompression with instrumented fusion and iliac crest bone graft to augment the local bone harvested during the laminectomy. Most often, we further extend bone graft volume with allograft supplement.

The patient would be placed prone on a four post Jackson table, paying particular attention to the

TABLE 18.1 Evidentiary Table: A Summary of the Quality of Evidence for Single-Level Lumbar Degenerative Spondylolisthesis with Stenosis.

Paper Author (Year)	Description	Summary of Results	Quality of Evidence
Fischgrund et al. (1997)	Prospective randomized	76 patients with symptomatic spinal stenosis associated with degenerative lumbar All patients underwent posterior decompression with concomitant posterolateral intertransverse process arthrodesis. Patients randomized to a segmental transpedicular instrumented or noninstrumented group. Clinical outcome was excellent or good in 76% of the patients in whom instrumentation was placed and in 85% of those in whom no instrumentation was placed ($p = 0.45$). Successful arthrodesis occurred in 82% of the instrumented cases vs. 45% of the noninstrumented cases ($p = 0.0015$).	High
Herkowitz and Kurz (1991)	Prospective study No control	50 patients with degenerative lumbar spondylolisthesis (L4-5). 25 patients treated with decompression and 25 treated with decompression and uninstrumented fusion. Patients with fusion had significant improvement in back and leg pain compared with decompression alone	High
Bjarke (2002)	Prospective randomized Control	129 patients with lumbar spondylolisthesis selected for either fusion with instrumentation or fusion alone. Patients with primary degenerative instability treated with instrumented fusion improved significantly compared to those treated with fusion alone ($p < 0.02$)	High
Ghogawala et al. (2004)	Prospective No control	34 patients with lumbar degenerative spondylolisthesis, Grade 1. Age 50–81. 20 patients underwent decompression alone, 14 patients underwent decompression and fusion. Both SF-36 scores and ODI scores demonstrated a significant and substantial improvement in fusion group as compared to decompression alone.	Low

padding of the chest, iliac crests, and ulnar nerve areas. An incision would be made spanning the spinous processes of L3-5. Care would be taken to avoid compromising the facet joints of L3-4 and L5-S1, while clearly exposing the transverse processes and pars of L4 and L5 bilaterally. Pedicle screws would then be placed in L4 and L5 bilaterally. A laminectomy and decompression would be performed across L4-5 with a total right-sided facetectomy. Attention would be focused on the right L4/L5 foramen and its compressed exiting fourth nerve root. Iliac crest bone graft would be harvested in the younger patient population (same incision), whereas local bone form the laminectomy would be supplemented with allograft in this particular patient. The rods would be placed in situ with no attempt at reduction. No brace would be used in the postoperative period.

GRADING THE EVIDENCE FOR THIS PLAN

In accordance with the method of grading recommendations set forth by Schunemann et al., our proposed treatment plan would be considered a strong recommendation.[31] In considering the existing evidence in the literature together with the risks and benefits of the proposed procedure, the proposed treatment plan offers the soundest approach to surgically treating a patient with lumbar stenosis and spondylolisthesis who has failed conservative treatment.

PREDICTING OUTCOMES

In the above discussion of conservative versus surgical treatment of lumbar stenosis, patients who underwent surgical treatment including decompression and fusion had better outcomes than similar groups treated nonoperatively at the 2-year mark.[15,16] Considering the operative approach, while Fischgrund et al. demonstrated no difference between patients treated with or without instrumented fusion at 2-year follow-up,[22] other studies have demonstrated improved outcomes in patients with instrumented fusions.[23,25]

In our personal experience, patients who have failed nonoperative therapy have obtained significant relief of symptoms and improvement in quality of life following the suggested procedure. Finally, in preoperatively counseling patients, it is of critical importance that the patient understands the different treatment options, both surgical and conservative. It is crucial that the patient understands the benefits as well as the risks of the treatment proposed.

REFERENCES

1. Katz JN, Harris MB. Clinical practice: lumbar spinal stenosis. N Engl J Med. 2008;358(8):818–825.
2. Amundsen T, Weber H, Lilleas F, et al. Lumbar spinal stenosis: clinical and radiologic features. Spine. 1995;20:1178–1186.
3. Katz JN, Dalgas M, Stucki G, et al. Degenerative lumbar spinal stenosis: diagnostic value of the history and physical examination. Arthritis Rheum. 1995;38(9):1236–1241.
4. Nizard RS, Wybier M, Laredo JD. Radiologic assessment of lumbar intervertebral instability and degenerative spondylolisthesis. Radiol Clin North Am. 2001;39(1):55–71, v–vi Review.
5. Boden SD, Davis DO, Dina TS, et al. Abnormal magnetic-resonance scans of the lumbar spine in asymptomatic subjects: a prospective investigation. J Bone Joint Surg Am. 1990;72(8):1178–1184.
6. Jensen MC, Brant-Zawadzki MN, Obuchowski N, et al. Magnetic resonance imaging of the lumbar spine in people without back pain. N Engl J Med. 1994;331(2):69–73.
7. Lurie JD, Tosteson AN, Tosteson TD, et al. Reliability of readings of magnetic resonance imaging features of lumbar spinal stenosis. Spine. 2008;33(14):1605–1610.
8. Amundsen T, Weber H, Nordal HJ, et al. Lumbar spinal stenosis: conservative or surgical management: a prospective 10-year study. Spine. 2000;25(2):197–203; discussions 203–204.
9. Simotas AC, Dorey FJ, Hansraj KK, et al. Nonoperative treatment for lumbar spinal stenosis. Clinical and outcome results and a 3-year survivorship analysis. Spine. 2000;25(2):197–203.
10. Cooper G, Lutz GE, Boachie-Adjei O, et al. Effectiveness of transforaminal epidural steroid injections in patients with degenerative lumbar scoliotic stenosis and radiculopathy. Pain Physician. 2004;7(3):311–317.
11. Botwin KP, Gruber RD, Bouchlas CG, et al. Fluoroscopically guided lumbar transformational epidural steroid injections in degenerative lumbar stenosis: an outcome study. Am J Phys Med Rehabil. 2002;81(12):898–905.
12. Landau WM, Nelson DA, Armon C, et al. Assessment: use of epidural steroid injections to treat radicular lumbosacral pain: report of the Therapeutics and Technology Assessment Subcommittee of the American Academy of Neurology. Neurology. 2007;69(6):614.
13. Cuckler JM, Bernini PA, Wiesel SW, et al. The use of epidural steroids in the treatment of lumbar radicular pain. A prospective, randomized, double-blind study. J Bone Joint Surg Am. 1985;67(1):63–66.
14. Rivest C, Katz JN, Ferrante FM, et al. Effects of epidural steroid injection on pain due to lumbar spinal stenosis or herniated disks: a prospective study. Arthritis Care Res. 1998;11(4):291–297.
15. Weinstein JN, Tosteson TD, Lurie JD, et al. Surgical versus nonsurgical therapy for lumbar spinal stenosis. N Engl J Med. 2008;358(8):794–810.
16. Malmivaara A, Slätis P, Heliövaara M, et al. Surgical or nonoperative treatment for lumbar spinal stenosis? A randomized controlled trial. Spine. 2007;32(1):1–8.
17. Atlas SJ, Keller RB, Wu YA, et al. Long-term outcomes of surgical and nonsurgical management of lumbar spinal

stenosis: 8 to 10 year results from the maine lumbar spine study. *Spine*. 2005;30(8):936–943.

18. Herkowitz HN, Kurz LT. Degenerative lumbar spondylolisthesis with spinal stenosis: a prospective study comparing decompression with decompression and intertransverse process arthrodesis. *JBJS*. 1991;73(6): 802–808.

19. Lombardi JS, Wiltse LL, Reynolds J, et al. Treatment of degenerative spondylolisthesis. *Spine*. 1985;10(9): 821–827.

20. Ghogawala Z, Benzel EC, Amin-Hanjani S, et al. Prospective outcomes evaluation after decompression with or without instrumented fusion for lumbar stenosis and degenerative Grade I spondylolisthesis. *J Neurosurg Spine*. 2004;1(3):267–272.

21. Matsudaira K, Yamazaki T, Seichi A, et al. Spinal stenosis in grade I degenerative lumbar spondylolisthesis: a comparative study of outcomes following laminoplasty and laminectomy with instrumented spinal fusion. *J Orthop Sci*. 2005;10(3):270–276.

22. Fischgrund JS, Mackay M, Herkowitz HN, et al. 1997 Volvo Award winner in clinical studies. Degenerative lumbar spondylolisthesis with spinal stenosis: a prospective, randomized study comparing decompressive laminectomy and arthrodesis with and without spinal instrumentation. *Spine*. 1997;22(24):2807–2812.

23. France JC, Yaszemski MJ, Lauerman WC, et al. A randomized prospective study of posterolateral lumbar fusion. Outcomes with and without pedicle screw instrumentation. *Spine*. 1999;24(6):553–560.

24. Booth KC, Bridwell KH, Eisenberg BA, et al. Minimum 5-year results of degenerative spondylolisthesis treated with decompression and instrumented posterior fusion. *Spine*. 1999;24(16):1721–1727.

25. Bjarke Christensen F, Stender Hansen E, Laursen M, et al. Long-term functional outcome of pedicle screw instrumentation as a support for posterolateral spinal fusion: randomized clinical study with a 5-year follow-up. *Spine*. 2002;27(12):1269–1277.

26. Rubin CT, Lanyon LE. Regulation of bone formation by applied dynamic loads. *J Bone Joint Surg Am*. 1984;66(3):397–402.

27. Yan DL, Pei FX, Li J, et al. Comparative study of PILF and TLIF treatment in adult degenerative spondylolisthesis. *Eur Spine J*. 2008;17(10):1311–1316.

28. Hosono N, Namekata M, Makino T, et al. Perioperative complications of primary posterior lumbar interbody fusion for nonisthmic spondylolisthesis: analysis of risk factors. *J Neurosurg Spine*. 2008;9(5):403–407.

29. DiPaola CP, Molinari RW. Posterior lumbar interbody fusion. *J Am Acad Orthop Surg*. 2008;16(3):130–139.

30. Dhall SS, Wang MY, Mummaneni PV. Clinical and radiographic comparison of mini-open transforaminal lumbar interbody fusion with open transforaminal lumbar interbody fusion in 42 patients with long-term follow-up. *J Neurosurg Spine*. 2008;9(6):560–565.

31. Schunemann HJ, Jaeschke R, Cook DJ, et al. ATS Documents Development and Implementation Committee. An official ATS statement: grading the quality of evidence and strength of recommendations in ATS guidelines and recommendations. *Am J Respir Crit Care Med*. 2006;174:605–614.

19 Single-Level Lumbar Degenerative Spondylolisthesis with Stenosis II

DON YOUNG PARK, MD AND EUGENE CARRAGEE, MD

EDITORS' CASE PRESENTATION

A 66-year-old man presents with complaints of low back pain and bilateral lower extremity pain for over 1 year. He reports calf pain and tightness when he walks. Symptoms are worse on the left than the right. He has had nonoperative treatment that included 8 weeks of physical therapy, from which he had minimal relief of his back or radicular pain. In addition, he has had three epidural injections, which only provided temporary relief. The man does not complain of numbness or tingling in the feet. Pain is worse with forward flexion and not necessarily relieved with extension. He does not have any bowel or bladder complaints, nor does he have balance issues.

Physical exam reveals that he can forward flex to touch his hands to his toes without pain. He can only extend to the neutral position. Motor, sensory, and reflex examination are normal. Straight leg test is negative.

Radiographic imaging studies are shown in Figures 19.1A–E and 19.2A–D.

INTERPRETATION OF CLINICAL PRESENTATION

This clinical vignette illustrates a male in his 60s with chronic low back pain and radicular complaints of the bilateral lower extremities with his left leg symptoms worse than the right. Thus far, nonoperative management

of physical therapy and epidural injections has not alleviated the patient's symptoms. At first glance, his complaints of calf pain and tightness with ambulation depict neurogenic claudication. Back pain is common in neurogenic claudication, as well as limited back motion as in this clinical scenario.[1] In this vignette, no vascular exam is given and it is not clear if the back pain or leg pain is worse with forward flexion. These are important points to clarify during the patient visit. Neurogenic claudication typically occurs with walking or standing and is usually relieved with sitting or bending. This type must be differentiated with vascular claudication, which is typically brought on by walking and relieved with standing upright but resting the legs. Pain relief with upright standing is so atypical with neurogenic claudication that it should be seen as a red flag to the spine surgeon when reported by a patient with spinal stenosis. Conversely, sensory symptoms, tingling, and dysesthetic sensations are highly atypical in vascular claudication.

Beyond lower extremity pulses, occasionally a more comprehensive vascular examination is required to be more certain there is not a distal ischemic component to his pain.[2] Functional testing with a treadmill or bicycle may be useful to differentiate vascular versus neurogenic claudication. A treadmill test may elicit typical symptoms with either vascular or neurogenic claudication; however, usually, vascular symptoms are more reliably reproducible. A bicycle test does not reproduce symptoms in neurogenic claudication since forward flexion of the spine while sitting forward would increase the central and foraminal space for the nerve roots involved.

The differential diagnosis for the patient's constellation of symptoms includes peripheral vascular disease, sciatic claudication, or insufficiency of the

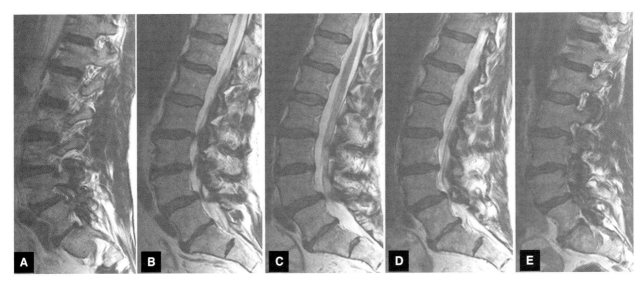

Figure 19.1.

inferior gluteal artery producing ischemia to the sciatic nerve, referred pain from the lumbar spine instability, hip or knee pathology, and psychological distress.[3] Sciatic claudication should be considered if there is no evidence of spinal stenosis or major vascular disease, but the symptoms seem more vascular. Referred pain from unstable spondylolisthesis may be present in different activities other than walking, such as bending as in this patient's situation. Psychosocial factors such as generalized somatization, compensation distress, or depression may amplify symptoms and contribute to the development of chronic back pain[4] but uncommonly have the typical stenosis and claudication history.

This patient does not have clear neurologic signs or symptoms. Straight leg testing is not typically provocative in neurogenic claudication. A relative increase in forward flexion compared with lumbar extension may be indicative of degenerative spondylosis and is seen in approximately 50% of patients with neurogenic claudication.[3]

The sagittal MRI images demonstrate grade 1 spondylolisthesis of L4 on L5 by the Meyerding classification with <25% of slippage seen. Lumbar lordosis is maintained and multilevel degenerative disk disease is seen, with prominent disc collapse at the L5-S1 level. Axial MRI images depict extensive facet joint arthropathy especially at L4-5 with medial facet fragmentation, joint effusion, and subluxation. There is mild subarticular stenosis seen at the L3-4 level and severe central and subarticular stenosis at L4-5 level. In addition, the L4-5 level has a large cystic lesion compressing the cauda equina, most significantly on the left side. The cystic lesion has a high-intensity signal with T2-weighted MRI sequences consistent with that of a synovial cyst. The majority of the canal impingement in this patient at L4-5 is due to the cysts. On the supine view of the MRI, despite the small listhesis, the canal subarticular space would be relatively patent without the synovial cysts.

There are no dynamic radiographs testing spinal instability. While there is some question of the importance of small degrees of motion in subjects with spondylolisthesis, gross instability may change the primary diagnosis in this case to a mainly deformity/instability problem with different treatment approaches. For the sake of this review, we will assume no instability was found on dynamic radiographs.

L3-4	L4-5	L5-S1

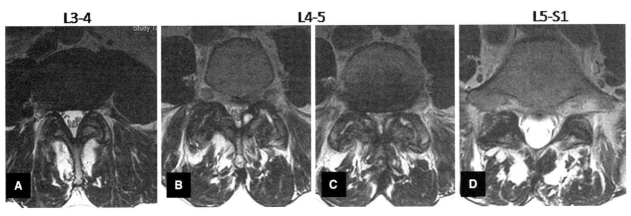

Figure 19.2.

Lumbar intraspinal synovial cysts (LISCs) usually arise from the zygapophyseal joint capsule of the lumbar spine and are also termed juxtafacet cysts based on their anatomic location.[5] Kao et al.[5] described and classified extradural intraspinal cysts into three groups: perineural cysts arising from the dorsal root ganglion, arachnoid cysts with pedicle attachment to spinal dura near the nerve root, and juxtafacet cysts that comprised of ganglion and synovial cysts attached to the facet joint capsule. Histologically, ganglion and synovial cysts differ primarily in that ganglion cysts do not have a synovial lining.[6–8]

LISCs typically occur in patients in their 7th decade of life as in this patient's case.[6] An unknown proportion of older persons with these findings are asymptomatic. When found in symptomatic patients, the presentation includes unilateral or bilateral radiculopathy occurring in 55% to 97% of patients, neurogenic claudication in 25% to 44% of patients with associated spinal stenosis, motor and sensory deficits in up to 40%, and cauda equina syndrome in up to 13% of patients in the literature.[7–9] Most LISCs are associated with facet joint arthropathy as seen in 75% to 90% of cases.[8,10] In addition, degenerative spondylolisthesis is seen in approximately 50% to 80% of symptomatic cases, and the L4-5 level, the level of greatest mobility in the lumbar spine, is most commonly identified as the location of LISCs.[6–11] The degenerative process and ensuing instability likely represent the pathogenic mechanism of LISCs. Degeneration may cause herniation of the synovial membrane through facet joint capsular defects, leading to the formation of a para-articular cavity filled with synovial fluid.[11] With concurrent spinal stenosis and progressive degenerative disease, an enlarging and expanding LISC can produce the constellation of symptoms experienced by this patient.

DECLARATION OF SPECIFIC DIAGNOSIS

This patient has neurogenic claudication and spinal stenosis primarily due to a large left-sided LISC. This problem is found in the context of multilevel degenerative disk disease, degenerative (and presumed stable) spondylolisthesis, facet joint arthropathy, and subarticular stenosis.

BRAINSTORMING: WHAT ARE THE TREATMENT GOALS AND THE SURGICAL OPTIONS?

The treatment goals are

1. Resolution of pain and symptoms
2. Avoiding neurological injury
3. Decompression of spinal canal and stenotic regions
4. Maintenance of spinal alignment and stability
5. Prevention of recurrence

The treatment options are

1. Nonoperative treatment consisting of bed rest, anti-inflammatory medications, analgesics, physical therapy, epidural or intra-articular steroid injections
2. Percutaneous cyst aspiration and rupture
3. Surgical cyst excision and decompression
4. "Minimally invasive techniques" for cyst excision and microdecompression
5. Lumbar fusion in addition to decompression surgery

EVALUATION OF THE LITERATURE

Utilizing Medline search methods, publications pertaining to LISCs were identified using MeSH (medical subject headings) and key words. The search criteria included keywords such as "lumbar intraspinal synovial cyst," "lumbosacral region," "synovial cyst," and "cyst." This led to 259 results utilizing this search strategy. One-hundred one English language abstracts and twenty-five full-text articles were reviewed.

DETAILED REVIEW OF PERTINENT ARTICLES

Close scrutiny of the pertinent publications regarding LISCs reveals poor quality of evidence with no level 1 prospective or randomized studies. Given the low incidence of synovial cysts with concomitant stenosis on CT and MRI studies,[12,13] a well-designed level 1 study may be difficult to perform with a large enough cohort in a short time frame. The vast majority of studies in the literature are comprised of retrospective reviews of small sample sizes as well as a multitude of small case series. The data from the literature suggest that operative treatment of LISCs is superior to nonoperative treatment in terms of pain relief and clinical outcome.

Nonoperative Treatment

Nonoperative treatment includes short-term bed rest, anti-inflammatory medications, analgesics, physical therapy, epidural or intra-articular steroid injections, and percutaneous cyst aspiration and rupture. These modalities led to a failure rate of 60% at 6 months and required all patients to undergo surgical treatment in a study of 77 patients.[14] Fluoroscopically guided cyst aspiration provided some pain relief for a period of 3.4 weeks, but 8/10 patients underwent surgery due to absence of sustained benefit.[6] Additional small case series have demonstrated similar results; however, their small sample sizes and the variety of various injection sites utilized significantly limit any veritable and worthwhile conclusions.[8,15–17] Upon review of nonsurgical treatment in the literature and pooling the results together with 149 total patients, nonsurgical treatment amassed a failure rate as high as 46.9%, with surgery being the ultimate endpoint.[6] This patient has failed nonsurgical treatment thus far and would not likely improve clinically without further intervention.

Recently, a retrospective review of 101 consecutive patients who underwent fluoroscopically guided percutaneous corticosteroid injection with attempted cyst rupture demonstrated successful cyst rupture in 81% with 54% requiring surgical intervention at a mean 0.70 years after the procedure.[18] Successful cyst rupture did not necessarily prevent the need for surgery and was associated with worse disability 3 years after the procedure. Another recent retrospective review of 32 patients undergoing a similar procedure aimed at contrast distention and cyst rupture demonstrated excellent pain relief in 72% of patients at a mean 1-year follow-up and 60% successful outcomes with no further treatment.[19] However, cyst recurrence occurred in 37.5% of patients and a second procedure 3 months later provided pain relief in only 45% of patients with 55% of these patients ultimately requiring surgical intervention. Potential causes of failure include inadequate cyst aspiration, rarity in cyst involution, inability to administer steroids into the correct site, inability to puncture the cyst, and cyst recurrence.[20]

Operative Treatment

Surgical treatment of LISCs has established high rates of successful outcomes as reported in cases series reports. In the largest retrospective review published thus far on surgical outcomes, 194 patients underwent lamina decompression and cyst resection with a mean follow-up of 26 months.[9] The surgeons' global assessment was that 91% of patients reported good or excellent relief of their preoperative radicular pain, with 82% and 79% of patients improving in their motor and sensory deficits, respectively. Another study detailing surgical outcomes followed 77 patients for a mean 42 months and compared the outcomes for patients with unilateral radiculopathy and bilateral neurogenic claudication.[14] The clinical results were similar for both groups with the authors reporting approximately 80% excellent and 15% good functional results postoperatively. Overall, 97.4% of patients had good to excellent results. Multiple smaller studies have corroborated these high rates of clinical success with short-term follow-up and fewer patients.[21–25]

Minimally invasive techniques have also been applied to surgically address LISCs, and similar clinical results are seen. A retrospective review of 46 patients with 9.7-year follow-up demonstrated 88% relief of preoperative pain and symptoms with 89% of patients reporting overall satisfaction with the surgery.[26] The authors reported 87% of patients reported resolution of numbness and 84% with resolution of weakness. In 28% of patients, new back pain developed after a period of initial improvement. A similar study utilizing minimally invasive techniques also demonstrated 94% good to excellent pain relief with only one patient with preexisting spondylolisthesis requiring spinal fusion.[27] However, the majority of surgical outcome studies in the literature were limited by the absence of well-validated outcome measures to better delineate clinical results, and the careful selection of patients for this treatment may limit generalization.

Fusion

The role of spinal fusion in surgical treatment of LISCs has been investigated since instability is regarded as part of the pathogenic process and may influence clinical results. A retrospective study of 39 patients demonstrated marginally better outcomes with spinal fusion, with 80% having good to excellent results versus 70% without fusion.[28] This patient population consisted of 82% of patients with degenerative spondylolisthesis, with 67% of patients requiring lateral spinal fusion with decompression and cyst excision. In contrast, no statistical differences were seen in clinical outcomes between patients requiring decompression alone versus patients with concomitant spinal fusion in a study with long-term (9.7 year) follow-up.[26] Three patients (6.5%) who were not fused at the initial surgery required eventual fusion due to instability. Lyons et al.[9] reported only 18 out of 194 patients (9.3%) required spinal fusion and only 4 out of 194 patients (2.1%) required delayed fusion for symptomatic spondylolisthesis. This patient population consisted of 50% Meyerding grade 1 degenerative spondylolisthesis. No statistical correlation was found between the development of symptomatic spondylolisthesis and the degree of laminectomy and facetectomy. However, an analysis was not performed in this study comparing clinical outcomes between patients with fusion versus without fusion.

Literature Inconsistencies

The largest inconsistency in the literature is the selection of patients for specific approaches. None of the articles reviewed gave defined entry and exclusion criteria and all of the retrospective studies accepted the clinicians' general impressions of the best treatment recommended and performed without clear definition. Important variables such as instability, facet orientation, disc height preservation, degree of spondylosis are rarely mentioned but likely contributed to enrollment.

Furthermore, treatment success may not be uniformly reported by patients and surgeons. Both surgeon and patient-based outcomes measures were utilized to evaluate results of decompressive laminectomies for synovial cyst excision in 45 patients with coexistent lumbar spinal stenosis and 35 patients with stenosis and degenerative spondylolisthesis.[29] After 2 years follow-up, surgeon-based outcomes data revealed 58% good to excellent results in the stenosis group and 63% good to excellent results in the spondylolisthesis group. Patient-based outcomes data utilized the SF-36 questionnaire that compared preoperative and postoperative responses. Somewhat more moderate improvements were seen in the Physical Function and Role-Emotional health scales in both groups. In this population, patients who demonstrated poorer outcomes had significant comorbidities, such as multiple sclerosis, tumors, spasticity, depression, recurrent disc herniation, and prior lumbar surgery. These comorbidities may have contributed to less favorable clinical results as compared to other studies in the literature. No primary fusions were performed in this study and subsequently 5 of 45 patients in the stenosis group and 11 of 35 patients in the spondylolisthesis group developed frank postoperative instability. This may indicate that primary fusion for synovial cysts, lumbar stenosis, and degenerative spondylolisthesis could improve the success rates. But again, the selection biases for these studies are difficult to assess.

EVIDENTIARY TABLE AND SELECTION OF TREATMENT METHOD

Based on the available evidence, this patient may benefit from surgical treatment since nonsurgical treatment has not provided improvement to this point. Although the rates of initial surgical success are consistently high and patients seem satisfied with surgery, the quality of evidence is poor with no prospective, randomized level 1 studies regarding LISCs. Table 19.1 summarizes the retrospective studies and case series in the literature regarding surgical intervention.

Percutaneous cyst aspiration and rupture is a reasonable option for the patient if he would like to exhaust all nonsurgical options, which has failed up to this point. Percutaneous treatment may provide sufficient symptomatic improvement so that the patient may possibly avoid surgery. However, the failure rate for this option can be as high as 60% and as high as 50% of patients will eventually require surgery despite experiencing temporary relief.[18,19] These

percutaneous procedures harbor definite risks, such as infection, bleeding, dural puncture, nerve root injury, and possible worsening of neurological deficit or pain, but these are not likely greater than surgical and anesthetic risks.[19] Patients should weigh these risks against the expected likelihood of temporary benefit of percutaneous treatment.

For more predictable clinical outcomes, surgical treatment may be necessary for this patient. Surgical treatment may include decompression and synovial cyst excision utilizing conventional or minimally invasive techniques. Minimally invasive techniques can spare the morbidity of larger open procedures with less muscle and soft-tissue disruption but may require specific expertise not generally available. Clinical results for minimally invasive LISC surgery are similar to conventional techniques,[26,27] as reported in these lower level evidence studies. Decompression of coexisting stenosis may also be necessary for optimal results. The most important aspect of the surgery is excision of the LISC to provide symptomatic relief, decompress the neural elements, and prevent recurrence.

Since the patient has grade 1 spondylolisthesis at L4-5, the level of maximum lumbar spine mobility, spinal fusion may treat the inherent instability that likely is contributing to the etiology of the synovial cyst. As discussed above, if gross instability were detected with preoperative flexion and extension radiographs, then concomitant fusion would likely improve the patient's clinical outcome. This decision for fusion should be specifically tailored to the patient's own situation with a thorough assessment of spinal stability, medical risks of a larger procedures, the patient's tolerance of a failure of the less invasive surgery, and the risks of a second anesthetic in high-risk patients.

DEFINITIVE TREATMENT PLAN

In our opinion, this patient should be best managed with surgical treatment of the left-sided LISC utilizing minimally invasive techniques, which we perform routinely. After proper positioning on the operating room table, the L4-5 level is identified using fluoroscopy and the dissection is taken down to ipsilateral lamina containing the synovial cyst. Using microscopy and minimally traumatic retractors, a laminotomy is performed and the ligamentum flavum is excised. Adequate exposure of the synovial cyst allows more complete excision. If the synovial cyst is adherent to the dura, careful blunt dissection may be necessary; however, overaggressive dissection may lead to a dural tear. The subarticular and foraminal zones are decompressed along with excision of the synovial cyst. A complete, wide

TABLE 19.1   Evidentiary Table.

Paper Author (Year)	Description	Summary of Results	Quality of Evidence
Lyons et al. (2000)	Retrospective, 194 patients, 6 mo follow-up	134/147 (91%) good-excellent (G-E) pain relief, 4/194 delayed fusion (2%), no recurrences	Low
Epstein et al. (2004)	Retrospective, 80 patients, (45 in cyst-stenosis group 1, 35 in cyst-spondylolisthesis group 2), 2 y follow-up	58% G-E results (group 1), 63% G-E results (group 2), SF-36 physical Function (group 1: + 44, group 2: + 38), Role-emotional (group 1: + 39, group 2: + 33), 4/80 (5%) delayed fusions, 2 recurrences	Low
Métellus et al. (2006)	Retrospective, 77 patients, 42 mo follow-up	75/77 (97.4%) G-E functional results, 1/77 (1%) delayed fusions, 1 recurrence	Low
Sabo et al. (1996)	Retrospective, 56 patients, 12 mo follow-up	52/53 (98%) G-E outcome, 1 recurrence	Low
Weiner et al. (2007)	Retrospective, 46 patients, 9.7 y follow-up	40/46 (88%)relief of preop pain/Sx, 41/46 (89%) overall satisfaction, 3/46 (6.5%) delayed fusions	Low
Khan et al. (2005)	Retrospective, 39 patients, 26 mo follow-up	22/24 (92%) G-E results, 80% G-E results with fusion, 2/39 (5%) delayed fusions, 1 recurrence	Low
Banning et al. (2001)	Retrospective, 29 patients, 24 mo follow-up	20/24 (83%) improved pain, 16/24 (67%) improved function, 2/29 (7%) delayed fusions, 2 recurrences	Low
Salmon et al. (2001)	Retrospective, 28 patients, 3 mo–10.5 y follow-up	21/28 (75%) complete resolution of symptoms, 1 recurrence	Very low
Trummer et al. (2001)	Retrospective, 19 patients, 23 mo follow-up	19/19 (100%) G-E pain relief, 1 recurrence	Low
Sandhu et al. (2004)	Retrospective, 17 patients, 13 mo follow-up	16/17 (94%) G-E pain relief, 1/17 (6%) delayed fusions	Low
Howington et al. (1999)	Case series, 28 patients, 40 mo follow-up	81% relief of LBP, 88% relief of radicular symptoms	Low
Freidberg et al. (1994)	Case series, 26 patients, 1 y follow-up	15/23 (65%) complete relief, 7/23 (30%) some residual symptoms, 1/26 (3.8%) delayed fusions	Very low
Boviatsis et al. (2008)	Case series, 7 patients, 12 mo follow-up	7/7 excellent outcomes	Very low
Jönsson et al. (1999)	Case series, 8 patients, 0.5–2 y follow-up	All radiculopathy improved, 5/8 pain free	Very low

decompression of stenotic levels may not be required to address his neurogenic claudication. If, intraoperatively, gross spinal instability is found (or created), then an instrumented posterolateral fusion, including facet joint fusion, is carried out.

The evidence to support the surgical treatment outlined is only moderate since the studies in the literature consist of retrospective clinical outcome studies or case series with relatively small sample sizes and the wide variety of outcome measures used.

In accordance with the method of grading recommendations set forth by Schunemann et al.,[21,31] our proposed treatment (compared to continued nonoperative care) would be considered a **strong recommendation**.

This recommendation is made despite the low quality of evidence in the literature since surgical intervention would more predictably improve the patient's pain and symptoms as compared to the nonsurgical options previously proposed. The potential benefit of surgical treatment would outweigh the risks and burdens of the intervention, especially in this patient with refractory pain and symptoms. However, this recommendation may change if the quality of evidence improves.

PREDICTING OUTCOMES

According to the literature, the patient would likely improve with surgical treatment in terms of his radicular pain, especially since the patient has failed nonsurgical interventions. Retrospective studies and case series demonstrated significant improvement in pain, motor and numbness symptoms, and satisfaction with surgical intervention. As previously mentioned, clinical results in the existing literature utilized various patient-based questionnaires and reported subjective patient satisfaction rates as measures of success. Better validated outcome measures would improve the quality of data and allow more confidence in the strength of our recommendation.

However, a definite pathologic abnormality is causing compression of already stenotic neural elements and decompression with cyst excision would allow the patient the best chances of clinical improvement and possible resolution of his leg symptoms and possible low back pain.[30] Our own clinical experience corresponds well with the results seen in the literature and provides weight to our recommendation for this patient. As always, the patient should be counseled that full resolution of pain and symptoms may not occur and the risks of surgery, such as dural tear, infection, epidural hematoma, and recurrence, are uncommon but definitely possible.

SUMMARY

In this case presentation, a 66-year-old man is discussed with chronic low back pain and bilateral lower extremity pain with neurogenic claudication and spinal stenosis and spondylolisthesis associated with a large LISC who has failed nonoperative treatment. The most appropriate treatment for this patient includes decompression with synovial cyst excision and possible fusion if clear instability is also present. Clinical improvement should be expected for this patient in terms of radicular pain relief and improvement in walking.

REFERENCES

1. Bell GR, Spinal stenosis. In: Chapman MW, ed; *Chapman's Orthopaedic Surgery.* 3rd ed. Philadelphia, PA: Lippincott Williams & Wilkins, 2001; 3817–3820, chap 147.
2. White C. Clinical practice. Intermittent claudication. *N Engl J Med.* 2007;356(12):1241–1250.
3. Porter RW. Spinal stenosis and neurogenic claudication. *Spine.* 1996;21(17):2046–2052.
4. Pincus T, Burton AK, Vogel S, et al. A systematic review of psychological factors as predictors of chronicity/disability in prospective cohorts of low back pain. *Spine.* 2002;27(5):E109–E120.
5. Kao CC, Winkler SS, Turner JH. Synovial cyst of spinal facet: case report. *J Neurosurg.* 1974;41(3):372–376.
6. Shah RV, Lutz GE. Lumbar intraspinal synovial cysts: conservative management and review of the world's literature. *Spine J.* 2003;3(6):479–488.
7. Howington JU, Connolly ES, Voorhies RM. Intraspinal synovial cysts: 10-year experience at the Ochsner Clinic. *J Neurosurg.* 1999;91(2 suppl):193–199.
8. Hsu KY, Zucherman JF, Shea WJ, et al. Lumbar intraspinal synovial and ganglion cysts (facet cysts). Ten-year experience in evaluation and treatment. *Spine.* 1995;20(1): 80–89.
9. Lyons MK, Atkinson JL, Wharen RE, et al. Surgical evaluation and management of lumbar synovial cysts: the Mayo Clinic experience. *J Neurosurg.* 2000;93(1 suppl):53–57.
10. Banning CS, Thorell WE, Leibrock LG. Patient outcome after resection of lumbar juxtafacet cysts. *Spine.* 2001;26(8):969–972.
11. Boviatsis EJ, Staurinou LC, Kouyialis AT, et al. Spinal synovial cysts: pathogenesis, diagnosis and surgical treatment in a series of seven cases and literature review. *Eur Spine J.* 2008;17(6):831–837.
12. Eyster EF, Scott WR. Lumbar synovial cysts: report of eleven cases. *Neurosurgery.* 1989;24(1):112–115.
13. Doyle AJ, Merrilees M. Synovial cysts of the lumbar facet joints in a symptomatic population: prevalence on magnetic resonance imaging. *Spine.* 2004;29(8):874–878.
14. Métellus P, Fuentes S, Adetchessi T, et al. Retrospective study of 77 patients harbouring lumbar synovial cysts: functional and neurological outcome. *Acta Neurochir (Wien).* 2006;148(1):47–54.
15. Parlier-Cuau C, Wybier M, Nizard R, et al. Symptomatic lumbar facet joint synovial cysts: clinical assessment of facet joint steroid injection after 1 and 6 months and long-term follow-up in 30 patients. *Radiology.* 1999;210(2): 509–513.
16. Slipman CW, Lipetz JS, Wakeshima Y, et al. Nonsurgical treatment of zygapophyseal joint cyst-induced radicular pain. *Arch Phys Med Rehabil.* 2000;81(7):973–977.
17. Bureau NJ, Kaplan PA, Dussault RG. Lumbar facet joint synovial cyst: percutaneous treatment with steroid injections and distention—clinical and imaging follow-up in 12 patients. *Radiology.* 2001;221(1):179–185.
18. Martha JF, Swaim B, Wang DA, et al. Outcome of percutaneous rupture of lumbar synovial cysts: a case series of 101 patients. *Spine J.* 2009;9(11):899–904.

19. Allen TL, Tatli Y, Lutz GE. Fluoroscopic percutaneous lumbar zygapophyseal joint cyst rupture: a clinical outcome study. *Spine J.* 2009;9(5):387–395.
20. Khan AM, Girardi F. Spinal lumbar synovial cysts. Diagnosis and management challenge. *Eur Spine J.* 2006;15(8):1176–1182.
21. Sabo RA, Tracy PT, Weinger JM. A series of 60 juxtafacet cysts: clinical presentation, the role of spinal instability, and treatment. *J Neurosurg.* 1996;85(4):560–565.
22. Salmon B, Martin D, Lenelle J, et al. Juxtafacet cyst of the lumbar spine. Clinical, radiological and therapeutic aspects in 28 cases. *Acta Neurochir (Wien).* 2001;143(2): 129–134.
23. Trummer M, Flaschka G, Tillich M, et al. Diagnosis and surgical management of intraspinal synovial cysts: report of 19 cases. *J Neurol Neurosurg Psychiatry.* 2001;70(1):74–77.
24. Jönsson B, Tufvesson A, Strömqvist B. Lumbar nerve root compression by intraspinal synovial cysts. Report of 8 cases. *Acta Orthop Scand.* 1999;70(2):203–206.
25. Freidberg SR, Fellows T, Thomas CB, et al. Experience with symptomatic spinal epidural cysts. *Neurosurgery.* 1994;34(6):989–993.
26. Weiner BK, Torretti J, Stauff M. Microdecompression for lumbar synovial cysts: an independent assessment of long term outcomes. *J Orthop Surg Res.* 2007;2:5.
27. Sandhu FA, Santiago P, Fessler RG, et al. Minimally invasive surgical treatment of lumbar synovial cysts. *Neurosurgery.* 2004;54(1):107–111.
28. Khan AM, Synnot K, Cammisa FP, et al. Lumbar synovial cysts of the spine: an evaluation of surgical outcome. *J Spinal Disord Tech.* 2005;18(2):127–131.
29. Epstein NE. Lumbar laminectomy for the resection of synovial cysts and coexisting lumbar spinal stenosis or degenerative spondylolisthesis: an outcome study. *Spine.* 2004;29(9):1049–1055.
30. Don AS, Carragee E. A brief overview of evidence-informed management of chronic low back pain with surgery. *Spine J.* 2008;8(1):258–265.
31. Schunemann HJ, Jaeschke R, Cook DJ, et al. ATS Documents Development and Implementation Committee. An official ATS statement: grading the quality of evidence and strength of recommendations in ATS guidelines and recommendations. *Am J Respir Crit Care Med.* 2006;174:605–614.

Lumbar Degenerative Spondylolisthesis with Multilevel Stenosis I

COLIN B. HARRIS, MD AND MICHAEL J. VIVES, MD

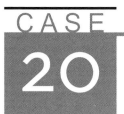

EDITORS' CASE PRESENTATION

A 65-year old woman presents to the clinic with a long-standing history of low back pain and left lower extremity pain. Her back pain is worse than her leg pain. However, she has no back pain at rest. Back pain is present when she stands for long periods of time and worse with ambulation, during which she uses a cane. Resting relieves her symptoms, after which she can resume walking. She reports no numbness and tingling. Nonoperative treatment has included three epidural steroid injections that produced some short-term relief for about 5 weeks. She has not had any exercise therapy. She has no bowel or bladder complaints.

On examination, she has pain that is exacerbated with extension. However, she can forward flex to touch her hands to her midshin. Her gait is stable with the use of a cane. Besides being overweight, she has no other pertinent positives. She is neurologically intact in the upper and lower extremities and demonstrates no positives to provocative tests.

Radiographic images are shown in Figures 20.1 and 20.2.

INTERPRETATION OF CLINICAL PRESENTATION

This case describes an adult patient of middle age who presents with complaints of both low back and leg pain. Her pain is described as absent at rest and exacerbated by long periods of standing and ambulation. This is consistent with neurogenic claudication, which is the most common clinical symptom of lumbar spinal stenosis.[1] Neurogenic claudication is typically characterized by lower extremity aching, burning, and paresthesias, radiates from proximal to distal, and is commonly associated with back pain. The lower extremity symptoms of neurogenic claudication must be differentiated from vascular claudication, which presents with calf tightness and lower extremity cramping made worse by exercise and improved with cessation of activity but not typically improved by flexion as in neurogenic claudication. Although this patient's symptoms are more typical of a neurogenic etiology, it is important to rule out vascular disease with a thorough physical examination and referral to a vascular surgeon for further evaluation if physical findings of significant peripheral vascular disease are found.[2] In addition, this patient reports no numbness or tingling in her lower extremities and denies any bowel or bladder involvement. This is also consistent with lumbar spinal stenosis, in which pain is often the presenting complaint and significant neurologic deficits are rare.

This patient's physical exam demonstrates pain exacerbated with extension and more ability to forward flex comfortably than to extend. This is typical of spinal stenosis in that flexion relieves discomfort and extension can worsen it. In this case, the gait is stable with the use of a cane. Although patients with spinal stenosis may be deconditioned and may lose strength and endurance, they will not typically have an unsteady gait or signs of hyperreflexia. The aforementioned are more typical of myelopathy and would prompt a search for compressive pathology more cephalad in the spinal axis. Furthermore, this patient is neurologically intact and demonstrates no tension signs on physical exam. This is consistent with spinal stenosis, as there is often no neurologic deficit or only subtle deficits in the lower lumbar or sacral nerve root distributions, with tension signs usually absent.[2]

The magnetic resonance imaging (MRI) sequences provided with this case include T2-weighted paramedian

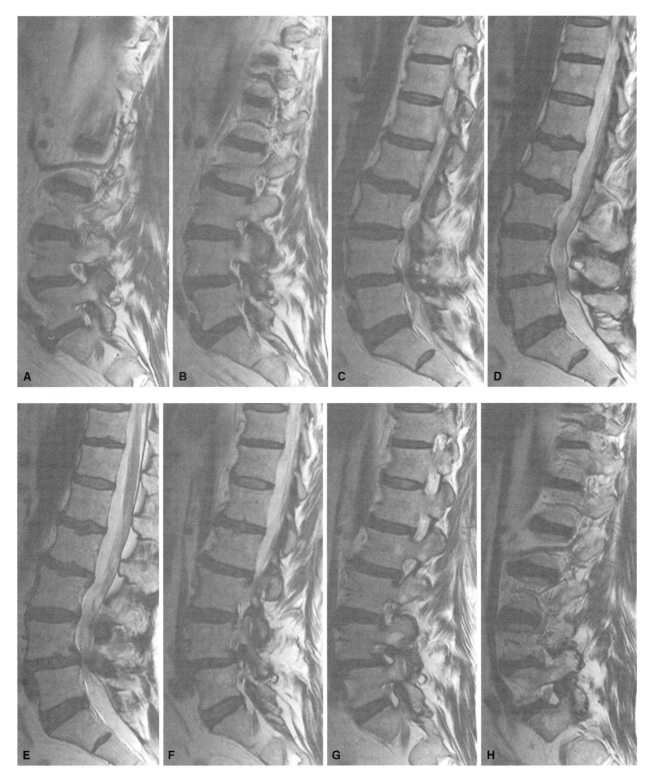

Figure 20.1

and median sagittal images of the lumbar spine as well as T2-weighted axial images through the level of the disc spaces from L2-3 to L5-S1. Figure 20.1D is a midline T2 sagittal image demonstrating multilevel degenerative disc disease with disc bulging at L2-3, L3-4, L4-5, and a 25% slip (Grade I spondylolisthesis) of L4 on L5.[3]

Stenosis of the spinal canal with buckling of the ligamentum flavum and compression of the thecal sac between the posterior elements and the disc can also be seen at the L4-5 level, although the axial cuts are more useful for defining the anatomic location of stenosis. Overall, sagittal alignment can also be seen on the sagittal

L2-3 L3-4 L4-5 L5-S1

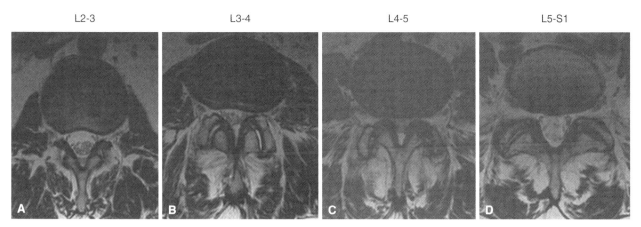

Figure 20.2

images, and loss of normal lordosis is seen in the mid to upper lumbar spine in Figure 20.1D and E. It should also be noted that in cases of previous lumbar surgery or spondylolisthesis, flexion/extension radiographs may be warranted in order to assess dynamic component to the slip as instability is difficult to assess on a static MRI or radiograph.

The paramedian images (Fig. 20.1A, B, F–H) demonstrate stenosis in both the subarticular zone and the foraminal zone to some degree at both L3-4 and L4-5. Figure 20.1B, a paramedian image through the patient's left side, shows foraminal stenosis at the L3-4 level, and to a lesser degree at the L4-5 level. This is seen also on the patient's right side at L4-5 and to lesser degrees at L3-4 in Figure 20.1F and G.

Representative axial images through the level of the disc spaces and facet joints are shown in Figure 20.2. The L2-3 level is relatively normal with a circular-shaped thecal sac and nerve roots that are evenly spaced, as shown in Figure 20.2A. In contrast, Figure 20.2B (demonstrating L3-4) shows a trefoil-shaped thecal sac with compression of the spinal canal by hypertrophic facet joints and ligamentum flavum posterolaterally and ventrally by a broad left-sided foraminal disc bulge. Similarly, the L4-5 level (shown in Fig. 20.2C) shows narrowing of the lateral recess and foraminal zones with disc bulging and prominent, hypertrophic facet joints. The next most caudal level, L5-S1, is shown in Figure 20.2D for comparison and appears normal without evidence of thecal sac compression.

DECLARATION OF SPECIFIC DIAGNOSIS

This patient has L4-5 degenerative spondylolisthesis with multilevel disc degeneration and lumbar spinal stenosis, most significant at the L3-4 and L4-5 levels.

BRAINSTORMING: WHAT ARE THE TREATMENT GOALS AND SURGICAL OPTIONS?

The treatment goals are

1. Relief of back and leg pain
2. Maintenance of normal alignment of the spine
3. Prevention of slip progression of the degenerative spondylolisthesis
4. Stabilization of all unstable motion segments

The treatment options are

1. Nonoperative treatment including physical therapy with or without additional lumbar epidural steroid injections
2. Decompression of all stenotic motion segments
3. Fusion of some or all of the decompressed levels
4. Instrumented or noninstrumented posterolateral fusion
5. Posterolateral fusion or with additional interbody fusion
6. Application of a motion sparing device

EVALUATION OF THE LITERATURE

In order to identify relevant articles, a Medline search was performed using the MeSH (medical subject headings) "lumbar spinal stenosis," "degenerative spondylolisthesis," and "lumbar spinal stenosis and degenerative spondylolisthesis." Searches were limited to articles published from 1950 to 2008, and only English language articles were read and their references further reviewed to identify additional pertinent articles. A total of 3,147 articles were identified, with 2,398 pertaining to lumbar spinal stenosis, 706 pertaining to degenerative spondylolisthesis, and 43 relevant to both lumbar spinal stenosis and degenerative spondylolisthesis. Out of these articles, 38 full-text papers were identified as most relevant to this case and were read in full. In addition, an evidence based medicine (EBM) review-Cochrane database search was performed, resulting in one relevant article entitled "Surgery for Degenerative Lumbar Spondylosis."[4]

DETAILED REVIEW OF PERTINENT ARTICLES

Operative or Nonoperative Treatment

Overall, there are few high-quality randomized controlled trials (RCTs) on the treatment of lumbar spinal stenosis with associated degenerative spondylolisthesis. While there are several studies that evaluate outcomes following lumbar decompression and fusion that have smaller subsets of patients with spinal stenosis and degenerative spondylolisthesis, only four RCTs specifically address this pathologic entity.[5–8] Three of these studies compare methods of surgical intervention,[5,6,8] while one[7] compares operative versus nonoperative treatment.

The first question in this case to be addressed is whether or not this patient will benefit from operative treatment. The Spine Patient Outcomes Research Trial (SPORT) was designed to compare the effectiveness of surgical and nonsurgical treatment for patients with lumbar disc herniation,[9,10] spinal stenosis,[11] and lumbar degenerative spondylolisthesis.[7] The results of the trial evaluating lumbar degenerative spondylolisthesis were published in 2007.[7] In 13 centers in the United States, patients with at least 12 weeks of symptoms were offered enrollment in a randomized cohort or an observational cohort. Treatment was decompressive laminectomy with or without fusion versus usual nonoperative care. High crossover rates (40% in each direction) in the randomized cohort presumably contributed to a failure to demonstrate significant effects on intent-to-treat analysis for the primary self-reported clinical outcome measures. As-treated analysis of the combined cohorts, however, showed a significant advantage for surgical treatment at 3 months that increased at 1 year and diminished only slightly at 2 years.

While the large amount of crossover diminished the true randomization effect, the baseline characteristics of both surgical and nonsurgical groups remained similar. The lack of a standardized nonoperative treatment regimen has also been criticized, despite the historical absence of widely accepted nonoperative treatment approaches. Despite these issues, this study provides

good evidence that operative treatment is superior to nonoperative treatment for this condition. In addition, the results of this study are consistent with the results demonstrated in the mixed-stenosis (those with and without degenerative spondylolisthesis) cohort of a nonrandomized trial, the Main Lumbar Spine Study.[12] Finally, an RCT of surgical versus nonoperative treatment of lumbar stenosis that was conducted in Finland included a subgroup of patients (42%) that had concomitant degenerative spondylolisthesis.[13] While the surgical group demonstrated greater improvement than the nonoperative group, separate analysis of those patients with degenerative spondylolisthesis was not performed.

Given the information presented, it is difficult to discern whether the patients' symptoms are predominantly a result of the pathology at the L4-5 level, the L3-4 level, or partly attributable to both. As such, the planned surgical intervention would include decompression of both levels, as failure rates as high as 27% have been reported due to recurrent same-level or adjacent-level stenosis.[14] The SPORT degenerative spondylolisthesis study included patients with multilevel stenosis (38% in the randomized cohort, 31% in the observational cohort) and subgroup analysis did not show significant effect modification.[7] This observation should be made with the awareness that the study was not designed, nor powered, to examine subgroup differences. The other RCTs evaluating surgical treatment of spinal stenosis[11–13,15] can be considered supporting evidence of the benefit of operative versus nonoperative treatment for the presented case.

The work of Schunemann et al.[16] has been widely cited as a useful framework for making clinical recommendations based on available evidence. In keeping with these guidelines, the evidence supporting operative treatment for this patient can be considered high quality, given the RCT for this condition, the consistency of results with other studies,[5,6,8] and the additional RCTs that indirectly evaluate this condition.[12,13,15] In addition to the quality of evidence supporting the efficacy of treatment, little evidence of harm was demonstrated from either surgical or nonsurgical care.[7] Given these two considerations, a strong recommendation for operative treatment can be made, assuming that the patient's pain and functional limitations would make her agreeable to such a recommendation.

EVIDENTIARY TABLE AND SELECTION OF TREATMENT METHOD

Although the best available evidence directs the patient in this clinical scenario toward operative treatment, this is stated under the assumption that the patient has failed at least 6 weeks of nonoperative treatment of some kind (medications, activity modification, physical therapy, or injections). The scenario suggests long-standing symptoms and partial relief for 5 weeks after injection treatments. Most studies looking at operative treatment require between 6 weeks and 3 months of failed nonoperative treatment of some form prior to surgery.[5–7,17] In order to evaluate the most *appropriate* surgical treatment, only articles pertaining to adult patients with surgical management of degenerative spondylolisthesis were critically examined. The highest-quality articles evaluating surgical treatment of this condition were examined in further detail, and the results are summarized in Table 20.1.

Fusion or no Fusion at the Time of Decompression

Once it is decided that operative treatment is superior and that a decompression should be performed, the next step is to determine whether this patient would benefit from a formal fusion and what levels should be included in the fusion. Three prospective studies have been performed comparing decompression with and without concomitant fusion for degenerative spondylolisthesis.[5,8,18] Bridwell et al.[8] prospectively compared three small subsets of patients undergoing surgical treatment of this condition (no fusion, noninstrumented posterolateral fusion without instrumentation,

and instrumented posterolateral fusion). They found that the fusion rate was higher in the instrumented fusion group, and the rate of spondylolisthesis progression was higher in both the unfused and noninstrumented fusion groups, although clinical outcomes scores were not available and a clear superiority of fusion could not be found. Herkowitz and Kurz performed a prospective RCT involving 50 patients who were alternatively assigned to either decompression or decompression with noninstrumented fusion, founding that the fusion group reported significantly improved back pain, leg pain, and had lower rates of progression of olisthesis than the unfused group.[5] Thirty-six percent of the fusion group developed pseudarthroses but still achieved good or excellent outcomes. The authors theorized that even a pseudarthrosis provided some degree of beneficial stability. More recently, Ghogawala et al.[18] performed a prospective comparative observational study of 34 patients who underwent decompression with and without fusion with autograft and pedicle screw instrumentation. They found that 1-year Oswestry Disability Index (ODI) and Short Form-36 (SF-36) scores were significantly better in the fusion group than in the unfused group, although both groups showed significant improvement from preoperative scores. While flaws in the methodology of the clinical trials (e.g., inadequate randomization) may warrant downgrading them to

| | TABLE 20 .1 | Evidentiary Table: A Summary of the Quality of Evidence for Surgical Treatment of Degenerative Spondylolisthesis with Lumbar Spinal Stenosis. | |

Paper Author (Year)	Description	Summary of Results	Quality of Evidence
Weinstein et al. (2007)	Prospective randomized and observational cohorts	304 patients in randomized cohort and 303 in observational cohort. Outcome measures included SF-36 and Oswestry scores. No difference in outcome in intent-to-treat analysis, but superior results in surgery group at 3 mo, 1 y, and 2 y in as-treated analysis.	High
Herkowitz and Kurz (1991)	Prospective study, patients alternately assigned	50 patients underwent decompression with or without posterolateral noninstrumented fusion Fusion group had significantly less back and leg pain and superior clinical outcome at 2 y follow-up despite 36% pseudoarthrosis rate	Moderate
Fischgrund et al. (1997)	Prospective randomized study	67 patients randomized to decompression and fusion with or without instrumentation Fusion rate 82% in instrumentation group vs. 45% in nonoperative group but no benefit in clinical outcome (76% good/excellent in instrumented group vs. 85% in noninstrumented group)	High
Ghogawala (2004)	Prospective, controlled observational study	34 patiens with degenerative spondylolisthesis, 20 underwent laminectomy, 14 underwent laminectomy and instrumented posterolateral fusion 1 y ODI and SF-36 scores significantly better in fusion group	Low

moderate-quality evidence, the overall agreement of these and the observational studies, plus the failure to demonstrate harm[7] with fusion, supports a strong recommendation for **decompression plus fusion.**

Instrumented Versus Noninstrumented Fusion

Although attempted fusion appears to improve clinical outcomes in most studies, the addition of instrumentation is more controversial. The only prospective, randomized study examining this issue specifically in patients with degenerative spondylolisthesis and spinal stenosis is that of Fischgrund et al, who reported clinical outcomes of 67 patients undergoing decompression with and without instrumentation at 2-year follow-up.[6] They found that although the fusion rate was significantly higher for the group undergoing instrumented fusion (82% vs. 45% in the noninstrumented group), this increased fusion rate did not predict better clinical outcomes, which was excellent or good in 76% of the instrumented group versus 85% in the noninstrumented group. The authors identified preoperative angular motion as the only variable that seemed to predict pseudoarthrosis; therefore, in this patient population, the addition of instrumentation would have added value. In a long-term (5–14 year) follow-up study of the noninstrumented patient groups from the previously cited studies of Herkowitz and Kurz[5] and Fischgrund et al.,[6] Kornblum et al.[17] demonstrated that the clinical outcome was significantly better in patients with radiographic and clinical evidence of a solid fusion than in patients with a pseudoarthrosis. While not directly comparing instrumented to noninstrumented fusion patients, the authors concluded that the beneficial effect of a solid fusion on clinical outcome at longer term follow-up supports the rationale for use of instrumentation at the index procedure.

In addition to the RCT described above, other comparative observational studies merit review. One prospective study looking at the clinical outcome of fusion performed with and without instrumentation included a smaller subgroup of patients with degenerative spondylolisthesis.[19] Fusion rates were higher in the rigid fixation group (86% fusion rate compared to 65% in the noninstrumented group and 50% of the semirigid fixation group), but clinical outcomes were not significantly different between the groups. Other retrospective case series have looked at clinical outcome following decompression and instrumented fusion and found satisfactory outcomes.[20,21] However, Booth et al.[20] noted that 12 of 41 patients had radiographic evidence of transition syndromes at adjacent levels, with 5 patients requiring reoperation or having the intention of undergoing reoperation. Bjarke-Christensen et al.[22] prospectively evaluated the outcome

of pedicle screw instrumentation for chronic low back pain and included a subset of patients with degenerative spondylolisthesis. They found that patients with degenerative spondylolisthesis had better results with instrumentation than those with grade 1 and 2 isthmic spondylolisthesis, although there was a 25% overall reoperation rate in the instrumentation group versus 14% in the noninstrumented posterolateral fusion group. Finally, as part of a systematic review, Martin et al. examined three observational studies[23–25] comparing instrumented and noninstrumented fusion for degenerative spondylolisthesis.[26] They felt there was no conclusive evidence at short-term follow-up of the clinical benefit of instrumented fusion over noninstrumented fusion. There was a significant trend, however, that the use of instrumentation increases the chance of achieving a solid fusion.

Given the conflicting results from the primary studies on the clinical benefit of instrumented fusion over noninstrumented fusion, the evidence supporting its use is graded as low to moderate quality. This is considered in concert with the authors' clinical expertise and presumed patient preferences. In the authors' experience, the addition of instrumentation adds an acceptable amount of additional operative time provided that there are no patient factors that would dictate otherwise. For example, if the patient has religious preclusions to accepting a blood transfusion, then this might alter the risk-benefit ratio of the additional blood loss during the placement of instrumentation. In the absence of such exceptions, the authors would offer the patient the option of instrumentation, with the assumption that the patient would prefer to maximize her chances for a satisfactory outcome over the long-term. Using the framework of Schunemann, et al.[16] this would constitute a strong recommendation for an **instrumented fusion.**

Number of Levels to be Fused

An additional dilemma here is whether to fuse only the level of the spondylolisthesis or to include the other decompressed levels as well. The authors were unable to locate any RCTs or even comparative observational studies that specifically addressed this issue. While the subject of adjacent segment degeneration has been extensively debated in the literature, relevant studies in patients with degenerative spondylolisthesis have focused on whether to include L5-S1 in the fusion if it demonstrates asymptomatic disc degeneration.[27–29] These have not found any adverse effect to fusing only the level of the degenerative spondylolisthesis. On careful review of the data presented in the SPORT degenerative spondylolisthesis study, 57% of the combined surgical cohort underwent multilevel decompression whereas only 23% underwent multilevel fusion.[7] Although not directly stated, this implies that a substantial number of patients underwent multilevel decompression with fusion only of the olisthetic level. On subgroup analysis, the number of stenotic levels did not significantly affect outcomes. This is an indirect observation, however, and the study was not powered to examine this issue. However, there is insufficient evidence to support extending the fusion an additional level. As a result, the authors recommend **fusing only the L4-5 level and not all of the decompressed levels** in this patient. Reasons for extending the fusion to adjacent levels might include evidence of instability on preoperative flexion-extension films or iatrogenic instability caused by aggressive resection of the facet joints during the decompression.

Role of Interbody Fusion

The addition of some type of interbody fusion has been advocated by some due to the important stabilizing role of the anterior column against compressive, torsion, and shear forces, the increased surface area available for fusion, and the higher fusion rate associated with circumferential fusion versus posterior and posterolateral fusions.[30] Several retrospective studies have looked at outcomes after either posterior lumbar interbody fusion (PLIF) or transforaminal lumbar interbody fusion (TLIF) in association with decompression for degencrative spondylolisthesis.[31–34] One retrospective study compared the addition of PLIF to posterolateral fusion in patient groups with and without instability at the level of spondylolisthesis, defined as >4 mm translation or >10-degree angulation on flexion/extension films.[34] They found no difference in outcomes among the patients in the stable group, but the unstable group with additional PLIF had significantly better clinical outcomes. Although the results of interbody fusion are favorable, there is **insufficient evidence to advocate the addition of an interbody fusion here**, since there are no prospective studies comparing either PLIF or TLIF to posterolateral lumbar fusion for this specific condition.

Motion-Sparing Technology

Several alternatives to posterolateral fusion have been proposed, including the use of dynamic posterior stabilization in place of rigid instrumentation.[35,36] Although no high-quality clinical evidence exists to support them, both the Graf flexible stabilization technique (INVISTA, Wichita, Kansas) and the Dynesys (Zimmer, Inc., Warsaw, Indiana) have been used in patients with degenerative spondylolisthesis with good short-term results.[35,36] Interspinous distraction devices prevent extension at the implanted level. The implant is intended for patients who report exacerbation of symptoms with extension and improvement with forward flexion (as our patient reports) since the implanted motion segment is placed in a position of relative flexion. In a recent randomized, controlled study, Anderson et al.[37] evaluated such an implant, the X-Stop (St. Francis Medical Technologies, Inc., Alameda, California), for use in patients with neurogenic claudication and degenerative spondylolisthesis. Patients were assigned to treatment with the X-Stop versus nonoperative treatment. At 2-year follow-up, 63% of the patients treated with X-Stop reported success compared with 13% treated nonoperatively. Another retrospective study, however, reported a 58% reoperation rate within 2 years after implantation in patients with degenerative spondylolisthesis.[38] Given the conflicting available evidence, and the lack of a direct comparative study between interspinous process devices and traditional surgical methods, the authors **would not recommend this option at this time.**

DEFINITIVE TREATMENT PLAN

This patient with an L4-5 degenerative spondylolisthesis with a 25% slip and multilevel lumbar spinal stenosis should be treated with a thorough decompression of the L3-4 and L4-5 levels, followed by posterolateral instrumented fusion with a pedicle screw and rod construct extending from L4 to L5. The procedure would begin with an exposure carried laterally to the tips of transverse processes. A posterolateral gutter should be developed with exposure down to the intertransverse membrane in anticipation of placing bone graft bilaterally from the L4 to the L5 transverse processes. Great care should be taken to preserve the L3-4 facet capsules. Laminectomy can be started in the midline and extended to the lateral recesses as far lateral as necessary to achieve an adequate decompression at L4-5. A chisel or osteotome can facilitate this process by thinning out the medial portion of the facet, requiring less forceful Kerrison bites. The traversing L5 nerve roots should be visualized in the lateral recesses and foraminotomies should be performed over the L4 and L5 nerve roots. A Woodson or Penfield-3 should easily pass through the foramen at the completion of the decompression. At L3-4, careful medial facetectomies should be performed in order to avoid destabilizing this level.

Pedicle screws can be placed at the appropriate levels either before or after the decompression is complete. The authors favor decortication of the transverse processes prior to pedicle screw insertion since the implants make this process more difficult later. The lateral portion of the L4-5 facet and the L4 and L5 pars regions should be rigorously decorticated. After the rods have been secured to the screws, morcelized autograft is packed over the decorticated posterolateral elements. The patient would be mobilized out of bed as tolerated starting on the first postoperative day.

Brace immobilization after an instrumented lumbar fusion has not been proven to have any mechanical stabilizing effect although it may have some psychological benefit.[39]

Grading the Evidence for this Plan

While the evidence to support decompression and fusion would be considered high quality since it is derived from RCTs, the evidence to support our selection for an instrumented fusion would be considered low since there are no prospective RCTs or comparative observational studies that directly demonstrate clinical benefit of instrumentation in this scenario. However, in accordance with the guidelines outlined by Schunemann et al.,[16] additional consideration is given to the potential benefits, harms, and burdens of the more controversial component of the proposed interventions (instrumentation). Given the low risk of harm and the anticipated superior long-term results of a solid fusion, our proposed treatment would be considered a **strong recommendation**.

PREDICTING OUTCOMES

Although clinical improvement can be expected following decompression and fusion in this clinical scenario, patients may have some persistent back pain despite radiographic evidence of fusion. Relief of neurogenic claudication and leg pain is more reliable following decompression.[7,11,17] However, most of the studies examining clinical outcome following decompression and fusion use visual analog scales for back and leg pain, and only the SPORT trials include validated outcome measures such as the SF-36 bodily pain and physical function scores, and the ODI.[7,11] Symptoms of stenosis, back pain, and leg pain were improved at 3 months, and these results persisted at 1 and 2 years, with significant differences at all time points in the as-treated analyses.

In addition, Kornblum et al.[17] studied 58 patients who underwent decompression and noninstrumented posterolateral fusion with autogenous bone graft and reported on 5-year clinical outcomes. Eighty-six percent of patients with a successful fusion had a good or excellent clinical outcome, while only 56% of patients with a pseudoarthrosis had a good or excellent result. In addition, 46% of patients with a solid fusion were able to walk 2 mile or more at final follow-up (vs. 8% in the pseudoarthrosis group) and 77% were community ambulators (vs. 24% of patients with a pseudoarthrosis).

While instrumented fusion appears to give patients the best chance of obtaining a solid fusion, patients must be given all treatment options in as thorough and unbiased a manner as possible and should be counseled that they will sustain a longer operation with increased blood loss and at considerably more expense should instrumentation be used.[40] As the role of biologics becomes increasingly important and new advances are made, which may significantly affect fusion rates, the best surgical treatment options for this clinical scenario may change. The roles for selected interbody fusion and motion-preserving devices will become better defined with further investigation.

SUMMARY

In this case, a 65-year old woman presented with degenerative spondylolisthesis at L4-5 with multilevel spinal stenosis at L3-4 and L4-5 and with complaints of back pain that was worse than her leg pain. After an appropriate trial of nonoperative treatment, this patient would benefit most from a bilateral posterior laminectomy from L3 to L5 followed by an instrumented posterolateral fusion with autograft at L4-5. Although she will need to be counseled that some back pain may persist and adjacent segment disease may occur, this procedure can be expected to reliably improve her symptoms of stenosis and leg pain and should improve her back pain to some extent.

REFERENCES

1. Spivak J. Current concepts review—lumbar spinal stenosis. *J Bone Joint Surg Am*. 1998;80:1053–1066.
2. Singh K, Samartzis D, Biyani A, et al. Lumbar spinal stenosis. *J Am Acad Orthop Surg*. 2008;16(3):171–176.
3. Meyerding HW. Spondylolisthesis. *Surg Gynecol Obstet*. 1932;54:371–377.
4. Gibson JNA, Waddell G. Surgery for degenerative lumbar spondylosis. *Cochrane Database Syst Rev*. 2005;(4):CD001352. DOI: 10.1002/14651858.CD001352.pub3.
5. Herkowitz H, Kurz L. Degenerative lumbar spondylolisthesis with spinal stenosis: a prospective study comparing decompression with decompression and intertransverse process arthrodesis. *J Bone Joint Surg Am*. 1991;73:802–808.
6. Fischgrund J, Mackay M, Herkowitz H, et al. 1997 Volvo Award Winner in clinical studies: degenerative lumbar spondylolisthesis with spinal stenosis: a prospective, randomized study comparing decompressive laminectomy and arthrodesis with and without spinal instrumentation. *Spine*. 1997;22(24):2807–2812.
7. Weinstein J, Lurie J, Tosteson T, et al. Surgical versus nonsurgical treatment for lumbar degenerative spondylolisthesis. *N Engl J Med*. 2007;356(22):2257–2270.
8. Bridwell K, Sedgewick T, O'Brien M, et al. The role of fusion and instrumentation in the treatment of

degenerative spondylolisthesis with spinal stenosis. *J Spinal Disord.* 1993;6(6):461–472.

9. Weinstein JN, Lurie JD, Tosteson TD, et al. Surgical vs. nonoperative treatment for lumbar disk herniation: the Spine Patient Outcomes Research Trial (SPORT) observational cohort. *JAMA.* 2006;296:2452–2459.

10. Weinstein JN, Tosteson TD, Lurie JD, et al. Surgical vs. nonoperative treatment for lumbar disk herniation: the Spine Patient Outcomes Research Trial (SPORT): a randomized trial. *JAMA.* 2006;296:2441–2450.

11. Weinstein J, Tosteson T, Lurie J, et al. Surgical versus nonsurgical therapy for lumbar spinal stenosis. *N Engl J Med.* 2008;358:794–810.

12. Atlas SJ, Deyo RA, Keller RB, et al. The Maine Lumbar Spine Study, Part III: 1-year outcomes of surgical and nonsurgical management of lumbar spinal stenosis. *Spine.* 1996;21:1787–1794.

13. Malmivaara A, Slatis P, Heliovaara M. Surgical or nonoperative treatment for lumbar spinal stenosis: a randomized controlled trial. *Spine.* 2007;32(1):1–8.

14. Caputy A, Luessenhop A. Long-term evaluation of decompressive surgery for degenerative lumbar stenosis. *J Neurosurg.* 1992;77:669–676.

15. Atlas S, Keller R, Wu Y, et al. Long-term outcomes of surgical and nonsurgical management of lumbar spinal stenosis: 8 to 10 year results from the Maine lumbar spine study. *Spine.* 2005;30(8):936–943.

16. Schunemann HJ, Jaeschke R, Cook DJ, et al. An official ATS statement: grading the quality of evidence and strength of recommendations in ATS guidelines and recommendations. *Am J Respir Crit Care Med.* 2006;174: 605–614.

17. Kornblum M, Fischgrund J, Herkowitz H, et al. Degenerative lumbar spondylolisthesis with spinal stenosis. A prospective long-term study comparing fusion and pseudoarthrosis. *Spine.* 2004;29(7):726–734.

18. Ghogawala Z, Benzel E, Amin-Hanjani S, et al. Prospective outcomes evaluation after decompression with or without instrumented fusion for lumbar stenosis and degenerative spondylolisthesis. *J Neurosurg.* 2004(3):267–272.

19. Zdeblick T. A prospective, randomized study of lumbar fusion: preliminary results. *Spine.* 1993;18:983–991.

20. Booth K, Bridwell K, Eisenberg B, et al. Mimimum 5-year results of degenerative spondylolisthesis treated with decompression and instrumented posterior fusion. *Spine.* 1999;24:1721–1727.

21. Nork S, Hu S, Workman K. Patient outcomes after decompression and instrumented posterior spinal fusion for degenerative spondylolisthesis. *Spine.* 1999;24(6): 561–569.

22. Bjarke Christensen F, Stender Hansen E, Laursen M, et al. Long-term functional outcome of pedicle screw instrumentation as a support for posterolateral spinal fusion. *Spine.* 2002;27(12):1269–1277.

23. Kakiuchi M, Ono K. Defatted, gas-sterilized cortical bone allograft for posterior lumbar interbody vertebral fusion. *Int Orthop.* 1998;22:69–76.

24. Mochida J, Suzuki K, Chiba M. How to stabilize a single level lesion of degenerative spondylolisthesis. *Clin Orthop.* 1999;368:126–134.

25. Kimura I, Shingu H, Murata M, et al. Lumbar posterolateral fusion alone or with transpedicular instrumentation in L4–5 degenerative spondylolisthesis. *J Spinal Disord.* 2001;14:301–310.

26. Martin CR, Gruszczynski AT, Braunsfurth HA, et al. The surgical management of degenerative lumbar spondylolisthesis: a systematic review. *Spine.* 2007;32(16): 1791–1798.

27. Ghiselli G, Wang J, Hsu W, et al. L5-S1 segment survivorship and clinical outcome analysis after L4–5 isolated fusion. *Spine.* 2003;28(12):1275–1280.

28. Miyakoshi N, Abe E, Shimada Y, et al. Outcome of one-level posterior lumbar interbody fusion for spondylolisthesis and postoperative intervertebral disc degeneration adjacent to the fusion. *Spine.* 2000;25:1837–1842.

29. Throckmorton T, Hilibrand A, Mencio G, et al. The impact of adjacent level disc degeneration on health status outcomes following lumbar fusion. *Spine.* 2003;28: 2546–2550.

30. Suk S, Lee C, Kim W, et al. Adding posterior lumbar interbody fusion to pedicle screw fixation and posterolateral fusion after decompression in spondylolytic spondylolisthesis. *Spine.* 1997;22:210–219.

31. Ha K, Na K, Shin J, et al. Comparison of posterolateral fusion with and without additional posterior lumbar interbody fusion for degenerative spondylolisthesis. *J Spinal Disord Tech.* 2008;21(4):229–234.

32. Lauber S, Schulte T, Liljenqvist U, et al. Clinical and radiologic 2- and 4-year results of transforaminal lumbar interbody fusion in degenerative and isthmic spondylolisthesis grades 1 and 2. *Spine.* 2006;31(15):1693–1698.

33. Zhao J, Wang X, Hoe T, et al. One versus two BAK fusion cages in posterior lumbar interbody fusion to L4-L5 degenerative spondylolisthesis. *Spine.* 2002;27(24): 2753–2757.

34. Yan DL, Pei FX, Li J, et al. Comparative study of PILF and TLIF treatment in adult degenerative spondylolisthesis. *Eur Spine J.* 2008;17(10):1311–1316.

35. Hashimoto T, Oha F, Shigenobu K, et al. Mid-term results of Graf stabilization for lumbar degenerative pathologies: a minimum 2-year follow-up. *Spine J.* 2001;1:283–289.

36. Grob D, Benini A, Junge A, et al. Clinical experience with the Dynesys semirigid fixation system for the lumbar spine. *Spine.* 2005;30(3):324–331.

37. Anderson PA, Tribus CB, Kitchel SH. Treatment of neurogenic claudication by interspinous decompression: application of the X Stop device in patients with degenerative spondylolisthesis. *J Neurosurg Spine.* 2006;4: 463–471.

38. Verhoof O, Bron J, Wapstra F, et al. High failure rate of the interspinous distraction device (X-Stop) for the treatment of lumbar spinal stenosis caused by degenerative spondylolisthesis. *Eur Spine J.* 2008;17:188–192.

39. Connelly P, Grob D. Bracing of patients after fusion for degenerative problems of the lumbar spine—yes or no? *Spine.* 1998;23(12):1426–1428.

40. Kuntz K, Snider R, Weinstein J. Cost-effectiveness of fusion with and without instrumentation for patients with degenerative spondylolisthesis and spinal stenosis. *Spine.* 2000;25(9):1132–1139.

Lumbar Degenerative Spondylolisthesis with Multilevel Stenosis II

JOHN R. DIMAR II, MD

EDITORS' CASE PRESENTATION

A 72-year-old woman with a history of hyperten-sion, diabetes mellitus, hypercholesterolemia, glaucoma, and gastroesophageal reflux presents with a complaint of bilateral thigh and buttock pain over the past 2½ years. She feels her symp-toms are better leaning forward or leaning on a shopping cart when she goes to the supermarket. Bowel and bladder functions are reportedly intact. The woman has had a course of nonoperative treatment that has included multiple epidural steroid injections and physical therapy, from which she has had only short-term relief. Since then, her pain has become unbearable and is substan-tially affecting her ability to function, as she can no longer walk long distances.

Physical exam demonstrates decreased exten-sion of the lumbar spine. Gait is fairly normal, though she does use a cane. Posture is stooped forward. She has intact strength and sensation bilaterally and no pain to palpation of the back. Reflexes are normal. Radiographic images are shown in Figures 21.1A–D and 21.2A–D.

INTERPRETATION OF CLINICAL PRESENTATION

This case demonstrates typical key features of symp-tomatic degenerative spondylolisthesis as it describes an elderly female with neurogenic claudication, mini-mal back pain complaints, positive sagittal balance, with involvement of the L4/5 level.[1-7] It also demon-strates the usual temporal progression of symptoms over a 2- to 3-year period as a result of worsening static stenosis combined with dynamic spinal stenosis.[8,9] The differential diagnoses to consider in elderly patients who complain of walking intolerance with referred pain down the buttocks and legs include peripheral vascular disease, spinal cord compression due to spon-dylosis, tumors proximal to the lumbosacral spine, degenerative joint disease or avascular necrosis of the hips and knees, metastatic disease to lower extremity osseous structures or the lumbosacral plexus, periph-eral neuropathy, and rare tumors of the peripheral nerves.[4] The etiology of spinal stenosis is multifactorial. There may be a component of preexisting congenital spinal stenosis as well as acquired spinal stenosis from gradual degeneration of discs and facet joints. Progres-sive instability of the spinal segment may result in spondylolisthesis.[7,8,10] As a result of progressive degen-eration, these patients tend to pursue a downward spiral of decreasing activity where increasing claudica-tion results in a more sedentary lifestyle resulting in significant deterioration of their core muscle strength.

Review of the available sagittal and axial magnetic resonance image demonstrates multilevel central and foraminal spinal stenosis at L2/3 (mild), L3/4 (mild), L4/5 (severe), and L5/S1 (mild). The Grade I spon-dylolisthesis at L4/5 appears to be the worst level of spinal stenosis, which is the result of a combination of posterior spondylosis, severe bilateral facet hypertro-phy, and ligamentum flavum thickening. The finding of severe static stenosis combined with the potential for additional dynamic stenosis that is frequently asso-ciated with a spondylolisthesis targets the L4/5 level as the likely source of this patient's spinal claudica-tion. No anteroposterior, lateral, or flexion-extension radiographs of the lumbar spine are available for review. Full-length 36-in anteroposterior and lateral radiographs may be helpful to further evaluate sagit-tal balance. A myelogram combined with a computed tomography (CT) scan can further delineate the degree

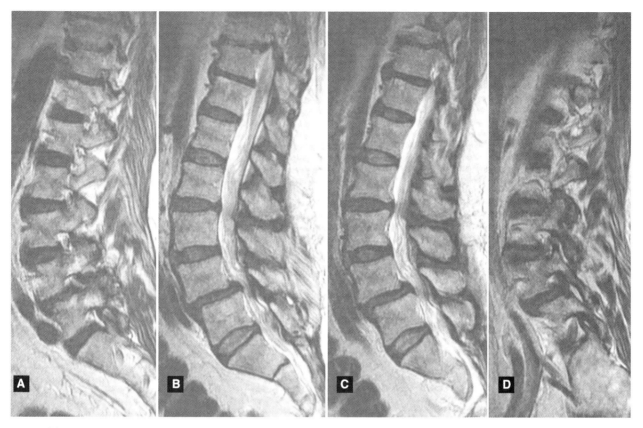

Figure 21.1.

of motion at the level of the spondylolisthesis and any weight-bearing-induced central or foraminal stenosis above or below the spondylolisthesis.[10–12]

DECLARATION OF SPECIFIC DIAGNOSIS

The case presented describes a patient with a potentially unstable grade 1 spondylolisthesis at L4/5 with associated severe spinal stenosis causing neurogenic claudication combined with mild adjacent central and foraminal stenosis at L2/3, L3/4, and L5/S1.

BRAINSTORMING: WHAT ARE THE TREATMENT GOALS AND SURGICAL OPTIONS?

The treatment goals are

1. Exhaust all reasonable conservative care and ensure the patient is medically fit for surgery.
2. Surgical treatment of the incapacitating spinal neurogenic claudication symptoms.
3. Restore long-term stability to the L4/5 spinal segment to prevent progression of slippage.

L2-3	L3-4	L4-5	L5-S1

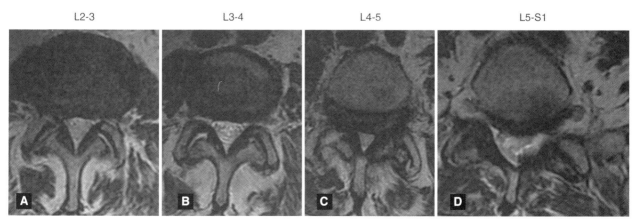

Figure 21.2.

4. Address any adjacent level central or foraminal stenosis only as absolutely necessary.

5. Maintain or improve the lumbosacral sagittal balance.

6. Improve quality of life (QOL) outcome measures to ensure meaningful improvement.

The treatment options are

1. Continue conservative care including NSAID, water aerobics, periodic epidural blocks, narcotic pain medications.

2. Surgical correction via posterior decompression of L4/5 and other required levels.

3. Surgical correction via posterior decompression, posterolateral spinal fusion (PLSF) in situ (no reduction).

4. Surgical correction via posterior decompression, PLSF with pedicle instrumentation with or without reduction of the spondylolisthesis.

5. Surgical correction via decompression, transforaminal lumbar interbody fusion (TLIF), posterior instrumentation, reduction of the spondylolisthesis, with or without a concurrent PLSF.

6. Surgical correction via an anterior lumbar interbody fusion (ALIF), PLSF, pedicle instrumentation, with or without a concurrent PLSF.

EVALUATION OF THE LITERATURE

Relevant articles addressing adult degenerative spondylolisthesis were identified by doing a computer search of MEDLINE, EMBASE, HealthSTAR, Cumulative Index to Nursing & Allied Health Literature, Cochrane Database of Systematic Reviews, ACP Journal Club, Database of Abstracts of Reviews of Effects, Cochrane Central Register of Controlled Trials, from the beginning of the databases up to January of 2008 using the search strategy outlined in Table 21.1. Five hundred and ninety article abstracts were identified.

DETAILED REVIEW OF PERTINENT ARTICLES

Operative Versus Nonoperative Treatment

Degenerative spondylolisthesis is a common diagnosis in the aging population in whom there is also a high incidence of concurrent comorbidities.[13] Therefore, because of the potentially high complication rate associated with surgery, physicians tend to exhaust all possible conservative modalities in the treatment of the

TABLE 21.1	Search Strategy.	
Results	Search Type	Display
1	spondylolisthesis {Including Related Terms}	761
2	child$.ti,ab.	718701
3	adolescent.ti,ab.	45555
4	pediatric.ti,ab.	98550
5	juvenile.ti,ab.	38413
6	infantile.ti,ab.	19398
7	isthmic.ti,ab.	1583
8	dysplastic.ti,ab.	9593
9	high.ti,ab.	1572065
10	trauma.ti,ab.	106239
11	cervical.ti,ab.	115569
12	6 or 11 or 3 or 7 or 9 or 2 or 8 or 4 or 10 or 5	2494255
13	1 not 11	717
14	limit 14 to humans	707
15	limit 15 to English language	590

elderly with spinal pathology.[14,15] These nonsurgical treatment methods are the same as for the treatment of low back pain and include activity modification, physical therapy, aquatic aerobics, nonsteroidal anti-inflammatory drugs, bracing, and epidural blocks. A recent systematic review of physiotherapy showed that specific exercise interventions alone or in combination with other treatments had a positive effect on low back pain due to spondylolisthesis; however, there were not enough studies that were similar enough to draw any conclusions.[16]

Although many patients temporarily respond to conservative care, approximately 15% of patients eventually undergo surgical intervention to increase the diameter of the spinal canal and restore stability.[4,9,17,18] Despite a course of nonoperative treatment including epidural steroid injections and physical therapy, the patient in the current case continues to have unbearable pain and can no longer walk long distances, diminishing her quality of life. Surgical decompression and stabilization of degenerative spondylolisthesis have been shown to reliably relieve a patient's symptoms and result in improved long-term outcome measures.[2,7,9,19–26] Surgery should only be considered if the patient's overall medical condition is stable enough to tolerate surgery, if the patient is aware of the risks associated with surgery, and the patient's perception of his or her QOL has deteriorated to such a degree that they are willing to undergo surgery.[27]

Weinstein et al.[9] recently reported the 2-year outcomes from the SPORT (Spine Patient Outcomes Research Trial) study where surgically treated patients showed substantially greater improvement of both pain and function compared to patients treated nonsurgically. The objective of surgical treatment is the relief of spinal claudication while ensuring a stable, balanced lumbosacral spine. Preoperative assessment should evaluate the potential risks and consider the unique features that affect success of the surgery. The slip grade, presence of osteopenia, positive sagittal imbalance, rotational and translational instabilities, and the severity of the stenosis all may affect the outcome of surgery.[8,9,24,28–30] Adequate decompression leads to rapid relief of the neurologic symptoms. Achieving a solid fusion has been associated with short- and long-term clinical improvement and patient satisfaction.[9,17,24,28–30] Studies demonstrate that when back and leg pain symptoms are severe enough, surgery offers substantially greater improvement of pain and function when compared to nonsurgical treatment.[6,9]

EVIDENTIARY TABLE AND SELECTION OF TREATMENT METHOD

The best available evidence was reviewed in order to develop a specific surgical treatment plan. This body of evidence is summarized in Table 21.2. The following is a description of pertinent data.

Decompression Alone Versus Fusion

There are two randomized clinical trials[29,31] and six observational cohorts[32–37] available that evaluated decompression alone versus decompression and fusion for degenerative spondylolisthesis. Except for one observational study,[35] all the studies showed better results with fusion compared to decompression alone.

Decompression with an Interspinous Spacer

There is one randomized clinical trial showing that decompression using an interspinous spacer leads to better clinical outcomes compared to nonoperative treatment in patients with a stable degenerative

TABLE 21.2	Evidentiary Table.		
Paper Author (Year)	**Description**	**Summary of Results**	**Quality of Evidence**
Weinstein et al. (2007)	RCT, nonoperative vs. operative treatment for degenerative spondylolisthesis	Patients treated surgically showed substantially greater improvement in pain and function during a period of 2 y than patients treated nonsurgically	High
Kornblum et al. (2004)	Long-term follow-up of patients with solid fusion and those with pseudarthrosis	Outcomes of patients with stable pseudarthrosis deteriorated over time; solid fusion achieved with instrumentation had better long-term results	Moderate
Fischgrund et al. (1997)	RCT, instrumented vs. noninstrumented fusion	Instrumented fusions had higher fusion rates, but outcomes were similar to noninstrumented fusions.	High
Montgomery and Fischgrund (1994)	Prospective study of passive reduction of spondylolisthesis on the operating room table	Postural reduction improves the degree of slippage	High
Herkowitz and Kurz (1991)	RCT, fusion vs. decompression alone	Patients who were fused had better outcomes and symptom relief even if they had a pseudarthrosis	High
Anderson et al. (2006)	RCT, interspinous spacer versus nonoperative care	Using an interspinous spacer leads to better clinical outcomes compared to nonoperative treatment	High

spondylolisthesis and symptomatic neurologic complaints.[38] The spacer has been shown to increase the interspinous distance and foraminal height, thus relieving nerve compression. This treatment may be extremely useful in patients who do not wish a more extensive surgical procedure or those with significant comorbidities that preclude a more extensive surgery.

Instrumented Versus Noninstrumented Fusion

Studies comparing instrumented versus noninstrumented fusions are available for posterolateral fusion techniques only. There are two randomized clinical trials[28,31] and three observational cohorts.[39–41] In these studies, higher rates of fusion were observed in patients who had instrumentation compared to those who were not instrumented. Long-term follow-up[30] has shown a correlation between achieving a solid fusion with instrumentation and improved clinical outcome and less pain. Instrumentation should be considered if there is documented listhesis >5 mm, the spondylolisthesis is more than 50%, or a previous wide laminectomy has been performed because of the potential to lead to further instability with just an isolated decompression.[7]

Interbody Fusion

An interbody technique via a posterior lumbar interbody fusion (PLIF) or TLIF may be indicated in higher grade spondylolistheses, significant segmental kyphosis, osteoporosis, or short transverse processes.[2,7,8,19,21,24,42] The placement of an interbody device through a posterior approach removes the morbidity of an anterior procedure and provides considerable support to the overall construct via load sharing. Interbody fusions have been shown to decrease the stress on the posterior pedicle instrumentation up to eighteen times.[43]

There are limited studies comparing instrumented posterolateral fusion alone versus the addition of an interbody fusion. Ha et al.[19] showed that the addition of PLIF to an instrumented posterolateral fusion improves outcomes in unstable spondylolistheses. In contrast, Inamdar et al.[20] showed better outcomes in patients with instrumented posterolateral fusion alone compared to those combined with PLIF. The study also showed better reduction but higher complications rates in patients who had PLIF. Observational cohorts[19,24] have shown improvement in outcome scores at follow-up compared to preoperative in patients who had TLIF or PLIF.

Anterior Interbody Fusion or Combined Anterior/Posterior Fusion

Certain authors have reported favorable results in observational cohorts with stand-alone ALIF with good restoration of disc space height, decompression of the foramen, and prevention of adjacent level degeneration.[44,45] There, however, were no differences in the amount of postoperative lordosis, percentage of slippage, improvement in outcome measures, or success of surgery when compared to a posterolateral fusion.[46]

Bone Grafting Options

There are a wide variety of bone graft materials available. Autograft demonstrates a fusion rate between 40% and 98%. A meta-analysis of all available fusion literature demonstrated an overall autograft fusion rate of 87%.[47] Demineralized bone matrix has also been shown to be useful as a bone graft extender in a recent study when combined with autograft.[48] Further studies have shown that use of the rhBMP's, with and without pedicle instrumentation, when compared to iliac crest bone graft (ICBG) significantly improves the chance of solid fusion and should be considered as adjunct treatment.[2,25,26,28,49–51]

Reduction of Spondylolisthesis

There is some controversy over whether or not a concurrent reduction should be performed in a grade 1 spondylolisthesis.[7] When there is documented instability on preoperative flexion and extension radiographs, the spondylolisthesis will usually reduce following muscle relaxation with positioning the patient in the prone position.[6,52] Additional posterior surgical maneuvers that facilitate reduction of the spondylolisthesis include the use of reduction screws, soft-tissue releases, facet osteotomies, and the PLIF or TLIF techniques that remove the disc and elevate the disc space while simultaneously effecting the interbody fusion.[21,24,42] However, a reduction should be abandoned in the instances where the spondylolisthesis is rigidly fixed or significant osteoporosis exists. In these instances, there is significant potential to lose fixation as a result of pedicle screw failure at the bone/screw interface or actual fracturing of the pedicle either acutely or in a delayed fashion.[53] Therefore, the general consensus is to use postural reduction and fuse in situ unless the patient's physiologic or chronologic age is such that reduction is mandatory to maintain good lordosis and prevent adjacent level degenerative disc disease.[6,7]

DEFINITIVE TREATMENT PLAN

Treatment is predicated on all reasonable nonoperative treatment modalities being exhausted prior to surgical consideration. Several different surgical techniques are available to address the grade I degenerative spondylolisthesis in his case. Based on the available evidence and the particular patient characteristics, the preferred treatment is a postural reduction or fusion in situ, followed by posterior decompression to address the spinal stenosis and a concurrent posterolateral fusion with pedicle instrumentation.

Grading the Evidence for this Plan

The evidence to support surgical treatment over continued nonoperative treatment would be considered high. The evidence to support fusion plus decompression over decompression alone would also be considered high. The evidence to support instrumented fusion rather than noninstrumented fusion would be considered low. However, given the reasonable risks and safety of the prescribed treatment, and the consistency of the data in general, the author considers the surgical plan as outlined to be a **strong recommendation**.

PREDICTING OUTCOMES

Predicting outcomes in an elderly population is difficult due to an extensive array of variables. These include the extensive differential diagnosis in the elderly, multiple comorbidities, and difficulty obtaining long-term follow-up. Prospective randomized trials and observational cohorts have shown improved outcomes in patients undergoing decompression and fusion for single-level degenerative spondylolisthesis.[28,29,54] Therefore, surgical intervention should reliably improve the patient's unremitting leg pain, instability, and the sagittal imbalance. Subsequent deterioration of the adjacent levels resulting in stenosis and the long-term effect on outcomes are controversial but may be an acceptable consequence in light of the patient's severe symptoms.

SUMMARY

This is a classic case example of a 72-year-old female with significant comorbidities who presents with a >2-year history of progressive spinal claudication. Having ruled out potential other etiologies of leg pain, she was treated with extensive conservative care including physical therapy and epidural blocks, neither of which has given her any lasting relief. She has pursued a typical downhill course of increasing symptoms that have severely affected her quality of life. If surgery is her choice to attempt to relieve her symptoms and she is medically fit enough to undergo surgery, then the surgical procedure that has the best supporting evidence is a posterior decompression and posterolateral fusion with instrumentation.

REFERENCES

1. Barrey C, Jund J, Perrin G, et al. Spinopelvic alignment of patients with degenerative spondylolisthesis. *Neurosurgery*. 2007;61(5):981–986.
2. Dimar JR, Djurasovic M, Carreon LY. Surgical management of degenerative and postsurgical spondylolisthesis. *Semin Spine Surg*. 2005;17:186–194.
3. Hosoe H, Ohmori K. Degenerative lumbosacral spondylolisthesis: possible factors which predispose the fifth lumbar vertebra to slip. *J Bone Joint Surg Br*. 2008;90(3): 356–359.
4. Hu SS, Tribus CB, Diab M, et al. Spondylolisthesis and spondylolysis. *Instr Course Lect*. 2008;57:431–445.
5. Jacobsen S, Sonne-Holm S, Rovsing H, et al. Degenerative lumbar spondylolisthesis: an epidemiological perspective: the Copenhagen Osteoarthritis Study. *Spine*. 2007;32(1):120–125.
6. Matsunaga S, Sakou T, Morizono Y, et al. Natural history of degenerative spondylolisthesis. Pathogenesis and naturalcourse of the slippage. *Spine*. 1990;15(11):1204–1210.
7. Sengupta DK, Herkowitz HN. Degenerative spondylolisthesis: review of current trends and controversies. *Spine*. 2005;30(6 suppl):S71–S81.
8. Iguchi T, Kanemura A, Kasahara K, et al. Lumbar instability and clinical symptoms: which is the more critical factor for symptoms: sagittal translation or segment angulation? *J Spinal Disord Tech*. 2004;17(4):284–290.
9. Weinstein JN, Lurie JD, Tosteson TD, et al. Surgical versus nonsurgical treatment for lumbar degenerative spondylolisthesis. *N Engl J Med*. 2007;356(22):2257–2270.
10. Jayakumar P, Nnadi C, Saifuddin A, et al. Dynamic degenerative lumbar spondylolisthesis: diagnosis with axial loaded magnetic resonance imaging. *Spine*. 2006;31(10): E298–E301.
11. Butt S, Saifuddin A. The imaging of lumbar spondylolisthesis. *Clin Radiol*. 2005;60(5):533–546.
12. Chaput C, Padon D, Rush J, et al. The significance of increased fluid signal on magnetic resonance imaging in lumbar facets in relationship to degenerative spondylolisthesis. *Spine*. 2007;32(17):1883–1887.
13. Rosenberg NJ. Degenerative spondylolisthesis: surgical treatment. *Clin Orthop Relat Res*. 1976;117:112–120.
14. Malmivaara A, Slätis P, Heliövaara M, et al. Surgical or nonoperative treatment for lumbar spinal stenosis? A randomized controlled trial. *Spine*. 2007;32(1):1–8.
15. Glassman SD, Schwab FJ, Bridwell KH, et al. The selection of operative versus nonoperative treatment in patients with adult scoliosis. *Spine*. 2007;32(1):93–97.
16. McNeely ML, Torrance G, Magee DJ. A systematic review of physiotherapy for spondylolysis and spondylolisthesis. *Man Ther*. 2003;8(2):80–91.
17. Martin CR, Gruszczynski AT, Braunsfurth HA, et al. The surgical management of degenerative lumbar spondylolisthesis: a systematic review. *Spine*. 2007;32(16):1791–1798.
18. Vibert BT, Sliva CD, Herkowitz HN. Treatment of instability and spondylolisthesis: surgical versus nonsurgical treatment. *Clin Orthop Relat Res*. 2006;443:222–227.
19. Ha KY, Na KH, Shin JH, et al. Comparison of posterolateral fusion with and without additional posterior lumbar

interbody fusion for degenerative lumbar spondylolisthesis. *J Spinal Disord Tech*. 2008;21(4):229–234.

20. Inamdar DN, Alagappan M, Shyam L, et al. Posterior lumbar interbody fusion versus intertransverse fusion in the treatment of lumbar spondylolisthesis. *J Orthop Surg (Hong Kong)*. 2006;14(1):21–26.

21. Lauber S, Schulte TL, Liljenqvist U, et al. Clinical and radiologic 2–4-year results of transforaminal lumbar interbody fusion in degenerative and isthmic spondylolisthesis grades 1 and 2. *Spine*. 2006;31(15):1693–1698.

22. Resnick DK, Choudhri TF, Dailey AT, et al. Guidelines for the performance of fusion procedures for degenerative disease of the lumbar spine. Part 9: fusion in patients with stenosis and spondylolisthesis. *J Neurosurg Spine*. 2005;2(6):679–685.

23. Schnake KJ, Schaeren S, Jeanneret B. Dynamic stabilization in addition to decompression for lumbar spinal stenosis with degenerative spondylolisthesis. *Spine*. 2006;31(4):442–449.

24. Sears W. Posterior lumbar interbody fusion for degenerative spondylolisthesis: restoration of sagittal balance using insert-and-rotate interbody spacers. *Spine J*. 2005;5(2):170–179.

25. Vaccaro AR, Anderson DG, Patel T, et al. Comparison of OP-1 Putty (rhBMP-7) to iliac crest autograft for posterolateral lumbar arthrodesis: a minimum 2-year follow-up pilot study. *Spine*. 2005;30(24):2709–2716.

26. Vaccaro AR, Patel T, Fischgrund J, et al. A pilot study evaluating the safety and efficacy of OP-1 Putty (rhBMP-7) as a replacement for iliac crest autograft in posterolateral lumbar arthrodesis for degenerative spondylolisthesis. *Spine*. 2004;29(17):1885–1892.

27. Hosono N, Namekata M, Makino T, et al. Perioperative complications of primary posterior lumbar interbody fusion for nonisthmic spondylolisthesis: analysis of risk factors. *J Neurosurg Spine*. 2008;9(5):403–407.

28. Fischgrund JS, Mackay M, Herkowitz HN, et al. 1997 Volvo Award winner in clinical studies. Degenerative lumbar spondylolisthesis with spinal stenosis: a prospective, randomized study comparing decompressive laminectomy and arthrodesis with and without spinal instrumentation. *Spine*. 1997;22(24):2807–2812.

29. Herkowitz HN, Kurz LT. Degenerative lumbar spondylolisthesis with spinal stenosis. A prospective study comparing decompression with decompression and intertransverse process arthrodesis. *J Bone Joint Surg Am*. 1991;73(6):802–808.

30. Kornblum MB, Fischgrund JS, Herkowitz HN, et al. Degenerative lumbar spondylolisthesis with spinal stenosis: a prospective long-term study comparing fusion and pseudarthrosis. *Spine*. 2004;29(7):726–733.

31. Bridwell KH, Sedgewick TA, O'Brien MF, et al. The role of fusion and instrumentation in the treatment of degenerative spondylolisthesis with spinal stenosis. *J Spinal Disord*. 1993;6(6):461–472.

32. Feffer HL, Wiesel SW, Cuckler JM, et al. Degenerative spondylolisthesis. To fuse or not to fuse. *Spine*. 1985;10(3):287–289.

33. Ghogawala Z, Benzel EC, Amin-Hanjani S, et al. Prospective outcomes evaluation after decompression with or without instrumented fusion for lumbar stenosis and degenerative Grade I spondylolisthesis. *J Neurosurg Spine*. 2004;1(3):267–272.

34. Lombardi JS, Wiltse LL, Reynolds J, et al. Treatment of degenerative spondylolisthesis. *Spine*. 1985;10(9):821–827.

35. Matsudaira K, Yamazaki T, Seichi A, et al. Spinal stenosis in grade I degenerative lumbar spondylolisthesis: a comparative study of outcomes following laminoplasty and laminectomy with instrumented spinal fusion. *J Orthop Sci*. 2005;10(3):270–276.

36. Satomi K, Hirabayashi K, Toyama Y, et al. A clinical study of degenerative spondylolisthesis. Radiographic analysis and choice of treatment. *Spine*. 1992;17(11):1329–1336.

37. Yone K, Sakou T. Usefulness of Posner's definition of spinal instability for selection of surgical treatment for lumbar spinal stenosis. *J Spinal Disord*. 1999;12(1):40–44.

38. Anderson PA, Tribus CB, Kitchel SH. Treatment of neurogenic claudication by interspinous decompression: application of the X STOP device in patients with lumbar degenerative spondylolisthesis. *J Neurosurg Spine*. 2006;4(6):463–471.

39. Kakiuchi M, Ono K. Defatted, gas-sterilised cortical bone allograft for posterior lumbar interbody vertebral fusion. *Int Orthop*. 1998;22(2):69–76.

40. Kimura I, Shingu H, Murata M, et al. Lumbar posterolateral fusion alone or with transpedicular instrumentation in L4-L5 degenerative spondylolisthesis. *J Spinal Disord*. 2001;14(4):301–310.

41. Mochida J, Suzuki K, Chiba M. How to stabilize a single level lesion of degenerative lumbar spondylolisthesis. *Clin Orthop Relat Res*. 1999;(368):126–134.

42. Potter BK, Freedman BA, Verwiebe EG, et al. Transforaminal lumbar interbody fusion: clinical and radiographic results and complications in 100 consecutive patients. *J Spinal Disord Tech*. 2005;18(4):337–346.

43. Polly DW Jr, Klemme WR, Cunningham BW, et al. The biomechanical significance of anterior column support in a simulated single-level spinal fusion. *J Spinal Disord*. 2000;13(1):58–62.

44. Inoue S, Watanabe T, Goto S, et al. Degenerative spondylolisthesis. Pathophysiology and results of anterior interbody fusion. *Clin Orthop Relat Res*. 1988;227:90–98.

45. Takahashi K, Kitahara H, Yamagata M, et al. Long-term results of anterior interbody fusion for treatment of degenerative spondylolisthesis. *Spine*. 1990;15(11):1211–1215.

46. Min JH, Jang JS, Lee SH. Comparison of anterior- and posterior-approach instrumented lumbar interbody fusion for spondylolisthesis. *J Neurosurg Spine*. 2007;7(1):21–26.

47. Bono CM, Lee CK. Critical analysis of trends in fusion for degenerative disc disease over the past 20 years: influence of technique on fusion rate and clinical outcome. *Spine*. 2004;29(4):455–463.

48. Cammisa FP Jr, Lowery G, Garfin SR, et al. Two-year fusion rate equivalency between Grafton DBM gel and autograft in posterolateral spine fusion: a prospective controlled trial employing a side-by-side comparison in the same patient. *Spine*. 2004;29(6):660–666.

49. Dimar JR, Glassman SD, Burkus KJ, et al. Clinical outcomes and fusion success at 2 years of single-level

instrumented posterolateral fusions with recombinant human bone morphogenetic protein-2/compression resistant matrix versus iliac crest bone graft. *Spine*. 2006;31(22):2534–2539.

50. Dimar JR, Glassman SD. The art of bone grafting. *Curr Opin Orthop*. 2007;18:226–233.

51. Singh K, Smucker JD, Gill S, et al. Use of recombinant human bone morphogenetic protein-2 as an adjunct in posterolateral lumbar spine fusion: a prospective CT-scan analysis at one and two years. *J Spinal Disord Tech*. 2006;19(6):416–423.

52. Montgomery DM, Fischgrund JS. Passive reduction of spondylolisthesis on the operating room table: a prospective study. *J Spinal Disord*. 1994;7(2):167–172.

53. Klineberg E, McHenry T, Bellabarba C, et al. Sacral insufficiency fractures caudal to instrumented posterior lumbosacral arthrodesis. *Spine*. 2008;33(16):1806–1811.

54. Nork SE, Hu SS, Workman KL, et al. Patient outcomes after decompression and instrumented posterior spinal fusion for degenerative spondylolisthesis. *Spine*. 1999;24(6):561–569.

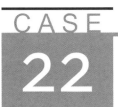
L5-S1 Slip and Herniation

WILLIAM C. WATTERS III, MS, MMS, MD

A 64-year-old woman with a history of hypertension, hypothyroidism, depression, gastroesophageal reflux, and anxiety presents with a primary complaint of low back pain and right lower extremity pain, numbness, and tingling. The onset of her pain was approximately 6 to 8 months ago. By history, low back pain started first followed by right leg symptoms. She feels the back pain is more significant than her leg pain. Right lower extremity pain radiates down to the plantar surface of the foot and is exacerbated with sneezing and coughing. Back pain is worse with forward flexion and somewhat relieved with extension. She can walk about ten minutes before the low back pain stops her. She has no bowel or bladder complaints. The patient has not undergone a formal course of physical therapy, but she has had three epidural steroid injections without relief.

Physical examination reveals pain with forward flexion, which is limited to touching her hands to her knees. Though extension is limited to about 15 degrees, there is little pain. Localized tenderness is present with palpation of the L5 spinous process. Sensation is intact. However, she has decreased strength in the quads and hamstrings bilaterally, seemingly secondary to pain. Straight leg raise test is negative. Reflexes are equal and intact bilaterally.

Radiographic imaging studies are shown in Figures 22.1 to 22.4.

INTERPRETATION OF CLINICAL PRESENTATION

This patient presents as a chronologically older though not elderly female with dominant lower back pain and with less intense radicular symptoms of right leg pain

as well as numbness and tingling to the plantar surface of her right foot. Her back pain is increased on forward flexion while she has little pain on extension. She has L5 spinous process tenderness on palpation and she has no clear-cut neurological changes. Potentially complicating her management is a history of hypertension, hypothyroidism, gastroesophageal reflux, depression, and anxiety.

Routine AP and lateral x-rays reveal a Grade I spondylolisthesis with >50% loss of disc height at the L5-S1 disc space (Fig. 22.1 A–C). The remaining lumbar discs are well preserved with minimal loss of height at L4-5, and there are few stigmata of degenerative spondylosis at these levels but some increased sclerosis of the sacroiliac joints. A lateral CT scan confirms a Grade I spondylolisthesis with severe loss of disc height and a central vacuum disc phenomenon (Fig. 22.2 A–C). This study suggests more spondylosis at other levels than the routine films, showing facet degenerative changes at L2-3 and L3-4 as well as the L4-5 and L5-S1 disc levels. T2 imaging on MRI shows generalized disc desiccation through the lumbar spine, worst at L4-5 and L5-S1. There are Schmoral nodes in the vertebral bodies of T11, T12, and L1 (Fig. 22.3 A,B). Transaxial views show a broad-based central disc protrusion at L4-5 with bilateral lateral stenosis though the lateral views of this same study suggest the lateral stenosis at L4-5 is only mild (Fig. 22.4 A–C). There is a Grade I spondylolisthesis at L5-S1 and a large herniated nucleus pulposus at L5-S1 as well, eccentric to the right producing central and bilateral, right greater than left lateral stenosis with nerve root impingement on the right. There are degenerative facet changes on the L3-4, L4-5, and L5-S1 images presented.

This patient's initial presentation demonstrating no progressive neurological deficits warranted a course of nonoperative care. The minimal physical findings included increased pain on forward flexion, a finding clinically felt to be consistent with discogenic pain, and spinous process tenderness clinically felt to be consistent with posterior element pain.[1] Her imaging

Figure 22.1.

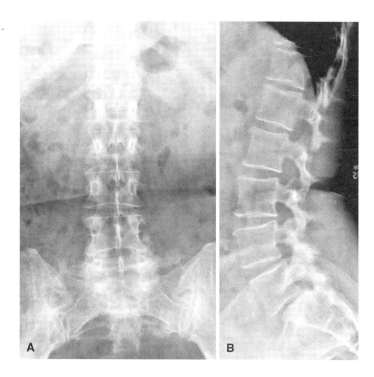

studies demonstrate mild bilateral, lateral stenosis at L4-5, and both a Grade I spondylolisthesis and an HNP on the right at L5-S1, the same side as her radicular symptoms. The potential for all of these conditions to respond favorably to conservative care is good. However, the presence of hypertension and, in particular, gastric reflux will seriously limit the use of oral anti-inflammatory medications, which would potentially be helpful for both axial and radicular pain.[2] With this limitation, continued attempts at conservative care are likely to be compromised.

We are further informed that the claimant has now undergone three epidural steroid injections without relief. We are not told whether these were targeted, transforaminal injections or simply interlaminar injections and also if any short-term relief, say for the

Figure 22.2.

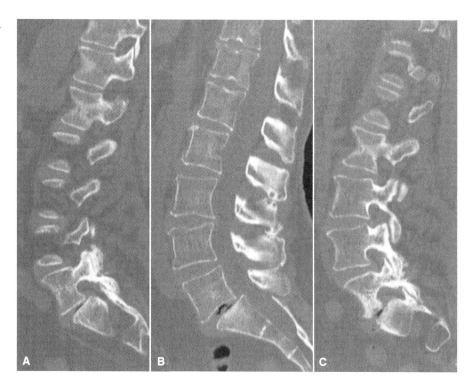

Figure 22.3.

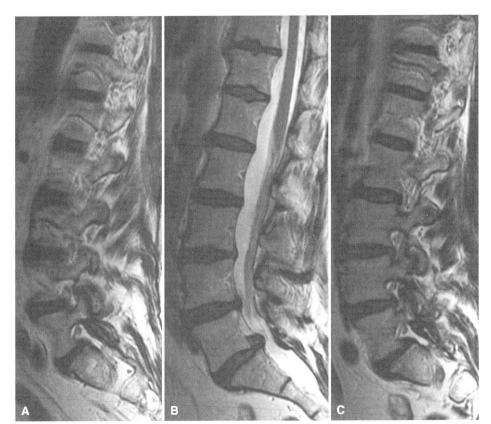

duration of the anesthetic, was achieved. We are also not told whether the claimant's leg pain was in fact improved with these injections, as would be expected,[3,4] to the point where now her back pain is dominant or whether the back pain was always the dominant complaint making the probability that lumbar epidural injections would help her far less likely.[5,6]

Finally, the claimant has not undergone a course of formal physical therapy. The role of physical therapy and other rehabilitation measures including bracing is not well described for degenerative lumbar spondylolisthesis, with or without an HNP, but there is a larger literature base for degenerative spinal stenosis, a pathologically similar condition. While physical therapy can be helpful in controlling back pain and radicular symptoms in degenerative spinal stenosis, a recent systematic review of the literature on the role of physical therapy and exercise yielded insufficient evidence to draw any conclusions on the long-term effectiveness of this treatment for the symptoms of degenerative spinal stenosis.[7] Thus, while a course of physical therapy certainly could be instituted in this patient, the likelihood of a successful and acceptable outcome is limited both by the evidence available in the literature on a similar condition, degenerative spinal stenosis, and by the patient's failure to improve over >8 months of nonsurgical care. Given the failure of appropriate nonsurgical measures on this patient and assuming her current clinical complaints are unacceptable to her, a surgical solution should be considered.

Figure 22.4.

L3-4	L4-5	L5-S1

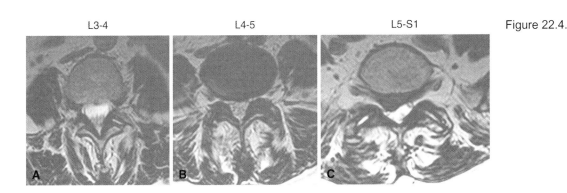

DECLARATION OF SPECIFIC DIAGNOSES

This patient has complaints of axial back pain greater than right leg radiculopathy associated and/or most likely attributable to Grade I L5-S1 degenerative spondylolisthesis and concomitant right-sided HNP at L5-S1.

BRAINSTORMING: WHAT ARE THE TREATMENT GOALS AND SURGICAL OPTIONS?

The treatment goals are

1. Long-term relief of or significant reduction in both axial and radicular complaints
2. Improved patient function in daily activities such as walking
3. Minimize the effects of medical comorbidities during treatment

The surgical treatment options are

1. Simple discectomy, open or minimally invasive, at L5-S1 on the right
2. Indirect decompression of the spinal canal by an interspinous process distraction device
3. Open decompression of spinal canal
4. Open decompression of the spinal canal with fusion
5. Open decompression of the spinal canal with fusion and internal fixation

EVALUATION OF THE LITERATURE

To identify relevant publications on the surgical treatment of degenerative lumbar spondylolisthesis (with or without HNP), PubMed was searched from 1966 to 2008 using both MeSH terms and key words. One search was performed addressing each of the surgical options listed for this patient. Key words included "lumbar disc herniation," "lumbar disc rupture," "lumbar HNP," "lumbar degenerative spondylolisthesis," "decompression," "laminectomy," "laminotomy," "foraminotomy," "fusion," "arthrodesis," "hardware," "instrumentation," and "pedicle screw." Electronic searches were also performed in answering Questions 4, 5, and 6 at the ACP Journal Club database, Cochrane Database of Systematic Reviews, Database of Abstracts of Reviews of Effectiveness (DARE), and Cochrane Central Register of Controlled Trials.

DETAILED REVIEW OF PERTINENT ARTICLES

Nonoperative Versus Operative Treatment

As previously discussed, this patient has been symptomatic for >8 months and has failed to improve significantly during a course of nonoperative care. She has not had a course of structured rehabilitative therapy, but a recent systematic review of the literature on degenerative spinal stenosis suggests that such treatment is at best useful for episodic relief only of symptom flair-ups and not useful for long-term treatment.[7] Furthermore, a recent large prospective controlled study presents moderate-level evidence that such a patient as this is likely to benefit more from surgical intervention than from continued nonsurgical care.[8] After a thoughtful and complete discussion with this patient and her family, the decision has been made to pursue a surgical solution to her problem. This decision was arrived at taking into account the three important components of evidence-based decision making: the patient's needs and desires, her treating physician's knowledge and experience, and the best evidence currently available in the clinical literature on her condition, which will be summarized below.

As noted above, one treatment goal in this 64-year-old patient is to minimize the effects of her medical comorbidities on the outcomes of her surgical treatment. The presence of both physical as well as psychological comorbidities can influence surgical outcomes in lumbar spinal surgery, and their presence appears to be additive.[9] This patient's history of hypertension, hypothyroidism, and gastrointestinal reflux has to be evaluated prior to any surgical intervention by a competent medical specialist. Assurances must be obtained that the patient can withstand not only the challenges of a possibly prolonged anesthesia and attendant blood loss and possible replacement but also the rigors of a potentially prolonged rehabilitation. The presence of depression and/or anxiety especially has been shown to be predictors of poor functional outcomes in lumbar spinal surgery for both back pain and radicular syndromes.[10–12] Thus, this patient should also be evaluated by a competent psychiatrist prior to surgery to assess her current status with respect to both her history of depression and anxiety. If significant depression and/or anxiety are present, these should be actively treated prior to surgery. The presences of either of these conditions could portend a poor functional outcome independent of choice of surgical intervention. Both the internist and the psychiatrist should be available for assistance in the postoperative management of this patient.

Simple Discectomy—Open or Minimally Invasive

This patient's axial back pain is felt by her to be more significant than her radicular symptoms. While a simple discectomy might further decrease this patient's radicular symptoms, the role of simple discectomy, either open or minimally invasive, in this patient is limited. A search of PubMed for the surgical treatment of lower back pain with or without radiculopathy by simple discectomy yielded 246 papers with only very low levels of evidence, primarily case series of various percutaneous procedures, suggesting that some patients can improve from solitary back pain with a variation of percutaneous discectomy. There is only very poor evidence supporting the limited use of simple discectomy for the relief of dominant axial lower back pain. Furthermore, this very poor evidence comes from reports of case series of relatively young patients, none of whom have the confounding problems that this patient does of degenerative lumbar spondylolisthesis and medical comorbidities. For this patient, a simple discectomy would appear to be a poor treatment option that would expose the patient to the risks of surgery with little or no chance that her main complaint, axial back pain, would be successfully treated.

Indirect Decompression of the Spinal Canal by an Interspinous Process Distraction Device

The use of an interspinous distraction device in both cadaver spines as well as in live patients with x-rays showing a Grade I degenerative spondylolisthesis similar to this patient has been promoted to unload the posterior facets and increase space available in the stenotic canal at the level of the implant.[13–15] Two randomized controlled trials (RCTs) with 2-year follow-up have been published comparing one commercially available device to nonoperative care, suggesting statistically improved functional outcomes for the interspinous device.[16–18] Three small case series have also been published suggesting a moderate effect for the same commercial device on a validated functional outcome measuring claudication, though one of these small trials saw a high failure rate of the device.[19–21] In summary, the data base is insufficient currently to strongly recommend for or against this device.

Even ignoring the fact that this claimant has an HNP in addition to her spondylolisthesis and in spite of the appearance of the remainder of this patient's imaging studies, she is not a candidate for consideration of one of these interspinous process distraction devices.[22] The critical historical prerequisite for use of this device is that forward flexion diminishes a patient's back pain. This maneuver can unload the posterior elements, theoretically increase the canal size and basically reproduce the intended action of spinous process distraction. The patient being discussed in this analysis actually has *increased* lower back pain on forward flexion, and thus, an interspinous distraction device might actually worsen her clinical complaints.

Open Decompression of the Spinal Canal Alone or with Fusion

If deciding to do a more aggressive surgery in this patient, the decision will have to be considered as to whether or not to add a simple, noninstrumented fusion to the surgical decompression and discectomy. Overall, the quality of evidence to make this decision is poor. An early and often quoted study by Herkowitz and Kurz[23] was a prospective comparative study of 50 patients with degenerative spondylolisthesis, 25 of whom underwent decompression only and 25 of whom underwent decompression and lateral transverse fusion. These patients were followed for 2 years with x-rays and a subjective (nonvalidated, nonfunctional) outcome scale. After 2 years, the authors reported statistically highly significant improvement in the subjective results for both leg and back pain in the patients who had a concomitant fusion with their decompression compared to those patients who underwent just a decompression. This study provides low levels of evidence that fusion improves patient outcomes when combined with decompression in the surgical treatment of symptomatic lumbar degenerative spondylolisthesis.

Mardjetko et al.[24] published a meta-analysis of papers published between 1970 and 1993 on the surgical treatment of degenerative lumbar spondylolisthesis. Twenty-five papers were identified with three presenting moderate levels of evidence and the remainder low levels of evidence. Over all, the Mardjetko et al., paper yielded low levels of evidence. Typical of papers from this period, none used validated functional outcome measures. Outcomes did include leg pain, back pain, and global outcome scores. In this meta-analysis, 11 papers reported patients who underwent decompression only, and of these, 69% of patients were reported to have a clinically satisfactory outcome by nonvalidated measures. In addition, six papers were identified that reported patients who underwent both a decompression and noninstrumented lateral transverse fusion with 90% of these patients reporting a clinically satisfactory outcome. When the clinical outcomes of these two groups, patients with decompression only versus patients with decompression and noninstrumented fusion, were compared in the meta-analysis, the decompression and fusion group was statistically highly significantly superior to the decompression only group.

Martin et al.[25] attempted to do a systematic review of higher level data by looking only at RCTs and comparative observational studies using surgery to treat degenerative lumbar spondylolisthesis from 1966 to 2005. Outcome measures utilized in the study included "clinical outcomes," reoperation rate and fusion status. An attempt was made to use only validated clinical outcomes measures, but because of the heterogeneity of the studies, comparisons could not be made across studies, and in the end, outcomes were reduced to a dichotomous scale of "satisfactory" or "unsatisfactory." Because of methodological problems in many of these studies, this systematic review actually yielded only moderate levels of evidence. Eight papers addressed decompression only versus fusion and decompression. When grouped data were analyzed, the authors reported a significantly higher probability of achieving a satisfactory clinical outcome when fusion was added to decompression. The significance deteriorated, however, if the only clinical measure was radiculopathy or claudication and did not also contain a measure of back pain.

Decompression and Fusion with or Without Internal Fixation

The evidence available appears to favor adding a fusion in this patient to a decompression for the treatment of her HNP and symptomatic degenerative lumbar spondylolisthesis. Would addition of internal fixation to the fusion improve her outcomes even further? In a follow-up publication to the Herkowitz and Kurz[23] publication noted above, Fischgrund et al., randomly assigned 76 patients with symptomatic degenerative lumbar spondylolisthesis to surgery with decompression and lateral transverse fusion or decompression with surgery and lateral transverse fusion and pedicle screw fixation.[26] Outcomes were pain on a 5-point VAS and examiner-assessed outcome based on pain and function along with fusion status on x-ray. The authors reported at 2-year follow-up that clinical outcomes were good or excellent in 76% of the instrumented patients and 82% of the non-instrumented patient, a nonsignificant difference. The fusion rate on routine x-rays was much higher for the instrumented group (82% vs. 45%), but there was no correlation between patient outcome and successful fusion, a finding noted in the original paper as well.[23] This study provides low levels of evidence that adding instrumentation to decompression and fusion for degenerative lumbar spinal stenosis does not improve patient outcomes.

Gibson and Waddell[27] found 8 RCTs of instrumented versus uninstrumented fusion for degenerative lumbar spondylolisthesis within a larger study of 31 RCTs for surgical treatment of lumbar spondylosis showing that instrumented lumbar fusions resulted in high fusion rates but with no correlation in clinical outcomes. Also suggested in these studies was a higher complication rate in the instrumented cases. Thus, these authors provided moderate levels of evidence that instrumenting a lumbar fusion does not lead to significantly improved patient outcomes.

The Mardjetko et al.[24] study discussed in the previous section also identified five studies in which patients underwent decompression with fusion and internal fixation for degenerative lumbar spondylolisthesis. When the patients in these five studies with decompression, fusion, and instrumentation were compared to the patients in the six studies who underwent decompression and simple uninstrumented fusion, there was no difference in outcomes. Thus, this meta-analysis provides low levels of evidence that adding instrumentation to a decompression and fusion for degenerative lumbar spondylolisthesis does not significantly improve patient outcomes.

Finally, the systematic review by Martin et al.[25] discussed in the last section also investigated patient outcomes in surgery for degenerative lumbar spondylolisthesis as a function of decompression and fusion with and without instrumentation. In this systematic review of higher levels of evidence, there were six studies addressing decompression and fusion versus decompression and fusion with instrumentation in the surgical treatment of degenerative lumbar spondylolisthesis. Three of these studies were RCTs. The authors found moderate levels of evidence that the addition of instrumentation significantly increased the probability of a solid arthrodesis but did not have any significant effect on clinical outcomes for the patients.

The role of reduction of the slip in addition to an instrumented fusion in the type of patient being discussed in this analysis remains ill defined with very low levels of evidence. Three case series have been published with incomplete follow-up at <2 years.[28–30] In all, outcomes were comparable to decompression or decompression and fusion except in one, in which 7% of the patients endured major complications.[28] There is insufficient evidence to support reduction of a Grade I lumbar degenerative spondylolisthesis as part of the surgical treatment of this condition.

EVIDENTIARY TABLE AND SELECTION OF TREATMENT METHOD

This patient has failed appropriate conservative care within the parameters of her medical condition. The best available evidence suggests that her clinical complaints and her functional status would best be improved by surgical intervention. This intervention would be provided in the context of an informed decision-making process including the patient's needs and desires as well as her physicians' and surgeon's experience and the knowledge of the best evidence available for her treatment decisions. The articles that best address the surgical decision-making process in this patient are listed in Table 22.1, and they address the respective roles of spinal decompression, spinal fusion, and spinal instrumentation.

TABLE 22.1 Evidentiary Table: A Summary of the Evidence for Decompression and Fusion Without Internal Fixation for Surgical Treatment of Symptomatic Degenerative Lumbar Spondylolisthesis with Lumbar HNP.

Paper Author (Year)	Description	Summary of Results	Quality of Evidence
Herkowitz and Kurz (1991)	Prospective cohort study Decompression vs decompression and uninstrumented fusion	25 patients with degenerative lumbar spondylolisthesis treated with decompression only and 25 patients treated with decompression and lateral transverse fusion. At 2 y, patient outcomes on a dichotomous scale were highly superior for the fusion group (Fisher exact test: $p < 0.0001$) independent of fusion status on x-ray	Low
Fischgrund et al. (1997)	Prospective, randomized comparative study Decompression and fusion vs decompression and instrumented fusion	76 patients were randomized to decompression and fusion alone or with pedicle fixation. Followup was at 2 y on 89% of patients with VAS and dichotomous outcome scale. Clinical outcome was good in 76% of instrumented patients and 82% of noninstrumented patients, a nonsignificant difference. Fusion rate was significantly higher among instrumented patients ($p = 0.0015$) but did not correlate with clinical outcomes ($p = 0.435$).	Low
Mardjetko et al. (1994)	Meta-analysis of literature on the surgical treatment of lumbar degenerative spondylolisthesis published between 1970 and 1993.	25 papers were identified encompassing 889 patients. Only three were prospective RCTs. Pain was the most frequently reported outcome with only 6 papers reporting function and only 2 papers patient-determined outcomes. 11 papers reported results of decompression only with 69% satisfactory outcomes. 6 papers were reported with decompression and fusion in which 90% had satisfactory results. 5 papers were reported with decompression and instrumented fusion in which 85% of the patients had satisfactory outcomes. Both uninstrumented ($p < 0.00001$) and instrumented ($p < 0.00001$) fusion patients had significantly better outcomes than those patients with decompression alone. There was no significant difference between the outcomes of the uninstrumented and instrumented fusion patients ($p = 0.08$)	Low
Martin et al. (2007)	Systematic review of RCTs and comparative studies examining the surgical management of degenerative lumbar spondylolisthesis	Clinical outcomes were recorded, but an attempt to compare patient-centered outcomes failed because of the heterogeneity of the study designs. Instead, outcomes were dichotomized into satisfactory and unsatisfactory. 8 studies, including 2 RCTs compared fusion to decompression alone. Fusion was found to contribute a significantly higher chance of a satisfactory outcome when compared to decompression alone ($p < 0.05$) but only if back pain was part of the symptoms. 6 studies looked at instrumented versus uninstrumented fusions of which 3 were RCTs. While the addition of instrumentation improved the probability of fusion ($p < 0.05$), there was no improvement in clinical outcomes from the surgery by the addition of instrumentation to the lumbar fusion.	Moderate
Gibson and Waddell (2005)	Systematic review of RCTs looking at surgical treatment of lumbar spondylosis	8 papers supported a higher fusion rate for instrumented vs. uninstrumented fusions but no differences in clinical outcomes were demonstrated between the 2 groups. Higher complications rates were noted with the instrumentation cases	Moderate

Open Decompression Alone or with Fusion

One small prospective cohort study and one meta-analysis on older clinical papers provide low levels of evidence for superior clinical outcomes with the addition of fusion to lumbar decompression.[23,24] In addition, one systematic review on higher levels of evidence provides moderate levels of evidence in favor of improved clinical outcomes from adding a fusion to lumbar decompression in this condition.[25] Thus, the best available evidence suggests that this patient's back pain and leg pain would best be treated by both a decompression (with discectomy) and lumbar fusion.

Open Decompression and Fusion with or Without Internal Fixation

One prospective, randomized comparative study of moderate size and one meta-analysis on older clinical papers provide low levels of evidence for improved fusion rates on x-rays with the addition of internal fixation but no improved patient outcomes by the addition of internal fixation to fusion in the treatment of degenerative lumbar spondylolisthesis.[24,26] Two systematic reviews of high level data provide moderate levels of evidence for the lack of improved patient outcomes by the addition of internal fixation to fusion procedures, though both papers suggest that improved rate of fusion on routine x-rays is seen.[25,27] One of these systematic reviews[27] suggests a higher complication rate occurs with internal fixation as well. Based on this best evidence, we have decided to treat this patient with a decompression and uninstrumented lateral intertransverse fusion.

DEFINITIVE TREATMENT PLAN

This patient with a Grade I L5-S1 spondylolisthesis and a right-sided L5-S1 HNP manifesting symptoms of dominant lower back pain worsened with exercise, forward flexion, and a right S1 radiculopathy should be taken to the operating room and undergo an L5-S1 decompression with bilateral foraminotomies and right-side discectomy. The option for a left-sided discectomy exists based on the MRI findings and would depend upon the findings at surgery. In addition, she should undergo a bilateral lateral transverse fusion with autograft. She would not undergo internal fixation as an adjunct to her fusion.

Grading the Evidence for this Plan

The evidence in support of the addition of a lateral transverse fusion to decompression and discectomy for this patient's condition is of a low level and is reflected in the first and third papers in Table 22.1. However, when back pain is a dominant symptom, as it is in this patient, the evidence is moderate that addition of a fusion will improve patient outcomes, as reflected in the fourth paper in Table 22.1.

The evidence in support of rejecting the addition of internal fixation as an adjunct to fusion in this patient is based on moderate levels of evidence as reflected in the fourth and fifth papers in Table 22.1, which demonstrate that, while rates of fusion are increased, clinical outcomes are not respectively improved by the addition of internal fixation and possibly complications are increased.

In accordance with the method of grading recommendations set forth by Schunemann, et al.,[31] our proposed treatment of decompression, discectomy, and lateral transverse fusion would be considered a **strong recommendation** based on low-quality evidence and the clinical situation in this patient that the benefits of this treatment outweigh its risks and burdens. Furthermore, according to these same grading of recommendations, our recommendation against the adjunctive use of internal fixation in the surgical treatment of this patient would be considered a **strong recommendation** based on moderate-quality evidence and the clinical situation in this patient that the benefits of this treatment do not outweigh its attendant risks and burdens.

PREDICTING OUTCOMES

Success in predicting surgical treatment outcomes on an individual patient is a process prone to extreme variance. These outcomes are influenced by patient factors including the patient's biological substrate or general condition as discussed in the introduction to this analysis as well and perhaps equally by the patient's psychological state, expectations, and trust in his or her surgeon. Surgeon factors that contribute to outcomes include, among others, expertise, experience, physical well being, and attitude toward and relationship with the patient. Finally, perhaps that which best can be assessed, outcomes can be predicted to some degree by the quality of the evidence available on the treatment choice. Unfortunately, the evidence base for the treatment choices in our patient contains few studies that rely on validated outcome measures and it is validated outcome measures that best predict surgical outcomes.

The statistical effects reported in the evidence base comparing decompression versus decompression with fusion strongly favor adding fusion in this patient's surgical treatment. The design of these studies, many of which are older, is lacking, however, in not employing validated outcome measures, and thus, the levels of evidence for adding fusion are low. On the other hand, the evidence base is stronger that the additional time of surgery and risk of complications along with the lack of improved patient outcomes validated, or otherwise, do not justify adding internal fixation to the procedure in this patient. From the standpoint of the surgeon in this case, my expertise and experience in treating similar cases match closely that of the literature reviewed and I would feel comfortable offering a decompression and fusion to this patient once she was properly cleared medically and psychologically for this surgery and once she and her family had an informed understanding of the evidence upon which the recommendation was being made.

SUMMARY

We have been presented a 64-year-old women with lower back pain greater than right leg radiculopathy, no neurological changes, and markedly reduced ambulatory ability all present for >8 months. Imaging has demonstrated a Grade I spondylolisthesis and right-sided HNP at L5-S1. The claimant has failed all reasonable nonoperative care but is noted to have several medical and psychological comorbidities. With appropriate adjunctive medical management of her comorbidities, the most appropriate surgical treatment of this patient's condition would be a decompression at L5-S1 with bilateral foraminotomies and an L5-S1 discectomy combined with an uninstrumented lateral transverse fusion with autograph. With good postoperative management of her medical condition and appropriate rehabilitative exercise, she can anticipate relief of her radiculopathy, a gradual reduction over several months of her back pain, and a significant increase in her walking and exercise endurance.

REFERENCES

1. Maigne R. Low back pain of thoracolumbar origin. *Arch Phys Med Rehabil*. 1980;61(9):389–395.
2. Chou R, Huffman LH. Medications for acute and chronic low back pain: a review of the evidence for an American Pain Society/American College of Physicians clinical practice guideline. American Pain Society; American College of Physicians. *Ann Intern Med*. 2007;147(7): 505–514.
3. Riew KD, Park JB, Cho YS, et al. Nerve root blocks in the treatment of lumbar radicular pain: a minimum five-year follow-up. *J Bone Joint Surg Am*. 2006;88(8):1722–1725.
4. Buttermann GR. Treatment of lumbar disc herniation: epidural steroid injection compared with discectomy: a prospective, randomized study. *J Bone Joint Surg Am*. 2004;86-A(4):670–679.
5. Buttermann GR. The effect of spinal steroid injections for degenerative disc disease. *Spine J*. 2004;4(5):495–505.
6. Resnick DK, Choudhri TF, Dailey AT, et al. Guidelines for the performance of fusion procedures for degenerative disease of the lumbar spine. Part 13: injection therapies, low-back pain, and lumbar fusion. *J Neurosurg Spine*. 2005;2(6):707–715.
7. Watters WC III, Baisden J, Gilbert TJ, et al. Degenerative lumbar spinal stenosis: an evidence-based clinical guideline for the diagnosis and treatment of degenerative lumbar spinal stenosis. *Spine J*. 2008;8(2):305–310.
8. Weinstein JN, Lurie JD, Tosteson TD, et al. Surgical versus nonsurgical treatment for lumbar degenerative spondylolisthesis. *N Engl J Med*. 2007;356(22):2257–2270.
9. Slover J, Abdu WA, Hanscom B, et al. The impact of comorbidities on the change in short-form 36 and Oswestry scores following lumbar spine surgery. *Spine*. 2006;31(17):1974–1980.
10. Sinikallio S, Aalto T, Airaksinen O, et al. Depression is associated with poorer outcome of lumbar spinal stenosis surgery. *Eur Spine J*. 2007;16(7):905–912; Epub 2007 Mar 30.
11. Edwards RR, Klick B, Buenaver L, et al. Symptoms of distress as prospective predictors of pain-related sciatica treatment outcomes. *Pain*. 2007;130(1–2):47–55; Epub 2006 Dec 6.
12. Trief PM, Ploutz-Snyder R, Fredrickson BE. Emotional health predicts pain and function after fusion: a prospective multicenter study. *Spine*. 2006;31(7):823–830.
13. Lindsey DP, Swanson KE, Fuchs P, et al. The effects of an interspinous implant on the kinematics of the instrumented and adjacent levels in the lumbar spine. *Spine*. 2003;28(19):2192–2197.
14. Wiseman CM, Lindsey DP, Fredrick AD, et al. The effect of an interspinous process implant on facet loading during extension. *Spine*. 2005;30(8):903–907.
15. Siddiqui M, Nicol M, Karadimas E, et al. The positional magnetic resonance imaging changes in the lumbar spine following insertion of a novel interspinous process distraction device. *Spine*. 2005;30(23):2677–2682.
16. Zucherman JF, Hsu KY, Hartjen CA, et al. A prospective randomized multi-center study for the treatment of lumbar spinal stenosis with the X STOP interspinous implant: 1-year results. *Eur Spine J*. 2004;13(1):22–31.
17. Zucherman JF, Hsu KY, Hartjen CA, et al. A multicenter, prospective, randomized trial evaluating the X STOP interspinous process decompression system for the treatment of neurogenic intermittent claudication: two-year follow-up results. *Spine*. 2005;30(12):1351–1358.
18. Anderson PA, Tribus CB, Kitchel SH. Treatment of neurogenic claudication by interspinous decompression: application of the X STOP device in patients with lumbar degenerative spondylolisthesis. *J Neurosurg Spine*. 2006;4(6):463–471.
19. Lee J, Hida K, Seki T, et al. An interspinous process distractor (X STOP) for lumbar spinal stenosis in elderly patients: preliminary experiences in 10 consecutive cases. *J Spinal Disord Tech*. 2004;17(1):72–77; discussion 78.
20. Kondrashov DG, Hannibal M, Hsu KY, et al. Interspinous process decompression with the X-STOP device for lumbar spinal stenosis: a 4-year follow-up study. *J Spinal Disord Tech*. 2006;19(5):323–327.
21. Verhoof OJ, Bron JL, Wapstra FH, et al. High failure rate of the interspinous distraction device (X-Stop) for the treatment

of lumbar spinal stenosis caused by degenerative spondylolisthesis. *Eur Spine J*. 2008;17(2):188–192.

22. Lauryssen C. Appropriate selection of patients with lumbar spinal stenosis for interspinous process decompression with the X STOP device. *Neurosurg Focus*. 2007;22(1):E5.

23. Herkowitz HN, Kurz LT. Degenerative lumbar spondylolisthesis with spinal stenosis: a prospective study comparing decompression with decompression and intertransverse process arthrodesis. *J Bone Joint Surg Am*. 1991;73(6):802.

24. Mardjetko SM, Connolly PJ, Shott S. Degenerative lumbar spondylolisthesis: a meta-analysis of literature 1970–1993. *Spine*. 1994;19(20 suppl):2256S–2265S.

25. Martin CR, Gruszczynski AT, Braunsfurth HA, et al. The surgical management of degenerative lumbar spondylolisthesis: a systematic review. *Spine*. 2007;32(16):1791–1798.

26. Fischgrund JS, Mackay M, Herkowitz HN, et al. 1997 Volvo Award winner in clinical studies. Degenerative lumbar spondylolisthesis with spinal stenosis: a prospective, randomized study comparing decompressive laminectomy and arthrodesis with and without spinal instrumentation. *Spine*. 1997;22(24):2807–2812.

27. Gibson JN, Waddell G. Surgery for degenerative lumbar spondylosis: updated Cochrane Review. *Spine*. 2005;30(20):2312–2320.

28. Bednar DA. Surgical management of lumbar degenerative spinal stenosis with spondylolisthesis via posterior reduction with minimal laminectomy. *J Spinal Disord Tech*. 2002;15(2):105–109.

29. Lee TC. Reduction and stabilization without laminectomy for unstable degenerative spondylolisthesis: a preliminary report. *Neurosurgery*. 1994;35(6):1072–1076.

30. Sears W. Posterior lumbar interbody fusion for degenerative spondylolisthesis: restoration of sagittal balance using insert-and-rotate interbody spacers. *Spine J*. 2005;5(2):170–179.

31. Schünemann HJ, Jaeschke R, Cook DJ, et al. An official ATS statement: grading the quality of evidence and strength of recommendations in ATS guidelines and recommendations. *Am J Respir Crit Care Med*. 2006;174(5):605–614.

23 L5-S1 Herniation

ANDREW J. SCHOENFELD, MD

A 32-year-old woman presents with a long-standing history of low back pain and, more acutely, left leg pain. Back pain started about 1 year ago, which was treated with physical therapy and epidural injections. Two months ago, she felt that she had an acute worsening of her back pain, at which time she also reported an onset of severe left leg pain. Currently, pain is worse with forward flexion, sneezing, and coughing. Since the exacerbation, she has continued with her home exercises as recommended by her physical therapist. She does not have any bowel or bladder complaints.

The physical exam demonstrates a positive left straight leg raise, point tenderness at the L5-S1 interspace, and decreased sensation in the L4 and S1 distributions on the left side compared to the right. Gait is normal. She can forward flex to touch her hands to her knees and extend past neutral, but both elicit pain. She has full strength otherwise and has no other pertinent positives.

Magnetic resonance imaging (MRI) studies are shown in Figures 23.1A–F and 23.2A–C.

INTERPRETATION OF CLINICAL PRESENTATION

The case scenario depicts a young woman with a 1-year history of prodromal back pain combined with radicular symptoms in the left lower extremity for 8 weeks' duration. Her complaints include left leg radicular pain, back pain localized to the L5-S1 interspace, and diminished sensation in the L4 and S1 dermatomal regions on the left side. Her pain appears to be exacerbated by activities that increase intradiscal pressure (forward flexion, Valsalva maneuver, etc.), but lumbar range of motion is not compromised.

She has no motor weakness, progressive neurologic deficits, or symptoms of cauda equina. She does have an ipsilateral positive straight leg raising sign. Her leg symptoms have persisted beyond 6 weeks despite a conservative course of home physical therapy exercises.

Her back pain localized to the L5-S1 region may be explained by paraspinal muscle spasm, although this finding is nonspecific and contributes little to the diagnosis. Alternatively, some of her back pain can be attributed to degenerative disc disease and/or the annular tear that potentiated the disc herniation. The posterior annulus is innervated by branches of the sinuvertebral nerve, and back pain in the setting of degenerative disc disease has been postulated to result from transmission along this pathway.[1,2] Jinkins et al.[3] have documented that back pain can result from disc herniations that do not enter the spinal canal or contact nerve roots.

The most significant findings in the physical examination are the pattern of radicular pain, the presence of paresthesias in an appropriate S1 distribution, and the ipsilateral positive straight leg raising sign. Pain and paresthesias in an S1 distribution are commonly the result of a disc herniation contacting the S1 nerve root. S1 radicular pain may involve the back of the calf but often extends into the dorsolateral aspect of the foot as well as the plantar surface. Compression of a noninflamed nerve has been found to produce sensory and motor deficits without pain, while pain occurs as a result of neural inflammation.[4,5] Nerve root inflammation may occur as a result of ischemia from prolonged mechanical compression, although neurochemical factors released from the herniated disc may play an important role.[6,7] Kang et al.[6] demonstrated that inflammatory factors, such as matrix metalloproteinase, nitric oxide, prostaglandin E_2, and interleukin-6, were present in herniated disc material inducing radiculopathy.

The straight leg raising test is a provocative examination and integral to the evaluation of patients with suspected lumbar disc herniations. Kosteljanetz et al.[8] reported that nerve root compression was present in 90% of individuals with a positive straight leg raise, and Xin et al.[9] documented an 88.5% correlation

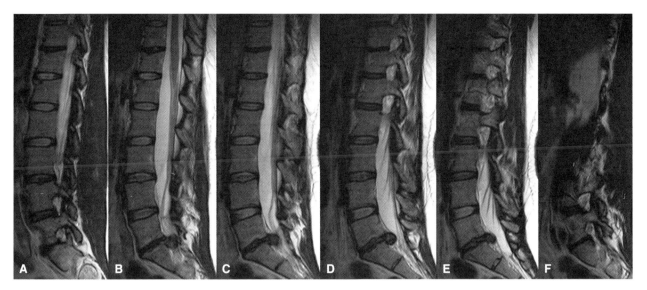

Figure 23.1.

between the presence of a positive straight leg raise and findings at time of discectomy. A recent prospective study by Majlesi et al.[10] found that the straight leg raise demonstrated 52% sensitivity for lumbar disc herniation and 89% specificity. In light of these findings, the authors suggested that, owing to a high specificity, the straight leg raise would be useful in identifying patients with a disc herniation requiring surgery.

The MR images available are representative fat-suppressed T2 weighted images. These include sagittal reformatted images (Fig. 23.1) as well as axial images through the L5-S1 level (Fig. 23.2). Paramedian and midline sagittal images (Fig. 23.1B–E) reveal mild disc degeneration throughout the lumbar spine with a severely degenerated disc at L5-S1 (Pfirrmann Grade 4-5).[11] There is mild evidence of endplate edema at this level. A large disc herniation can also be appreciated at the L5-S1 disc space (Fig. 23.1C). The herniation appears to be of the extruded type according to the classification of Spengler et al.[12] Axial sections of the MRI (Fig. 23.2) indicate that the disc herniation is large and occupies portions of the central zone as well as the lateral recess. This corresponds to a paracentral disc herniation as described by Knop-Jergas et al.[13] The disc fragment is large (>6 mm in anteroposterior diameter)[14] and appears to be impinging on the left S1 nerve root. There is no evidence of compression on the cauda equina, nor is there evidence of other osseous or intramedullary findings (i.e., tumor, infection, or hematoma) that could adequately explain the patient's symptoms.

DECLARATION OF SPECIFIC DIAGNOSIS

This patient has an L5-S1 disc herniation preferentially impacting the left S1 nerve root. This is associated with radiculopathy in an appropriate S1 nerve distribution.

BRAINSTORMING: WHAT ARE THE TREATMENT GOALS AND SURGICAL OPTIONS?

The treatment goals are

1. Eliminate radicular pain symptoms.
2. Improve sensation in the S1 distribution in the patient's left lower extremity.
3. Accelerate rehabilitation and healing.
4. Return patient to normal activities of daily living.

The treatment options are
1. Continued conservative management with formal physical therapy and/or epidural steroid injection

Figure 23.2.

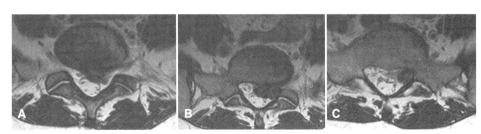

2. Open discectomy
3. Minimally invasive discectomy or microdiscectomy

EVALUATION OF THE LITERATURE

To facilitate an evidence-based analysis of the existing literature, a formal search was performed using the PubMed and Medline databases. A Medline search was conducted using both medical subject headings and key words. The initial step entailed a focused search using "intervertebral disc displacement" as the medical subject heading. This was followed by key word searches using "lumbar disc herniation" and "lumbar disc displacement." Results of these searches were combined with a focused search for publications regarding "lumbar spine." Pertinent articles identified in this initial Medline search were accessed and their references used to identify further publications of interest. This search strategy revealed 6,338 potential publications between 1950 and 2008. A similar approach was applied to PubMed, revealing 2,256 potentially relevant articles. One-hundred sixteen abstracts were reviewed, and 50 full text articles were read.

DETAILED REVIEW OF PERTINENT ARTICLES

Operative or Nonoperative Treatment

Until recently, the quality of evidence pertaining to operative versus nonoperative management of lumbar disc herniations was poor. In the last few years, a number of higher quality, scientifically rigorous studies have been published on this topic.[15–23] Unfortunately, due to difficulties with methodology, many of these studies have not yielded the definitive conclusions that the scientific community hoped they would and controversy still persists.[24] Some of the disagreement results from the fact that the natural history of lumbar disc herniations remains incompletely described, but the number of poor quality, retrospective studies in the current literature obfuscates the issue as well.

Support for nonoperative intervention is largely derived from studies that have treated patients using nonoperative modalities alone[25] or from nonoperative arms of operative versus nonoperative investigations.[15–20,22,23,26] The most widely quoted study used to support nonoperative treatment of disc herniations is that of Saal and Saal.[25] In this retrospective investigation, 58 patients treated conservatively for lumbar disc herniation were followed for an average of 31 months. Nonoperative treatment consisted of spinal stabilization exercises, flexibility training, and epidural injections as indicated. Using this protocol, the authors reported that 90% of patients were found to have good or excellent outcomes at the time of final follow-up. Ninety-two percent of patients in this study were able to return to work. Concerns about this study include the fact that 10% of the initial cohort received surgery and that the 58 patients included represent a small proportion of the 347 patients initially identified for enrollment.[25] Based on these factors, it is possible that the study of Saal and Saal represents a "best-case scenario" and overestimates the beneficial effects of nonoperative management for the average patient with a lumbar disc herniation.

Indeed, the nonoperative arms of many case-control investigations do not substantiate the findings reported by Saal and Saal. For example, the 10-year results of the prospective Maine Lumbar Spine Study endorse a 56% satisfaction rate, 61% improvement in predominant symptom, and 40% resolution of low back issues in patients managed nonoperatively.[20] The 4-year results of the SPORT trial document similar results, with only 51.7% of nonoperatively managed patients reporting major improvement in symptoms.[17] In the 2-year results of a prospective randomized controlled trial (PRCT) conducted by Peul et al.[23] the authors cite a 56% success rate for nonoperative management, with the ability to avoid surgery used as the measure.

Several cohort studies support satisfactory outcomes for patients with lumbar disc herniations treated surgically.[12,18–20,27–35] Spengler et al.[12] documented a good result in 77% of patients treated with open discectomy. In a prospective series of 203 patients undergoing discectomy, Guilfoyle et al.[28] observed continued relief of symptoms and substantial overall health gains at an average of 2 years after surgery.

In one of the most extensive studies on the topic conducted to date, the Maine Lumbar Spine Study Group prospectively followed patients with lumbar disc herniations for a period of 10 years after index presentation.[18–20] More than 500 patients were enrolled in this investigation, with the decision regarding treatment determined by patients' wishes. At 1-year follow-up 71% of surgically treated patients reported resolution of their back or leg symptoms as compared to 43% of those managed conservatively.[18] Seventy percent of those patients in the surgical group reported continued relief of symptoms at the 5-year time point, compared to 56% in the nonoperative group.[19] In the study's 10-year analysis, 69% of surgical patients maintained symptom relief, while 61% of conservatively treated patients experienced symptom resolution. In terms of level of satisfaction, however, significantly more patients who had received surgery were satisfied compared with their nonoperative counterparts (71% vs 56%, $p = 0.002$).[20]

The major critique regarding the above-cited studies is that some were not prospective and all were not randomized. Within the last decade, the randomized controlled trial has come to be accepted by the orthopaedic and neurosurgical communities as the most valid and conclusive manifestation of scientific research. Of the 50 full-text articles reviewed for this chapter, only 6 were prospective randomized trials regarding the treatment of lumbar disc herniations.[15,21-23,26,36] Two of these, however, involved the same cohort of patients, reporting outcomes at 1[22] and 2 years[23] following randomization.

Weber's classic study consisted of three groups: one requiring surgery, one without indications for surgery, and one where the benefit of surgery was felt to be unclear.[26] Only this "undecided" group was randomized to receive surgery. The other, more modern investigations, randomized patients to receive either surgery or conservative management.[15,21-23,36] In one instance, conservative treatment was under the direction of the patient's primary care practitioner.[22,23] In the SPORT trial, nonoperative management included physical therapy, education, and nonsteroidal drugs, but treatment was individually tailored to each patient.[15,37] In Buttermann's investigation, patients were randomized to receive either surgery or epidural steroid injections.[36]

The main difficulty encountered in all of these randomized investigations was a significant degree of crossover, or lack of adherence to randomized treatment, between groups. In all of the studies, there was crossover from the nonoperative to the operative group in more than one third of the randomized patients (Table 23.1). Among patients assigned to surgery, there was generally good adherence except in the SPORT trial, which experienced 40% crossover from the surgical group.[15] The difficulty with these randomized studies lies in the fact that all sought to conduct intent-to-treat analyses, where patients were evaluated according to the treatment they were initially assigned and not according to the intervention received. In intent-to-treat analysis, demonstrating significant differences between groups becomes difficult once 50% of patients refuse assigned treatment.[24] As a result, although the majority of the randomized trials reported some advantage for surgery, particularly in regard to early relief of symptoms and functional improvement, most findings were not statistically significant.[15,21-23,36] Weber documented significantly better results for the surgically treated group at 1-year follow-up only.[26] At 4-year evaluation, although the surgical group continued to exhibit better results, the differences between the operative and nonoperative groups were no longer statistically significant.

In a review of the randomized controlled literature regarding treatment of lumbar disc herniations, Anderson et al.[24] maintained that in light of increasing crossover, the randomized investigations did not validly address the interventions under study. Furthermore, Anderson et al.[24] maintained that the randomized controlled trial was an inappropriate research model, incapable of answering the question of optimal treatment in the setting of a herniated lumbar disc. "...(Statistical) techniques based on null hypothesis testing and (p) values make valid subgroup analyses difficult...limiting the amount of relevant data that can be obtained from...(randomized controlled trials)...." These authors maintain that in the absence of intent-to-treat analysis, the effect of surgical intervention would have been more substantial.

Supporting this contention, the observational arm of the SPORT trial demonstrated significantly greater treatment effects following surgery at 3-month, 1-year, and 2-year time-points.[16] Similarly, the as-treated analysis of 4-year results in the SPORT documented significantly improved results in the surgical group for all outcome measures at every time-point in the study.[17]

TABLE 23.1 Comparison of Crossover Rates in Randomized Controlled Trials for Treatment of Lumbar Disc Herniation.

Investigation	% Crossover Conservative	% Crossover Surgery
Weber (1983)	35	2
Buttermann (2004)	54	0
Osterman et al. (2006)	39	0
SPORT (2006)	45	40
Peul et al. (2007)[a]	39	11
Peul et al. (2008)[a]	44	11

[a]Represents the same cohort of patients followed for 1 (2007) and 2 (2008) years, respectively.

EVIDENTIARY TABLE AND SELECTION OF TREATMENT METHOD

Because of the large number of studies relevant to this topic, inclusion in the evidentiary table was limited to high-quality level I and II studies available in the literature.[38] Some of these investigations, such as that of the Maine Lumbar Spine Study, were published in multiple installments over the course of several years.[18–20] In such instances, a single level of evidence was assigned to the whole study based on analyses performed at the various time-points, as well as at the study's conclusion. The qualities of evidence for the studies are presented in Table 23.2.

Due to the large crossover effects, the qualities of evidence for most of the randomized trials were downgraded to moderate.[15,21–23,36] The study conducted by Weber had a smaller percentage of crossovers and reported a statistically significant finding at the 1-year time-point.[26] Based on these facts, this study was felt to provide high-quality evidence. The prospective case-control trials of the Maine Lumbar Spine Study and the observational/as-treated arms of the SPORT provide moderate-quality evidence.[16–20] This results from the fact that the treatment effects in these studies were not large enough to warrant the appellation of high-quality evidence.

In the case under consideration, based on the patient's age, radicular symptoms, positive straight leg raise, and MRI findings, the best available evidence supports a surgical intervention. The surgery would entail a discectomy performed using standard open techniques or with the assistance of an operative microscope.[29,35,39–41] Recently, minimally invasive techniques for discectomy, including tubular retractors or the use of an endoscope, have also gained popularity.[42–46]

There are numerous studies that support performing a discectomy using any of the techniques mentioned above.[15–20,29,34,35,41,47] Although there are many who maintain that superior results are achieved with microscopic or minimally invasive techniques, such findings are not borne out in the literature. Kahanovitz et al.[41] documented decreased hospital stays for patients treated with microdiscectomy but were unable to demonstrate any other benefit. In a comparative

TABLE 23.2	Evidentiary Table: Summary of the Quality of Evidence Available in Level I or II Studies Regarding Treatment of Lumbar Disc Herniation.		
Investigation	**Description**	**Summary of Results**	**Quality of Evidence**
Weber (1983)	PRCT	Significantly improved results for surgery at 1 y but not after 4.	High
Maine Lumbar Spine Study (1996–2005)	Prospective case-control study	More patients with pain relief and higher satisfaction levels in the operative group.	Moderate
Buttermann (2004)	PRCT	Greater success rate for surgery. Large crossover effect.	Moderate
Osterman et al. (2006)	PRCT	No clinically significant differences between treatment groups over 2 y. Large crossover effect.	Moderate
SPORT RCT (2006)	PRCT	No clinically or statistically significant differences between treatment groups. Large crossover effect.	Moderate
SPORT Observational (2006)	Prospective case-control study	Significantly improved outcomes for surgical group at 3-mo, 1-y, and 2-y time-points.	Moderate
Peul et al. (2007–2008)	PRCT	Early significant benefit to surgery in terms of relief of leg pain. Benefit of surgery no longer significant after 6 mo. Large crossover effect.	Moderate
SPORT As Treated (2008)	Prospective case-control study	Significantly improved results in the surgical group for all outcome measures at every time-point in the study.	Moderate

review, McCulloch,[29] arguably one of the founders and strongest proponents of microdiscectomy surgery, affirmed that no advantage for the procedure could be supported by the available literature, with success rates documented from 80% to 96% regardless of technique. The rate of complications following microdiscectomy also approximates that of open procedures,[48] although higher rates of infection have been reported.[32,49]

Similarly, multiple studies have attempted to contrast results following standard discectomy with those obtained using tubular, or endoscopically assisted, procedures.[43,44,45] While results are comparable, no study has been able to demonstrate a clinical advantage for minimally invasive discectomy. A recent study by Arts et al.,[46] however, calls into question the purported advantages of tubular discectomy techniques. In a randomized controlled trial comparing outcomes of patients treated with microdiscectomy or tubular discectomy in 328 patients, Arts et al.[46] reported inferior results following tubular discectomy in terms of degree of leg and back pain relief and level of recovery.

DEFINITIVE TREATMENT PLAN

The patient presented in this case should be treated with an open discectomy procedure at L5-S1 performed on a Jackson table with Wilson frame, or an Andrews surgical table.[34,39,50] The surgery should be conducted with the use of surgical loupes and an operative headlight.[34,50] Laminotomy, or hemilaminectomy, can be utilized as necessary to allow removal of the ligamentum flavum and sufficient exposure of the interlaminar window. A Love nerve root retractor is employed to protect the thecal sac and traversing S1 nerve root, while the herniated disc is removed with a pituitary rongeur. Exploration of the disc space may be necessary if the herniated fragment is not readily apparent within the canal. Aggressive curettage of the disc space is not supported.[51,52]

Grading the Evidence for this Plan

The proposed surgical intervention in this patient would be considered a **strong recommendation** based on **moderate-quality evidence** according to the grading recommendations of Schünemann et al.[53] The literature supports benefits of more reliable reduction of leg pain, earlier return to function, and increased satisfaction for as long as 10 years following intervention.[17–20,24,26,36,39,54] The benefits of surgery in this patient outweigh the potential harms, and a recommendation for surgery would apply to most other patients of similar age, with like findings on physical examination and radiographic evidence of a lumbar disc herniation. The technical

aspects of the open discectomy procedure, and the decision to use open discectomy over other techniques, are considered **strong recommendations** based on **low-quality evidence** from mostly retrospective case series.

PREDICTING OUTCOMES

The literature supports reliable outcomes following discectomy in numerous level I–IV investigations.[15–24,26,29–32,34–36,40,41,47,48,50,54,55] The most important factors in terms of predicting outcomes appear to be strict adherence to preoperative selection criteria, predominance of leg symptoms, and location and size of the herniation.[17–20,26,29,36,50] In the case scenario, the patient has a large disc fragment (>6 mm) located in the paracentral region, or lateral recess. Carragee and Kim[14] demonstrated that herniated discs with an intracanalicular component greater than 6 mm in size were predictive of good outcomes following surgery. Similarly, Knop-Jergas et al.[13] found that patients with paracentral disc herniations achieved the greatest benefit following surgical interventions. The recent report of Pearson et al.[54] also supports such findings. Based on the available evidence, the patient would most likely experience relief of her leg pain following surgery and return to full activities earlier than if she was treated conservatively.

Especially in light of the fact that many prospective investigations do not show a demonstrable benefit for surgery, however, the desires of the patient are paramount in making the decision to perform an elective discectomy.[23] In light of the equivocal findings present in their study, Peul et al.[22,23] advocated that surgeons should educate their patients on the current state of the literature, helping them to decide which treatment option best meets their needs. Preoperative discussion must include the potential risks of surgery as well as the anticipated benefits, including earlier relief of leg pain, accelerated recovery, and greater level of satisfaction. It is also wise to counsel this patient that the discectomy would not likely positively impact her level of back pain, although many investigations support a concomitant reduction in back-related symptoms following discectomy.[16–20,54]

Results presented here are aligned with what I have experienced in my own clinical practice as a spine surgeon. A predominance of back pain in a patient with absence of radicular symptoms and no reproducible findings on physical examination, such as a positive straight leg raise, would lead to a more conservative recommendation of nonoperative management. Ultimately, however, the decision for surgical intervention rests with the patient and her desires following a frank discussion with a spine surgeon.

SUMMARY

This case presents a 32-year-old woman with a 2-month history of radicular symptoms in her left leg. The patient presents with radicular pain in a dermatomal distribution, hypesthesia, and a positive straight leg raising sign on physical exam. MRI findings are concordant with her presentation and demonstrate a large, paracentral, L5-S1 disc herniation. Based on her young age, physical examination findings, and the presence of radicular pain for more than 6 weeks, the most appropriate treatment option for this individual would be surgical intervention. Resolution of her radicular pain following surgery can be expected. She should also be able to return to full activities of daily living following a brief convalescence. A reduction in her back pain, while less predictable, may also be anticipated following surgery.

REFERENCES

1. Grönblad M, Weinstein JN, Santavirta S. Immunohistochemical observations on spinal tissue innervation: a review of hypothetical mechanisms of back pain. *Acta Orthop Scand*. 1991;62:614–622.
2. Peng B, Hou S, Wu W, et al. The pathogenesis and clinical significance of a high-intensity zone (HIZ) of lumbar intervertebral disc on MR imaging in the patient with discogenic low back pain. *Eur Spine J*. 2006;15:583–587.
3. Jinkins JR, Whitmore AR, Bradley WG. The anatomic basis of vertebrogenic pain and the autonomic syndrome associated with lumbar disc extrusion. *Am J Roetgenol*. 1989;152:1277–1289.
4. Smyth MJ, Wright VJ. Sciatica and the intervertebral disc: an experimental study. *J Bone Joint Surg Am*. 1958;40:1401–1418.
5. Howe JF, Loeser JD, Calvin WH. Mechanosensitivity of dorsal root ganglia and chronically injured axons: a physiological basis for the radicular pain of nerve root compression. *Pain*. 1977;3:25–41.
6. Kang JD, Stefanovic-Racic M, McIntyre LA, et al. Toward a biochemical understanding of human intervertebral disc degeneration and herniation. Contributions of nitric oxide, interleukins, prostaglandin E2, and matrix metalloproteinases. *Spine*. 1997;15:1065–1073.
7. Spiliopoulou I, Korovessis P, Konstantinou D, et al. IgG and IgM concentration in the prolapsed human intervertebral disc and sciatica etiology. *Spine*. 1994;19:1320–1323.
8. Kosteljanetz M, Espersen JO, Halaburt H, et al. Predictive value of clinical and surgical findings in patients with lumbago-sciatica: a prospective study (Part I). *Acta Neurochir (Wien)*. 1998;140:120–125.
9. Xin SQ, Zhang QZ, Fan DH. Significance of the straight-leg-raising test in the diagnosis and clinical evaluation of lower lumbar intervertebral-disc protrusion. *J Bone Joint Surg Am*. 1987;69:517–522.
10. Majlesi J, Togay H, Unalan H, et al. The sensitivity and specificity of the slump and the straight leg raising tests in patients with lumbar disc herniation. *J Clin Rheumatol*. 2008;14:87–91.
11. Pfirrmann CW, Metzdorf A, Zanetti M, et al. Magnetic resonance classification of lumbar intervertebral disc degeneration. *Spine*. 2001;26:1873–1878.
12. Spengler DM, Ouellette EA, Battie M, et al. Elective discectomy for herniation of a lumbar disc: additional experience with an objective method. *J Bone Joint Surg Am*. 1990;72:320–327.
13. Knop-Jergas BM, Zucherman JF, Hsu KY, et al. Anatomic position of a herniated nucleus pulposus predicts the outcome of lumbar discectomy. *J Spinal Disord*. 1996;9:246–250.
14. Carragee EJ, Kim D. A prospective analysis of magnetic resonance imaging findings in patients with sciatica and lumbar disc herniation: correlation of outcomes with disc fragment and canal morphology. *Spine*. 1997;22:1650–1660.
15. Weinstein JN, Tosteson TD, Lurie JD, et al. Surgical vs nonoperative treatment for lumbar disk herniation: the Spine Patient Outcomes Research Trial (SPORT): a randomized trial. *JAMA*. 2006;296:2441–2450.
16. Weinstein JN, Lurie JD, Tosteson TD, et al. Surgical vs nonoperative treatment for lumbar disk herniation: the Spine Patient Outcomes Research Trial (SPORT) observational cohort. *JAMA*. 2006;296:2451–2459.
17. Weinstein JN, Lurie JD, Tosteson TD, et al. Surgical versus nonoperative treatment for lumbar disc herniation: four-year results for the Spine Patient Outcomes Research Trial (SPORT). *Spine*. 2008;33:2789–2800.
18. Atlas SJ, Deyo RA, Keller RB, et al. The Maine Lumbar Spine Study, Part II. 1-year outcomes of surgical and nonsurgical management of sciatica. *Spine*. 1996;21:1777–1786.
19. Atlas SJ, Keller RB, Chang Y, et al. Surgical and nonsurgical management of sciatica secondary to a lumbar disc herniation: five-year outcomes from the Maine Lumbar Spine Study. *Spine*. 2001;26:1179–1187.
20. Atlas SJ, Keller RB, Wu YA, et al. Long-term outcomes of surgical and nonsurgical management of sciatica secondary to a lumbar disc herniation: 10 year results from the Maine Lumbar Spine Study. *Spine*. 2005;30:927–935.
21. Osterman H, Seitsalo S, Karppinen J, et al. Effectiveness of microdiscectomy for lumbar disc herniation: a randomized controlled trial with 2 years of follow-up. *Spine*. 2006;31:2409–2414.
22. Peul WC, van Houwelingen HC, van den Hout WB, et al. Surgery versus prolonged conservative treatment for sciatica. *N Engl J Med*. 2007;356:2245–2256.
23. Peul WC, van den Hout WB, Brand R, et al. Prolonged conservative care versus early surgery in patients with sciatica caused by lumbar disc herniation: two year results of a randomised controlled trial. *Br Med J*. 2008;336:1355–1358.
24. Anderson PA, McCormick PC, Angevine PD. Randomized controlled trials of the treatment of lumbar disk herniation: 1983–2007. *J Am Acad Orthop Surg*. 2008;16:566–573.

25. Saal JA, Saal JS. Nonoperative treatment of herniated lumbar intervertebral disc with radiculopathy: an outcome study. *Spine*. 1989;14:431–437.

26. Weber H. Lumbar disc herniation: a controlled, prospective study with ten years of observation. *Spine*. 1983;8:131–140.

27. Robinson JS. Sciatica and the lumbar disk syndrome: a historic perspective. *South Med J*. 1983;76:232–238.

28. Guilfoyle MR, Ganesan D, Seeley H, et al. Prospective study of outcomes in lumbar discectomy. *Br J Neurosurg*. 2007;21:389–395.

29. McCulloch JA. Focus issue on lumbar disc herniation: macro- and microdiscectomy. *Spine*. 1996;21:45S–56S.

30. Dewing CB, Provencher MT, Riffenburgh RH, et al. The outcomes of lumbar microdiscectomy in a young, active population: correlation by herniation type and level. *Spine*. 2008;33:33–38.

31. Smorgick Y, Floman Y, Millgram MA, et al. Mid- to long-term outcome of disc excision in adolescent disc herniation. *Spine J*. 2006;6:380–384.

32. Wilson DH, Harbaugh R. Microsurgical and standard removal of the protruded lumbar disc: a comparative study. *Neurosurgery*. 1981;8:422–427.

33. Watters WC III, McGirt MJ. An evidence-based review of the literature on the consequences of conservative versus aggressive discectomy for the treatment of primary disc herniation with radiculopathy. *Spine J*. 2009;9:240–257.

34. Schoeggl A, Maier H, Saringer W, et al. Outcome after chronic sciatica as the only reason for lumbar microdiscectomy. *J Spinal Disord Tech*. 2002;15:415–419.

35. Schoeggl A, Reddy M, Matula C. Functional and economic outcome following microdiscectomy for lumbar disc herniation in 672 patients. *J Spinal Disord Tech*. 2003;16:150–155.

36. Buttermann GR. Treatment of lumbar disc herniation: epidural steroid injection compared with discectomy. *J Bone Joint Surg Am*. 2004;86:670–679.

37. Birkmeyer NJ, Weinstein JN, Tosteson AN, et al. Design of the Spine Patient outcomes Research Trial (SPORT). *Spine*. 2002;27:1361–1372.

38. Obremskey WT, Pappas N, Attallah-Wasif E, et al. Level of evidence in orthopaedic journals. *J Bone Joint Surg Am*. 2005;87:2632–2638.

39. McCulloch JA, Snook D, Kruse CF. Advantages of the operating microscope in lumbar spine surgery. *Instr Course Lect*. 2002;51:243–245.

40. Tulberg T, Isacson J, Weidenhielm L. Does microscopic removal of lumbar disc herniation lead to better results than the standard procedure? Results of a one-year randomized study. *Spine*. 1993;18:24–27.

41. Kahanovitz N, Viola K, McCulloch J. Limited surgical discectomy and microdiscectomy: a clinical comparison. *Spine*. 1989;14:79–81.

42. Wu CG, Li YD, Li MH, et al. Prospective evaluation of transabdominal percutaneous lumbar discectomy for L5-S1 disc herniation: initial clinical experience. *J Neurosurg Spine*. 2008;8:321–326.

43. Wu X, Zhuang S, Mao Z, et al. Microendoscopic discectomy for lumbar disc herniation: surgical technique and outcome in 873 consecutive cases. *Spine*. 2006;31:2689–2694.

44. Righesso O, Falavigna A, Avanzi O. Comparison of open discectomy with microendoscopic discectomy in lumbar disc herniations: results of a randomized controlled trial. *Neurosurgery*. 2007;61:545–549.

45. Ruetten S, Komp M, Merk H, et al. Full-endoscopic interlaminar and transforaminal lumbar discectomy versus conventional microsurgical technique: a prospective, randomized, controlled study. *Spine*. 2008;33:931–939.

46. Arts MP, Brand R, van den Akker ME, et al. Tubular diskectomy vs conventional microdiskectomy for sciatica: a randomized controlled trial. *JAMA*. 2009;302:149–158.

47. Abramovitz JN, Neff SR. Lumbar disc surgery: results of the Prospective Lumbar Discectomy Study of the Joint Section on Disorders of the Spine and Peripheral Nerves of the American Association of Neurological Surgeons and the Congress of Neurological Surgeons. *Neurosurgery*. 1991;29:301–308.

48. Goffin J. Microdiscectomy for lumbar disc herniations. *Clin Neurol Neurosurg*. 1994;96:130–134.

49. Wilson DH, Kenning J. Microsurgical lumbar discectomy: preliminary report of 83 consecutive cases. *Neurosurgery*. 1979;4:137–140.

50. An HS, Simpson JM, Stein R. Outpatient laminotomy and discectomy. *J Spinal Disord*. 1999;12:19–26.

51. Carragee EJ, Spinnickie AO, Alamin TF, et al. A prospective controlled study of limited versus subtotal posterior discectomy: short-term outcomes in patients with herniated lumbar intervertebral discs and large posterior anular defect. *Spine*. 2006;31:653–657.

52. Balderston RA, Gilyard GG, Jones AA, et al. The treatment of lumbar disc herniation: simple fragment excision versus disc space curettage. *J Spinal Disord*. 1991;4:22–25.

53. Schünemann HJ, Jaeschke R, Cook DJ, et al. An official ATS statement: grading the quality of evidence and strength of recommendations in ATS guidelines and recommendations. *Am J Respir Crit Care Med*. 2006;174:605–614.

54. Pearson AM, Blood EA, Frymoyer JW, et al. SPORT lumbar intervertebral disk herniation and back pain: does treatment, location, or morphology matter? *Spine*. 2008;33:428–435.

55. Spangfort EV. The lumbar disc herniation: a computer-aided analysis of 2504 operations. *Acta Orthop Scand (Suppl)*. 1972;142:1–95.

Isthmic Spondylolisthesis

HAREL ARZI, MD AND PAUL M. ARNOLD, MD, FACS

A 34-year-old man has a primary complaint of low back pain and a secondary complaint of left leg pain greater than right leg pain. Symptoms began after a work injury 2 years ago. However, worker's compensation refuses to claim responsibility for his injury, so he has sought care under his private insurance carrier. Because of his pain, he has not worked since the injury. His back pain is worse with extension, though he does have some pain with flexion. He has no bowel and bladder complaints. He has failed three courses of physical therapy as well as multiple epidural and transforaminal steroid injections.

Physical examination demonstrates that he is neurologically intact to motor, sensory, and reflex testing. He has tenderness primarily over the L5-S1 interspace with midline palpation. He has pain that is provoked with extension more than flexion. His gait is normal and is not overweight. A straight leg test produces back pain but not leg pain.

Radiographic imaging studies are shown in Figure 24.1.

INTERPRETATION OF CLINICAL PRESENTATION

The clinical scenario describes a young man suffering with low back pain after a work injury. The pain is getting worse with movement and thus can be described as "mechanical" pain. The pain is greater in extension than in flexion. Radicular pain that is greater in extension usually indicates nerve root compression that might be correlated to foraminal or central spinal stenosis, but back pain that worsens with extension is more typical of spondylolysis or spondylolisthesis. The patient complains of leg pain greater on the left but his straight leg raising (SLR) test is negative,

so severe nerve root compression is less likely to be present. The intact motor, sensory, and reflex testing further support absence of severe nerve or dural sac compression as well as the absence of bowel and bladder complaints. The tenderness over L5-S1 noted on physical examination supports a bony lesion at that level, as other nonbony degenerative and developmental disease processes will not usually produce tenderness upon palpation.

The T2-weighted magnetic resonance images (MRI) presented include one midline sagittal (Fig. 24.1B), three paramedian (Fig. 24.1A, C, and D), and three axial images at the level of L4-5 disc space (Fig. 24.1E), L5 body (Fig. 24.1F), and L5-S1 disc space (Fig. 24.1G). In Figure 24.1A, a paramedian cut shows a bony lesion at the pars interarticularis of L5 with a mild degree of anterior displacement of L5 over S1 and posterior bulging of the intervertebral disc annulus with narrowing of the L5 foramen and possible nerve root compression. Figure 24.1C and D shows a similar picture on the other side but with a somewhat higher degree of anterior displacement of the vertebral body and less foraminal narrowing. Figure 24.1B demonstrates a minimal degree of anterior displacement of the body of L5 over S1 (Meyerding Grade 0),[1] mild bulging of the intervertebral disc annulus with no significant compression of the dural sac, very few bony degenerative signs, and a relatively low signal intensity at the intervertebral disc indicative of possibly an early degenerative process in the disc. The disc height is moderately decreased.

Although best measured using a plain lateral radiograph, the slip angle measured on the median sagittal MRI cut is not kyphotic and measures <30 degrees. Figure 24.1E shows minimal facet joint hypertrophy with no significant disc bulging and no neural element compression. Figure 24.1F demonstrates the bony lesion at the pars interarticularis with abundant soft tissue surrounding it, indicating nonunion of the pars lesion. Figure 24.1G shows mild L5-S1 disc bulging with possible compression on the exiting nerve root, worse on the left. Several reports emphasize a possible correlation between isthmic

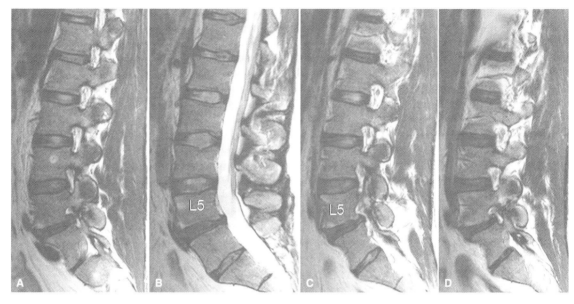

Figure 24.1.

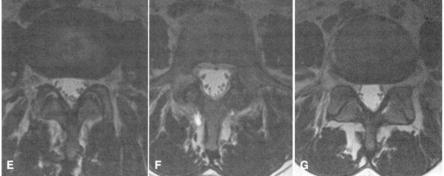

| L4-5 | L5 Body | L5-S1 |

spondylolisthesis (IS) and spina bifida occulta,[2] but no evidence for that pathology was found on this patient's MRI.

The imaging studies correlate well with the patient's complaints of back pain due to the spondylolysis and leg pain greater on the left as a result of the foraminal stenosis of L5-S1 on the left. Of the several types of spondylolysis described, this case is best described as isthmic spondylolisthesis, Wiltse subtype A (fatigue fracture of the pars with complete bony separation).[3] Signs of high-grade dysplastic spondylolisthesis, such as a trapezoid shape of the vertebral body of L5 or domed-shaped S1 upper end plate, are not found on the current imaging studies and therefore will be further classified as a developmental low dysplastic slip with lysis, according to Marchetti and Bartolozzi.[4]

DECLARATION OF SPECIFIC DIAGNOSIS

This patient has a symptomatic isthmic spondylolysis and spondylolisthesis with foraminal stenosis greater on the left.

BRAINSTORMING: WHAT ARE THE TREATMENT GOALS AND SURGICAL OPTIONS?

IS is a defect of the pars interarticularis in the posterior column of the lumbar spine. It can cause back pain due to mechanical instability of the spinal segment, degenerative disc changes, or direct pressure on the thecal sac. Foraminal stenosis caused by the fibrous tissue at the defect site or compression by the free laminar fragment or the bulging intervertebral disc can cause radicular symptoms, including thigh and leg pain and nerve root compression signs such as SLR or Lasegue sign. Both neurological deficit and proof of advancing slip are uncommon in low-grade IS, and thus the first line of treatment for most patients with low-grade IS will be nonoperative. As per history, this patient has failed a comprehensive trial of nonoperative treatment.

The treatment goals are

1. Relief of back pain
2. Relief of leg pain

3. Return to previous occupation and sport activities

4. Prevention of disc degeneration and slip progression

The treatment options are

1. Direct pars defect repair

2. Decompression of dural sac and/or nerve roots alone

3. Posterolateral fusion with possible instrumentation and reduction

4. Lumbar interbody fusion, anterior or posterior, with or without posterolateral fusion

EVALUATION OF LITERATURE

A Medline search was conducted in order to identify the relevant literature regarding the surgical treatment of symptomatic adult IS. The terms "adult" and "isthmic" were used as key words, and the term "spondylolisthesis" was used both as a keyword and as a MeSH (Medical Subject Heading) with the sub-headings of "surgery" and "therapy." A search strategy combining the terms above resulted in 215 citations. A similar strategy was utilized for searching the archives of specific journals, including but not limited to *Spine, JBJS American, JBJS British, European Spine Journal*, and the *Journal of Neurosurgery: Spine*. References were screened to identify pertinent articles. Search strings for specific treatment options were used to identify relevant publications. After limiting the scope for English language results and eliminating articles overtly irrelevant by title, patient population, or surgical technique, 152 abstracts and 55 full-text articles were reviewed.

DETAILED REVIEW OF PERTINENT ARTICLES

Operative versus Nonoperative

Only articles regarding operative treatment were reviewed for the discussion of this case, as it is clear from the case description that nonoperative treatment had failed.

Types of Operative Treatment

An extensive body of literature concerning the surgical treatment of symptomatic spondylolisthesis in adults was reviewed. The vast majority of this literature was comprised of uncontrolled cohort studies and other studies that were either nonrandomized comparative studies or had historical controls.

Direct Pars Repair

Direct pars repair is usually indicated for the adolescent and very young adult population and is not widely used for adult patients. No comparative studies or cohort studies with sufficient number of patients were found to support such a treatment in the nonpediatric population, and therefore, this option is not currently recommended.[5]

Decompression without Fusion

Formal laminectomy, foraminotomy, and removal of the free laminar fragment (Gill procedure) have all been used for the treatment of IS. A report by Gill[6] shows satisfactory results in long-term follow-up after Gill procedure despite worse radiographic findings. Many methodological shortcomings render the quality of these conclusions very low. In the opinion of many authors, decompression of the affected spinal segment could adversely influence the structural stability of the spinal segment and thus increase the likelihood of increasing slippage and mechanical symptoms related to instability, as well as accelerated disc degeneration.[7] Decompression without fusion is not currently recommended for adult spondylolisthesis.

Spinal Fusion

Spinal fusion of the involved segment is the mainstay of treatment for symptomatic adult IS. Fusion can be achieved through a posterior approach via a transverse process fusion (TPF), an anterior approach via interbody fusion (anterior lumbar interbody fusion, ALIF), or a posterior approach to interbody fusion (posterior lumbar interbody fusion, PLIF, or transforaminal lumbar interbody fusion, TLIF). In order to promote union even further, combinations of two fusion methods can be utilized, that is, posterior instrumentation plus ALIF or posterior instrumentation plus PLIF. Each of the approaches has its advantages and drawbacks.

The posterior approach is most commonly utilized by spine surgeons for the treatment of different lumbar spine pathologies. As such, no access surgeon is needed. The complications related to the surgical exposure are minimal; however, stripping of the paravertebral muscles can be a cause of postoperative back pain, though it is rarely prolonged. The posterior approach enables internal fixation using pedicle screws but does not address the issue of anterior column stability and disc degeneration, which, as shown by Barrick et al.,[8] can result in significant symptoms despite solid fusion.

Posterior fusion can be performed with or without the addition of instrumentation, most commonly pedicle screws. While most surgeons will use posterior instrumentation to achieve immediate stabilization and enhance fusion, the literature is not definitive about the influence of instrumentation on fusion rate.

Several randomized controlled studies have tested the question of instrumentation for spinal fusion. Some studies favor instrumentation for better fusion rates, prevention of further slip, and better clinical results.[9,10] Others have shown no benefit to fusion rates with instrumentation, nor lower reoperation rates or improved clinical results.[11,12] No difference was found in a prospective randomized study by Thomsen et al.[13] with more blood loss and longer operative time in the instrumentation group and minor functional improvement in functional results only when combined with decompression. Ekman et al.[14] did not find a significant difference in any of the clinical outcome measures used in their randomized controlled study from 2005.[14]) The reasons for the different results may be associated with the use of heterogeneous patient groups with variable degrees of slip, different outcome measures, different methods for assessing nonunion, and the use of different questionnaires to assess postoperative results. Posterior spine instrumentation has become a standard of practice, but its clinical efficacy is yet to be fully determined.

Yet another question is whether posterior decompression has a role in addition to fusion in the treatment of IS. While some surgeons will argue that a patient with complaints related to spinal canal or foraminal stenosis should have an adequate decompression of these elements in order to alleviate symptoms, others will state that the decompression is a factor of instability added to an already unstable spine segment and that back and leg pain relief is achieved by solid fusion without decompression.[7,15] Several uncontrolled studies have been published and the results are mixed, with some showing satisfactory clinical outcome without fusion.[16] Other comparative nonrandomized studies found no clinical and radiographic differences between fusion alone and fusion with decompression.[17,18] A prospective randomized study by Carragee[15] in 1997 found that removal of the free lamina and decompression of the nerve root in patients undergoing spine fusion for IS were associated with higher rates of nonunion and unsatisfactory results. In the absence of neurological compromise or severe central or foraminal stenosis, current data lead to a strong recommendation against decompression when added to spine fusion in low-grade IS[19] (Table 24.1).

To a similar extent, reduction of IS is debatable. In the patient case discussed, however, the degree of slip is minimal and near-complete reduction is expected with prone patient positioning alone.[20] Whether such reduction occurs or not, in-situ fusion will be recommended.

The anterior approach to the lumbar spine enables direct access to the disc space, and thus, a complete discectomy can be performed. Reduction of slip and correction of sagittal spinal alignment are best done using the anterior approach. Further, intervertebral fusion can be achieved using the largest surface area and largest size graft or implant possible. Stripping of the paravertebral muscles is avoided and so is the resultant pain, but other significant structures are placed at risk. Decompression occurs as a result of disc height restoration.[21] Catastrophic complications can occur as a result of a major vascular or other retroperitoneal structure injury, but even a minor vascular injury can lead to a significant blood loss necessitating transfusion. Retrograde ejaculation is a result of a sympathetic injury, usually at L5-S1 level, and should be carefully taken into consideration when counseling a young male regarding the surgical options. Many will use an access surgeon to complete the transperitoneal or retroperitoneal approach. Although restoration of the disc space height may open the foramen and minimize foraminal stenosis, direct dural sac and nerve root decompression cannot be completed using an anterior approach alone.

Both PLIF and TLIF will enable stabilization of the anterior spinal column and avoid the risks of an anterior approach. Near-complete discectomy and interbody instrumentation can be performed using a posterior approach. Restoration of disc space height and greater bone surface for bone fusion are the mechanical advantages of these techniques.[22,23] PLIF and TLIF are more technically demanding procedures than TPF alone, and operation time is longer; in addition, special implants are commonly used, thus increasing procedure costs.

Numerous studies have been published addressing the question of posterior, anterior, or combined approaches for IS. Most of them are retrospective or prospective cohort studies, each evaluating a different treatment option such as anterior,[21,24] posterior,[12,25] PLIF or TLIF,[23,26] or combined anterior and posterior surgery.[27–29] All authors report good clinical, functional, and radiographic outcomes.[30] Nonrandomized controlled studies comparing TPF with or without PLIF have had varied results. Some have found better fusion with PLIF and equal clinical outcome,[31] others found better fusion, better reduction and worse clinical outcome with PLIF,[32] and yet others indicated equal clinical outcome at 2 years[33] or better results for posterior instrumentation with PLIF in higher grades of slip with equal results on the lower grades.[34] A nonrandomized controlled study comparing TPF with or without ALIF found that the ALIF group had better clinical results in the short-term only (up to 2 years).[35] A retrospective comparison between PLIF and ALIF found no significant clinical difference but less adjacent-segment degeneration in the ALIF group.[36] One randomized controlled study compared posterior lumbar instrumentation with TPF versus PLIF.[37] The PLIF group showed better reduction, but the TPF group had better clinical and subjective outcomes. Both groups

TABLE 24.1 Evidentiary Table.

Paper Author (Year)	Description	Summary of Results	Quality of Evidence
Carragee (1997)	Prospective randomized study	• 42 patients with LGIS • 18 fusion w/ decompression, 24 fusion w/o decompression • mean f/u 4.5 y • Clinical: 6/18 unsatisfactory results vs. 1/24 • Fusion: 4/18 nonunion vs. 0/24	High
La Rosa et al. (2003)	Retrospective controlled study	• 35 patients with IS Grade II–III decompression, 18 PLF 17 PI + PLIF. • Clinical results: equal • Fusion results: PI + PLIF better	Low-moderate
Madan and Boeree (2002)	Retrospective controlled study	• 44 patients with IS Grade I–II decompression, 21 PLF 23 PI + PLIF • Fusion: PLIF better • Clinical: PLF better	Low-moderate
Dehoux et al. (2004)	Prospective nonrandomized controlled study	• 52 patients with IS Grade I–III Decompression, 25 PLF 27 PI + PLIF • Fusion: PLIF better • Clinical: Grade I equal, Grade II–III PLIF better	Moderate-high
Ekman et al. (2007)	Prospective study with historical controls	• 163 patients with IS Grade I–III decompression for sciatica only, 77 PLF 86 PLIF • Clinical: PLF = PLIF • Fusion: N/A	Low
Swan et al. (2006)	Prospective controlled study	• 93 patients with IS Grade I–II no decompression 47 PLF + ALIF 46 PLF only • Clinical: better for ALIF + PLF up to 2 y • Increased minor complications at ALIF + PLF	Moderate
Kwon et al. (2005)	Systematic literature review	• 4 RCT 30 case series • Decompression: Trend toward worse results. • Instrumentation: Better clinical and radiographic results. • Comparing approaches: • Clinical results: ALIF and combined give better results than PLF • Fusion results: combined better than ALIF or PLF	Low-moderate
Jacobs et al. (2006)	Systematic literature review	• 8 RCT 21 case series • Decompression and fusion do not improve outcome. • Cumulative outcome • 80% good or excellent results PLF and ALIF groups • 80% fusion rate PLF and PLIF groups	Low-moderate

LGIS, low-grade IS; PI, posterior instrumentation; RCT, randomized controlled trial.

had 100% fusion rates. Shortcomings of this study were the small treatment groups of ten patients each and a short follow-up time of <2 years.

Two systematic literature reviews were found that evaluated this large body of literature. The first included 34 studies, the majority of which were retrospective uncontrolled studies. Fusion rates for combined procedures were significantly higher than anterior or posterior alone, with a nonsignificant trend toward better fusion for TPF when compared to ALIF.

However, posterior spine fusion had inferior clinical results to both ALIF and combined treatment groups. Differences in the complication rate could not be determined. Covariate analysis revealed better radiographic and clinical results for instrumented fusion over noninstrumented fusion. Patients who underwent laminectomy showed a trend toward worse results.[38]

The second systematic review included 29 studies, most of which were retrospective cohort studies and case series. Eight randomized controlled studies were identified, all evaluating different techniques of posterior lumbar fusion. Decompression and instrumentation did not appear to improve outcome, and no conclusion could be drawn regarding the best treatment method. Good or excellent outcome was found in more than 80% of posterior lumbar fusion and ALIF studies. The complication rate was highly variable. Fusion rate was 80% for PLF and PLIF and 60% for ALIF.[39]

The reasons for the different outcomes in the different studies may be a combination of various factors. There is no comprehensive and homogeneous method to evaluate both clinical and functional outcomes. The evaluation of radiographic outcome is even more inconsistent, making comparison of results from different studies somewhat challenging. Some authors performed decompression that included complete laminectomy and foraminotomy in all cases, while others used it only in selected cases. Some authors used partial decompression, and others did not use decompression at all. This heterogeneity alone could contribute to the variation in results. The group of patients who underwent decompression might benefit more from aggressive stabilization, that is, adding interbody fusion to posterior lumbar fusion, as decompression is believed to contribute to segmental instability. The grade of spondylolisthesis and the methods of measurement were not standardized across the different studies. Significant variations can be found in patient selection and inclusion criteria in both clinical variables and indication for surgical treatment.

EVIDENTIARY TABLE AND SELECTION OF TREATMENT METHOD

After reviewing the articles described above, an evidentiary table was constructed (Table 24.1). Utilizing these data, the following treatment plan was developed.

Posterior fusion remains the mainstay of surgical treatment for symptomatic low-grade IS. No clear evidence was found for better results after an instrumented procedure, yet the possible immediate stability and avoidance of any cast or brace make instrumentation a favorable option. Decompression was found to be ineffective in the absence of other compressive lesion or neurological deficit, and some data show that

outcome will be compromised, especially regarding the development of nonunion. Decompression is therefore not recommended for this case.

Adding PLIF, TLIF, or anterior approach to the posterior lumbar fusion did not prove to be efficacious in improving clinical results when compared to posterior lumbar fusion alone in IS and particularly in low-grade IS. Those procedures can be performed with a reasonable degree of reproducibility and safety, but the clinical outcome does not seem to justify the added cost of implants and extended operative time as well as the additional rare though significant complications.

Many of the studies reviewed had no information regarding the type of bone graft used. Among the studies that specified the graft type, the majority used iliac crest bone graft taken through the same or a separate incision[11,16,25,35] or spinous process with bone substitute.[37] Autologous iliac crest autograft is indeed the "gold standard" for posterior spine fusion, but donor site morbidity[40] and evidence of good results with the use of allograft[41] with or without the addition of demineralized bone matrix[42] make these other options viable. These recommendations are also consistent with the Scoliosis Research Society Committee on Spondylolisthesis published in 2005.[43]

In summary, the evidence suggests that the selected treatment plan for this particular patient would be instrumented posterior fusion with no decompression.

DEFINITIVE TREATMENT PLAN

The patient in the scenario presented had failed a comprehensive course of nonoperative treatment, and, therefore, operative treatment is indicated. Positioning of the patient for surgery in a prone or jack-knife position can facilitate complete reduction of the minimal slip shown on imaging studies. We use a posterior approach to the lower lumbar spine with midline skin incision and exposure of the entry points for screw insertion and transverse processes bilaterally. Stabilization is effected using bilateral pedicle screws at L5 and S1 with a rod-based system. Meticulous decortication of facet joints and transverse process followed by implantation of allograft or bone substitute at the lateral gutter will complete the fusion.

Early mobilization is initiated in the early postoperative period with instructions to avoid extreme range of motion and physical exercise. Physical therapy can be started after surgery.

Grading the Evidence for this Plan

Evidence reviewed to support our treatment plan varies in quality. Most studies reviewed were prospective or retrospective cohort studies, and thus rated low or very low quality according to Schünemann et al. However, many studies found were randomized, controlled studies or upgraded observational studies graded moderate or high quality[44] (Table 24.1).

In accordance with the method of grading set forth by Schünemann et al., the recommendation to perform posterior spine fusion and refrain from decompression and PLIF in this case are **strong**. The recommendation to perform instrumented fusion is **weak** considering the mixed results and the disadvantages of the high cost of implants and prolonged surgery time as compared to the advantages of early stabilization and low complication rate.

PREDICTING OUTCOMES

Reported bony fusion rates vary from 60% to 100%[15,31–35] across the studies reviewed with no correlation to the type of bone graft or instrumentation used. Predicting radiographic outcome is very inconsistent across studies evaluating posterior spine fusion, and even more so with the presence of metal implants in the involved segment. Fusion rates have not been shown to correlate well with clinical outcome.

Clinical and functional outcomes ranged from 65% to 90% good or excellent results, with 70% to 95% of improvement in back pain and similar results in alleviating leg pain. Despite encouraging clinical results, return to preoperative work status occurred in only 50% to 60% of the patients undergoing posterior spine fusion for low-grade IS.[15,31–35]

SUMMARY

A 34-year-old patient presents with complaints of back and leg pain unresponsive to conservative treatment. The imaging studies show low-grade IS. The selected treatment option is instrumented posterior spine fusion without decompression. A significant improvement in back and leg pain is expected as well as improved back-pain-related quality of life.

REFERENCES

1. Meyerding H. Spondylolisthesis. *Surg Gynecol Obstet.* 1932;54:371–377.
2. Hammerberg KW. New concepts on the pathogenesis and classification of spondylolisthesis. *Spine.* 2005 Mar 15;30(6 suppl):S4–S11.
3. Wiltse LL, Newman PH, MacNab I. Classification of spondylolysis and spondylolisthesis. *Clin Orthop Relat Res.* 1976;117:23–29.
4. Marchetti PG, Bartolozzi P. Classification of spondylolisthesis as a guideline for treatment. In: Bridwell KH,

DeWald RL, eds. *The Textbook of Spinal Surgery.* 2nd ed. Philadelphia, PA: Lippincott-Raven, 1997:1212.
5. Schlenzka D, Remes V, Helenius I, et al. Direct repair for treatment of symptomatic spondylolysis and low-grade isthmic spondylolisthesis in young patients: no benefit in comparison to segmental fusion after a mean follow-up of 14.8 years. *Eur Spine J.* 2006 Oct;15(10):1437–1447.
6. Gill GG. Long-term follow-up evaluation of a few patients with spondylolisthesis treated by excision of the loose lamina with decompression of the nerve roots without spinal fusion. *Clin Orthop Relat Res.* 1984 Jan–Feb;182:215–219.
7. Kwon BK, Albert TJ. Adult low-grade acquired spondylolytic spondylolisthesis: evaluation and management. *Spine.* 2005 Mar 15;30(6 suppl):S35–S41.
8. Barrick WT, Schofferman JA, Reynolds JB, et al. Anterior lumbar fusion improves discogenic pain at levels of prior posterolateral fusion. *Spine.* 2000;25:853–857.
9. Zdeblick TA. A prospective, randomized study of lumbar fusion: preliminary results. *Spine.* 1993;18:983–991.
10. Bridwell KH, Sedgewick TA, O'Brien MF, et al. The role of fusion and instrumentation in the treatment of degenerative spondylolisthesis with spinal stenosis. *J Spinal Disord.* 1993;6:461–472.
11. Moller H, Hedlund R. Instrumented and noninstrumented posterolateral fusion in adult spondylolisthesis: a prospective randomized study: part 2. *Spine.* 2000;25:1716–1721.
12. Bjarke CF, Stender HE, Laursen M, et al. Long-term functional outcome of pedicle screw instrumentation as a support for posterolateral spinal fusion: randomized clinical study with a 5-year follow-up. *Spine.* 2002;27:1269–1277.
13. Thomsen K, Christensen FB, Eiskjaer SP, et al. 1997 Volvo Award winner in clinical studies. The effect of pedicle screw instrumentation on functional outcome and fusion rates in posterolateral lumbar spinal fusion: a prospective, randomized clinical study. *Spine.* 1997 Dec 15;22(24):2813–2822.
14. Ekman P, Möller H, Hedlund R. The long-term effect of posterolateral fusion in adult isthmic spondylolisthesis: a randomized controlled study. *Spine J.* 2005 Jan–Feb;5(1):36–44.
15. Carragee EJ. Single-level posterolateral arthrodesis, with or without posterior decompression, for the treatment of isthmic spondylolisthesis in adults. A prospective, randomized study. *J Bone Joint Surg Am.* 1997 Aug;79(8):1175–1180.
16. Butt MF, Dhar SA, Hakeem I, et al. In situ instrumented posterolateral fusion without decompression in symptomatic low-grade isthmic spondylolisthesis in adults. *Int Orthop.* 2008 Oct;32(5):663–669.
17. Garreau de Loubresse C, Bon T, et al. Posterolateral Fusion for Radicular Pain in Isthmic Spondylolisthesis. *Clin Orthop Rel Res.* 1996;323:194–201.
18. Adam FF. Surgical management of isthmic spondylolisthesis with radicular pain. *Int Orthop.* 2003;27(5):311–314.
19. Hu SS, Tribus CB, Diab M, et al. Spondylolisthesis and spondylolysis. *Instr Course Lect.* 2008;57:431–445.
20. Montgomery DM, Fischgrund JS. Passive reduction of spondylolisthesis on the operating room table: a prospective study. *J Spinal Disord.* 1994;7:167–172.

21. Ishihara H, Osada R, Kanamori M, et al. Minimum 10-year follow-up study of anterior lumbar interbody fusion for isthmic spondylolisthesis. *Spinal Disord*. 2001 Apr;14(2):91–99.

22. Molinari RW, Bridwell KH, Lenke LG, et al. Anterior column support in surgery for high-grade, isthmic spondylolisthesis. *Clin Orthop Relat Res*. 2002 Jan;(394):109–120.

23. Lauber S, Schulte TL, Liljenqvist U, et al. Clinical and radiologic 2–4-year results of transforaminal lumbar interbody fusion in degenerative and isthmic spondylolisthesis grades 1 and 2. *Spine*. 2006 Jul 1;31(15): 1693–1698.

24. Kim NH, Lee JW. Anterior interbody fusion versus posterolateral fusion with transpedicular fixation for isthmic spondylolisthesis in adults. A comparison of clinical results. *Spine*. 1999 Apr 15;24(8):812–816; discussion 817.

25. Wenger M, Sapio N, Markwalder TM. Long-term outcome in 132 consecutive patients after posterior internal fixation and fusion for Grade I and II isthmic spondylolisthesis. *J Neurosurg Spine*. 2005 Mar;2(3):289–297.

26. Molinari RW, Sloboda JF, Arrington EC. Low-grade isthmic spondylolisthesis treated with instrumented posterior lumbar interbody fusion in U.S. servicemen. *J Spinal Disord Tech*. 2005 Feb;18(suppl):S24–S29.

27. Spruit M, Pavlov PW, Leitao J, et al. Posterior reduction and anterior lumbar interbody fusion in symptomatic low-grade adult isthmic spondylolisthesis: short-term radiological and functional outcome. *Eur Spine J*. 2002 Oct;11(5):428–433.

28. Spruit M, van Jonbergen JP, de Kleuver M. A concise follow-up of a previous report: posterior reduction and anterior lumbar interbody fusion in symptomatic low-grade adult isthmic spondylolisthesis. *Eur Spine J*. 2005 Nov;14(9):828–832.

29. Lee SH, Choi WG, Lim SR, et al. Minimally invasive anterior lumbar interbody fusion followed by percutaneous pedicle screw fixation for isthmic spondylolisthesis. *Spine J*. 2004 Nov–Dec;4(6):644–649.

30. L'Heureux EA Jr, Perra JH, Pinto MR, et al. Functional outcome analysis including preoperative and postoperative SF-36 for surgically treated adult isthmic spondylolisthesis. *Spine*. 2003;28:1269–1274.

31. La Rosa G, Conti A, Cacciola F, et al. Pedicle screw fixation for isthmic spondylolisthesis: does posterior lumbar interbody fusion improve outcome over posterolateral fusion? *J Neurosurg*. 2003;99:143–150.

32. Madan S, Boeree NR. Outcome of posterior lumbar interbody fusion versus posterolateral fusion for spondylolytic spondylolisthesis. *Spine*. 2002 Jul 15;27(14): 1536–1542.

33. Ekman P, Möller H, Tullberg T, et al. Posterior lumbar interbody fusion versus posterolateral fusion in adult isthmic spondylolisthesis. *Spine*. 2007 Sep 15;32(20): 2178–2183.

34. Dehoux E, Fourati E, Madi K, et al. Posterolateral versus interbody fusion in isthmic spondylolisthesis: functional results in 52 cases with a minimum follow-up of 6 years. *Acta Orthop Belg*. 2004 Dec;70(6):578–582.

35. Swan J, Hurwitz E, Malek F, et al. Surgical treatment for unstable low-grade isthmic spondylolisthesis in adults: a prospective controlled study of posterior instrumented fusion compared with combined anterior-posterior fusion. *Spine J*. 2006 Nov–Dec;6(6):606–614.

36. Min JH, Jang JS, Lee SH. Comparison of anterior- and posterior-approach instrumented lumbar interbody fusion for spondylolisthesis. *Neurosurg Spine*. 2007 Jul;7(1):21–26.

37. Inamdar DN, Alagappan M, Shyam L, et al. Posterior lumbar interbody fusion versus intertransverse fusion in the treatment of lumbar spondylolisthesis. *J Orthop Surg (Hong Kong)*. 2006 Apr;14(1):21–26.

38. Kwon BK, Hilibrand AS, Malloy K, et al. A critical analysis of the literature regarding surgical approach and outcome for adult low-grade isthmic spondylolisthesis. *J Spinal Disord Tech*. 2005 Feb;18 (suppl):S30–S40.

39. Jacobs WC, Vreeling A, De Kleuver M. Fusion for low-grade adult isthmic spondylolisthesis: a systematic review of the literature. *Eur Spine J*. 2006 Apr;15(4):391–402.

40. Younger EM, Chapman MW. Morbidity at bone graft donor sites. *J Orthop Trauma*. 1989;3:192–195.

41. Aurori BF, Weierman RJ, Lowell HA, et al. Pseudarthrosis after spinal fusion for scoliosis: A comparison of autogeneic and allogeneic bone grafts. *Clin Orthop*. 1985;199:153–158.

42. Lee KJ, Roper JG, Wang JC. Demineralized bone matrix and spinal arthrodesis. *Spine J*. 2005 Nov–Dec; 5(6 suppl):217S–223S.

43. Mardjetko S, Albert T, Andersson G, et al. Spine/SRS spondylolisthesis summary statement. *Spine*. 2005 Mar 15;30(6 suppl):S3.

44. Schünemann HJ, Jaeschke R, Cook DJ, et al.; ATS Documents Development and Implementation Committee. An official ATS statement: grading the quality of evidence and strength of recommendations in ATS guidelines and recommendations. *Am J Respir Crit Care Med*. 2006 Sep 1;174(5):605–614.

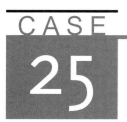
Two-Level Degenerative Slip with Stenosis

RAJA RAMPERSAND, MD, FRCSC AND OMA PERSAUD, MSc

◼ EDITORS' CASE PRESENTATION

A 73-year-old diabetic man presents with complaints of back and leg pain. He reports increased ambulation tolerance with leaning on a shopping cart. In general, he describes more right leg pain than left leg pain. However, he feels his back pain is worse than his leg pain. He has had physical therapy and two epidural steroid injections but has not had substantial relief. He does not have any bowel or bladder complaints.

Physical examination reveals that he is overweight for his body habitus. Neurological examination is normal except that he has absent patella tendon and Achilles tendon reflexes. He has no pain to palpation of the low back. Besides being slow to rise from a chair, his gait is normal.

Radiographic imaging studies are shown in Figures 25.1A–D and 25.2A–D.

INTERPRETATION OF CLINICAL PRESENTATION

The clinical scenario describes a 73-year old, overweight, diabetic male with back and leg pain that is relieved by forward flexion. Relief of symptoms by forward flexion suggests pseudoclaudication, that is, neurogenic claudication. However, this patient has back dominant pain that is also presumably relieved by flexion and thus suggests that the facets could be a major source of his back pain. Further history as to the degree of mechanical versus constant nonmechanical symptoms would be helpful in determining whether this patient has any evidence of constant chronic low back pain. In addition, a history of significant back pain while in a seated position may suggest a concomitant discogenic source of back pain. These important factors that are determined by a detailed pain history would help elucidate whether there is a component of multifactorial back pain. There are no reported symptoms to suggest any urgent neurological issues. He has failed reasonable conservative treatment.

There are no sensory or motor deficits on physical examination. However, his absent reflexes may suggest the possibility of diabetic peripheral neuropathy. Consequently, further detailed neurologic examination, electromyography/nerve conduction studies, and a medical assessment of his glucose control would be advised.

Sagittal and paramedian T2-weighted magnetic resonance imaging (MRI) in Figure 25.1 demonstrates multilevel degenerative changes throughout the entire visible thoracolumbar spine. A degenerative, grade 1 spondylolisthesis is noted at L3-5 and to a lesser extent at L4-5. There is foraminal narrowing at multiple levels that is worse in the left L3-4 and right L5-S1 foramina; however, there is still space for the nerve roots at these and all other visible levels. From the history provided, it is undetermined whether he has any indication of an L3 pattern of pain on the left or L5 pattern on the right. Consequently, these findings may not be clinically significant. There is also significant disc space collapse throughout the lumbar spine with near bone-on-bone collapse at L2-3 and L5-S1. Figure 25.2A shows an axial image of L2-3 demonstrating some facet arthrosis on the right side. The left facet is not visible. Figure 25.2B is an axial image of L3-4 demonstrating significant central and bilateral lateral recess stenosis. There is a small amount of fluid in the facet joints bilaterally, and both facets are more sagittally oriented. Figure 25.2C is an axial image of L4-5 demonstrating significant bilateral lateral recess stenosis with some fluid in the facet joints and normally orientated facets. Figure 25.2D is an axial image of L5-S1 demonstrating early bilateral lateral recess stenosis but no significant or obvious compression of the S1 roots bilaterally.

From a clinical perspective, the stenosis noted at L3-4 and L4-5 correlates with the history of claudicant

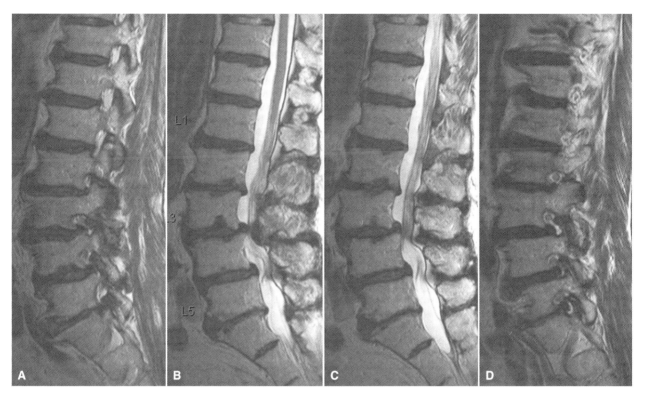

Figure 25.1.

type symptoms presented in this scenario. If there is a clear pattern of L3 or L5 radicular pain on the left and right, respectively, then the foraminal stenosis at the respective foramina may be clinically significant. The facet arthrosis at L3-4 and L4-5 is also likely related to the mechanical low back pain that is dominant in this individual. Furthermore, the presence of facet fluid can signify greater instability than is demonstrated on the recumbent unloaded MRI.[1–3] As such, standing plain radiographs including flexion extension views would be strongly recommended in this case to rule out any further translation of L3-4 and/or L4-5. For these reasons, the senior author routinely uses standing plain radiographs in this type of clinical scenario.

The significant multilevel degenerative disc changes cannot be ignored in this individual. These findings may be incidental as they are commonly seen in asymptomatic individuals and often poorly correlate in symptomatic patients.[4–8] Consequently, the pain history is the most important tool used to make this important distinction. Obviously, if his multilevel degenerative disc plays a significant role in his back dominant complaint, then interventions targeted at his spondylolisthesis alone will not adequately address his primary complaint and limited surgical expectations need to be considered. The authors feel that this is a crucial piece of information for surgical decision making as it relates to a specific structural diagnosis. In this scenario, we would perform

| L2-3 | L3-4 | L4-5 | L5-S1 |

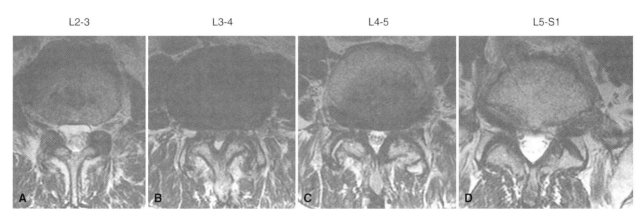

Figure 25.2.

facet injections at L3-4 and L4-5 to ascertain the degree of back pain that is coming from his spondylolisthesis levels.

DECLARATION OF SPECIFIC DIAGNOSIS

This patient has two levels of degenerative spondylolisthesis with back and leg pain. The clinical scenario suggests neurogenic claudication; however, there exists the possibility of multifactorial back pain. For the purposes of this case, a presumption going forward will be made that the majority of symptoms are indeed from the two level degenerate spondylolisthesis and the evidentiary review as well as the clinical decision making will be performed in this regard only.

BRAINSTORMING: WHAT ARE THE TREATMENT GOALS AND SURGICAL OPTIONS?

The treatment goals are

1. Relief of leg symptoms
2. Relief of the back pain that is most likely from the degenerative spondylolisthesis (DS)

The treatment options are

1. Continue conservative care, including flexion exercises
2. Decompression alone at L3-4 and L4-5
3. Decompression and fusion
4. Indirect decompression with interspinous spacer at L3-4 and L4-5

EVALUATION OF THE LITERATURE

To identify relevant publications on two-level DS with stenosis, a PubMed search was performed. A significant number of articles exist regarding DS and spinal stenosis. In a quantitative systematic review performed by Martin et al.,[9] the authors found that sufficient comparative evidence existed on DS patients that a review restricted to comparative data only is possible for this population. From 1923 possible studies, the authors utilized 13 studies (randomized studies and comparative observational studies) published between 1966 and June 2005. In our own review of these studies, we further excluded one additional study. These 12 studies were used as part of the current systematic review.

For additional publications, a search of PubMed using the search term "degenerative spondylolisthesis" was performed. Since the relevant studies identified by

Martin et al. were reviewed, this search was limited to the time frame of 2005 to 2009. This yielded 226 additional titles, which were reviewed for relevance to the current systematic review and further narrowed down to 43 abstracts. The inclusion criteria (which were studies that compared surgery versus nonsurgical treatment, two or more different surgical strategies, spinal stenosis with and without spondylolisthesis, and in which the outcome of the subgroup of spondylolisthesis patients could be analyzed) were applied to these abstracts to yield 25 studies that were then reviewed in detail. Of these, seven met the criteria for inclusion and were used for the evidentiary table. Combined with the aforementioned twelve articles, a total of nineteen comparative articles[10-28] were utilized (Table 25.1).

DETAILED REVIEW OF PERTINENT ARTICLES

The overall quality of evidence for DS is reasonable. However, only a few studies with a clearly defined DS cohort specifically denote the presence of two-level DS (see second column of Table 25.1). Furthermore, of the studies that mention two-level DS, the outcome is not differentiated from one-level DS. Consequently, a presumption is being made that the evidence available for predominantly single-level DS can be extrapolated to two-level DS. This presumption is based on expert opinion, and the authors feel that based on their own clinical experience the presumption is reasonable.

Regarding the quality of the evidence, there were 6 moderate, 2 low, and 11 very low quality papers that met our inclusion criteria. Although there were seven randomized studies, all were flawed for a variety of reasons (Table 25.1). The data presented represent the best available comparative evidence that pertains to the current treatment goals and clinical decisions. How best to manage the specific patient will be based on thoughtful analysis of three factors: patient factors, literature evidence, and clinical expertise specifically related to nonsurgical versus surgical management and the best surgical option for this specific patient.

Patient Factors

This patient has several issues to consider. Any significant end-organ disease from his diabetes as well as the degree of obesity may play a significant role in increased perioperative risk of complications. Within the context of overall decision making, an appropriately informed patient and surgeon must obviously consider the impact that medical comorbidities may have on operative risk and clinical outcomes.[29] Assuming that this patient is medically fit to proceed with elective surgical intervention, the presence of multilevel degenerative changes and dominant back pain

TABLE 25.1	Evidentiary Table: A Summary of the Quality of Evidence for DS.		
Paper Author (Year)	**Description**	**Summary of Results**	**Quality of Evidence**
Feffer et al. (1985)	Retrospective cohort study. Number of spinal levels: unable to determine.	19 patients with DS; 8 patients—DNF-PL and 11-D (laminectomy). DNF-PL group: Mean follow-up 42 mo (12–72). 5 graded (patient reported) results as good, 3 fair. No nonunions based on flexion-extension radiographs. D group: mean follow-up of 25 mo (12–60). 5: good, 3: fair, and 3: poor. 4 in this group developed instability.	Very low
Lombardi et al. (1985)	Retrospective cohort study. Number of spinal levels: one-level DS, 1 patient with two-level DS (outcomes not differentiated).	47 patients with grade I–II—DS: Group 1—wide decompression sacrificing the articular processes, Group 2—facet preserving midline decompression, Group 3—facet preserving decompression and with fusion (DNF-PL). Mean follow-up 32.4 mo (2–7 y). Patient-graded outcome: Group 1 (n = 6)—33% good to excellent, one revision to fusion; Group 2 (n = 20)—80% good to excellent, 2 revisions to fusion; Group 3 (n = 21)—90% good to excellent, 2 nonunion (1 revised, the other patient refused further surgery and had a poor result).	Very low
Herkowitz and Kurz (1991)	Prospective pseudorandomized study Number of spinal levels: one-level DS	50 patients with grade I—DS (n = 25) DNF-PL and n = 25, had decompression (laminectomy) alone (D). At 3 y (2.4–4) mean follow-up, fusion patients had significantly better relief of back and leg pain (VAS).	Moderate
Satomi et al. (1992)	Retrospective cohort study. Number of spinal levels: one and two (12%) level DS (outcomes not differentiated).	41 patients with grade I—DS. Group A—Anterior interbody fusion—n = 27, Group B (n = 14) posterior decompression (mixed techniques—laminotomy or laminectomy, n = 4 fusion [3 DNF-PL/1 with Luque rods]). Mean follow-up—3 y. Mean improvement in JOA scores: group A—5.5, degree of improvement—77%; Group B 4.5, degree of improvement 55.7%.	Very low
Bridwell et al. (1993)	Prospective randomized study with unclear randomization process. Number of spinal levels: one to two level disease, 1 with two level DS.	44 patients with DS randomized to 3 treatment groups: group I—D (n = 9); group II—DNF-PL (n = 10); and group III—DIF-PL (24 patients, 18 one-level pedicle fixation and 6 two-level fixation). D = facet preserving in all cases. A higher fusion rate in group III vs. group II (p = 0.002). Greater spondylolisthesis progression in groups I and II vs. III (p = 0.001). More patients without progression of DS reported they were helped by the surgery than those with progression (p < 0.01).	Moderate
Yone et al. (1996)	Retrospective cohort study. Number of spinal levels: one to two level disease,	34 stenosis patients, 17 patients with DS. 10—DIF-PL (mean follow-up 3 y [2–6 y]) and 7—D-laminotomy (mean follow-up 3.2 y [2–5 y]). Outcome with JAO-back	Very low

(Continued)

TABLE 25.1	Evidentiary Table: A Summary of the Quality of Evidence for DS. (*Continued*)

Paper Author (Year)	Description	Summary of Results	Quality of Evidence
	unable to determine one vs. two level DS.	scores: DIF—80% good-to-excellent, D—29% good-to-excellent ($p < 0.05$). One nonunion occurred.	
Fischgrund et al. (1997)	Prospective randomized study. Number of spinal levels: one level DS	76 patients with grade I—DS ($n = 35$) DIF-PL, $n = 33$ DNF-PL. 67 patients available for 2-y follow-up. No difference in clinical outcome (back and leg pain VAS, activity level; $p = 0.45$). Arthrodesis occurred in 82% of the DIF-PL cases vs. 45% of the DNF-PL cases ($p = 0.0015$). Fusion did not influence patient outcome ($p = 0.435$).	Moderate
France et al. (1999)	Prospective study with undocumented randomization process. Number of spinal levels: one to three level disease, unable to separate DS group regarding levels.	83 patients with mixed diagnoses. 10 patients with DS, underwent DIF-PL ($n = 5$) or DNF-PL ($n = 5$). The DIF group reported better outcomes (patient reported) in 4/5 vs. 2/5 in the DNF group ($p > 0.1$ due to small sample).	Very low
Mochida et al. (1999)	Retrospective cohort study. Number of spinal levels: one level DS.	102 patients with grade I–II—DS. Group 1—DIF-PL-ligament (artificial ligament stabilization)—33, Group 2—DIF-PL-screws—34, Group 3—DNF-PL—35. Outcomes: JOA score at 2 y, 82% success in ligament group, 91% in screw group, and 71% in the noninstrument group. Radiographs showed 4 delayed fusion, 2 nonunion in the ligament group, 2 delayed fusions and 1 nonunion in the screw group, and 7 delayed fusions and 5 nonunion in the noninstrumented group.	Very low
Kimura et al. (2001)	Retrospective cohort study. Number of spinal levels: one level DS.	60 patients with grade I–II—DS. Group A—DNF-PL—29 and group B—DIF-PL—28. Outcomes: Improvement rate (JOA scores) was Group A—72% at a mean 6 y follow-up and Group B—82% at a mean of 3 y follow-up. Fusion rate was 82.8% Group A and 92.8% in Group B. No significant clinical difference in outcome of the non-fused vs. fused patients. Higher complication and reoperation rate in DIF group.	Very low
Ghogawala et al. (2004)	Prospective cohort study. Number of spinal levels: one level DS.	34 patients with grade I—DS (without gross instability <mm motion on flex-ex). D—midline facet preserving—20, DIF-PL—14. Outcomes: improvement in ODI and SF-36 PCS was greater for the fusion group (ODI—27.5 vs. 13.6, $p = 0.02$); PCS—15.9 vs. 6.5, $p = 0.003$). 1-y fusion rate was 93%. At 1 y, no revisions for the DIF vs. 3 (fusion for instability) D alone group. Both forms of surgery independently improved outcome compared with baseline status.	Low

(*Continued*)

TABLE 25.1	**Evidentiary Table: A Summary of the Quality of Evidence for DS.** *(Continued)*		
Paper Author (Year)	**Description**	**Summary of Results**	**Quality of Evidence**
Matsudaira et al. (2005)	Retrospective cohort study. Number of spinal levels: one level DS.	53 patients with grade I—DS. Group 1—DIF-PL—19, Group 2: D—facet and midline persevering laminotomy—18, Group 3—Conservatively (refused surgery)—16. Outcomes: JOA-scores at 2 y showed extent of improvement was significantly greater in groups 1 and 2 than in group 3, but no significant difference was noted between groups 1 and 2. Radiographic—Increase slip in group 2 and 3, greater incidence of adjacent segment degeneration in group 1.	Very low
Anderson et al. (2006)	Randomized controlled study (subgroup analysis of larger multicentered study). Number of spinal levels: one and two level DS (outcomes not differentiated).	75 patients with grade I—DS. Group 1—interspinous process decompression (IPD—X-Stop)—44 and group 2—nonoperative care. Outcomes measured at 2 y (Zurich claudication questionnaire, patient satisfaction, SF-36, additional surgery rate): Significant improvement compared to baseline scores was seen in all intervals in IPD group, whereas essentially no change in baseline score was observed in the control patients. Overall success was 63.4% in the IPD group compared to 12.9 in the control. Five patients in the X-Stop device treatment and four patients in the control groups eventually required laminectomy or laminectomy and fusion.	Moderate
Martin et al. (2007)	Retrospective cohort study—Administrative database (state registry) analysis. Number of spinal levels: indeterminate.	24,882 patients undergoing primary lumbar surgery between 1990–1993. Spondylolisthesis: Group 1: D—143 and group 2—Fusion. The 11-y cumulative incidence of reoperation was lower with fusion than with decompression alone (17.1% vs. 28.0%). *Due to the nature of this study, it was not possible to differentiate between types of spondylolisthesis or fusion techniques; however, a reasonable presumption can be made that those undergoing decompression alone (D) were likely DS; thus this study was graded as very low evidence as it pertains to the question of this chapter.*	Very low
Weinstein et al. (2007)	Randomized clinical trail and prospective observational cohort study.	601 patients with DS (undifferentiated grade)—combined randomized and observational as-treated cohorts. Group I—surgical—368 and group 2—nonsurgical—233. Outcomes (ODI, SF-36 [BP and PF]) at 2 y: a significant advantage for surgery was seen at all intervals. There was little evidence of harm from either treatment. 5% and 21% of the surgical cohort had decompression alone and DIF with the remaining having a DIF-PL. Subgroup analysis for difference in surgical treatment was not performed.	Moderate

(Continued)

TABLE 25.1	Evidentiary Table: A Summary of the Quality of Evidence for DS. *(Continued)*		
Paper Author (Year)	**Description**	**Summary of Results**	**Quality of Evidence**
Ha et al. (2008)	Retrospective cohort study. Number of spinal levels: one level DS.	40 patients with grade I—DS. All had DIF and were divided into 4 subgroups: Stable slip (S): S-DIF-PL—13 and S-DIF-PLIF—11. Unstable slip (U): U-DIF-PL—8 and U-DIF-PLIF—8. Outcomes (ODI/VAS) at a minimum follow-up of 2 y (mean 4.5 y): The unstable, PLIF group demonstrated greater clinical improvement compared to the PL group. There was no difference in the stable groups. In the stable group, the fusion rates were 92% in the PL group and 100% in the PLIF group. In the unstable group, the fusion rates were 88% in the PL group and 100% in the PLIF group ($p = 1.0$).	Very low
Sasai et al. (2008)	Retrospective cohort study. Number of spinal levels: one level DS, on patient had two level DS.	48 patients, 23 with grade I—DS (1 patient had grade II). All patients had midline/facet preserving bilateral decompression from a unilateral approach. Group 1 with DS—23 and group 2—stenosis only—25. Outcomes (ODI, neurogenic claudication outcome score) at a minimum 2 y follow-up showed no significant differences between the 2 groups including overall satisfaction. No additional surgeries in either group. There was a mean of 1.7% increase in slip in the DS group ($p = 0.03$).	Very low
Vaccaro et al. (2008)	Randomized controlled trial. Number of spinal levels: one level DS.	36 patients with grade I–II DS. All patients had DNF. Group 1—OP 1–24 and group 2—autograft—12. Outcomes (ODI, SF-36) at a minimum of 4 y: Comparable clinical outcomes, and overall success was noted between groups (group 1—16 patients and group 2—6 patients). Radiographic successes were 69% for group 1 and 50% for group 2 ($p > 0.05$).	Moderate
Yan et al. (2008)	Retrospective cohort study. Number of spinal levels: one level DS.	176 patients with grade I–II—DS. Group 1—DIF-PLIF—85 and group 2—DIF-TLIF—91. Outcomes (VAS, JOA) at minimum 2 y (mean 29 mo): Clinical outcomes were not significantly different between groups. Both groups achieved 84% excellent to good outcomes on JOA scores. There was no difference in radiographic parameters. There was no difference in complication rate.	Low

All studies had radiographic outcome assessment;
DIF-PL, decompression and instrumented fusion—posterolateral; DNF-PL, decompression and noninstrumented fusion—posterolateral; ODI, Oswestry Disability Index.

is, perhaps, the biggest concern as it may predict a poorer outcome.[29] However, specific discussion and evidentiary review around this dilemma are beyond the scope of this chapter. Although implicit, it must be specifically noted that the patient must feel that their symptoms are impacting their quality of life significantly enough to consider surgical intervention and the possible associated risk.

Operative or Nonoperative Treatment

The best evidence in this regard is provided by the SPORT study of DS comparing operative to nonoperative management.[24] Validated patient-reported outcomes data from the as-treated analysis of this multicenter study showed superiority of surgical treatment for up to 2 years. Satisfaction with residual symptoms was 70% in the surgical group versus 32% in the nonsurgical group. The investigators did, however, note that there was "little evidence of harm for either treatment," and as such, an appropriate trial of conservative treatment should always precede the choice of surgical intervention (unless intractable symptoms or objective neurological findings dictate otherwise). Two smaller studies of lower quality evidence have also shown a similarly poor response to conservative treatment in the symptomatic DS population.[21,22] It must be emphasized, again, that these are patients with a diagnosis of DS who typically are symptomatic enough to consider surgical intervention.

Operative Treatment
Decompression Alone Versus Decompression and Fusion

When taking all factors into consideration, patient outcomes,[10–14] increasing degree of listhesis (instability),[10,12,14,21] and reoperation rates,[11,20,23] the literature would suggest that decompression and fusion are more successful compared to decompression alone. However, it must be noted that the greatest number of patients come from series where a traditional laminectomy was performed.[9–12,30] A traditional laminectomy does not preserve the midline structures and may not be facet preserving. As such, this technique may have a higher likelihood of increased postoperative instability in patients with DS. However, several small series in which a facet and midline preserving technique was used suggest that fusion was still superior.[11,14,15,20]

There are only two comparative studies that are contradictory to these findings. In a small study, Matsudaira et al.[21] demonstrated no difference in outcome between midline, facet preserving decompression and fusion in patients with DS. In a more recent study, Sasai et al.[26] demonstrated that the outcomes of midline, facet-preserving decompression in the DS group were similar to those with spinal stenosis without DS. In a recent study,[31] the

senior author (RR) has demonstrated similar findings. At a minimum of 2 years following microdecompression alone, the authors demonstrated preoperative and postoperative ODI of 48% to 18.7% for patients with no spondylolisthesis when compared to 48% to 24.6% for those with stable spondylolisthesis (less than 4 mm of motion on supine to standing imaging or standing flexion-extension radiographs, leg dominant symptoms).

Several noncomparative case series also suggest decompression alone can be effectively performed in selected patients with DS.[32–42] However, these series typically involve stenosis patients with and without DS, for which the outcome for DS patents is not differentiated and hence a positive outcome is typically inferred. Inconsistencies among the above studies may be due to patient selection and different surgical techniques.[11,14,15,20,21,26] Specifically variable facet anatomy, grade and stability of the listhesis, and differences in surgical technique, which cannot be distinguished from a literature review, may account for these inconsistencies. Specific to this patient, there would be concerns regarding the right L3-4 facet that appears very thin and sagittally oriented (Fig. 25.2B).

Indirect decompression using an interspinous spacer device to block terminal extension may help both this patient's stenosis and facet symptoms. Given its minimal operative morbidity, this technique may be ideally suited to a higher risk patient such as in this scenario, though the success of this technique has been shown to be only 63% by one study of moderate quality.[22] Furthermore, no comparative studies to other operative techniques or studies with DS and back dominant pain are available. In addition, a recent small case series has reported very poor outcomes in the DS population.[43]

Instrumented Versus Noninstrumented Fusion

Evidence regarding this question is dependent on what is used to determine success: radiographic fusion, reoperation rate, or clinical outcomes. Clinical outcomes clearly have the most patient impact and should be weighed most heavily. The current available comparative evidence does show a significantly greater fusion rate with instrumented fusion.[14,16,18]

Reoperation rates in the current available evidence are poorly documented. The clinical outcome data are variable. Of the relevant papers, the highest quality study suggests no difference in clinical outcome at the 2-year mark.[16] No difference in longer term outcome was also reported by Kimura et al.[19] Studies by Bridwell et al., France et al., and Mochida et al., however, suggest that decompression with instrumented fusion has a greater impact on clinical outcome in addition to radiographic outcome compared to noninstrumented fusion.[32–42] These studies, however, report outcomes on a very small number of DS subjects[14,17] or are of very low quality.[18] To date, this inconsistency remains controversial and many experts argue that the outcomes in the patient populations with radiographic nonunion will likely decline in time. This also reflects the bias of the senior author. However, albeit plausible, there are no moderate- or greater quality comparative data to strongly support this premise.

The study by Kornblum et al.[44] is often quoted as support of this premise. In this study, the authors report the outcomes of 47 patients who had undergone decompression with noninstrumented fusion from 2 previous randomized studies.[12,16] At a mean of 7 years and 8 months follow-up (5–14 years), the authors noted that solid fusion was associated with a significantly better clinical outcome and lower reoperation rate. As there is significant evidence that demonstrates instrumentation results in a significantly greater fusion rate, the inference that is made from this study is that instrumentation should also result in a greater clinical outcome. Although the follow-up in this study is commendable, the authors did not follow up or contact the instrumented fusion group from the available cohort in order to compare outcomes in reoperation rate of those in the instrumented group.

A similar finding was also noted in a more recent case series by Tsutsumimoto et al.[45] The authors reported on 42 DS patients who had undergone noninstrumented fusion with a mean follow-up of 9.5 years (minimum of 8 years). Patients with a fusion (nonunion rate was 26%) demonstrated superior clinical outcomes (Japanese Orthopaedic Association [JOA] scores). Using stepwise regression, the authors noted that fusion status and the presence of comorbid disease were predictors of the percent recovery as assessed by JOA scores.[45] Nevertheless, as demonstrated in the multicenter SPORT study, fusion with instrumentation is by far the preferred treatment (instrumented fusion was performed in 74% of the patients) for symptomatic DS and reflects current expert opinion, including that of the senior author on this particular question. The inconsistency in the current literature is likely reflective of the available evidence being underpowered.

Assumptions

The greatest assumption specific to this case as it relates to the current literature is the presence of back dominant complaints. From the evidence reviewed, it was not possible to objectively extract data in a meaningful way that was specific to the back dominant pain patient population. Overall, the evidence supports that surgical intervention results in significant improvement of both leg and back pain. Based on clinical expertise and the literature, it is reasonable to assume that the majority of patients undergoing surgical intervention for DS have a history of neurogenic claudication and likely had both back and leg pain.[24] In addition, the treatment effect of surgical intervention tends to be greater for leg symptoms compared to back symptoms.[24,29]

EVIDENTIARY TABLE AND SELECTION OF TREATMENT METHOD

The best available evidence dictates that the current patient should be treated operatively. All evidence, including several moderate-quality paper, shows significant superiority for those who have failed reasonable nonoperative treatment. The evidence also dictates that this patient should have a decompression and fusion versus a decompression alone. Data regarding the use of an interspinous spacer in the DS population are very limited and are not supported at this time. Based on the available evidence, expert opinion, and patient-specific factors (both clinical and anatomical), decompression and instrumented fusion are best supported. The evidence regarding this specific treatment option is supported by a higher fusion rate with a neutral effect on clinical outcome at 2 years and possibly superior effect in the long-term. In this scenario, patient and surgeon preference play an important role in the decision-making process. The possibility of a poor outcome with increased back pain or a nonunion and subsequent higher likelihood of reoperation with decompression alone or noninstrumented fusion would likely be higher given this particular patient with back dominant pain. In addition to patient and surgeon preference, issues regarding cost and societal preference may also influence the decision in this case.[46]

Although decompression alone will alleviate this patient's leg symptoms, a fusion in this scenario is targeted at stabilization and elimination of motion at the spondylolisthesis levels and is more likely to address this patients' dominant complaint. Given the challenging anatomy of the right L3-4 facet and the fact that decompression alone is unlikely to significantly influence back pain, it is the author's opinion that this individual would not be a good candidate for a midline, facet-sparing decompression. It must be noted that the senior author routinely performs decompression alone for patients with leg dominant symptoms and grade 1, stable DS. Although not borne out by the evidence specifically, expert opinion would suggest a fusion is more likely to address his back pain (presuming the degenerative discs are not the dominant source of his pain). Although not the focus of this chapter, the risk of adjacent segment disease and the increased risk of at least ongoing residual back pain or greater back pain down the road must also be part of the informed consent process for this specific patient.

DEFINITIVE TREATMENT PLAN

The specific options for instrumented fusion are numerous (bilateral posterolateral instrumented fusion, posterior interbody fusion with posterior fixation, lateral interbody fixation with or without posterior instrumentation, and anterior lumbar interbody with or without poster instrumentation performed by open or minimal access approaches). It is the first author's personal preference to perform a minimal axis decompression and instrumented fusion through a posterior paramedian muscle splitting approach. However, there is no comparative evidence comparing MIS versus open techniques in the specific patient population and a review of the available case series is out of the scope of this chapter. The majority of the available literature would suggest that there are no significant differences between the different types of instrumented techniques and as such, patient, surgeon, institutional, and societal preferences typically influence the decision as to the specific type of instrumented fusion.[25,28,47]

Following appropriate preoperative workup and anesthesia clearance and informed consent, this patient would be taken to the operating room. He would be positioned prone on a radiolucent table with a Wilson frame. The L3-5 levels would be localized using intraoperative image intensifier or computer-assisted surgery (the latter is the preference of the senior author). Bilateral 3 cm incisions would be made about 4 to 5 cm from the midline. A transforaminal lumbar interbody fusion (TLIF) approach would be performed via a 22 mm fixed tubular retractor. This would be performed on the more symptomatic right side. Beginning at L3-4, complete removal of the facet including decompression of the lateral lamina of L4 with complete removal of the ligamentum flavum will be performed. This will achieve a central, as well as foraminal and lateral recess decompression on the right side. The disk space would then be entered and the disk sequentially distracted until good annular tension was achieved. Distraction also provides indirect (bilateral) foraminal decompression. The disc space would then be prepared by complete discectomy including removal of the cartilaginous endplate from right to left. The appropriate size interbody device would be filled with local decompression bone graft, and the remaining bone (with our without graft augmentation) would be packed into the disc space. This procedure would be repeated at the L4-5 level. Distraction of the disc space typically decompresses the contralateral side; however, the senior author routinely inspects the contralateral side by means of a unilateral, subspinous process, epidural approach and will remove the contralateral ligamentum flavum as required. Prior to performing the ipsilateral decompression or interbody work, the senior author would typically place instrumentation on the contralateral side using a percutaneous technique with image guidance. The contralateral instrumentation is used to temporarily maintain distraction after intradiscal distraction using endplate distraction techniques. This enables adequate working space for preparation of the disc. Once the interbody cages are placed, the contralateral instrumentation is compressed. Instrumentation would then be placed on the ipsilateral side and also compressed. Final intraoperative live fluoroscopic images are taken to confirm the final position of the instrumentation, and the wounds are closed. The patient would be mobilized on postoperative day 1 and discharged as per our institutions protocol. Routine clinical and radiographic follow-up are performed at 6, 12, 26, 52 weeks as well as annually thereafter.

Grading the Evidence for this Plan

In accordance with the method of grading recommendations set forth by Schunemann et al.[48] a **strong recommendation** based on moderate-quality evidence would be given to operative treatment compared to nonoperative treatment in this scenario. The specific proposed treatment (decompression and instrumented fusion) would be considered **a weak recommendation** based on overall low (very low to moderate)-quality evidence. The grading paradigm utilized is necessary because it not only considers the quality of evidence but also addresses the benefits, harms, and burdens of the proposed interventions. As a variety of other reasonable treatment options exist, a weak recommendation is given for the specific proposed surgical treatment. In addition, it is likely that further research or other patient-specific factors may have an important impact on the decision making in this case and are also likely to change the estimated outcomes.

PREDICTING OUTCOMES

Based on the best available comparative literature, this patient will most likely have a 70% to 90% chance of a good to excellent clinical outcome with greater than a 70% satisfaction rate with the proposed surgical plan. Specifically, as reported in the SPORT study, a mean improvement of 24% in the Oswestry Disability Index, which represents a substantial clinical improvement, can be expected.[24] Comparatively, there would be a very low likelihood of a significant improvement with continued nonoperative treatment. Given the preexisting significant degenerative changes throughout this patient's lumbar spine, there is certainly a possibility that he may develop significant symptoms from progressive degeneration adjacent to the proposed fusion levels. The available literature would suggest a 10% to 20% reoperation rate in the short- and long-term.[9,24]

These results are in keeping with my experience as a spine surgeon. As a variety of other reasonable treatment options exist for the general patient population with DS, the process and evidence presented in this chapter should drive the clinician to be selective with the specific type of surgical treatment.

Patient preference is an important component of evidence-based medicine.[49] Preoperative counseling requires a frank discussion of the treatment options and their inherent risks, benefits, potential outcomes, and associated burdens. The information conveyed must contain the best available evidence and expert opinion. Importantly, the delivery must consider the fact that the patient is not cognizant of the scientific evidence and is often relying on the surgeon to advocate the choice that will most likely provide them with the best outcome and the least risk. As previously stated, the presence of significant multilevel degenerative changes and back dominant pain in this individual would also necessitate discussion around the limitations related to treatment of his back pain in both the short- and long-term and comprehension of limited expectations in this regard. If, in this scenario, the patient had leg dominant pain and could tolerate his back pain, then given all the other issues associated with this case, an argument for decompression alone would have been recommended.

SUMMARY

We are presented with a diabetic male with back dominant pain as well as leg pain resulting from spinal stenosis and DS at L3-4 and L4-5. The most appropriate treatment for this patient's symptoms would be a decompression and instrumented fusion at L3-5. A sustained and substantial degree of leg pain relief with likely some degree of persistent back pain can be expected.

REFERENCES

1. Schinnerer KA, Katz LD, Grauer JN. MR findings of exaggerated fluid in facet joints predicts instability. *J Spinal Disord Tech*. 2008 Oct;21(7):468–472.
2. Chaput C, Padon D, Rush J, et al. The significance of increased fluid signal on magnetic resonance imaging in lumbar facets in relationship to degenerative spondylolisthesis. *Spine*. 2007 Aug 1;32(17):1883–1887.
3. Rihn JA, Lee JY, Khan M, et al. Does lumbar facet fluid detected on magnetic resonance imaging correlate with radiographic instability in patients with degenerative lumbar disease? *Spine*. 2007 Jun 15;32(14):1555–1560.
4. Beattie PF, Meyers SP, Stratford P, et al. Associations between patient report of symptoms and anatomic impairment visible on lumbar magnetic resonance imaging. *Spine*. 2000 Apr 1;25(7), 819–828.
5. Boden SD, Davis DO, Dina TS, et al. Abnormal magnetic-resonance scans of the lumbar spine in asymptomatic subjects. A prospective investigation. *J Bone Joint Surg Am*. 1990 Mar;72(3):403–408.
6. Boos N, Rieder R, Schade V, et al. The diagnostic accuracy of magnetic resonance imaging, work perception, and psychosocial factors in identifying symptomatic disc herniations. *Spine*. 1995 Dec 15;20(24);2613–2625.
7. Buirski G, Silberstein M. The symptomatic lumbar disc in patients with low-back pain. Magnetic resonance imaging appearances in both a symptomatic and control population. *Spine*. 1993 Oct 1;18(13):1808–1811.
8. Modic MT, Ross JS. Lumbar degenerative disk disease. *Radiology*. 2007;245(1):43–61.
9. Martin CR, Gruszczynski AT, Braunsfurth HA, et al. The surgical management of degenerative lumbar spondylolisthesis: a systematic review. *Spine*. 2007 Jul 15;32(16):1791–1798.
10. Feffer HL, Wiesel SW, Cuckler JM, et al. Degenerative spondylolisthesis. To fuse or not to fuse. *Spine*. 1985 Apr;10(3):287–289.
11. Lombardi JS, Wiltse LL, Reynolds J, et al. Treatment of degenerative spondylolisthesis. *Spine*. 1985 Nov;10(9):821–827.
12. Herkowitz HN, Kurz LT. Degenerative lumbar spondylolisthesis with spinal stenosis. A prospective study comparing decompression with decompression and intertransverse process arthrodesis. *J Bone Joint Surg Am*. 1991 Jul;73(6):802–808.
13. Satomi K, Hirabayashi K, Toyama Y, et al. A clinical study of degenerative spondylolisthesis. Radiographic analysis and choice of treatment. *Spine*. 1992 Nov;17(11):1329–1336.
14. Bridwell KH, Sedgewick TA, O'Brien MF, et al. The role of fusion and instrumentation in the treatment of degenerative spondylolisthesis with spinal stenosis. *J Spinal Disord*. 1993 Dec;6(6):461–472.
15. Yone K, Sakou T, Kawauchi Y, et al. Indication of fusion for lumbar spinal stenosis in elderly patients and its significance. *Spine*. 1996 Jan 15;21(2):242–248.
16. Fischgrund JS, Mackay M, Herkowitz HN, et al. Degenerative lumbar spondylolisthesis with spinal stenosis: a prospective, randomized study comparing decompressive laminectomy and arthrodesis with and without spinal instrumentation. *Spine*. 1997 Dec 15;22(24):2807–2812.
17. France JC, Yaszemski MJ, Lauerman WC, et al. A randomized prospective study of posterolateral lumbar fusion. Outcomes with and without pedicle screw instrumentation. *Spine*. 1999 Mar 15;24(6):553–560.
18. Mochida J, Suzuki K, Chiba M. How to stabilize a single level lesion of degenerative lumbar spondylolisthesis. *Clin Orthop Relat Res*. 1999 Nov;(368):126–134.
19. Kimura I, Shingu H, Murata M, et al. Lumbar posterolateral fusion alone or with transpedicular instrumentation in L4-L5 degenerative spondylolisthesis. *J Spinal Disord*. 2001 Aug;14(4):301–310.
20. Ghogawala Z, Benzel EC, Amin-Hanjani S, et al. Prospective outcomes evaluation after decompression with or without instrumented fusion for lumbar stenosis and degenerative Grade I spondylolisthesis. *J Neurosurg Spine*. 2004 Oct;1(3):267–272.
21. Matsudaira K, Yamazaki T, Seichi A, et al. Spinal stenosis in grade I degenerative lumbar spondylolisthesis: a comparative study of outcomes following laminoplasty and laminectomy with instrumented spinal fusion. *J Orthop Sci*. 2005 May;10(3):270–276.
22. Anderson PA, Tribus CB, Kitchel SH. Treatment of neurogenic claudication by interspinous decompression:

application of the X STOP device in patients with lumbar degenerative spondylolisthesis. *J Neurosurg Spine*. 2006 Jun;4(6):463–471.

23. Martin BI, Mirza SK, Comstock BA, et al. Reoperation rates following lumbar spine surgery and the influence of spinal fusion procedures. *Spine*. 2007 Feb 1;32(3):382–387.

24. Weinstein JN, Lurie JD, Tosteson TD, et al. Surgical versus nonsurgical treatment for lumbar degenerative spondylolisthesis. *N Engl J Med*. 2007 May 31;356(22):2257–2270.

25. Ha KY, Na KH, Shin JH, et al. Comparison of posterolateral fusion with and without additional posterior lumbar interbody fusion for degenerative lumbar spondylolisthesis. *J Spinal Disord Tech*. 2008 Jun;21(4):229–234.

26. Sasai K, Umeda M, Maruyama T, et al. Microsurgical bilateral decompression via a unilateral approach for lumbar spinal canal stenosis including degenerative spondylolisthesis. *J Neurosurg Spine*. 2008 Dec;9(6):554–559.

27. Vaccaro AR, Whang PG, Patel T, et al. The safety and efficacy of OP-1 (rhBMP-7) as a replacement for iliac crest autograft for posterolateral lumbar arthrodesis: minimum 4-year follow-up of a pilot study. *Spine J*. 2008 May–Jun;8(3):457–465; Epub 2007 May 25.

28. Yan DL, Pei FX, Li J, Soo CL. Comparative study of PILF and TLIF treatment in adult degenerative spondylolisthesis. *Eur Spine J*. 2008 Oct;17(10):1311–1316; Epub 2008 Aug 7.

29. Aalto TJ, Malmivaara A, Kovacs F, et al. Preoperative predictors for postoperative clinical outcome in lumbar spinal stenosis: systematic review. *Spine*. 2006 Aug 15;31(18):E648–E663.

30. Mardjetko SM, Connolly PJ, Shott S. Degenerative lumbar spondylolisthesis. A meta-analysis of literature 1970–1993. *Spine*. 1994 Oct 15;19(20 suppl):2256S–2265S.

31. Kelleher MO, Timlin M, Persaud O, Rampersaud YR. Success and failure of minimally invasive decompression for focal lumbar spinal stenosis in patients with and without deformity. *Spine* (Philadelphia, PA, 1976). 2010 Apr 9. [Epub ahead of print]

32. Khoo LT, Fessler RG. Microendoscopic decompressive laminotomy for the treatment of lumbar stenosis. *Neurosurgery*. 2002 Nov;S146–S154.

33. Podichetty VK, Spears J, Isaacs RE, et al. Complications associated with minimally invasive decompression for lumbar spinal stenosis. *J Spinal Disord Tech*. 2006 May;161–166.

34. Palmer S, Turner R, Palmer R. Bilateral decompression of lumbar spinal stenosis involving a unilateral approach with microscope and tubular retractor system. *J Neurosurg*. 2002;213–217.

35. Palmer S, Turner R, Palmer R. Bilateral decompressive surgery in lumbar spinal stenosis associated with spondylolisthesis: unilateral approach and use of a microscope and tubular retractor system. *Neurosurg Focus*. 2002 July;E4.

36. Guiot BH, Khoo LT, Fessler RG. A minimally invasive technique for decompression of the lumbar spine. *Spine*. 2002 Feb 15;432–438.

37. Cavusogul H, Kaya RA, Türkmenoglu ON, et al. Mid-term outcome after unilateral approach for bilateral decompression of lumbar spinal stenosis: 5-year prospective study. *Eur Spine J*. 2007 Dec;16:133–142.

38. Thome C, Zevgaridis D, Leheta O, et al. Outcome after less-invasive decompression of lumbar spinal stenosis: a randomized comparison of unilateral laminotomy, bilateral laminotomy, and laminectomy. *J Neurosurg Spine*. 2005 Aug;3:129–141.

39. Mackay DC, Wheelwright EF. Unilateral fenestration in the treatment of lumbar spinal stenosis. *Br J Neurosurg*. 1998 Dec;12:556–558.

40. Weiner BK, Walker M, Brower RS, et al. Microdecompression for lumbar spinal canal stenosis. *Spine*. 1999 Nov 1;24:2268–2272.

41. McCulloch JA. Microdecompression and uninstrumented single-level fusion for spinal canal stenosis with degenerative spondylolisthesis. *Spine*. 1998 Oct 15; 2243–2252.

42. Ikuta K, Tono O, Oga M. Clinical outcome of microendoscopic posterior decompression for spinal stenosis associated with degenerative spondylolisthesis–minimum 2-year outcome of 37 patients. *Minim Invasive Neurosurg*. 2008 Oct;51(5):267–271; Epub 2008 Oct 14.

43. Verhoof OJ, Bron JL, Wapstra FH, et al. High failure rate of the interspinous distraction device (X-Stop) for the treatment of lumbar spinal stenosis caused by degenerative spondylolisthesis. *Eur Spine J*. 2008 Feb;17(2):188–192; Epub 2007 Sep 11.

44. Kornblum MB, Fischgrund JS, Herkowitz HN, et al. Degenerative lumbar spondylolisthesis with spinal stenosis: a prospective long-term study comparing fusion and pseudarthrosis. *Spine*. 2004 Apr 1;726–733.

45. Tsutsumimoto T, Shimogata M, Yoshimura Y, et al. Union versus nonunion after posterolateral lumbar fusion: a comparison of long-term surgical outcomes in patients with degenerative lumbar spondylolisthesis. *Eur Spine J*. 2008 Aug;17(8):1107–1112; Epub 2008 Jun 7.

46. Tosteson AN, Lurie JD, Tosteson TD, et al; SPORT Investigators. Surgical treatment of spinal stenosis with and without degenerative spondylolisthesis: cost-effectiveness after 2 years. *Ann Intern Med*. 2008 Dec 16;149(12):845–853.

47. Bono CM, Lee CK. Critical analysis of trends in fusion for degenerative disc disease over the past 20 years: influence of technique on fusion rate and clinical outcome. *Spine*. 2004 Feb 15;29(4):455–463; discussion Z5.

48. Schunemann HJ, Jaeschke R, Cook DJ, et al. ATS Documents Development and Implementation Committee. An official ATS statement: grading the quality of evidence and strength of recommendations in ATS guidelines and recommendations. *Am J Respir Crit Care Med*. 2006 Sep1;174:605–614.

49. Fisher CG, Wood KB. Introduction to and techniques of evidence-based medicine. *Spine*. 2007 Sep 1; 32(suppl):66–72.

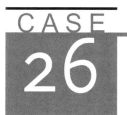

CASE
26

Low Back Pain with Degenerative Disc Disease

DANIEL K. RESNICK, MD, MS

EDITORS' CASE PRESENTATION

A 40-year-old man is referred from a physiatrist with a complaint of persistent and unabating low back pain after a 6-month course of nonoperative treatment that has included physical therapy and epidural injections. He states that his pain is worse with flexion than extension. He is still working, though with difficulty.

On physical examination, he has flexion to about 15 to 20 degrees and extension to about 5 to 10 degrees through the lumbar spine. He has decreased sensation in the right anterolateral aspect of the thigh, lateral leg, and dorsum of the foot. He has negative straight leg raise tests bilaterally. Strength is equal and full bilaterally, though testing is inhibited by some volitional reluctance because of pain. He has tenderness that is generally localized to the L4-5 level.

The patient has had a recent discogram that produced concordant pain at the L4-5 level but was negative at the L3-4 level. L5-S1 could not be accessed.

Radiographic imaging studies are shown in Figures 26.1A–C and 26.2.

INTERPRETATION OF CLINICAL PRESENTATION

This patient presents with a diagnosis of chronic low back pain that has not responded to physical therapy and epidural injections. An MRI of the lumbar spine was provided. These images reveal mild degenerative changes at L4-5 with a central disc bulge and minimal foraminal stenosis. A discogram was performed that produced concordant pain at L4-5 and was negative at L3-4. The patient's examination revealed some decreased sensation in what may be the L5 distribution, back tenderness, and reluctance to cooperate with strength testing in the lower extremities.

It is difficult to reconcile an L5 radicular pattern of sensory loss to the imaging findings provided. There is no evidence of compression of the L5 nerve root on the images provided. There may be minimal foraminal stenosis at L4-5, but this would be expected to affect the L4 root (with sensory loss along the medial border of the foot). While there is some individual variation in dermatomal representation, any discordance between imaging findings and examination findings raised a red flag when considering invasive treatments for benign axial back pain. Similarly, reluctance to participate in a full strength examination and tenderness to palpation of the low back may be considered signs of somatization and represent negative predictive factors for relief of pain following surgical intervention.[1,2] The discogram results, while consistent with the hypothesis that the mild degenerative changes at L4-5 are responsible for the low back complaints, are not definitive both because of the inherent limitations of discography for the diagnosis of low back pain[3,4] and because of the failure to obtain two negative control levels.

Assessment for issues related to secondary gain, particularly the presence or absence of workplace related issues, would be an essential component to any further decision making in this particular patient.

DECLARATION OF SPECIFIC DIAGNOSIS

This patient has chronic low back pain likely due to degenerative disc disease at L4-5.

236

Figure 26.1.

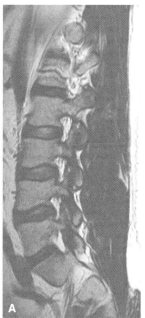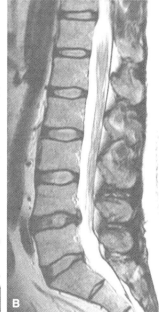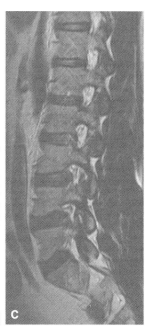

BRAINSTORMING: WHAT ARE THE TREATMENT GOALS AND THE SURGICAL OPTIONS?

Treatment goals:

1. Reducing low back pain
2. Improving functional outcome

Surgical options:

1. None
2. L4-5 fusion
   a. Noninstrumented
   b. Instrumented

    i. Posterolateral
   ii. Interbody
      1. ALIF
      2. TLIF/PLIF
      3. Circumferential
3. Lumbar disc arthroplasty

EVALUATION OF THE LITERATURE

A computerized search of the medical literature from 1966 to October 2008 was performed using the PubMed search engine with the search terms "low back pain" and "randomized controlled trial" and "human." This yielded 48 references. A second search included the terms "lumbar fusion" and "randomized controlled trial" and "human." This yielded 227 references. A third search included the terms "lumbar arthroplasty" and "randomized controlled trial" and "human." This search yielded 60 references. The titles and abstracts of each of these references were reviewed. In addition, the bibliographies of selected references as well as previously published guidelines on the surgical management of low back pain were used to identify supplemental references. After discarding duplicates, nonrandomized studies, studies evaluating nuances of technique, irrelevant studies (such as trials of tuberculosis chemotherapy or induction techniques), and small pilot studies or preliminary reports, 33 remaining references were felt to provide important information relevant to the clinical question. Of these, five provided primary information directly relevant to the question "what is the best treatment for a patient with low back pain and mild degenerative changes at L4-5." The aspect of this question that we will address with

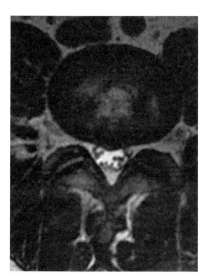

Figure 26.2.

regard to this particular patient is whether or not any surgical intervention is appropriate. Three references were directly related to the question of whether fusion is indicated and two references were directly related to the question of whether disc arthroplasty is a viable alternative to fusion for this patient.

DETAILED REVIEW OF PERTINENT ARTICLES AND EVIDENTIARY TABLE

Five papers were relevant to the current clinical scenario. A brief description of each of these papers appears in the evidentiary table (Table 26.1), with a more in-depth discussion below.

Operative Versus Nonoperative Treatment

When using evidence-based medicine techniques to guide patient care, it is important to consider the strength of the evidence, the nature of the evidence, and whether or not the evidence applies to your patient. The strength of the evidence is related to the study design and findings of the index studies. The nature of the evidence is related to the results of the index studies and the consistency of those results. The applicability of the evidence is related to the degree of similarity between your patient and the patients treated in the index studies.

TABLE 26.1	Evidentiary Table: Randomized Studies of Fusion Versus Nonoperative Management of Chronic Low Back Pain and Lumbar Disc Arthroplasty Versus Fusion.		
Paper Author (Year)	**Description**	**Summary of Results**	**Quality of Evidence**
Fritzell et al. (2001)	Level 1 "no surgery vs fusion for chronic axial back pain" Randomized controlled trial (RCT) comparing fusion vs standard nonoperative care for patients with recalcitrant low back pain due to degenerative disease at one or two levels. Treatment groups were 72 patients per group. Valid outcomes measures were used. Surgical interventions were well described. Follow-up was 2 y and was achieved in 98% of patients.	Patients treated with fusion did better in terms of pain, functional outcome, return to work, and overall success than patients treated with standard nonsurgical management.	Strong
Brox et al. (2003)	Level 1 instrumented PLF vs structured physical and cognitive therapy for chronic axial back pain RCT involving patients with chronic low back pain due to degenerative disease at one or two levels with 32 patients per group. The study compared instrumented posterolateral lumbar fusion to cognitive therapy with intensive physical therapy. Surgical as well as nonsurgical interventions were well described. Follow-up was 2 y and was achieved in 97%.	Lumbar fusion and intensive structured physical therapy with cognitive therapy both resulted in improved outcomes. Benefits of lumbar fusion included better back and leg pain relief. Benefits of cognitive therapy included improved fear avoidance behavior. Benefit of surgery for improved functional outcome did not reach significance.	Strong
Fairbank et al. (2005)	Level 4 Structured physical and cognitive therapy vs a variety of surgical procedures (fusion and nonfusion) for chronic axial back pain RCT comparing same protocol as Brox to a variety of surgical interventions in a large but poorly described patient population with back pain for >1 y. Significant crossover, lost to follow-up rate, poorly described patient selection criteria and variety of surgical procedures preclude the ability to draw meaningful conclusions.	Patients randomized to surgery had better outcomes on the Oswestry but this difference was small. Significant issues with crossover and follow-up limit utility of study.	Weak

(Continued)

TABLE 26.1	Evidentiary Table: Randomized Studies of Fusion Versus Nonoperative Management of Chronic Low Back Pain and Lumbar Disc Arthroplasty Versus Fusion. *(Continued)*		
Paper Author (Year)	**Description**	**Summary of Results**	**Quality of Evidence**
Blumenthal et al. (2005)	Level 2 lumbar disc arthroplasty vs stand-alone ALIF (downgraded due to choice of control group and non-generalizability due to select patient population).	Charite LDA provides results comparable or slightly better than ALIF in a highly select patient population.	Moderate
Zigler et al. (2007)	Level 2 lumbar disc arthroplasty vs circumferential fusion (downgraded due to choice of control group and nongeneralizability due to select patient population). RCT involving 236 patients comparing ProDisc LDA with circumferential fusion. Patients treated with LDA did somewhat better. Significant concerns regarding definitions of success, choice of control, and generalizability of results.	ProDisc LDA provides results that are comparable or perhaps slightly better than circumferential fusion in a highly select patient population.	Moderate

In the present case, the best data regarding the question as to whether or not this patient would benefit from an operation come from the three randomized trials that compared operative versus nonoperative treatment for patients with low back pain. The first study published, by Fritzell et al.,[5] was a randomized controlled study comparing several different fusion techniques to what would probably be standard nonoperative care in most North American practices. Patients selected for the study were required to have had symptoms for at least 2 years and had to have been on disability for at least 1 year prior to randomization. Patients were required to have degenerative disease at L4-5 and/or L5-S1 levels diagnosed via radiograph, CT, or MRI and the randomizing physician had to be convinced that the degenerative disc was the pain generator. Patients with psychiatric diagnoses, confounding hip degeneration, symptoms of nerve compression, deformity, spondylolysis, or evidence of other pathological processes were excluded.

Once patients were randomized, they received one of three fusion procedures (noninstrumented posterolateral fusion [PLF], instrumented PLF, or a circumferential interbody fusion) or received standard nonoperative treatment consisting of physical therapy, injections, and medications. Patients entered into the study actually had very long durations of symptoms, averaging 8 years of failed nonoperative management and 3 years of disability. Results were reported based on an intent-to-treat analysis and there was an approximate 10% crossover rate and a 98% follow-up rate at 2 years.[5] At 2 years, patients treated surgically had significantly less back and leg pain, significantly decreased disability scores, significantly better scores on the General Function Scale (GFS), and significantly better Million scores than patients treated nonoperatively.[5] Sixty-three percent of surgical patients considered themselves "much better" or "better" compared to 29% of the nonsurgical group, a statistically significant difference.[5]

The authors of the Fritzell study described their results as supporting fusion for chronic low back pain in carefully selected patients. These conclusions were criticized because the patients who did not receive fusion procedures did not receive any treatment that they had not already failed. Two other groups performed randomized studies comparing various surgical procedures to a specific and highly intensive program of physical and cognitive therapy, which had previously been shown to be more effective than standard medical management of low back pain.[6,7]

Brox et al.[6] randomized a smaller group of patients to receive either an instrumented PLF or the highly intensive regimen described above. Sixty-four patients were randomized to the two groups and were followed for 1 year. Inclusion criteria were similar to the Fritzell study described above in that all patients with psychiatric conditions or evidence of neurological compression syndromes were excluded from the study. An important difference is the less stringent requirement for duration of symptoms and severity as the Brox group required only 1 year of symptoms recalcitrant to standard management and no requirement for disability. Patients were required to have spondylosis limited to one or two levels diagnosed by either radiograph, CT, or MRI.[6]

Twenty-seven patients were randomized to the rehabilitation program and thirty-seven to surgery. There was an approximate 10% crossover rate and 97% follow-up rate. Patients in both groups did very well with significant improvements in all measured outcomes. Patients treated with surgery did significantly better with regard to leg pain and tended to do better in terms of back pain, Oswestry disability scores, General Function Score, emotional distress, life satisfaction, and overall satisfaction with their treatment. Patients treated with the physical and cognitive rehabilitation programs did significantly better in terms of fear avoidance behavior and fingertip to floor distance.[6] The authors reported an 18% complication rate in the surgical group, comprised of two wound infections, two "bleedings," one dural tear (apparently without CSF leak), and one deep venous thrombosis. The authors concluded that the benefits in the surgical group were not substantial enough to recommend surgery given the risk of complications of surgery.[6]

Several issues regarding conclusions drawn from the Brox paper are worth brief consideration. First, the rehabilitation program described is not available outside of a few European institutions, limiting the generalizability of the results of the study. Second, the study was very small, meaning that the differences in outcomes favoring surgery may well be found to be significant in a larger study. To be fair, the magnitude of many of the differences favoring surgery was not large and the issue of clinically relevant differences in some scales is a valid concern.[10] Third, the stated goal of surgery is to relieve back and leg pain, not to improve fingertip to floor distance. Finally, there were no long-term complications, and while wound infections and the occasional dural tear are inevitable complications of surgery, they are usually insignificant in the long run.

In 2005, Fairbank et al.[7] published the results of a larger clinical trial evaluating the effectiveness of lumbar fusion for chronic low back pain compared to an intensive rehabilitation program similar to the one described by Brox. Research therapists were employed at multiple centers and recruited 349 patients who were randomized into two cohorts. One cohort received an intensive outpatient rehabilitation program, and the other cohort received some sort of surgical intervention. The main outcomes measures were the Oswestry disability index and shuttle walking. An intent-to-treat analysis was planned. Overall results favored surgery, with a statistically significant yet small improvement in the Oswestry disability index and a nonsignificant improvement in shuttle walking compared to the rehabilitation group. Patients in the surgical cohort enjoyed a 17.6 point mean improvement in the Oswestry as opposed to an 11.4 point mean improvement on the rehabilitation arm. No assessment of back or leg pain was made. The authors concluded that "no clear evidence emerged that primary spinal fusion surgery was more beneficial than intensive rehabilitation using principles of cognitive and behavioral therapy."

The Fairbank study is highly flawed, and the conclusions stated by the authors are misleading. First of all, the patients were recruited by therapists, not surgeons. Very few surgeons rely on other physicians to choose their operative patients for them. Second, the surgical procedures employed varied widely and included anterior approaches, posterior approaches, variable use of instrumentation, and even the use of "dynamic stabilization," a nonfusion procedure in 15% of surgical patients. This wide variety of approaches clearly indicates a very heterogeneous patient population and surgical opinion and lacks diagnostic specificity. Third, the statistical evaluation was done as an intent-to-treat analysis with imputation (investigator assigned values based on historical data) of missing data points. Thirty-seven patients (21% of cohort) randomized to surgery never had surgery as seven crossed over to the rehabilitation group and the rest left the study. Twenty-two patients randomized to rehabilitation never received the rehabilitation program with ten patients switching to the surgical cohort, and twelve leaving the study. Following the rehabilitation program, an additional 38 patients went on to have fusion surgery. Therefore, of the 173 patients randomized to rehabilitation, 48 (28%) actually were treated with surgery and 7% never received any therapy. This degree of crossover significantly biases the study toward the null hypothesis (that the groups are equivalent since the study is de facto comparing groups that are receiving a combination of surgery and rehabilitation to each other). Furthermore, between 16% and 32% of patients were lost to follow-up, further decreasing the power of the study to detect differences between groups.[7] The fact that the surgical group achieved better outcomes in this scenario is remarkable and is not consistent with the authors' conclusions.

There are a number of prospective series with long-term follow-up indicating that spinal surgery is associated with durable long-term outcomes in various patient populations.[11,12] With regard to individual surgical techniques to achieve fusion, there are a large number of randomized and prospective studies comparing different techniques with each other.[13–24] The reader is encouraged to review this literature when making an informed decision regarding which fusion technique to use in an individual patient. These studies confirm the hypothesis that the chronic low back pain population is heterogeneous, and that different approaches are warranted in different patients. These studies are not extremely helpful in determining whether or not a patient should have a fusion in the first place.

Several systematic reviews were identified dealing with the issue of fusion versus nonoperative management of chronic low back pain.[25–29] There is some variation regarding the studies included in each review, the methods by which the review was performed, and the ultimate conclusions reached by the authors. Gibson and Waddell, writing for the Cochrane Review, concluded that no firm conclusions could be reached based on the available literature. Resnick et al., in a review performed prior to the publication of the Fairbank study, concluded that the literature did support fusion for the management of low back pain in carefully selected patients. Mirza et al. concluded that the literature was too flawed to allow any firm conclusions regarding the North American patient population. Ibrahim et al. performed a meta-analysis and found that the overall results of the included studies favored surgery but reported that the benefit may be outweighed by complications.[25–29] It is important to consider the outcomes measures deemed important by the authors of the primary studies as well as the systematic reviews. Focusing on back and leg pain tends to improve the apparent benefit of surgery, whereas focusing on behavioral measures (such as fear avoidance) tends to favor therapies that are specifically geared toward ameliorating those behaviors.

Disc arthroplasty has emerged as a treatment option in patients with chronic low back pain. No prospective studies comparing outcomes of patients treated with arthroplasty versus patients treated nonsurgically were identified in the literature search described above and the author is aware of no such studies. Two randomized controlled studies of arthroplasty compared to fusion for chronic low back pain were identified.[8,9] Blumenthal et al. published the results of a large randomized trial comparing disc arthroplasty with the Charite device to anterior interbody fusion performed with BAK cages. Three hundred and four patients were randomized in a 2:1 arthroplasty/fusion fashion in order to establish the noninferiority of arthroplasty compared to fusion. Patient selection criteria excluded patients with spondylosis, spondylolisthesis, or facet joint arthrosis (among other exclusion criteria) and allowed patients with relatively mild symptoms (Oswesty ≥ 30, VAS ≥ 40) to enroll. Success was defined as a 25% improvement in preoperative Oswestry score with no major device-related complication or neurologic injury.[8]

The authors achieved approximately 90% follow-up at 2 years and reported roughly equivalent "success rates" between the two groups (64% arthroplasty vs 57% control). Many patients in both groups were still using narcotics at 24-month follow-up (64% and 80% respectively). This paper establishes that the use of arthroplasty is not inferior to a single

level stand-alone ALIF in a young healthy patient population with minimal degenerative changes. The study has been criticized because of the select patient selection criteria. Many surgeons would never have offered such patients fusion surgery.[30] In addition, the choice of the control procedure may not be considered ideal. The stability of the ALIF construct is dependent upon tensioning of the annulus through distraction of a collapsed (spondylotic) disc space. Inadequate tensioning of the annulus through placement of too small of a cage or placement of a cage into a normal disc space is associated with poor results and complications, as pointed out by one of the authors of the Charite study.[31] The relatively poor results (compared to contemporaneous series of similar procedures in different patient populations[32]) seen in both groups are likely related to the patient selection criteria and choice of control group.

Zigler et al.[9] reported the results of another noninferiority study involving the ProDisc arthroplasty device. These authors randomized 236 patients to receive either arthroplasty (n = 161) or circumferential fusion (n = 75). Patients were again highly selected and with relatively normal spinal anatomy as facet arthrosis, stenosis, or lytic spondylolisthesis were exclusion criteria. Patients were followed for 2 years and excellent follow-up was achieved in both groups (>97%). At 2 years, there were no significant differences between groups with regard to mean Oswestry disability scores, VAS pain scores, or changes in narcotic usage. Using a dichotomous rating scheme of success incorporating ten aspects of device, radiographic, and clinical factors, the authors report a greater percentage of success in the arthroplasty group compared to the fusion group (53% vs 41%). Six of the ten aspects related to radiographic features and the device aspect related to survival of the device. Claims of superiority are not warranted, however, given the study design and the fact that patients who enrolled in the study with a desire to receive an arthroplasty procedure were not blinded to the procedure, potentially biasing the functional outcomes measures. It also should be noted that the six device failures in the investigational group involved migration, displacement, or malposition of the device, all of which required reoperation. The two "device failures" in the fusion group were considered device failures only because the patient complained of persistent pain and not because of any failure of the device. Reoperation rates also reflect the author's practice of routine device removal following fusion by some participating surgeons.

In any case, the Charite and Prodisc studies described above do indicate that for certain very highly selected patients, disc arthroplasty is not inferior to lumbar fusion. The nature of the selection criteria and the overall poor results seen may indicate that these patients are not good candidates for fusion in the first place and that a more relevant comparison would be nonoperative management.

DEFINITIVE TREATMENT PLAN

A weak recommendation (with moderate-quality evidence) for fusion (regardless of technique) for patients with disabling and persistent low back pain due to degenerative changes at L4-5 would be supported by the literature. However, I personally do not feel that this particular patient is a candidate for fusion based upon the information provided in the case study and would not offer him a lumbar fusion procedure. The degenerative changes shown are minimal at best and the disc space height is preserved. The duration of symptoms is short in relation to that required in the randomized studies supporting fusion. Findings such as "volitional weakness" and tenderness to palpation of the back are red flags in my practice. I do not trust the discogram results both because of the technical inadequacy of the study and the notorious unreliability of the findings of even well-performed discography.

Because of the minimal MRI findings and absence of facet arthropathy, this patient may be one who fits the inclusion criteria for a disc arthroplasty procedure. However, the literature evidence supporting the performance of disc arthroplasty versus nonoperative treatment is nonexistent. The best available data derived from the two large randomized trials comparing arthroplasty to fusion in very highly select populations indicate that while arthroplasty is not inferior to fusion, the overall results are less than stellar.

In my opinion, the reported success rates (especially given the definitions of success) do not warrant the risks, hassles, and expense of such surgery. In my practice, this patient would be sent to one of my rehabilitation colleagues for further work on pain management and coping strategies coupled with an exercise-based therapy program and perhaps some changes in medication and injection therapy (for temporary amelioration of symptoms to facilitate participation in the overall program). If his pain persisted for another 6 months despite these treatments, I would reevaluate him at that time. The passage of sufficient time for an exercise and behavioral-based treatment regimen to work, a new assessment of secondary gain issues, and a new physical examination would be used to establish potential candidacy for surgical intervention at that time.

Grading the Evidence for this Plan

In accordance with the method of grading recommendations set forth by Schunemann et al., a **weak**

recommendation for nonoperative treatment would be made based on poor- to high- quality evidence.

SUMMARY

The literature indicates that there is moderate evidence to support the performance of lumbar fusion in select patients with low back pain due to degenerative changes at one or two levels. Other treatment strategies (such as intensive rehabilitation as described above) may also provide acceptable results and should be considered when available. There is strong evidence to support the noninferiority of lumbar disc arthroplasty compared to stand-alone ALIF or circumferential fusion in a small subset of patients considered to be candidates for surgery despite minimal radiographic signs of degeneration.

REFERENCES

1. Manchikanti L, Fellows B, Singh V, et al. Correlates of non-physiological behavior in patients with chronic low back pain. *Pain Physician*. 2003;6:159–166.
2. Waddell G, Main CJ, Morris EW, et al. Chronic low-back pain, psychologic distress, and illness behavior. *Spine*. 1984;9:209–213.
3. Carragee EJ, Chen Y, Tanner CM, et al. Provocative discography in patients after limited lumbar discectomy: a controlled, randomized study of pain response in symptomatic and asymptomatic subjects. *Spine*. 2000;25: 3065–3071.
4. Resnick DK, Choudhri TF, Dailey AT, et al. Guidelines for the performance of fusion procedures for degenerative disease of the lumbar spine. Part 6: magnetic resonance imaging and discography for patient selection for lumbar fusion. *J Neurosurg*. 2005;2:662–669.
5. Fritzell P, Hagg O, Wessberg P, et al. 2001 Volvo Award Winner in Clinical Studies: lumbar fusion versus nonsurgical treatment for chronic low back pain: a multicenter randomized controlled trial from the Swedish Lumbar Spine Study Group. *Spine*. 2001;26:2521–2532; discussion 2532–2524.
6. Brox JI, Sorensen R, Friis A, et al. Randomized clinical trial of lumbar instrumented fusion and cognitive intervention and exercises in patients with chronic low back pain and disc degeneration. *Spine*. 2003;28:1913–1921.
7. Fairbank J, Frost H, Wilson-MacDonald J, et al. Randomised controlled trial to compare surgical stabilisation of the lumbar spine with an intensive rehabilitation programme for patients with chronic low back pain: the MRC spine stabilisation trial. *Br Med J (Clin Res Ed)*. 2005;330:1233.
8. Blumenthal S, McAfee PC, Guyer RD, et al. A prospective, randomized, multicenter Food and Drug Administration investigational device exemptions study of lumbar total disc replacement with the CHARITE artificial disc versus lumbar fusion: part I: evaluation of clinical outcomes. *Spine*. 2005;30:1565–1575; discussion E1387–E1591.

9. Zigler J, Delamarter R, Spivak JM, et al. Results of the prospective, randomized, multicenter Food and Drug Administration investigational device exemption study of the ProDisc-L total disc replacement versus circumferential fusion for the treatment of 1-level degenerative disc disease. *Spine*. 2007;32:1155–1162; discussion 1163.

10. Hagg O, Fritzell P, Nordwall A. The clinical importance of changes in outcome scores after treatment for chronic low back pain. *Eur Spine J*. 2003;12:12–20.

11. Andersen T, Videbaek TS, Hansen ES, et al. The positive effect of posterolateral lumbar spinal fusion is preserved at long-term follow-up: a RCT with 11–13 year follow-up. *Eur Spine J*. 2008;17:272–280.

12. Bjarke Christensen F, Stender Hansen E, Laursen M, et al. Long-term functional outcome of pedicle screw instrumentation as a support for posterolateral spinal fusion: randomized clinical study with a 5-year follow-up. *Spine*. 2002;27:1269–1277.

13. Christensen FB, Hansen ES, Eiskjaer SP, et al. Circumferential lumbar spinal fusion with Brantigan cage versus posterolateral fusion with titanium Cotrel-Dubousset instrumentation: a prospective, randomized clinical study of 146 patients. *Spine*. 2002;27:2674–2683.

14. Dimar JR, Glassman SD, Burkus KJ, et al. Clinical outcomes and fusion success at 2 years of single-level instrumented posterolateral fusions with recombinant human bone morphogenetic protein-2/compression resistant matrix versus iliac crest bone graft. *Spine*. 2006;31:2534–2539; discussion 2540.

15. Gibson S, McLeod I, Wardlaw D, et al. Allograft versus autograft in instrumented posterolateral lumbar spinal fusion: a randomized control trial. *Spine*. 2002;27:1599–1603.

16. Kim KT, Lee SH, Lee YH, et al. Clinical outcomes of 3 fusion methods through the posterior approach in the lumbar spine. *Spine*. 2006;31:1351–1357; discussion 1358.

17. Linovitz RJ, Pathria M, Bernhardt M, et al. Combined magnetic fields accelerate and increase spine fusion: a double-blind, randomized, placebo controlled study. *Spine*. 2002;27:1383–1389; discussion 1389.

18. McKenna PJ, Freeman BJ, Mulholland RC, et al. A prospective, randomised controlled trial of femoral ring allograft versus a titanium cage in circumferential lumbar spinal fusion with minimum 2-year clinical results. *Eur Spine J*. 2005;14:727–737.

19. Mooney V. A randomized double-blind prospective study of the efficacy of pulsed electromagnetic fields for interbody lumbar fusions. *Spine*. 1990;15:708–712.

20. Sasso RC, Kitchel SH, Dawson EG. A prospective, randomized controlled clinical trial of anterior lumbar interbody fusion using a titanium cylindrical threaded fusion device. *Spine*. 2004;29:113–122; discussion 121–112.

21. Schofferman J, Slosar P, Reynolds J, et al. A prospective randomized comparison of 270 degrees fusions to 360 degrees fusions (circumferential fusions). *Spine*. 2001;26:E207–E212.

22. Vaccaro AR, Anderson DG, Patel T, et al. Comparison of OP-1 Putty (rhBMP-7) to iliac crest autograft for posterolateral lumbar arthrodesis: a minimum 2-year follow-up pilot study. *Spine*. 2005;30:2709–2716.

23. Videbaek TS, Christensen FB, Soegaard R, et al. Circumferential fusion improves outcome in comparison with instrumented posterolateral fusion: long-term results of a randomized clinical trial. *Spine*. 2006;31:2875–2880.

24. Zdeblick TA. A prospective, randomized study of lumbar fusion. Preliminary results. *Spine*. 1993;18:983–991.

25. Gibson JN, Waddell G. Surgery for degenerative lumbar spondylosis: updated Cochrane Review. *Spine*. 2005;30:2312–2320.

26. Ibrahim T, Tleyjeh IM, Gabbar O. Surgical versus nonsurgical treatment of chronic low back pain: a meta-analysis of randomised trials. *Int Orthop*. 2008;32:107–113.

27. Mirza SK, Deyo RA. Systematic review of randomized trials comparing lumbar fusion surgery to nonoperative care for treatment of chronic back pain. *Spine*. 2007;32:816–823.

28. Resnick DK, Choudhri TF, Dailey AT, et al. Guidelines for the performance of fusion procedures for degenerative disease of the lumbar spine. Part 7: intractable low-back pain without stenosis or spondylolisthesis. *J Neurosurg*. 2005;2:670–672.

29. Schafer J, O'Connor D, Feinglass S, et al. Medicare Evidence Development and Coverage Advisory Committee Meeting on lumbar fusion surgery for treatment of chronic back pain from degenerative disc disease. *Spine*. 2007;32:2403–2404.

30. Wong DA, Annesser B, Birney T, et al. Incidence of contraindications to total disc arthroplasty: a retrospective review of 100 consecutive fusion patients with a specific analysis of facet arthrosis. *Spine J*. 2007;7:5–11.

31. McAfee PC, Cunningham BW, Lee GA, et al. Revision strategies for salvaging or improving failed cylindrical cages. *Spine*. 1999;24:2147–2153.

32. Burkus JK, Gornet MF, Dickman CA, et al. Anterior lumbar interbody fusion using rhBMP-2 with tapered interbody cages. *J Spinal Disorders Tech*. 2002;15:337–349.

Recurrent Disc Herniation

DAVID KAYE I., BS AND ALOK D. SHARAN, MD

EDITORS' CASE PRESENTATION

A 42-year-old woman presents with a complaint of low back pain and right lower extremity pain. She has had a previous discectomy 1-year prior, after which she had some relief of her leg pain for 2 months. Insidiously, back more than leg pain returned since 2 months after the surgery. Pain is worse with coughing, sneezing, and lying flat. She does not have any left leg pain. The patient has had conservative treatment including physical therapy and epidural injections. She has no bowel or bladder complaints. She does have a history of depression.

Her physical exam demonstrates that she is somewhat overweight. She can flex her lumbar spine to touch her knees and extend to neutral, but both movements are painful. She has pain with palpation over the L5-S1 interspace. Sensation and motor testing are normal, and she has a negative straight leg raise test.

Radiographic imaging studies are shown in Figures 27.1 and 27.2.

INTERPRETATION OF CLINICAL PRESENTATION

The clinical vignette describes a middle-aged woman who has experienced lower back pain for the past 10 months that radiates to her right lower limb. One year earlier, she had undergone a discectomy, but the pain returned after only 2 months. T2-weighted magnetic resonance (MR) sagittal and axial sequences are given, which demonstrate a right-sided herniation at L5-S1 with lateral recess and foraminal stenosis at that level. Figure 27.1C–E shows the disc herniation on the

sagittal sequences. Figure 27.1D and E demonstrates contact of the disc herniation with the exiting L5 nerve root. Figure 27.2C is an axial sequence through the L5-S1 segment demonstrating the herniation resulting in lateral recess and foraminal stenosis. The laminotomy defect is best appreciated in Figure 27.2C.

Previous papers have categorized pain returning within 6 months after the index surgery as a failed surgery rather than a recurrence of radiculopathy associated with a recurrent disc herniation (RDH). According to these papers, the strict definition of a RDH indicates the presence of herniated disc material at the same level, ipsi- or contralateral, in a patient who has experienced a pain-free interval of at least 6 months since surgery. Clinically, the more relevant definition may be disc herniation at the previously operated site, regardless of the time interval since surgery. In the case example, the patient here would be classified as suffering from a RDH. In fact, some of her reported history seems to point to a RDH. Jonsson et al.[1] reported that the presence of pain on coughing, a severely reduced walking capacity, and a straight leg raise test <30 degrees were indicative of a RDH. Similarly, Rubinstein claims that for a consistent overall diagnosis, emphasis should be placed on the response to pain with coughing, sneezing, and straining, a feeling of coldness in the legs, and urinary incontinence.[2]

The patient has several conflicting symptoms which make a likely diagnosis based on her symptoms and physical exam alone more difficult. While she has pain with coughing and flexing her lumbar spine, as well as experiences pain over the L5-S1 interspace, her straight-leg test (SLR) was negative and she has no motor or sensory deficits. An evaluation of the accuracy of the tests used for her physical exam and more information regarding the prevalence of her specific symptoms in other cases of recurrent lumbar disc herniation are necessary.

Rubinstein and Tulder[2] searched the PubMed version of MEDLINE from 1997 until present for

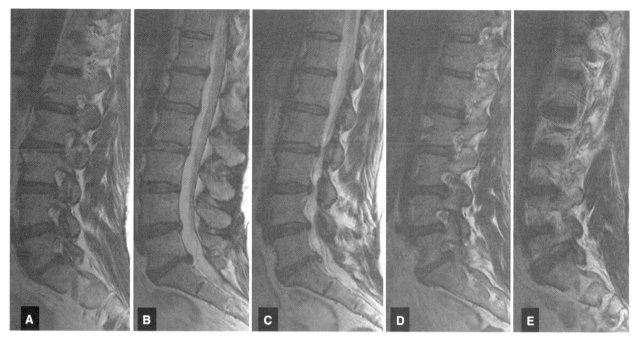

Figure 27.1.

systematic reviews and relevant primary studies on diagnostic procedures for neck and low-back pain. They aimed to present the best evidence on the principal tools available to the clinician for establishing a correct working diagnosis, including the history, physical examination, and special studies together with diagnostic imaging. They concluded largely based on a 1999 review by Vroomen et al.[3] that with regard to the physical examination, the straight-leg raise is the only sign consistently reported to be sensitive for radiculopathy due to disc herniation but is limited by its low specificity. According to their paper, the diagnostic accuracy of other neurological signs and tests is unclear. However, Wera et al.,[4] in a review of 1,320 patients, found that each of the 14 patients with a RDH had documented motor or neurological deficits, including root tension signs.

With regard to spinal palpation, Hestbaek et al.[5] concluded that tests for palpation had acceptable results, but motion palpation tests were not reliable. Another systematic review found that the reliability of most commonly used examination procedures by clinicians in patients with low-back pain was poor.[6] The review by Vroomen et al. of 37 studies of subjects suspected of sciatica due to disc herniation found pain distribution to be the only useful history item. Morgan[7] found that the odds ratio for a recurrence was 1.96 for a herniation at the L5/S1 level over L4/5 level. Ultimately, Vroomen concludes that many studies have demonstrated that the physical examination serves primarily to confirm suspicions raised during the history but not to serve as a basis for diagnosis itself.

Based on a review of the diagnostic procedures for evaluating a RDH, Vroomen concluded that the level

Figure 27.2.

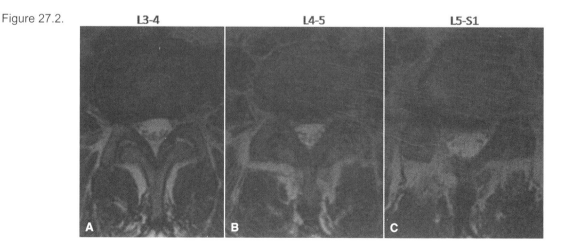

of the patient's pain is the only reliable measure, which is consistent with a RDH.[3] Therefore, combined with evidence that recurrence is more common at the L5/S1 interspace and other positive signs associated with a RDH (e.g., pain on coughing), even in the face of a negative SLR and no other neurological deficits, further workup is warranted. The next step in management is obtaining a gadolinium-enhanced magnetic resonance imaging (MRI) to attempt to visualize any recurrence of disc herniation. If a RDH can easily be visualized, modalities of treatment must be discussed.

The epidemiology of RDHs warrants discussion. The recurrence of back or sciatic pain after primary discectomy can be caused by a true recurrence of disc herniation, new disc herniation at a different level, epidural fibrosis, local arachnoiditis, symptomatic arthritis of the small intervertebral joints (facet syndrome), secondary spinal stenosis, instability, and spondylitis or spondylodiscitis.[8] Recurrent lumbar disc herniation, a relatively common disease process, has been noted to occur in 5% to 15% of cases surgically treated for primary lumbar disc herniation.[8–11]

Most of the literature deals with recurrences of radiculopathy returning after 6 months from the index surgery. However, little has been written about recurrent lumbar disc herniations that occur within 2 months following surgery. The rates of such recurrences are low. In one series of 152 patients, the rates of reherniation within the first year were reported to be 0.7% at 6 months and 5.5% at 12 months after fragment excision alone.[12] Wera et al.[4] specifically addressed cases of RDH within 1 year from the initial discectomy. They identified fourteen patients with recurrent lumbar disc herniations within 1 year after the index procedure. All had radicular pain and weakness prior to and complete relief of radiculopathy after the index procedure. All reherniations occurred at the same level as the index procedure, but eight occurred in a different direction than the original herniation. They concluded that patients who undergo reoperation because of early recurrent lumbar disc herniation can have clinical outcomes comparable with those of patients undergoing an uncomplicated subtotal lumbar discectomy.

DECLARATION OF SPECIFIC DIAGNOSIS

While the patient has some findings that are consistent with an RDH, epidural fibrosis may present similarly. The need to distinguish one from the other preoperatively for surgical considerations and for predicting outcomes is crucial. Numerous studies have shown that a scar does not benefit from reoperation and in fact may result in worse outcomes.[13] Gadolinium-enhanced MRI is thought to be the best modality to differentiate between the two diagnoses.[14–17] In one study,[18] the sensitivity of MR as verified by reoperation was found to be over 90% and this diagnostic tool was recommended for making the differential diagnosis of RDH.[19–21] Enhancement is best seen within 5 minutes of contrast administration. It is important to be able to properly identify normal post-op appearances as they may look like a recurrent or retained disc.

BRAINSTORMING: WHAT ARE THE TREATMENT GOALS AND SURGICAL OPTIONS?

The treatment goals are

1. Relief of back pain
2. Relief of leg pain

The treatment options are

1. Observation with aggressive medical management
2. Revision microdiscectomy
3. Revision microdiscectomy with posterolateral fusion
4. Anterior lumbar interbody fusion (ALIF)

EVALUATION OF THE LITERATURE

A Medline search was performed to identify studies that have examined the various treatment options for a RDH. The keywords "recurrent disc herniation" was entered, which yielded 19 results, of which only 2 articles were relevant to the topic. A search was also conducted using three MeSH (medical subject headings) categories: intervertebral disc displacement, reoperation, and recurrence. The first heading was combined with the second and third headings individually. This yielded 247 and 222 results, respectively. The individual articles were reviewed, and the references for these articles were also reviewed. Many of the studies were either case series or retrospective reviews. There were no randomized, prospective studies comparing the various treatment options for a RDH.

DETAILED REVIEW OF PERTINENT ARTICLES

There have been many articles written on treatment options for a primary lumbar disc herniation. Most recently, an NIH-sponsored, prospective, randomized, multicenter trial was conducted examining the role of surgery versus nonsurgical options for a lumbar disc herniation.[22] Unfortunately, there has been no detailed investigation performed of patients with a RDH. Many of the studies that have been conducted are retrospective case control or observational cohorts.

In deciding the various treatment options for a RDH, it is important to remember that many patients will benefit from appropriate nonoperative interventions. If these measures are not successful, surgical intervention is considered. The main debate in the literature has been in regard to performing a revision discectomy versus a lumbar fusion (using either a posterolateral, TLIF, or ALIF approach). There have been no trials that have directly compared the three methods of fusion. Only one study in the literature has compared fusion versus revision discectomy.[33] In selecting the appropriate surgical intervention, it is important to compare the risks and benefits for each procedure and counsel the patient regarding future risks or benefits.

Observation with Aggressive Medical Management

Many studies have found that lumbar disc herniations show a favorable response to conservative treatment even in the presence of a neurological deficit. These studies discussed primary herniation[23–25] which are more likely to resorb over time;[24,25] whether this occurs with RDH is not clear. Alternatively, some studies have shown that as the number of revision surgeries increases, so does the possibility for fibrosis and long-term complications.[18,25] Erbayraktar et al.[18] noted that the rate of epidural fibrosis and spinal instability increases to >60% in multiple revision patients and the outcome significantly worsens. Morgan et al.[7] claims that a protracted conservative regimen in the presence of severe radicular symptoms should be avoided since waiting increases morbidity and reduces the chances of a successful outcome.

Revision Microdiscectomy

Revision laminotomy and discectomy are the most commonly performed surgical treatments for RDH. The surgical principles are to start in an area known to be intact, find landmarks, begin medially, and then work out laterally to locate the pathological entity. The literature analysis suggests that revision surgery provides satisfactory results comparable to those achieved after the initial surgery.[4,18,26–31]

Cinotti et al.[20,32] examined patients who had ipsilateral as well as contralateral disc herniations at the same level. In both groups, patients who underwent revision microdiscectomy had results comparable to patients who underwent a primary discectomy. The majority of the spine surgeon community considers microdiscectomy to be the gold standard of operative treatment for lumbar disc herniation and probably also for recurrent herniation that is not adequately responding to conservative treatment.

Revision Microdiscectomy and Fusion

The success of a revision microdiscectomy has been noted in multiple studies in the literature. Some authors have advocated complete removal of the disc and fusion across the interspace. Proponents of this theory claim that fusion would eliminate any pathologic motion in the degenerated disc, thus reducing pain and risk of RDH.

In an attempt to determine the best treatment option for patients with a RDH, Fu et al.[33] performed a retrospective analysis of 61 patients in whom either a revision microdiscectomy or a posterolateral fusion was performed. The authors selected patients in whom a RDH was noted on imaging studies and was confirmed during surgery. Cases in which there was a concomitant instability or stenosis were excluded so that only cases with a documented RDH were noted. Outcomes were assessed using the Japanese Orthopedic Association (JOA) score. Clinical outcome improved in both groups, with 78.3% of patients in the nonfusion group achieving good to excellent outcomes compared to 83.3% of patients in the fusion group. The difference between the two groups was not statistically significant.

Anterior Lumbar Interbody Fusion

In 2001, Vishteh and Dickman[34] reported on a series of six patients in whom they performed an ALIF for RDH. All six patients had a RDH at the same level as their index procedure. The patients were followed for a mean of 14 months. Standardized outcome measures were not used to assess results of surgery. In this study, all six patients had complete resolution of their radicular symptoms. By direct visualization as well as postoperative imaging studies, the authors confirmed that the herniated fragments were removed via this approach.

Choi et al.[35] retrospectively examined a cohort of 22 patients in whom an ALIF was performed for a RDH. Outcomes were measured by surveys that measured pain (a five point scale for back and leg pain) and functional outcomes. Successful outcomes were defined as an improvement in two levels in pain and functional scores. The patients were followed for a minimum of 2 years with a mean follow-up period of 35 months. 86% of the patients achieved successful outcomes in regard to their leg pain whereas 77% of patients achieved a successful outcome in regard to their back pain. Functional improvement occurred in 82% of their patients, and 86.3% of patients stated they would undergo the same surgery again. Although these results were not compared to patients who underwent alternate procedures, this paper established that an ALIF can yield satisfactory results for a reherniation.

Comparing Treatments

While there are numerous techniques and methods available for surgery, the studies available are hard to compare. Suk reported on the retrospective results in 28 patients treated by standard revision discectomy with a 71% success rate.[36] The results were measured using a visual analog scale and no other standard outcome measures. Morgan-Hough[7] reported on open revision discectomies in 42 patients with a 19.1% complication rate including two chest-infections after general anesthesia, 14% dural tears, and one pseudo-meningocele. Jonsson and Stromqvist[27] reported on a 2-year follow-up after redecompressions in 19 reherniations, 16 excellent results without specification of the scoring criteria. Cinotti et al.[20] used a 100-point system to assess the clinical outcome following revision microdiscectomy, including pain, functional status, patient satisfaction, and physical examination. They found that the clinical outcome was satisfactory in 85% of patients in the study group and 88% of the control group. Haglund[37] reviewed 55 patients retrospectively after second microdiscectomy over a 4-year period and reported 86% complete or partial relief of all symptoms. In terms of efficacy, the superiority of one procedure over the other cannot be determined with an appropriate level of confidence due to the various methods used to compare outcomes.

DEFINITIVE TREATMENT PLAN

Before proceeding with any treatment plans, a gadolinium-enhanced MRI of her spine must be obtained to check for visible signs of herniation. If evidence of reherniation is present, a revision surgery is in order. Haglund[37] noted that those with the most favorable outcomes after a revision surgery fell into a bimodal distribution of the time between operations (<6 or >24 months) suggesting that earlier evaluation and repeat microdiscectomy upon return of symptoms may prevent development of the long-term effects of nerve root injury and also limit the progressive negative psychosocial aspects of chronic pain syndromes.

The patients with early reoperation also had a significantly better outcome than the patients with a later reoperation. The relief of leg pain was significantly better when the patients underwent their second reoperation earlier, and a clear trend was established for a better outcome from earlier repeat surgery in relief of back pain, but it did not reach significance.

Erbayraktar et al.[18] found that the majority of patients whose symptoms had recurred within 1 year had a RDH. Furthermore, superior results were achieved in this group confirming that among patients with disc herniations, those developing early recurrent sciatica seem to offer better results. Coupled with the overwhelming evidence that a revision surgery provides results similar to those achieved after an index surgery, surgery for our patient is warranted.

Keeping in mind to have the surgery performed earlier rather than later, we recommend a revision microdiscectomy. The herniation can be approached through the same incision. An appropriate plane should be developed between the scar tissue and the lamina. Proper identification of the nerve root should be performed, and the nerve should be mobilized medially. Removal of the herniated disc can be performed with a combination of curettes, pituitaries, and kerrisons. A partial foraminotomy may be necessary to ensure complete decompression of the nerve root.

Grading the Evidence for this Plan

Based on guidelines published by Schunemann et al.[38] the evidence for revision microdiscectomy would be considered low. To be considered moderate to high would require a prospective randomized controlled trial. None of the studies mentioned have examined the treatment choices in this fashion. Although the quality of the evidence is low, using Schunemann's criteria, this treatment recommendation would be considered strong with low-quality evidence. The benefits of a revision microdiscectomy clearly outweigh the harms and burdens of nonoperative treatment. Since very few articles have mentioned fusion as an alternative, a recommendation cannot be made on the quality of evidence or the strength of the recommendation.

PREDICTING OUTCOMES

There have been studies that have attempted to predict outcomes of a revision microdiscectomy. Many of the studies have compared the results of revision to patients undergoing primary microdiscectomy. Unfortunately, there has not been a uniform method to compare the outcomes of these groups. Papadopoulos et al.[31] used the MODEMs instrument and found no major differences between the two groups. The only statistically significant difference was demonstrated in an increased back pain and leg numbness in the revision group. Dai et al.[30] retrospectively examined JOA scores and found that the majority of patients achieved good to excellent outcomes scores. Based on these and other studies, the evidence indicates that the patient in this case scenario has a reasonable chance of an improvement in symptoms comparable to her index procedure.

In counseling this patient regarding the various treatment options, it is important to emphasize the expected benefit of any surgical intervention. In the literature, a microdiscectomy has been shown to improve leg pain symptoms greater than back pain.

The results of a microdiscectomy for back pain are not as predictable. Recently, the Spine Patient Outcomes Research Trial (SPORT) was completed, and it examined the relief in back pain among patients treated surgically versus nonoperative methods for a lumbar disc herniation.[39] In this study, patients who underwent surgery had greater relief in both their back and leg pain than patients who continued with nonoperative treatment. It is important to remember that the relief in back pain was in patients who had a demonstrated nerve root compression from a disc herniation. For this patient, it is important to clarify which pain is significantly affecting her quality of life and what the predicted result can be from a revision microdiscectomy.

SUMMARY

In summary, this is a 42-year-old female with a reherniation of the L5-S1 intervertebral disc. She had previously undergone a microdiscectomy for similar symptoms. The patient reports back pain and right leg pain, with the back pain greater than her leg pain. There is a strong recommendation for this patient, after she has exhausted nonoperative measures, to proceed with a revision microdiscectomy. The patient is expected to have greater relief in her leg pain than her back pain after surgery.

REFERENCES

1. Jonsson B, Stromqvist B. Clinical characteristics of recurrent sciatica after lumbar discectomy. *Spine*. 1996;21: 500–505.
2. Rubinstein SM, Tulder MV. A best-evidence review of diagnostic procedures for neck and low-back pain. *Best Pract Res Clin Rheumatol*. 2008;22:471–482.
3. Vroomen PC, de Krom MC, Knottnerus JA. Diagnostic value of history and physical examination in patients suspected of sciatica due to disc herniation: a systematic review. *J Neurol*. 1999;246(10):899–906.
4. Wera GD, Marcus RE, Ghanayem AJ, et al. Failure within one year following subtotal lumbar discectomy. *J Bone Joint Surg (Am)*. 2008;90:10–15.
5. Hestbaek L, Leboeuf-Yde C. Are chiropractic tests for the lumbo-pelvic spine reliable and valid? A systematic critical literature review. *J Manipulative Physiol Ther*. 2000;23(4):258–275.
6. May S, Littlewood C, Bishop A. Reliability of procedures used in the physical examination of non-specific low back pain: a systematic review. *Aus J Physiother*. 2006;52(2): 91–102.
7. Morgan-Hough CVJ, Jones PW, Eisenstein SM. Primary and revision lumbar discectomy: a 16 year review from one centre. *J Bone Joint Surg Br*. 2003;85-B:871–874.
8. Crock HV. Observation on the management of failed spinal operations. *J Bone Joint Surg Br*. 1976;58:193–199.
9. Connolly ES. Surgery for recurrent lumbar disc herniation. *Clin Neurosurg*. 1992;39:211–216.
10. O'Sullivan MG, Connolly AE, Buckley TF. Recurrent lumbar disc protrusion. *Br J Neurosurg*. 1990;4:319–325.
11. Hu RW, Jaglal S, Axcell T, et al. A population-based study of reoperations after back surgery. *Spine*. 1997;22: 2265–2270.
12. Carragee EJ, Han MY, Yang B, et al. Activity restrictions after posterior lumbar discectomy. A prospective study of outcomes in 152 cases with no postoperative restrictions. *Spine*. 1999;24:2346–2351.
13. Grane P, Tullberg T, Rydberg J, et al. Postoperative lumbar MR imaging with contrast enhancement: comparison between symptomatic and asymptomatic patients. *Acta Radiol*. 1996;37:366–372.
14. Babar S, Saifuddin A. MRI of the post-discectomy lumbar spine. *Clin Radiol*. 2002;57:969–981.
15. Barrera MC, Alustiza JM, Gervas C, et al. Post-operative lumbar spine: comparative study of TSE T2 and turbo-FLAIR sequences vs contrast-enhanced SE T1. *Clin Radiol*. 2001;56:133–137.
16. Ross JS. MR imaging of the postoperative lumbar spine. *Magn Reson Imaging Clin N Am*. 1999;7:513–524.
17. Van de Kelft EJ, van Goethem JW, de La Porte C, et al. Early postoperative gadolinium-DTPA-enhanced MR imaging after successful lumbar discectomy. *Br J Neurosurg*. 1996;10:41–49.
18. Erbayraktar S, Acar F, Tekinsoy B, et al. Outcome analysis of reoperations after lumbar discectomies: a report of 22 patients. *Kobe J Med Sci*. 2002;48:33–41.
19. Canavach S, Stevens J, Johnson JR. High-resolution MRI in the investigation of recurrent pain after lumbar discectomy. *J Bone Joint Surg Br*. 1993;75:524–528.
20. Cinotti G, Roysam GS, Eisenstein SM, et al. Ipsilateral recurrent lumbar disc herniation: a prospective, controlled study. *J Bone Joint Surg Br*. 1998;80:825–832.
21. Frank AM, Trappe AE, Allgayer B. Diagnosis of recurrent intervertebral disk prolapse with nuclear magnetic resonance tomography. *Neurochirurgica (Stuttg)*. 1993;36: 141–147.
22. Weinstein JN, Tosteson TD, Lurie JD, et al. Surgical vs nonoperative treatment for lumbar disc herniation. The Spine Patient Outcomes Research Trial (SPORT): a randomized trial. *JAMA*. 2006;296:2441–2445.
23. Weber H. Lumbar disc herniation: a controlled, prospective study with ten years of observation. *Spine*. 1983;8:131–140.
24. Bush K, Cowan N, Katz DE, et al. The natural history of sciatica associated with disc pathology: a prospective study with clinical and independent radiological follow-up. *Spine*. 1992;17:1205–1212.
25. Weinstein JN, Lurie JD, Tosteson TD, et al. Surgical vs nonoperative treatment for lumbar disk herniation The Spine Patient Outcomes Research Trial (SPORT) Observational Cohort. *JAMA*. 2006;296:2451–2459.
26. Fiume D, Sherkat S, Callovini GM, et al. Treatment of the failed back surgery syndrome due to lumbo-sacral epidural fibrosis. *Acta Neurochir Suppl (Wien)*. 1995;64:116–118.
27. Jonsson B, Stromqvist B. Repeat decompression of lumbar nerve roots: a prospective two-year evaluation. *J Bone Joint Surg Br*. 1993;75:894–897.

28. Laus M, Alfonso C, Tigani D, et al. Failed back syndrome: a study on 95 patients submitted to reintervention after lumbar nerve root decompression for the treatment of spondylotic lesions. *Chir Organi Mov*. 1994;79:119–126.

29. Fritsch EW, Heisel J, Rupp S. The failed back surgery syndrome: reasons, intraoperative findings, and long-term results: a report of 182 operative treatments. *Spine*. 1996;21:626–633.

30. Dai LY, Zhou Q, Yao WF, et al. Recurrent lumbar disc herniation after discectomy: outcome of repeat discectomy. *Surg Neurol*. 2005;64(3):226–231.

31. Papadopoulos EC, Girardi FP, Sandhu HS, et al. Outcome of revision discectomies following recurrent lumbar disc herniation. *Spine*. 2008;31:1473–1476.

32. Cinotti G, Gumina S, Giannicola G, et al. Contralateral recurrent lumbar disc herniation: results of discectomy compared with those in primary herniation. *Spine*. 1999;24(8):800–806.

33. Fu TS, Lai PL, Tsai TT, et al. Long-term results of disc excision for recurrent lumbar disc herniation with or without posterolateral fusion. *Spine*. 2005;30:2830–2834.

34. Vishteh AG, Dickman CA. Anterior lumbar microdiscectomy and interbody fusion for the treatment of recurrent disc herniation. *Neurosurgery*. 2001;48:334–337.

35. Choi JY, Choi YW, Sung KH. Anterior lumbar interbody fusion in patients with a previous discectomy minimum 2-year follow-up. *J Spinal Disord Tech*. 2005;18:347–352.

36. Suk KS, Lee HM, Moon SH, et al. Recurrent lumbar disc herniation: results of operative management. *Spine*. 2001;26:672–676.

37. Haglund M, Moore A, Marsh H, et al. Outcome after repeat lumbar micro-discectomy. *Br J Neurosurg*. 1995;9:487–495.

38. Schunemann HJ, Jaeschke R, Cook DJ. An official ATS statement: grading the quality of evidence and strength of recommendations in ATS guidelines and recommendations. *Am J Respir Crit Care Med*. 2006;174: 605–614.

39. Pearson AM, Blood EA, Frymoyer JW, et al. SPORT lumbar intervertebral disk herniation and back pain dose treatment, location, or morphology matter. *Spine*. 2008;33(4):428–435.

THORACOLUMBAR DEFORMITY

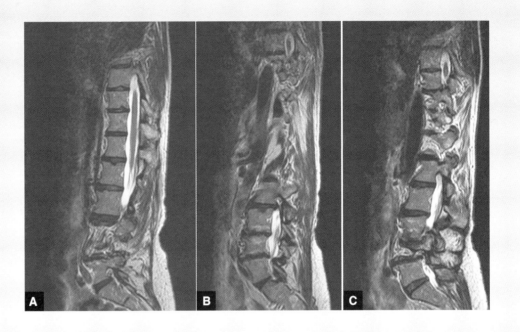

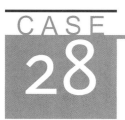

Multilevel Degeneration with Back and Leg Pain

EERIC TRUUMEES, MD

A 57-year-old woman with a history of fibromy-algia presents with a complaint of low back and right foot pain. She had a number of right foot surgeries for presumed intrinsic foot pathology; however, her pain has continued. The lower extremity pain radiates to the lateral aspect of her foot and is associated with numbness and tingling in the same distribution. She does not have any thigh pain as her pain begins at the knee and radiates distally. Nonoperative treatment has included physical therapy and epidural injections, which have given her only short-term relief. She complains of increased pain with flexion but also states that she is not able to extend her low back. She has no bowel or bladder complaints or sub-jective weakness.

Physical examination reveals localized ten-derness upon palpation of the L4-5 and L5-1 interspaces. Provocatively, she has pain that is worse with extension than flexion of her lumbar spine. She cannot extend past neutral. She has decreased sensation in the right L4, L5, and S1 dermatomes. In addition, she has a positive straight leg raise on the right side but a negative femoral stretch test. Reflexes are normal.

Radiographic imaging studies are shown in Figures 28.1A–C and 28.2A–C.

INTERPRETATION OF CLINICAL PRESENTATION

As is common in clinical practice, this patient forces us to face a number of confounding and overlapping clinical issues. In particular, we have a patient with back pain and distal lower extremity pain in a setting of fibromyalgia. Each element of her history, physical examination, and MRI may have one meaning, no meaning, or multiple meanings.

This patient complains of low back pain of indefi-nite chronicity. Back pain is common in the community at large but certainly more likely in patients with fibro-myalgia or even those with disrupted gaits due to foot pathology. She is tender over the L4-5 and L5-S1 inter-spaces, but this is a nonspecific finding. She complains of increased pain with flexion, but, on exam, her pain worsens more with extension than flexion. She is not able to actively extend her back.

While worse pain could relate to foraminal steno-sis, the history cannot confirm this. No clear discogenic or muscular pattern is established with the history and exam as provided.

Our patient reports radiating right leg pain. It is unclear if the back pain is more debilitating than the leg pain. By history, the pain begins at the knee and radi-ates distally to the lateral aspect of the foot. She does not exhibit classical dermatomal features in that sev-eral dermatomes are involved, but only distally. This pattern could reflect peripheral nerve dysfunction.

This patient reports multiple foot surgeries with no benefit suggesting her true pain generator was not identified. The physical examination offers some local-izing findings including a sciatic nerve tension sign on the right with numbness in the L4-S1 dermatomes. No other clear radicular findings are offered: her reflexes are normal and there is no weakness.

At the time of presentation, this patient had attempted nonoperative management in the form of physical therapy and epidural injections. The injections provided her short-term relief. It is not clear which ele-ments of this management were more or less helpful. In fibromyalgia patients, diffuse pain and a failure to respond to physical therapy are quite common.[1]

Advanced spinal imaging is available in the form of an MRI. On the MRI, we see slight loss of lumbar lordosis with hypotrophic to normal extensor mus-culature. The psoas and quadratus lumborum appear small but with little fatty infiltration. Certainly, mild

Figure 28.1.

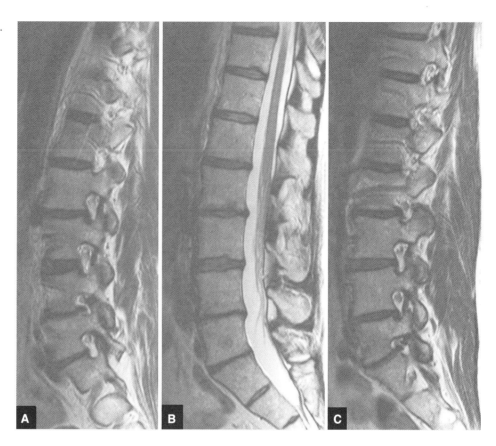

fatty replacement is seen in the lower lumbar spine. Only very mild facet joint degeneration is seen without evidence of joint fluid signal or redundancy of the capsule or the ligamentum flavum.

While no standing or bending films are available, there is no evidence of segmental instability, kyphosis, or translation. Disc degeneration is seen at virtually every level including disc height loss, desiccation, and mild endplate irregularities. On the T2 sagittal views available, little in the way of endplate reaction (Modic change) is evident, nor are there any high-intensity zones or other features that, reputedly, assist in the identification of axial "pain generators."[2]

Our patient's sagittal images include left foraminal, midline, and right foraminal sections (from left to right). Certainly, there is no central stenosis seen on either the axial or sagittal images. At the L4-5 level, mild foraminal stenosis is seen on the left greater than right side. At the lumbosacral junction, foraminal and "far-out" stenosis are seen on the right side, with clear compression of the L5 nerve. There is no clear compression of the S1 root to account for lateral foot pain. In this setting, plain film assessment looking for a transitional vertebra or an assessment of a postfixed lumbar plexus could resolve the discrepancy. Any of these changes can be seen in asymptomatic patients.[3]

Occasionally, response to treatment offers additional, diagnostic information. Epidural steroid injections appear to have had an impact on this patient's pain, which may favor a radicular origin.[4] We are given little information as to whether the pain relief included the back, the leg, or both and how long it lasted. In

Figure 28.2.

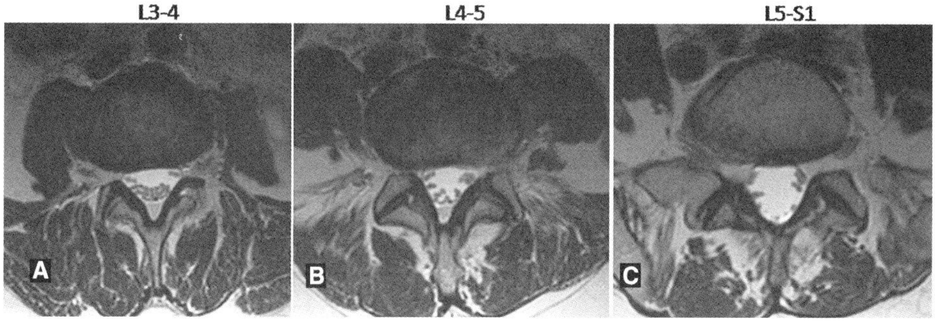

L3-4   L4-5   L5-S1

this case, the compression is foraminal and may be beyond the reflection of the dura around the DRG.[5] This reflects the difference between a transforaminal ESI and a selective nerve root block (SNRB). The SNRB has to be extraforaminal so that it does not contact the epidural space and medication does not flow into the canal, where additional roots could be affected.[4]

The literature gives us little guidance in interpreting this patient's response to spinal injection therapy. Using OVID Medline, 3,780 references included dorsal root ganglion and another 581 for epidural steroid injections. Combining these sets yielded 39 references, most of which were review articles. In one meta-analysis of the hundreds of LESI studies, 12 met review criteria and only 4 were found to be methodologically sound.[6] Significant variability is seen in dispersion of the injectate with greater flow in the posterior canal than the anterior and far less flow into the foraminal regions unless a transforaminal route is selected.[7,8]

We are not told how long the physical therapy was carried out and if it included traction or other occasionally diagnostically helpful modalities.[9] It would appear, based on the limited range of motion, that this patient has not maintained a home therapy program. She remains weak and stiff.

Unlike trauma, tumor, or infection, back pain conditions in the context of degenerative change require a close assessment of what the patient *doesn't* have. We should exclude the "red flags" that demand either further workup or treatment. While our patient has symptoms that could reflect radiculopathy, there is no high-grade neural compression or evidence of cauda equina symptoms. There is no weakness or bowel or bladder change. There are no symptoms or signs consistent with upper motor neuron involvement. From a neurological perspective, therefore, there is no indication for urgent intervention.

We are not offered a timeline for symptoms, but these symptoms appear to be longstanding. This implies a nonmalignant etiology. With these "red flags" excluded, we are free to look for one or several "pain generators" and offer opinions as to which treatments might be effective.

This search for "pain generators" requires correlation of the patient's symptoms to available imaging and physical exam findings. The greater the concordance of these elements, the more effective the treatment offered. Unfortunately, while this patient has a number of "findings," there is more overlap in potential causes for each of her findings than the findings overlapping in pointing to a single diagnosis.[10]

Many of this patient's findings are common in both fibromyalgia and spondylotic low back pain. For example, while pain with extension may correlate with symptom severity in foraminal stenosis,

focal, decreased spinal range of motion is common in fibromyalgia as well.[11,12]

The imaging findings presented here are not uncommon in patients in their 6th decade. As with mechanical low back pain, the severity of radiographic degenerative changes does not predict pain levels in fibromyalgia. In a group of 53 chronic low back pain (CLBP) patients followed for 18 years, 25% went on to develop fibromyalgia and most of those had degenerative changes on imaging. Female gender was the greatest predictor of developing fibromyalgia.[13]

There is little agreement as to the degree of foraminal narrowing required to constitute clinically significant stenosis between centers and individual practitioners.[14]

DECLARATION OF SPECIFIC DIAGNOSIS

This patient has axial back pain in the context of lumbar degeneration and fibromyalgia and distal right lower extremity pain in the context of foraminal narrowing and multiple foot surgeries.

BRAINSTORMING: WHAT ARE THE TREATMENT GOALS AND THE SURGICAL OPTIONS?

This patient has no evidence of spinal instability or impending neurological disaster. The goals, therefore, are to further elaborate the diagnosis, improve function, and decrease pain. Both the patient's multilevel degeneration and fibromyalgia predict for poor surgical results in terms of axial pain. Operative intervention could be considered for the lower extremity symptoms but only after further investigation and careful deliberation with the patient.[15] The relative patency of the central canal and lateral recess limits the benefit of a CT myelogram. There is little evidence that discography would benefit this patient.[16,17]

If the patient clearly reported improvement, however short-lived, with the epidurals, an EMG could be obtained to further assess nerve irritability and to exclude peripheral nerve issues causative of or stemming from the multiple foot surgeries. Given this patient's history of multiple foot operations, the possibility of a double crush phenomenon or even ongoing, primary peripheral compression cannot be excluded. The lateral plantar nerve, affected in tarsal tunnel syndrome, gets twigs from L4, L5, S1.[18] Which is more likely, given the distal nature of her complaints, spinal irritation of three nerves, or peripheral entrapment of one nerve that has feeders from multiple lumbar radicular levels?

"Failed" peripheral nerve decompression should be considered because 7% of posterior tibial nerves branch before they reach the tarsal tunnel, proximal migration of symptoms is common, and specific diagnosis in peripheral entrapment syndromes is as clouded by fibromyalgia as are spinal pathologies.[19,20] At this point, we do not know results of specific foot exam. Does she get symptoms with foot eversion or inversion, compression of tarsal tunnel, or with a Tinel's along posterior tibial nerve?

EVALUATION OF THE LITERATURE

To identify relevant publications on the effectiveness of surgery in patients with lumbar spondylosis and fibromyalgia, Medline and OVID searches were performed. Search strategies included the use of MeSH (medical subject headings) and key words. Key words included "foraminal stenosis," "fibromyalgia," "degenerative disc disease," "low back pain," and "spinal fusion" *or* "laminectomy." After I completed the search, it was repeated by the medical librarian at my institution with similar results. We do not have an Embase subscription, but an outsourced request using even broader search terms failed to identify additional articles.

A focused search of "lumbar spondylosis" with subheadings of classification, complications, radiography, rehabilitation, surgery, and therapy was performed. The results for "spinal stenosis" were then combined with fibromyalgia or chronic widespread musculoskeletal pain. Journals were hand searched, and references were reviewed to identify pertinent articles. This search strategy, date limited to 1950–2009 revealed no potential publications. Medline "in process" and nonindexed citations were searched as was EBM reviews-Cochrane database.

Given the limited results when search terms were combined (zero), the terms were examined two at a time. The level one studies discussed this patient's diagnoses only obliquely. No relevant surgical studies were recovered. I therefore analyzed the few level II and level III studies assessing foraminal stenosis, focal lumbar, and radicular symptoms in fibromyalgia patients. There were 312 English language abstracts that were reviewed and 47 full-text articles were read.

DETAILED REVIEW OF PERTINENT ARTICLES

On the surface, this patient appears to present with a complex and individual set of complaints. None of her individual problems are rare, however. In one epidemiologic study, 59 million people were found to have low back pain over a 3-month period; 10% of them had fibromyalgia.[21] Looking at this another way, a German study found that low back pain was the single most common complaint in fibromyalgia.[22] In another study of CLBP and WMP (widespread musculoskeletal pain) patients, 76% were women and most were, like this patient, middle aged.[23] In a 7-year prospective study of 538 fibromyalgia patients, subjects had about one health care visit per month.[24] When compared to controls, the fibromyalgia patients had high rates of back and neck surgery.

Given the frequency with which these problems are seen together, the dearth of literature assistance in selecting treatment is startling. This is not a problem, common to clinical practice guidelines, in which poor quality or limited evidence can too easily be construed as "no evidence." Rather, this case represents a situation in which there really is no evidence.

The active practice of EBM as it relates to this patient is stymied in all of the standard five steps:

1. Defining question or problem. The exact delineation of the "pain generator" is never easy in spine surgery. But, in this patient, the process is made more complex by a history of lower extremity problems on the symptomatic side, the presence of fibromyalgia, and the absence of true concordance between history, imaging, and examination findings. One series described the difficulty ascribing back and leg symptoms to either spondylosis or widespread musculoskeletal pain syndromes.[23] The authors recommended early testing for fear-avoidance behavior, depression, anxiety, balance, and endurance.

2. Searching for evidence. While there is ample, though often low quality, literature discussing outcomes of surgery for spinal stenosis, considerably less attention has been paid to foraminal stenosis. Similarly, I was unable to identify outcome studies that specifically addressed a subgroup of stenosis patients with fibromyalgia. Even examining the larger side of the equation first, there are few and low-quality papers describing outcomes of spinal surgery in fibromyalgia patients.

3. Critically appraising literature. Given the complete absence of quality literature mapping to this patient's pathologies, critical appraisal of the literature requires extrapolation of the data that we do have. That is, selecting papers that offer more oblique guidance as to management of this patient's condition.

4. Applying results. In our patient, applying the results of a critical appraisal of the literature leaves us in the position of counseling conservative, nonoperative management.

In principle, "first, do no harm." Surgery can only be legitimately recommended if it can be shown to improve on the natural history of the disease state being explored. In this case, we have no such evidence.

5. Auditing outcome. We do not have outcomes information for this patient. If the patient failed a given treatment, which aspect of her condition failed to improve (or both)? Exclusion of fibromyalgia and other chronic pain disorders is central to the evaluation of Failed back syndrome.[25]

6. But, additional testing may be useful to further delineate her pain generators and the relative impact of each. For example, a selective nerve root injection may allow us to identify that portion of her pain that is actually coming from her foraminal stenosis. Good, but temporary relief of her leg pain may predict for better results of surgical decompression, but even here, the data are lacking.

Optimally, EBM integrates the best available evidence with clinical expertise and patient preference. In this patient scenario, a couple of issues come to mind: (a) In my experience, even if I can improve a fibromyalgia patient's leg pain with surgical decompression, their postoperative satisfaction often remains lower because of ongoing back pain issues. (b) The more radiographically impressive the neurocompression, the higher degree of postoperative relief. (c) Patients who have failed to improve after surgery elsewhere tend to have less favorable results after spinal surgery.

EVIDENTIARY TABLE AND SELECTION OF TREATMENT METHOD

When assessing outcomes, one "systematic review" found that many of the papers failed to give clear details about subgroups, like fibromyalgia.[27] There was little evidence of effectiveness of one program over another. While the data remain general, pharmacotherapy remains the foundation of much care in fibromyalgia and chronic radiculopathy patients.[28] Reasonable recommendations for early return to activity and exercise can also be made in most LBP groups.[29,30] In particular, fibromyalgia patients have been shown to have weaker core muscles (Table 28.1).[31]

A number of papers warn against elective surgery in fibromyalgia patients. If surgery is offered, there is little literature guidance as to whether a decompression alone or decompression and fusion should be offered. If a fusion is performed, a posterolateral, anterior, or anterior-posterior procedure must be selected. In one 5-year RCT, a small group of 44 patients was divided into three groups: decompression, decompression and PL fusion, or TLIF. While almost all patients were improved at 5 years, the authors concluded that "no significant additional benefit" arose from the more complex surgery.[26]

TABLE 28.1	Evidentiary Table: A Summary of the Quality of Evidence for Nonoperative Management of Back and Leg Pain in Patients with Fibromyalgia.			
Paper Author (Year)	**Description**	**Summary of Results**	**Quality of Evidence**
Van der Westhuizen et al. (2003)[41]	Patients with fibromyalgia undergoing spine surgery	80% still had pain postoperatively, 10% believed surgery had alleviated their problems	Very low
Ostelo et al. (2005)[42]	Patients with chronic widespread pain undergoing primary spine surgery	Fibromyalgia and similar diseases had a "markedly detrimental" effect on final outcomes	Very low
Velanovich (2003)[43]	Quality of Life analysis of chronic pain syndrome patients undergoing surgery	In the control group, patient satisfaction was 93%; in the chronic pain group, satisfaction was only 25%	Very low
Hallet et al. (2007)[26]	Comparison of three surgical cohorts treated for foraminal stenosis	A small group of 44 patients was divided into decompression alone, decompression and fusion, and transforaminal lumbar interbody fusion groups. More complex surgery did not confer significant benefits in outcomes	Low

DEFINITIVE TREATMENT PLAN

Given the absence of level I or II data for this complex patient, in accordance with Schuneman et al.'s grading system, best available evidence has a limited role in treatment recommendations. Unfortunately, there is little evidence to support *any* specific course of action. A **strong** recommendation can be made to avoid surgery in this patient, at this time.

Until better evidence and a more conclusive diagnosis are reached, sound, conservative treatment principles should be followed (e.g., first, do no harm). Rather than outlining surgical steps, therefore, I would outline additional workup that could allow this patient better pain control and improved function.

While patient preference *not* to have surgery must always be respected, especially when confronting elective spinal problems, a preference *for* surgery should always be tempered by the surgeon's sense that he can, indeed, help the patient. In this setting, a patient "demanding" surgery should be offered additional opinions.

A number of factors diminish surgical results including depression, worker's compensation, prior surgeries, and fibromyalgia. It is not clear why fibromyalgia increases pain. However, surgery has been shown to have three effects:

1. It may cause so-called secondary fibromyalgia.
2. In standing cases, it may increase fibromyalgia symptoms.
3. It decreases the portion of a patient's pain that is actually arising from the target of the surgical intervention. In that only a smaller part of their pain is being addressed, outcomes are bound to suffer.

While some surgeries are necessary on an urgent or emergent basis to save life and limb, many spinal operations for degenerative indications are elective. They can be justified only if they can be shown to improve on the natural history of the condition in question and, further, if the benefits outweigh the risks of the intervention. When outcomes are challenged by comorbidities, surgery should be undertaken rarely and only after careful and extensive deliberation with the patient and other caregivers.

If surgery were performed, the decompression of the lumbar roots between L4 and S1 on the right side would be undertaken. For some surgeons, this approach would include decompression and fusion, often with interbody support, partly to increase foraminal height. There is little literature evidence for this approach. A **weak** recommendation could be made, in the absence of segmental instability, to avoid fusion in this patient. Surgery would not likely address her back pain.

PREDICTING OUTCOMES

If surgery were to be undertaken in this patient, reported outcomes vary widely. Often, improvements in back pain and leg pain are considered separately. Despite years of study, the benefits of spinal surgery for mechanical low back pain remain controversial.

In case series, excellent outcomes have occasionally been described for multilevel spondylosis. When effective, fusion or disc replacement is most useful in patients with single level disease and in the absence of confounding variables.[32] Some authors have reported that fusion procedures yield more pain relief in patients with spondylolisthesis than in those with degeneration alone.[33,34]

In isolated series, the diagnosis of fibromyalgia did not impact the surgical result.[35] More typically fibromyalgia patients report extended postoperative recoveries. Postoperative pain management is usually difficult, and final results are suboptimal.[36] Preoperative identification of these patients remains difficult. One study of 62 patients sought to predict postoperative pain syndromes using preoperative assessment of diffuse noxious inhibitory control (DNIC). Patients with higher inhibitory control values had lower risk of postoperative pain syndromes. Fibromyalgia patients tend to have very poor DNIC.[37] Other clinical factors to assess include fear avoidance behavior (such as this patients inability to extend her spine), deficits of endogenous pain inhibition, and high levels of psychological distress.[38–40]

A few papers specifically examine the impact of fibromyalgia on surgical outcomes. None of these are carefully controlled, level one papers. Aside from being listed as a "comorbidity," the impact of fibromyalgia is not specifically recorded in the SPORT study. Between January 1999 and December 2000, 82 previous spinal surgery patients diagnosed with fibromyalgia. Postoperatively, 10% believed that surgery had alleviated their neck or back symptoms; 62% were unhappy with the results of surgery. Before surgery, 82% had chronic pain, and after surgery, 80% still had pain. There was no significant difference in preoperative and postoperative evaluations of quality of life, and the impact of spinal surgery on function was negative. The authors concluded that spinal surgery neither ameliorates the symptoms nor improves the poor quality of life of fibromyalgia patients.[41]

In a study of 105 patients undergoing first time disc surgery, fibromyalgia and other diseases affecting perceived recovery had a significant detrimental impact on final outcomes.[42]

What evidence we have suggests that fibromyalgia dominates outcomes relative to any other diseases a patient may have. For example, one study found that quality of life subgroup measures for bodily pain and vitality were lower in fibromyalgia patients than in COPD, AIDS, and prostate cancer.[43] Often poor patient reported outcomes (relative to physician measured results) are attributed to catastrophizing and a high rate of comorbid but often undiagnosed, depression.[44]

In one controlled cohort analysis, 93% of the control patients were satisfied with the surgery, whereas only 25% of the chronic pain syndrome patents were. While health-related quality of life improved in both groups, the extent of the improvement was much higher in the control group ($p < 0.001$).[36] WA Macrae examined the literature regarding postoperative pain and found that, particularly in spinal disorders, it was of poor quality. Very little could be said about outcomes of surgery in fibromyalgia patients other than they are significantly worse compared to unaffected patients.[45]

These predictions from the literature are in keeping with my clinical experience. At one point in training, I was taught that surgery in this patient population merely "redefines what 10 out of 10 pain really means." For fibromyalgia patients with clear radiculopathy, favorable outcomes can be achieved but are typically hard-fought even in minimally invasive decompression procedures. Larger fusion operations are associated with lengthy recovery intervals and poor results.

If, in fact, this patient's foot pain can clearly be attributed to her foraminal compression, she may see some improvement here. The lumbar complaints, on the other hand, are less likely to improve, sadly, more likely to worsen after surgery.[15]

As a result, I would continue to explore the exact nature of this patient's foot pain. If additional testing, such as EMG, was consistent with radiculopathy, selective nerve root blocks could be considered. Repeat evaluation with strict concordancy of history and examination findings, increased collapse with upright radiographs might favor operative intervention at some point in the future.

Until then, this patient is best served with ongoing, multidisciplinary management, including psychological help with coping mechanisms, rheumatologic evaluation, encouragement toward increased aerobic exercise and core strengthening, and, perhaps, pre-Gabalin or a similar agent.[46] Narcotics should be avoided.

SUMMARY

We are presented with a 57-year-old female with fibromyalgia and multiple prior right foot surgeries presenting with low back and right foot pain. While this patient has a tension sign on the right side and numbness in what could represent a dermatomal distribution, the MRI reveals only limited foraminal com-

pression. In the absence of red flags, we give a strong recommendation for nonsurgical care.

In any patient with multilevel disc degeneration, no surgery reliably relieves back pain. This is especially true in fibromyalgia patients, in whom the risk for worsening pain is high. Operative intervention for her leg pain is a closer call. However, with multiple prior foot surgeries and diffuse nonclassically dermatomal symptoms, decompressive surgery also risks failure to provide significant relief. At this time, surgery cannot be recommended. In the absence of solid evidence supporting surgical intervention, a conservative approach is strongly recommended.[47]

REFERENCES

1. Mayer TG, Towns BL, Neblett R, et al. Chronic widespread pain in patients with occupational spinal disorders: prevalence, psychiatric comorbidity, and association with outcomes. *Spine*. 2008;33:1889–1897.
2. Modic MT, Ross JS. Magnetic resonance imaging in the evaluation of low back pain. *Orthop Clin North Am*. 1991;22:283–301.
3. Jensen MC, Kelly AP, Brant-Zawadzki MN. MRI of degenerative disease of the lumbar spine. *Magn Reson Q*. 1994;10:173–190.
4. Gajraj NM. Selective nerve root blocks for low back pain and radiculopathy. *Reg Anesth Pain Med*. 2004;29:243–256.
5. Hasue M, Kikuchi S, Sakuyama Y, et al. Anatomic study of the interrelation between lumbosacral nerve roots and their surrounding tissues. *Spine*. 1983;8:50–58.
6. Koes BW, Scholten RJPM, Mens JMA, et al. Efficacy for epidural steroids for low back pain and sciatica: a systematic review of randomized clinical trials. *Pain*. 1995;63:279–288.
7. Vad VB, Bhat AL, Lutz GE, et al. Transforaminal epidural steroid injections in lumbosacral radiculopathy. *Spine*. 2002;27:11–16.
8. Weiner B, Fraser R. Foraminal injection for lateral lumbar disc herniation. *J Bone Joint Surg Br*. 1997;79:804–807.
9. Jenis L, An H. Foraminal stenosis. *Spine*. 2000;25(3): 389–394.
10. Deng XL, Liu XY, Xu N. Comparative study on low back pain misdiagnosed as spondyloarthropathy. *Clin Rheumatol*. 2009;28:893–898.
11. Lyles KW, Gold DT, Shipp KM, et al. Association of osteoporotic vertebral compression fractures with impaired functional status. *Am J Med*. 1993;94:595–601.
12. Muller W, Kelemen J, Stratz T. Spinal factors in the generation of fibromyalgia syndrome. *Z Rheumatol*. 1998;57(suppl 2):36–42.
13. Lapossy E, Maleitzke R, Hrycaj P, et al. The frequency of transition of chronic low back pain to fibromyalgia. *Scand J Rheumatol*. 1995;24:29–33.
14. Attias N, Hayman A, Hipp JA, et al. Assessment of magnetic resonance imaging in the diagnosis of lumbar spine foraminal stenosis—a surgeon's perspective. *J Spinal Disord Tech*. 2006;19:249–256.

15. Gibson JN, Waddell G. Surgery for degenerative lumbar spondylosis. *Cochrane Database Syst Rev.* 2005:CD001352.

16. Carragee EJ, Alamin TF, Miller JL, et al. Discographic, MRI and psychosocial determinants of low back pain disability and remission: a prospective study in subjects with benign persistent back pain. *Spine J.* 2005;5:24–35.

17. Scuderi GJ, Brusovanik GV, Golish SR, et al. A critical evaluation of discography in patients with lumbar intervertebral disc disease. *Spine J.* 2008;8:624–629.

18. Bailie DS, Kelikian AS. Tarsal tunnel syndrome: diagnosis, surgical technique, and functional outcome. *Foot Ankle Int.* 1998;19:65–72.

19. Raikin SM, Minnich JM. Failed tarsal tunnel syndrome surgery. *Foot Ankle Clin.* 2003;8:159–174.

20. Shookster L, Falke GI, Ducic I, et al. Fibromyalgia and Tinel's sign in the foot. *J Am Podiatr Med Assoc.* 2004;94:400–403.

21. Lawrence RC, Felson DT, Helmick CG, et al. Estimates of the prevalence of arthritis and other rheumatic conditions in the United States. Part II. *Arthritis Rheum.* 2008;58:26–35.

22. Hauser W, Akritidou I, Felde E, et al. Steps towards a symptom-based diagnosis of fibromyalgia syndrome: symptom profiles of patients from different clinical settings. *Z Rheumatol.* 2008;67:511–515.

23. Friedrich M, Hahne J, Wepner F. A controlled examination of medical and psychosocial factors associated with low back pain in combination with widespread musculoskeletal pain. *Phys Ther.* 2009;89:786–803.

24. Wolfe F, Anderson J, Harkness D, et al. A prospective, longitudinal, multicenter study of service utilization and costs in fibromyalgia. *Arthritis Rheum.* 1997;40:1560–1570.

25. Hsu K, Zucherman J, Shea W, et al. High lumbar disc degeneration: incidence and etiology. *Spine.* 1990;15:679–682.

26. Hallett A, Huntley JS, Gibson JN. Foraminal stenosis and single-level degenerative disc disease: a randomized controlled trial comparing decompression with decompression and instrumented fusion. *Spine.* 2007;32:1375–1380.

27. Mior S. Exercise in the treatment of chronic pain. *Clin J Pain.* 2001;17:S77–S85.

28. Rao SG, Bennett RM. Pharmacological therapies in fibromyalgia. *Best Pract Res Clin Rheumatol.* 2003;17:611–627.

29. Borenstein D. Epidemiology, etiology, diagnostic evaluation, and treatment of low back pain. *Curr Opin Rheumatol.* 1996;8:124–129.

30. Sculco AD, Paup DC, Fernhall B, et al. Effects of aerobic exercise on low back pain patients in treatment. *Spine J.* 2001;1:95–101.

31. Okumus M, Gokoglu F, Kocaoglu S, et al. Muscle performance in patients with fibromyalgia. *Singapore Med J.* 2006;47:752–756.

32. Guyer RD, McAfee PC, Banco RJ, et al. Prospective, randomized, multicenter Food and Drug Administration investigational device exemption study of lumbar total disc replacement with the CHARITE artificial disc versus lumbar fusion: five-year follow-up. *Spine J.* 2009;9:374–386.

33. Bono CM, Lee CK. The influence of subdiagnosis on radiographic and clinical outcomes after lumbar fusion for degenerative disc disorders: an analysis of the literature from two decades. *Spine.* 2005;30:227–234.

34. Glassman SD, Carreon LY, Djurasovic M, et al. Lumbar fusion outcomes stratified by specific diagnostic indication. *Spine J.* 2009;9:13–21.

35. Bernstein RM. Injections and surgical therapy in chronic pain. *Clin J Pain.* 2001;17:S94–S104.

36. Velanovich V. The effect of chronic pain syndromes and psychoemotional disorders on symptomatic and quality-of-life outcomes of antireflux surgery. *J Gastrointest Surg.* 2003;7:53–58.

37. Yarnitsky D, Crispel E, Eisenberg Y, et al. Prediction of chronic post-operative pain. Pre-operative DNIC testing identifies patients at risk. *Pain.* 2009;138:22–29.

38. Julien N, Goffaux P, Arsenault P, et al. Widespread pain in fibromyalgia is related to a deficit of endogenous pain inhibition. *Pain.* 2005;114:295–302.

39. Roelofs J, Sluiter JK, Frings-Dresen MH, et al. Fear of movement and (re)injury in chronic musculoskeletal pain: evidence for an invariant two-factor model of the Tampa Scale for Kinesiophobia across pain diagnoses and Dutch, Swedish, and Canadian samples. *Pain.* 2007;131:181–190.

40. Verbunt JA, Pernot DH, Smeets RJ. Disability and quality of life in patients with fibromyalgia. *Health Qual Life Outcomes.* 2008;6:8.

41. van der Westhuizen FD. The impact of spinal surgery on patients with fibromyalgia. *J Bone Joint Surg.* 2003;85-B:147–148.

42. Ostelo R, Vlaeuen J, van den Brandt P, et al. Residual complaints following lumbar disc surgery: prognostic indicators of outcome. *Pain.* 2005;114:177–185.

43. Schlenk E, Erlen J, Dunbar-Jacob J, et al. Health related quality of life in chronic disorders: A comparison across studies using the MOS SF-36. *Qual Life Res.* 1998;7:57–65.

44. Hassett A, Cone J, Patella S, et al. The role of catastrophizing in the pain and depression of women with fibromyalgia syndrome. *Arthrit Rheumatism.* 2000;43:2493–2500.

45. Macrae W. Chronic pain after surgery. *Br J Anesthesia.* 2001;87:88–98.

46. Fishbain DA, Lewis J, Cole B, et al. Multidisciplinary pain facility treatment outcome for pain-associated fatigue. *Pain Med.* 2005;6:299–304.

47. Sypert GW. Low back pain disorders: lumbar fusion? *Clin Neurosurg.* 1986;33:457–483.

Thoracic Stenosis

SHIVEINDRA JEYAMOHAN, MD, CIRO G. RANDAZZO, MD, MPH, AND JAMES S. HARROP, MD

EDITORS' CASE PRESENTATION

A 53-year-old woman presents after she had undergone uncomplicated cervical spine decompression for symptoms that appear to have been related to cervical myelopathy. While her upper extremity pain, numbness, and tingling have improved substantially since the surgery, she has had persistent imbalance and frequent falls. In addition, she complains of pain in her thoracic region that radiates from her back to the umbilicus. She has had previous lumbar spine surgery many years ago, from which she still has some mild low back and leg pain. She has not had any physical therapy since her cervical surgery but reports little neck pain and a functional range of motion.

Physical examination demonstrates a wide-based gait. She is slightly forward stooped with ambulation. Reflexes in the upper and lower extremities are diffusely brisk (3+), but bilaterally equal. She has a positive Hoffman test on the right. There are four beats of clonus in the right foot, while there is no clonus in the left foot. Toes are downgoing bilaterally. She has tenderness to palpation at the thoracolumbar junction. Strength is normal in the upper and lower extremities. Sensation is decreased in the right lower extremity in a nondermatomal pattern.

Cervical spine films demonstrate adequate decompression and fusion with no signs of pseudoarthrosis. Flexion-extension films demonstrate no movement through the fusion. A cervical MRI shows adequate canal and foraminal decompression.

Radiographic images are shown in Figure 29.1A–F.

INTERPRETATION OF CLINICAL PRESENTATION

The clinical scenario portrays a middle-aged woman presenting with imbalance, a wide-based gait, falls, radicular pain within the thoracic dermatomes, right foot clonus, and nonspecific right lower extremity pain. There is a recent history of cervical decompression for myelopathy and remote lumbar spine surgery with residual back and leg pain.

These symptoms can be attributed to cervical and/or thoracic myelopathy; with prior surgery, consideration of residual cervical stenosis or irreversible pathology should be given. Residual stenosis was ruled out with a cervical MRI. The clinician at this point should be concerned that the symptoms of isolated lower extremity weakness, decreased sensation in the thoracic dermatomes, thoracic back pain radiating around the flank to the abdomen, and nondermatomal unilateral lower extremity sensory loss are more specific to thoracic pathology. This individual's forward stoop with ambulation could be indicatory of Scheuermann kyphosis, which has been reported in conjunction with congenital thoracic stenosis. Scheuermann kyphosis, however, is usually a disease of adolescent males and typically does not develop in middle age. In the presence of congenital thoracic stenosis, the onset of symptoms can be abrupt even with the slightest of insults, including small disc herniations that can produce significant neurologic deficits.[1] Clinical signs of thoracic stenosis include paraparesis, hyperactive lower extremity reflexes, thoracic sensory level, cross-abductor signs, Babinski sign, clonus, gait dysfunction, loss of proprioception, and point tenderness in the thoracic region.

The patient's minimal neck pain and decreased range of motion are most consistent with residual discomfort from her previous cervical fusion and not typical of thoracic stenosis. The clinical relevance of

Figure 29.1.

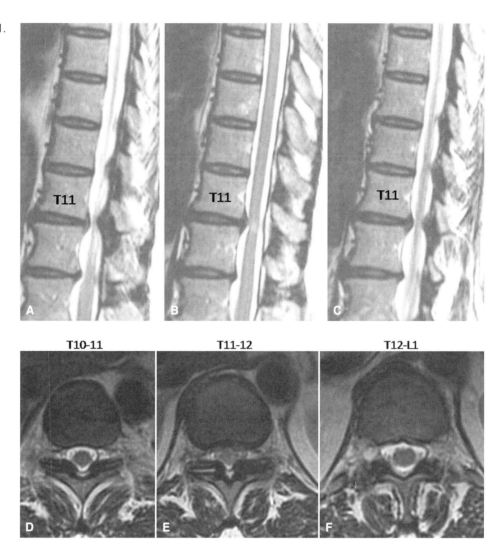

the presence of Hoffman sign is debatable in this case. Glaser et al.[2] found this an unreliable test in the diagnosis of cervical cord compression. However, since the patient had a documented cervical myelopathy, the unilateral Hoffman sign most likely represents a residual upper tract sign. The majority of cervical myelopathic reflexes do not resolve despite successful cervical decompression. Decreased sensation in the patient's right leg does not follow a dermatomal pattern and therefore makes a radicular process unlikely. Thoracic lesions typical sensory findings are bilateral in the lower extremities, and unilateral symptoms are more suggestive of a lumbar nerve root injury or rarely an intracranial process. Unilateral lower extremity sensory loss can be seen due to a lateral disc herniation or thoracic stenosis. Some patients with tandem spinal cord injuries (cervical and thoracic) can have extension of symptoms as a result of their previous injury. The clonus in the patient's foot is likely a long tract sign attributable to her thoracic stenosis or residual from cervical stenosis.

Etiologies that should be included in the differential diagnosis for a patient with thoracic myelopathy include thoracic stenosis, multiple sclerosis (MS), congenital abnormalities that demonstrate upper motor neuron signs in the lower extremities, spinal cord tumors, and cervical and lumbar stenosis or disc herniations. MS is less likely in this case given the focal sensory and motor abnormalities without ocular complaints, seizures, or other neurological disturbances. To assist in excluding a diagnosis of MS, an MRI of the brain would be useful to evaluate for intracranial white matter lesions. A congenital etiology such as congenital spinal stenosis may be a component given the patient's extensive spine surgery history and her related symptoms.

The patient's MRI, Figure 29.1A–F, is consistent with the radiographic appearance of thoracic stenosis. The sagittal T2 MRI images (Fig. 29.1A–C) show a disk protrusion ventral to the spinal cord at the T11-12 disk space, which abuts the thecal sac and causes narrowing of the canal. In addition, further canal stenosis is evident, on the sagittal MRI, as posterior canal narrowing due to thickening and buckling of the ligamentum flavum. In addition, the axial MRI imaging demonstrates significant tricompartmental stenosis at the T11-12 disk space in Figure 29.1E as compared to the disk spaces above and below, Figure 29.1D and F. This patient's thoracic stenosis therefore is due to

1. A ventral disc protrusion
2. Thickening of the ligamentum flavum posteriorly
3. Facet joint hypertrophy and lateral recess stenosis
4. A developmentally stenotic canal due to short pedicles

DECLARATION OF SPECIFIC DIAGNOSIS

This patient has a thoracic myelopathy due to spine stenosis at T11-T12.

BRAINSTORMING: WHAT ARE THE TREATMENT GOALS AND THE SURGICAL OPTIONS?

Treatment goals

1. Decompression of neural elements
2. Prevention of further deterioration
3. Thoracic back pain relief

Treatment options

1. Nonoperative management
2. Posterior decompression with thoracic laminectomy and partial medial facetectomy
3. Posterolateral thoracic decompression
4. Anterior thoracic decompression
5. Instrumented fusion following anterior and/or posterior approach decompression

EVALUATION OF THE LITERATURE REVIEW

The authors posed to answer the question, "What is the optimal treatment for thoracic myelopathy?" In order to obtain relevant literature, a MEDLINE search was performed. Search strategies included use of MeSH (medical subject headings) and keywords. Keywords included "thoracic vertebrae" and "spinal stenosis." Each search was performed separately and coinciding results were extracted by combining the two searches.

When limited to the English language, 103 articles were located published between 1950 and 2008, in which all abstracts were reviewed and relevant manuscripts were obtained and read. In addition, literature was further supplemented with references from the initial query as well as from the authors' personal knowledge. Because thoracic myelopathy is rare, level one studies were not anticipated.

DETAILED REVIEW OF PERTINENT ARTICLES

Only three articles met inclusion exclusion criteria and all three were low-quality evidence. Nonoperative options typically include physical therapy with core strengthening exercises. Chang et al.,[3] however, demonstrated that patients with symptom duration >2 years had worse outcomes after surgery, suggesting that prolonged nonoperative care could have a negative impact on outcome. Therefore, patients with symptomatic thoracic myelopathy from thoracic spinal stenosis should consider undergoing early surgical decompression.

Palumbo et al.,[4] in 2001, reported a retrospective series of 12 patients who underwent operative decompression of the thoracic spine, with an average follow-up just over 5 years. Of these 12 patients, 8 underwent a posterior decompression and 4 underwent anterior decompression. There were no combined procedures. In patients with preoperative motor deficit as measured by the Eismont system, improvement occurred in 80%. Of the 11 patients with gait disturbance as measured by the Japanese Orthopaedic Association (JOA) scoring system, 65% improved. Sixty-six percent of patients had improvement in pain. Interestingly in five patients who had early improvement there was subsequent deterioration secondary to recurrent stenosis or progressive deformity. Therefore, careful assessment of the degree of spinal instability or potential instability, especially in the setting of deformity, should be done and if necessary a concomitant fusion done.

Chang et al.[3] reported on 28 patients with thoracic stenosis and a mean follow-up of 30.6 months. Twenty-four patients underwent a posterior decompression with laminectomy and bilateral medial facetectomy. The remaining four patients underwent an anterior decompression through a thoracotomy due to a prominent ventral spur and/or ossification of the posterior longitudinal ligament (OPLL). One patient underwent a costotransversectomy for a preexisting compression fracture and one for OPLL. A combined anterior, or transpedicular, approach and posterior decompression was performed in one patient with a disc herniation and concurrent thickened yellow ligament. This series reported neurological improvement in 16 patients with an average improvement in Nurick grade from 3.3 to 1.8. The authors noted a statistically significant improvement when symptoms were present for <2 years; there was sufficient decompression and no additional proximal stenosis. The authors concluded that thoracic myelopathy could be reversed with appropriate decompression and timing of procedure.

Matsumoto et al.[5] in 2008 reported a retrospective multicenter study of outcomes for patients with thoracic ossification of the OPLL who underwent surgical decompression. The study included 154 patients at 34 institutions who underwent either anterior and/or posterior decompression with approximately 1/3 undergoing concurrent instrumented fusion. Mean follow-up was 3 years. The authors reported a mean improvement of JOA score of 36.8% at final follow-up. They also reported neurologic function, as measured by a modified Frankel classification, improved by one grade in 69.5%, unchanged in 24.7%, and deteriorated by at least one grade in nine patients (5.8%). Matsumoto et al. reported no statistically significant difference in outcome among patients treated by different surgical methods; however, they noted ossification at the upper thoracic spine and use of spinal instrumentation to be significantly related to favorable surgical outcomes.

In this case presentation, imaging illustrates a focal stenosis at the T11-12 level. Decompression would appear to be indicated without fusion. In Chang's study, the average posterior decompression group had 2.2 levels of stenosis with 3.6 levels decompressed, whereas the anterior decompression group had 1.8 stenotic segments with 1.2 decompressed segments.[3] In Palumbo's trial, an average 1.8 levels were decompressed, similar to Chang's.[3,4] Here, they cited that levels included were determined by radiologic evidence of compression correlating with patients' signs and symptoms. Kalfas performed a review of the literature on thoracic stenosis and detailed the use of a laminectomy procedure for which he concluded that a posterior approach was the most appropriate surgical approach for concentric narrowing of the canal or for patients with a primarily posterior component to their stenosis and no abnormal kyphotic deformity. Kalfas also recommended a posterolateral or anterior thoracic approach for patients with a ventral component of epidural encroachment in their stenosis.[1]

The above referenced studies are all retrospective case series (class III) of decompression for thoracic spinal cord stenosis. There is no high-quality evidence for determining the most appropriate surgical management of thoracic stenosis. There are no studies on nonoperative management or natural history. Thus, at this time, careful evaluation of patient symptoms, signs, and imaging must be integrated with sound clinical judgment in selecting the appropriate surgical management.

Resolving Literature Inconsistencies

The systematic review concerning optimal treatment for thoracic stenosis was consistent. Each series demonstrated a postoperative improvement in patients who underwent surgical decompression. Palumbo et al. reported the possibility of further neurologic deterioration over time and their series included 5-year follow-up. The existence of concurrent proximal spinal stenosis resulted in poorer clinical outcomes, thus leading the authors to recommend an examination for cervical stenosis prior to operative treatment of thoracic stenosis.[4]

EVIDENTIARY TABLE AND SELECTION OF TREATMENT METHOD

In this particular case, the patient has symptomatic thoracic myelopathy confirmed by imaging. Utilizing the best available evidence (Table 29.1), a laminectomy with partial medial facetectomy would be most appropriate. However, an anterior approach and decompression with a T11-12 discectomy to relieve cord impingement are also supported by the literature.[1,3–5] The literature suggests short-term improvement in myelopathy, thoracic back pain, and possibly gait; however, the duration of this improvement is unclear.

TABLE 29.1 Evidentiary Table of Studies About Surgical Treatment of Thoracic Myelopathy.

Paper Authors (Year)	Description	Summary of Results	Quality of Evidence
Matsumoto et al. (2008)	Retrospective, multi-institutional 154 patients	Posterior decompression and fusion for OPLL at the upper thoracic spine is relatively safe and effective	Low
Palumbo et al. (2001)	Retrospective 12 patients	Thoracic decompression can give early satisfactory outcomes in thoracic stenosis	Low
Chang et al. (2001)	Series 28 patients	Myelopathy from thoracic stenosis can be reversible with appropriate decompression	Low

DEFINITIVE TREATMENT PLAN

The described patient has circumferential compression of the spinal cord due to loss of disc height, degenerative posterior element disease, and ligamentous hypertrophy. Although an anterior or posterior decompression would be appropriate, an isolated posterior decompression may have the lowest overall surgical morbidity and the greatest chance for success. The posterior laminectomy and lateral recess decompression should remove the posterior and lateral osseous and ligamentous elements. This decompression should resolve the canal stenosis and thus provide an indirect decompression of the anterior disc and osteophyte complex. In cases where there is significant anterior compression or ventral mass effect, this indirect decompression will not suffice and an anterior decompression may be required. The additional issue of performing an arthrodesis should be considered if there is a deformity over the area of decompression or instability is created due to significant removal of the facet complex.

With an uncommon condition, literature is going to be of low quality. Results of this systematic review confirm this, but the results are consistent throughout the studies.[6] Despite the limited strength of the literature, the patient's progressive decline in neurologic function, myelopathic features, and imaging evidence of spinal cord compression favor operative treatment.

PREDICTING OUTCOMES

A systematic review of the literature suggests that immediately postoperatively the patient will experience at least short-term relief of her myelopathic features and radiculopathy. Gait dysfunction improvement is influenced by numerous components including recovery of proximal leg strength and recovery of light touch and proprioception.[1,3–5] Therefore, gait recovery is unpredictable but may be facilitated by a rehabilitation program. The long-term outcomes are uncertain as she is at risk for progressive or recurrent stenosis, thoracolumbar instability subsequent to surgery, or progression of any preexisting deformity.

In Palumbo et al.'s series, 10 of 12 patients had motor deficits prior to intervention. Postoperatively 8 illustrated clear motor improvement as classified by the Eismont grading scale, whereas 2 had no change.[4] Of the remaining 2 without deficit, one experienced deterioration secondary to an operative complication, whereas the other remained stable. Ambulatory status or gait improved in 7 of the 11 patients with altered ambulation, 2 remained unchanged, and 2 worsened. On average, ambulatory function improved 1.3/4 to 2.3/4 as measured by the JOA grading system at 2 to 9 years. Eight of 12 patients experienced improvement in pain, with the other 4 remaining unchanged. Thus, it appears that the decompression procedure did not aggravate any condition. Five-year follow-up showed pain to be characterized as moderate in 5 patients, mild in 4, and none in three patients, thus questioning the overall outcome as a procedure for pain symptoms. Four patients had urinary/bowel incontinence preoperatively of which 2 resolved completely, one resolved for 10 months but eventually recurred, and one with no recovery.

Chang et al.[3] also reported a high incidence of improvement: 79% experienced motor function improvement, while 57% had sensory improvement and 22% had pain improvement. In 4 cases, functional grade worsened from posterior decompression. The only significant positive prognostic factors reported in this series were the absence of proximal stenosis, sufficient decompression, and duration of initial symptoms <2 years.

Predicting this patient's outcome from the experiences of the above authors, she will likely have short-term improvement after surgery provided a sufficient decompression is achieved. However, prior to surgery, an evaluation of her cervical and thoracic spine should be performed to rule out more proximal stenosis. It is also important to review duration of the patient's symptoms when discussing postoperative expectations.

Preoperative evaluation for the patient with thoracic stenosis should include a full discussion of surgical risks and benefits. Surgical risks include persistence or worsening of pain, further deterioration of neurological function, bowel/bladder dysfunction, cerebrospinal fluid leak, hematoma formation, wound dehiscence, infection, progressive spinal deformity, DVT, need for reoperation, and other such risks associated with spinal surgery. Further risks include instability of the thoracolumbar junction, although Kalfas notes such subsequent iatrogenic spinal instability is a rare complication.

In addition, it is important to inform the patients that their neurologic condition as well as pain symptoms may not improve. For example, the current patient should be informed that her neck pain and range of motion will not improve with surgery. Also, her low back pain and right leg pain may or may not improve and in fact may worsen. She should also be informed that failure to intervene could result in progressive myelopathy, worsening of gait with increased hyperreflexia, and possible loss of continence to bowel and bladder function if her stenosis progresses or if she experiences an event such as a trauma that precipitously exacerbates her thoracic stenosis.

SUMMARY

In summary, a 53-year-old woman with a prior cervical decompression for myelopathy and low back surgery with residual pain is now presenting with a wide-based gait, falls, thoracic radicular pain, right foot clonus, and nonspecific right lower extremity pain. She has radiographic evidence of thoracic spinal stenosis from T10 to T12 with an associated T11-12 disc herniation. Imaging of her cervical spine shows no residual cervical spinal cord compression. A detailed systematic review illustrates sparse, low-quality literature on this topic. Based on this evidence and clinical experience, the most reasonable treatment plan would include a posterior decompression utilizing laminectomy with partial medial facetectomy. An alternative algorithm would be an anterior decompression to include a T11-12 discectomy. Short-term improvement could be expected in her radiating back pain and myelopathic features including her gait, with long-term beneficial results less certain.

REFERENCES

1. Kalfas IH. Laminectomy for thoracic spinal stenosis. *Neurosurg Focus*. 2000;9(4):e2 16833245.
2. Glaser JA, Cure JK, Bailey KL, et al. Cervical spinal cord compression and the Hoffman sign. *Iowa Orthop J*. 2001;21:49–52.
3. Chang UK, Choe WJ, Chung CK, et al. Surgical treatment for thoracic spinal stenosis. *Spinal Cord*. (2001);39: 362–369.
4. Palumbo AM, Hilibrand AS, Hart RA, et al. Surgical treatment of thoracic spinal stenosis: a 2- to 9-year follow-up. *Spine*. 2001;26(5):558–566.
5. Matsumoto M, Chiba K, Toyama Y, et al. Surgical results and related factors for ossification of posterior longitudinal ligament of the thoracic spine: a multi-institutional retrospective study. *Spine (Phila Pa 1976)*. 2008;33(9): 1034–1041.
6. Schünemann HJ, Jaeschke R, Cook DJ. An official ATS statement: grading the quality of evidence and strength of recommendations in ATS guidelines and recommendations. *Am J Respir Crit Care Med*. 2006;174:605–614.

Adult Scoliosis I

PETER G. PASSIAS, MD, GANG LI, MD,
AND KIRKHAM B. WOOD, MD

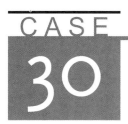

EDITORS' CASE PRESENTATION

A 68-year-old woman has a complaint of progressive deformity of the back and low back pain that she first noticed 5 years ago. She feels that her pain and symptoms have been getting worse recently. She has no complaints of numbness, tingling, or weakness in the upper or lower extremities. She does feel, however, that her ability to perform her daily functions is substantially limited. She has a concomitant history of depression, ischemic heart disease, arrhythmias, and smoking. She has had a long course of nonoperative treatment that has included pain medication and therapy.

Physical examination reveals a thin, but not frail, elderly woman. Her gait is slow, but symmetric. Inspection of her back shows a severe coronal imbalance with a shift of her center of gravity to the left. Side inspection shows a sagittal imbalance with forward shift of her center of gravity. Upon manipulation, her curve has moderate flexibility. She is neurologically intact.

Radiographic imaging studies are shown in Figures 30.1 to 30.5.

INTERPRETATION OF CLINICAL PRESENTATION

The clinical scenario describes an elderly woman with chronic low back pain, deformity with malalignment, and significant limitations in her ability to perform her daily functions. She denies any history of experiencing trauma. This combination of symptoms makes the diagnosis of adult scoliosis (AS) likely.[1] The prevalence of AS has been estimated to be between 2% and 32%[2–5] and has been shown to increase with age,

with rates exceeding 60% in populations older than 65 years.[6] AS is broadly defined as any curvature of the spine that either presents or requires treatment during adulthood. AS curves are divided into two general types based on when the curve develops. Adult idiopathic scoliosis develops before skeletal maturity, and de novo, or degenerative, scoliosis develops later in life long after skeletal maturity. De novo scoliosis, although most commonly of degenerative etiology, can also result from osteoporosis, prior trauma, and postsurgical changes. It is important to note that these two categories are principally descriptive and have not been shown to be helpful in guiding treatment, as the principles regarding their treatment are similar.

It is not surprising that this patient presents with a chief complaint of low back pain. It is estimated that 90% of AS patients present with pain as their chief complaint,[7,8] and among those who go on to require surgical intervention, back pain is responsible for approximately 85% of presenting complaints.[9–11] In addition, this patient's advanced age makes her more likely to experience low back pain associated with her scoliosis, as the incidence of symptomatic scoliosis also increases with age.[6] It is also likely that her curvature is substantial, given the association that has been established between the presence of back pain and scoliosis curves >45 degrees.[12]

The presence of significant functional limitations and depression is also consistent with her diagnosis. Based on information obtained using the Medical Outcomes Study 36-Item Short Form (SF-36), AS patients were found to have worse psychosocial well-being in 7 of the 8 categories when compared to the general population.[13,14] Her symptoms have significantly progressed over the past 5 years. Prior to this we are not given any information. It is not clear whether this represents a case of AS of idiopathic or de novo degenerative etiology, although it is more likely the former given the characteristics of her curvature which will be discussed later.[7,8,15]

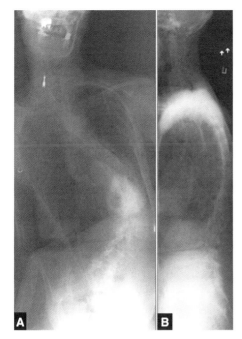

Figure 30.1.

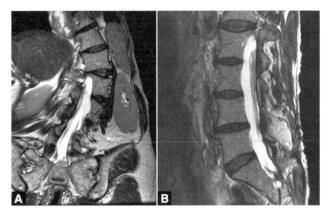

Figure 30.3.

A thorough neurological examination is important in all cases of AS. Although the lack of a neurologic deficit is not uncommon, particularly in younger patients with AS, neurogenic claudication and radicular pain can occur secondary to concurrent stenosis, especially in the presence of a secondary degenerative changes that may develop.[16] Neurogenic symptoms in AS become progressively more common in patients beyond the age of 50 years and especially in AS curves of a degenerative etiology.[16]

There are several other components to her history that are pertinent. If surgery is considered, her medical comorbidities put her at higher risk of poor functional outcomes and increased surgical complication rates, including depression,[17] ischemic heart disease,[18,19] and certain arrhythmias.[18,19] Another aspect of her history that is concerning is her advanced age.

Elderly patients are more likely to have multiple medical comorbidities, poor nutritional status, and reduced activity demands.[20] Her elderly status places her at increased risk of morbidity or even mortality with surgical intervention.[21] Finally, her smoking status also places her at an increased risk of being osteoporotic, as well as for developing a pseudarthrosis if she undergoes a fusion.[22]

Figure 30.1A is a full-length (36-in) posterior-anterior (PA) image presumably taken in the standing position. From the PA view, we use the Cobb method to determine the magnitude of the curve and its superior and inferior extent. In this patient, a right-sided thoracolumbar curve is seen extending from T10-L3 measuring 82 degrees. There is also a small compensatory thoracic curve measuring 33 degrees. The characteristics of her curve most likely reflect an idiopathic curvature with secondary degenerative changes. These plain films can also give us an idea of the risk of further curve progression. Some of the established radiographic parameters associated with progression of an

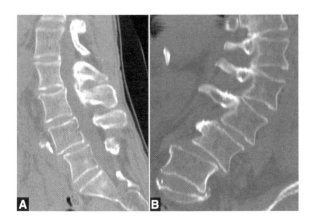

Figure 30.2.

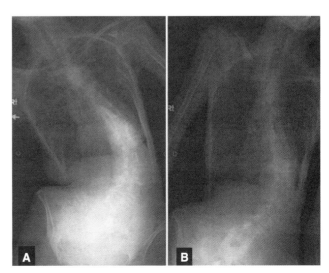

Figure 30.4.

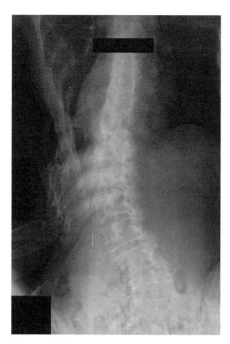

Figure 30.5.

AS curve that are present in this patient include severe rotation of the apical vertebrae, large curves (thoracic curves ≥50–60 degrees, lumbar >40 degrees), and lateral vertebral translation of 6 mm or more.[23–25] This view also allows us to assess the coronal balance. Measuring from the central sacral vertical line (CSVL) the distance to the C7 body measures 6 cm. Coronal imbalance >4 cm has been shown to be a risk factor for curve progression and to be associated with deterioration in pain and function scores for AS patients who have not undergone surgery.[26]

Figure 30.1B is a full-length lateral image. A principle utility of the lateral view is for the assessment of sagittal balance. Sagittal balance is the most reliable predictor of clinical symptoms in AS patients.[26] Obtaining sagittal balance is the critical goal in spinal reconstructive surgery.[26] Sagittal balance is measured from a plumb line from the mid-C7 vertebral body to the posterosuperior S1 vertebral body on the lateral x-ray. In this patient the sagittal balance is positive and measures 6 cm. Sagittal imbalance more than 5 cm has been shown to be associated with increased energy requirements for ambulation, pain and fatigue, and diminished overall health.[27] The lateral view also enables us to evaluate the degree of thoracic kyphosis, lumbar lordosis, and signs of degeneration, including spondylosis, disc space collapse, and spondylolisthesis. In this patient the lumbar lordosis measures only 9 degrees. Schwab et al. have found the loss of lumbar lordosis to be strongly correlated with preoperative symptoms and clinical improvement following surgical intervention in AS.[1,6,13,15,28] This loss of lumbar lordosis and her positive sagittal imbalance are likely the two most important factors that are contributing to her pain and functional limitations.[13,29] The thoracic kyphosis measures 45 degrees in this patient. This number is important to keep in mind, for although this falls within the normal range, there is evidence that a sagittal Cobb angle difference between lumbar lordosis and thoracic kyphosis of >20 degrees (higher lumbar lordosis) is advisable to achieve optimal sagittal balance.[30]

Preoperative bending films are useful, particularly when surgical treatment is considered, in order to determine curve flexibility. Figure 30.4A shows a right bending demonstrating the T10-L3 curvature measured at 75 degrees, while on left bending this curve decreases to 45 degrees. Collectively, they reveal that the curvature is moderately flexible. Rigid curves are more common in adults, and they tend to make any coronal and/or sagittal balance less well tolerated.[27,31,32] Figure 30.5 demonstrates a traction view with correction of the curvature to 32 degrees. This increased flexibility seen with traction views is expected, as curves >50 degrees show greater flexibility with traction views, while those <50 degrees show greater flexibility with side bending because of different responses to axial/transverse loading patterns.[33,34] In AS patients, traction radiographs have also been shown to be highly predictive of postoperative reduction of stiff (<35% reduction of curve) thoracic and thoracolumbar curves that are treated by segmental instrumentation, with the postoperative result estimated within a margin of error of ±7 degrees.[35]

The computed tomography (CT) scan images available include a median sagittal cut of the lumbar spine (Fig. 30.2A) as well as a coronal cut of the lumbar spine through the vertebral bodies (Fig. 30.2B). These images reveal several common characteristics of ADS curves. The degenerative changes are more pronounced in the lower lumbar segments, in particular at the lumbosacral junction. In addition, rotatory subluxation and obliquity as seen in this patient are commonly found at the L4-5 segment, although the former is more frequently seen at the L3-4 segment.[36] The lateral and anterior listhesis translation seen at the L4-5 segment is also an indication of relative instability at this segment and the need to include the fusion distal to this level. In addition, coupled with the obliquity and the degeneration present at the lumbosacral junction, fusion to the pelvis should also be performed. Lastly, it is important to note that CT scans are useful for evaluating pedicle morphology should pedicle screws be used.

In cases of ADS, MRI scans are helpful for evaluating sites of neural compression as well as assessing potentially painful degenerative changes in the disc. Representative fat-suppressed T2-weighted images in the coronal (A) and sagittal (B) planes are shown in Figure 30.3. Although this patient has no symptoms that can be attributed to stenosis or nerve root impingement, the intervertebral disc at the L2-3 and

L4-5 levels reveal a loss of disc height with disc bulging and loss of signal intensity, although these findings are not necessarily related to her symptoms. Additional studies, including discography and facet blocks, may be useful in evaluating the contribution of these radiographic findings to her symptoms of LBP, but are controversial.

DECLARATION OF SPECIFIC DIAGNOSIS

This patient has AS of the thoracolumbar spine, likely of idiopathic etiology.

BRAINSTORMING: WHAT ARE THE TREATMENT GOALS AND SURGICAL OPTIONS?

The treatment goals are

1. Improving low back pain
2. Restoring sagittal and coronal balance
3. Stabilizing the curve and alignment
4. Preservation of neural elements
5. Early mobilization
6. Rehabilitation and healing

The treatment options are

1. Observation
2. Repeating conservative modalities
3. Percutaneous/minimally invasive instrumentation
4. Posterior, anterior, or combined spinal fusion
5. Extending fusion to the pelvis

EVALUATION OF THE LITERATURE

To identify relevant publications on AS of the thoracolumbar spine, a MEDLINE search was performed. Search strategies included the use of MeSH (medical subject headings) and keywords. Keywords included "adult," "scoliosis," and "surgical procedures, operative" within three words of "scoliosis," and "fusion," "pelvis," and "outcomes" within three words of "scoliosis." A focused search of "adult scoliosis" with subheadings of degenerative, idiopathic, mortality, classification, complications, radiography, rehabilitation, surgery, and therapy was performed. The results for "scoliosis" were then combined with thoracolumbar or lumbar scoliosis to identify patients within larger heterogeneous studies on spinal deformity. Journals were hand searched and references were reviewed to identify pertinent articles. The search strategy revealed 382 potential publications after limiting from 1990 to 2008. The same search strategy was applied to EMBASE and revealed 208 results. MEDLINE "in process" and nonindexed citations were searched as was EBM reviews-Cochrane database. There were 121 English language abstracts that were reviewed and 35 full-text articles were read.

DETAILED REVIEW OF PERTINENT ARTICLES

Operative Versus Nonoperative Treatment

Presently, there is no consensus on the indications for the operative treatment of AS, particularly in patients over 65. Several studies have examined the surgical treatment of AS using "Harrington generation" instrumentation,[32,37–41] but more limited data are available on newer segmental techniques. To date, there have been no randomized prospective studies and no reports published directly comparing the outcomes of operative and nonoperative treatment for AS patients specifically older than 65 years of age. Nevertheless, these studies in addition to numerous case series represent the best available evidence. As such, for the purpose of this chapter, the decisions concerning how to manage this patient will be based on the three components of evidence-based medicine: patient factors, best available evidence, and clinical expertise.

This patient has several medical comorbidities that need to be considered when choosing treatment. Entities such as ischemic heart disease and arrhythmias need to be thoroughly evaluated, in order to determine her operative risk. In addition, her age places her at a higher risk of experiencing a surgical complication, should such treatment be chosen. There are several nonoperative treatment options for this patient, including physical therapy, medical management, and spinal orthoses. A recent systematic review of the literature, however, revealed the evidence for using conservative care to be minimal, with only level IV evidence existing for physical therapy, chiropractic care, and bracing and level III evidence for injections.[42] Although the use of spinal orthoses has been shown to improve back pain in some patients,[24] they are unable to prevent the progression of adult scoliotic curves and have high rates of skin breakdown, muscle atrophy, and deconditioning in this population.[23] This patient has failed medical treatment and physical therapy thus far, and further attempts at conservative management are unlikely to be helpful in alleviating her symptoms. We would not recommend conservative treatment at this point if her preoperative evaluation demonstrates her to be a reasonable surgical candidate.

Most scoliosis classification attempts have focused on adolescent idiopathic scoliosis and have not been found to be helpful at guiding treatment or predicting outcomes in AS patients.[43–46] In this population, we have been limited by unclear relationships between many traditional radiographic parameters and clinical outcomes.[15] There have been several attempts to classify AS specifically. The Aebi classification is a simplistic approach based on etiology.[47] The SRS classification, although richly descriptive, is difficult to apply and does not take into account clinical parameters.[48] Although not as descriptive as the SRS classification, the most clinically relevant system available may be that developed by Schwab et al.[49] Using data collected in a multicenter prospective study,[49] the authors developed a classification for AS based on the apical level of scoliotic deformity, the degree of lumbar lordosis, and the maximal intervertebral subluxation as seen on frontal and sagittal plane standing radiographs.[15] A fourth modifier, sagittal balance, was later added and applied to treatment and outcomes.[28] All of the factors used in the classification have individually been shown to be correlated with self-reported pain and disability prior to treatment.[13,15,26] In this patient, the apical level of the deformity (L1) would place her in category IV (thoracolumbar major curve; apex T11-L1). In the initial series, this category had the highest surgical rate.[49] Her lumbar lordosis measures 9 degrees, which would place her in the moderate (B) category, while her maximal subluxation is >7 mm, which would make her a ++. Lastly, her positive sagittal balance further increases her classification grade according to the later modification. The lumbar lordosis and subluxation modifiers offer a stratification of patients into clinical groups.[49] Higher grades are tied to increasing disability and pain by the SRS-22 and ODI outcomes tools.[49] This classification system has been shown to have value in predicting the requirement for surgical treatment, with higher surgical rates seen with higher curvature types.[28] It also has predictive value for the surgical approach and procedure used.[28] Lastly, higher grade curves appear to benefit the most from surgical intervention.[28] Long-term follow-up data for the application of this classification system have yet to be published. In addition, future analysis that is prospectively being obtained by the Spinal Deformity Study Group on pelvic parameters, sagittal alignment, and the lumbosacral junction will undoubtedly help us to predict which AS patients benefit the most from surgical intervention.

In order to offer clinical recommendations, it is suggested that the clinician considers the quality of the evidence in addition to the perceived benefits, harms, and burdens of the interventions. On an individual level, patient preference will influence the variables considered above. However, without specific knowledge of the weight of various outcomes or risks from his or her perspective, the clinician must be the patient's surrogate. From retrospective case series, nonoperative treatment has a more unpredictable outcome with respect to efficacy and radiographic deterioration. For this particular patient, **operative treatment is selected** because of proven benefit, risk of progression, moderate risk, and fewer treatment-related burdens, such as brace wear and closer radiographic follow-up due to the greater potential for deformity progression. The results of the studies in Table 30.1, which utilized modern spinal instrumentation, demonstrate that surgical treatment results in acceptable disease-specific outcome scores and health-related quality of life (HrQoL) outcome scores. Furthermore, surgical complications and radiographic failure are controlled in properly selected individuals.[50]

Literature Inconsistencies

The literature is inconsistent regarding certain aspects of this case. Two areas are particularly concerning and will be discussed in depth in later sections of this chapter. From an indications standpoint, the operative treatment of AS individuals older than 65 years is particularly deficient, as will be discussed in the outcomes section. From a technical standpoint, the literature is similarly inconsistent regarding the proximal and distal fusion levels, which will be discussed in the treatment sections.

EVIDENTIARY TABLE AND SELECTION OF TREATMENT METHOD

The best available evidence dictates that the patient presented in the clinical scenario should be treated operatively. In order to evaluate the most appropriate surgical treatment, only articles pertaining to adult patients with thoracolumbar scoliosis treated with modern spinal instrumentation were critically examined. These results are summarized in Table 30.1.

Open or Percutaneous (Minimally Invasive Surgery) Correction and Stabilization

Minimally invasive surgery (MIS) techniques are appealing because they have the potential to reduce the extensive soft-tissue trauma and large blood losses that are frequently associated with AS surgery. Schwab et al.[51] performed an anterior release and thoracoplasty using endoscopic techniques, followed by posterior spinal fusion, successfully in nine patients. More recently, Anand et al.[52] conducted a prospective evaluation of 12 patients undergoing surgery for lumbar degenerative scoliosis and reported good results using various combinations of MIS techniques supplemented with percutaneous posterior pedicle screw instrumentation. Presently, there is not enough evidence to support this

TABLE 30.1   **Evidentiary Table.**

Paper Author (Year)	Description	Summary of Results	Quality of Evidence
Bradford et al. (1999)	A retrospective study	With a minimum 2-y follow-up, 17 patients who underwent extension of a previous idiopathic scoliosis fusion to the sacrum via a combined approach had improvement in the Oswestry Disability Index from an average preoperative score of 40 to an average postoperative score of 28.	Level III
Kim et al. (2008)	A retrospective study Outcomes compared between groups	Forty-eight adult patients with lumbar scoliosis (average age at surgery 49.6 y, average follow-up 3.7 y) who underwent posterior segmental spinal instrumentation and fusion (PSSIF) were analyzed. Twenty-three patients underwent an anterior apical release of the lumbar curve via a thoracoabdominal approach followed by PSSIF (group I). The remaining 25 patients underwent a PSSIF of the lumbar curve followed by anterior column support at the lumbosacral region through an anterior paramedian retroperitoneal or posterior transforaminal approach (group II). At the ultimate follow-up, there were no significant differences in major Cobb angle, C7 plumbline to the center sacral vertical line ($p= 0.17$), C7 plumbline to the posterior superior endplate of S1 ($p = 0.44$), and sagittal Cobb angles at the proximal junction ($p = 0.57$), T10-L2 ($p = 0.24$) and T12-S1 ($p = 0.51$). There were 4 pseudarthroses in Group I and one in group II ($p = 0.02$) (anterior combined posterior paramedian retroperitoneal or posterior transforaminal approach). Postoperative total normalized SRS outcome scores at ultimate follow-up were significantly higher in Group II (69% vs. 79%, $p = 0.01$)	Level III
Anand et al. (2008)	Prospective evaluation No control group	Twelve patients underwent circumferential fusion. The age range of these patients was 50–85 y (mean of 72.8 y). All patients underwent direct lateral transpsoas approach for discectomy and fusion with polyetheretherketone cage and rh-BMP2. All fusions to the sacrum included L5-S1 fusion with the Trans1 Axial Lumbar Interbody Fusion technique. Mean number of segments operated on was 3.64 (range: 2–8 segments). Mean blood loss for anterior procedures (transpsoas discectomy/fusion and in some cases L5-S1 interbody fusion) was 163.89 mL (SD 105.41) and for posterior percutaneous pedicle screw fixation (and in some cases L5-S1 interbody fusion) was 93.33 mL (SD 101.43). Mean surgical time for anterior procedures was 4.01 h (SD 1.88) and for posterior procedures was 3.99 h (SD 1.19). Mean Cobb angle preoperatively was 18.93 degrees (SD 10.48) and postoperatively was 6.19 degrees (SD 7.20). Mean preoperative VAS score was 7.1; mean preoperative TIS score was 56.0. At mean follow-up of 75.5 d, mean VAS was 4.8; TIS was 28.0. A combination of 3 MIS techniques allows for correction of lumbar degenerative scoliosis.	Level III

(Continued)

TABLE 30.1   **Evidentiary Table.** *(Continued)*

Paper Author (Year)	Description	Summary of Results	Quality of Evidence
Kuhns et al. (2007)	A retrospective long-term follow-up study	31 patients with an average age of 45 y (range, 20–62 y) were fused from the thoracic spine to L5 and were evaluated at a mean follow-up of 9.4 y (range, 5–20.1 y). 2 out of 31 patients had preoperative advanced degeneration of the L5-S1 disc (Weiner grade 2–3). Three additional patients had an early revision to the sacrum secondary to sagittal imbalance not thought to be related to SAD. 26 out of 31 patients were assessed as "healthy discs" preoperative (Weiner grade 0–1) and were evaluated for subsequent advanced degeneration (SAD). By latest follow-up, L5-S1 SAD developed in 18 of these 26 patients (69%). Risk factors for the development of SAD included long fusions extending into the upper thoracic spine down to L5 ($p = 0.02$) and having a circumferential lumbar fusion ($p = 0.02$). Although preoperative sagittal balance was not significantly different between the "healthy" and SAD group, sagittal balance at follow-up was C7 plumb >5 cm in 67% of SAD patients and only 13% of "healthy" disc patients ($p = 0.009$).	Level III
Kim et al. (2007)	A retrospective comparison study	A clinical and radiographic assessment in addition to revision prevalence of 125 adult lumbar deformity patients who underwent long segmental posterior spinal instrumented fusion from the distal thoracic/upper lumbar spine (T9-L2) to L5 or S1 with a minimum 2-y follow-up were compared as influenced by T9-10 (group 1, $n = 37$), T11-12 (group 2, $n = 49$), and L1-2 (group 3, $n = 39$) proximal fusion levels. Three groups demonstrated nonsignificant differences in the prevalence of proximal junctional kyphosis (group 1 51% vs. group 2 55% vs. group 3 36%, $p = 0.20$) and revision (group 1 24% vs. group 2 24% vs. group 3 26%, $p = 0.99$) at the ultimate follow-up. Subsequent proximal junctional angle and sagittal vertical axis changes between the ultimate follow-up and preoperative ($p = 0.10$ and 0.46 respectively) were not significantly different.	Level III
Schwab et al. (2006)	Multicenter, prospective, consecutive clinical series	To establish and validate classification of scoliosis in the adult, higher intervertebral sublaxation were detected a total of 947 adults with spinal deformity had radiographic analysis: frontal Cobb angle, deformity apex, lumbar lordosis, and intervertebral subluxation. Mean maximal coronal Cobb was 46 degrees and lumbar lordosis 46 degrees. Mean maximal intervertebral subluxation (frontal plane) was 4.2 mm (sagittal plane, 1.2 mm). In thoracolumbar/lumbar deformities, the loss of lordosis/higher subluxation was associated with lower Scoliosis Research Society pain/function and higher Oswestry Disability Index scores. Across the study group, lower apex combined with lower lordosis led to higher disability. Higher surgical rates with decreasing lumbar lordosis and higher intervertebral subluxation were detected.	Level III

technique for this patient and we would perform **open correction and stabilization**.

Anterior Versus Posterior Fusion

Anterior approaches for the treatment of scoliosis are particularly helpful in younger patients with thoracolumbar or lumbar curves without neurologic symptoms. When combined with posterior surgery, anterior surgery can improve the amount of correction, reduce the number of segments included, and allow for greater improvement in lumbar lordosis.[39,53,54] Other potential advantages include lower infection rates and higher fusion rates.[39,53,54] However, anterior surgery in older patients is generally limited to certain clinical scenarios, including revisions of failed posterior fusions, rigid curves that require anterior release, significant thoracolumbar or thoracolumbar kyphosis, and long fusions that extend to the sacrum.[39,53,54] In addition, anterior procedures also are associated with significant risks in an older population including respiratory compromise and prolonged surgical times.[53,54] Isolated anterior approaches are also unable to extend to the L5 level or sacrum and do not allow for adequate release when significant degenerative changes or disc space collapse is present. Several studies have evaluated the ability of anterior or posterior approaches for the treatment of AS; however, there have been none directly comparing the two approaches and the majority have been retrospective series. Hamzaoglu et al.[55] retrospectively studied 15 AS patients with severe scoliosis that were treated with posterior-only release and pedicle screw instrumentation with intraoperative halo-femoral traction and found that they were able to achieve and maintain good balance and correction without anterior releases. In their retrospective series, Deviren et al.[56] followed 15 adults treated with anterior release and fusion, concluding that ASF was a good option for adults with flexible, moderate thoracolumbar/lumbar curves. However, they cautioned that flexibility significantly decreased with increased age and curve magnitude and careful patient selection was critical.[56] Although no direct comparison is available, a posterior approach would enable our surgical goals to be accomplished and would minimize respiratory complications, particularly in a long-time smoker. In this clinical scenario, the evidence favors the use of a **posterior approach and fusion** and anterior augmentation only at the lower lumbar segments as will be discussed below in the section "Fusion to the Pelvis."

Anterior Release

Anterior release has been used in the past for rigid curves. Several studies have evaluated the addition of anterior apical release and fusion for AS, citing possible improvements in correction, fusion rates, and lumbar lordosis.[39,53,54] However, the need for this is thought to have been lessened with modern instrumentation techniques. In their retrospective series, Kim et al.[57] compared 25 patients who underwent posterior segmental spinal instrumentation and anterior augmentation at the lumbosacral junction with 23 patients who underwent an anterior apical release of the lumbar curve via a thoracolumbar approach followed by PSSIF. They found that posterior segmental spinal instrumentation and fusion without anterior release of lumbar curves demonstrated better total SRS outcome scores and no differences in radiographic parameters without differences in clinical complications.[57] Given the available evidence, **anterior apical release** is not required for this patient.

Proximal Extent of Fusion

The ideal level of the proximal fusion in thoracolumbar/lumbar curves is unclear given the existing evidence. Based strictly on the characteristics of her curve in the coronal plane, her thoracic curve is minor, is not structural, and therefore does not need to be included in the fusion. Given this, Kim et al.[58] published the only comparative analysis of postoperative sagittal plane change and revision prevalence according to the three different proximal fusion levels at the thoracolumbar junction (T9-10 vs. T11-12 vs. L1-2). They found that the three different proximal fusion levels did not demonstrate significant radiographic and clinical outcomes or revision prevalence after surgery.[58] Although not supported by the available literature, based on our experience, we would recommend proximal extension of the fusion to the upper thoracic spine in this patient for several reasons. Her curve is a thoracolumbar curve likely of idiopathic etiology and not a degenerative lumbar curve. In addition, taking the sagittal plane characteristics into account, her stable vertebral level and the apex of her kyphosis are located at T7 and it would allow for better correction of her sagittal imbalance to extend her fusion to the proximal thoracic spine. Lastly, her anticipated poor bone quality would make us more inclined to seek more proximal fixation points.

Fusion to the Pelvis

This patient's curvature extends to the L3 level. The topic of whether to fuse to L5 or include the sacrum and/or the remaining pelvis remains somewhat controversial. The literature is still unclear as to whether or not fusion to the sacrum results in higher complication rates and lower patient satisfaction compared to stopping at L5.[59–64] In a matched cohort analysis of 95 patients, Edwards et al.[65] found that long fusions to the sacrum required more procedures and had a higher frequency of complications than similar fusions to L5, although subjacent disc degeneration was common in this group. Kuhns et al.[66] retrospectively looked at 31 AS patients who underwent long fusions to L5 with 5- to 15-year follow-up and found advanced L5-S1 degenerative changes in 69% of patients, although not all of these patients experienced clinical symptoms as a result. There are several factors that are frequently used as indications for extending the fusion past the distal extent of the curve to include the pelvis, including the following: the presence of a rigid unbalanced lumbosacral curve, significant pelvic obliquity, severe symptomatic degenerative changes at the lumbosacral junction, spondylolisthesis at the L5-S1 level, spinal stenosis, or the requirement for decompression below a lumbar fusion. In our clinical scenario, there is evidence of degenerative changes in her lower lumbar spine below her curvature. Although further diagnostic testing is indicated, these likely contribute to her LBP symptoms. In addition, given her sagittal and coronal imbalance, extension of the fusion to the pelvis will allow for better correction. Lastly, because of her osteoporosis, we anticipate that **fusion to the pelvis would likely be appropriate**. Prior to surgical intervention, however, further diagnostic testing, such as discography and DEXA, may be helpful for more detailed surgical planning.

If one is considering extending the fusion distal to L5, biomechanical studies performed in animals have shown that iliac screws provide a significant reduction in S1 screw strain and the lowest rates of catastrophic failure at the lumbosacral junction.[67] In addition, bicortical sacral fixation and larger diameter screws can also be used in order to enhance fixation depending on intraoperative insertional torque. In our clinical scenario, because of the length of the posterior fusion required and her probable osteoporotic bone, **extension to the ileum** is indicated to maximize sagittal balance correction and minimize the risk of late sacral fractures.[62,63]

Pseudarthrosis rates can reach 40% to 60% when long posterior fusions are extended to the sacrum.[62,63] Anterior column support in the form of anterior grafts, additional points of sacral fixation, and extension to the ileum have all been shown to reduce the stress on the sacral pedicle screws and increase the rate of fusion. Anterior column augmentation most likely increases the fusion rate secondary to increased fusion surface area under compressive forces.[67] Interbody reconstruction also provides the potential to increase lumbar lordosis that has been lost, thereby improving sagittal balance and indirectly decompressing stenosis by restoring intervertebral height. Newer techniques have been described to provide anterior column support through posterior or extreme lateral approaches[68]; however, there is evidence that separate anterior approaches allow for a better discectomy, thus facilitating fusion.[69] In our patient, **anterior column support** should be carried out. Although the literature is unclear, a separate anterior approach is our preference because of the theoretical advantage of allowing for a more complete discectomy and maximizing the surface area for a fusion.

Osteoporosis Influence

Osteoporosis is a common comorbidity in AS patients. This patient has several risk factors (Caucasian, female, smoking, elderly), and further preoperative testing is indicated. This is an important consideration because of its potential to weaken the strength of pedicle screw fixation.[70–72] Several options do exist to enhance spinal instrumentation in this population, such as additional sublaminar wires,[72] or augmenting the weakened trabecular bone with polymethylmethacrylate cement[73] or calcium phosphate.[74] The clinical data supporting such techniques are limited and we do not anticipate the need for such techniques in this patient. **Cross-links** have also been shown to increase the stiffness of long fusions while adding minimal morbidity and time to the procedure; however, their utility in long pedicle screw constructs has been shown to be minimal.[75]

Graft Options

Obtaining a solid fusion is essential for achieving and maintaining stabilization in AS. This can be particularly challenging in an adult population as pseudarthrosis rates can be as high as 24%.[30] In addition, this patient has several additional risk factors for this including a sagittal balance >5 cm, smoking, and an age >55 years.[30] In addition to technical factors such as optimizing spine mechanics and providing adequate surface area for fusion, choosing the appropriate graft is also important. Although the details of bone grafting are beyond the scope of this chapter, autografting with iliac crest remains the gold standard and would be used in this patient.[16] Newer techniques, such as the use of bone morphogenic proteins, have anecdotal evidence to support their use in long posterior fusions[76] but are not approved for such use, and the complications[77,78] of using such products as well as their long-term effects are not presently well-defined.

DEFINITIVE TREATMENT PLAN

The patient in this clinical scenario should be managed operatively because of the severity of her symptoms and her failed attempts at conservative management. We would supplement our posterior fusion to the sacrum with anterior structural interbody grafting at L5-S1 and also at the L4-5 segment. Our preference would be to perform this through a separate anterior approach (midline retroperitoneal) prior to performing the posterior fusion in order to maximize lumbar lordosis, although evidence to support this sequence is lacking. We perform the posterior portion first only in cases of significant segmental instability. Obtaining anterior column support at these levels using newer techniques (TLIF, PLIF, DLIF) is an alternative option.

The patient is then positioned supine on a radiolucent Jackson frame (Orthopaedic Systems, Union City, California). We would then perform an open midline posterior approach to expose all levels that will be included in the fusion. It is important to preserve the supraspinous ligament, intraspinous ligament, and the ligamentum flavum at the proximal adjacent level, in order to minimize the risk of developing degenerative changes and subsequent junctional kyphosis. In this case there is no neurologic deficit and therefore no requirement for operative decompression. We also do not anticipate a need for an osteotomy to achieve global balance. Given her moderate sagittal imbalance and flexibility, standard techniques should be sufficient to achieve these goals. Following exposure, a segmentally instrumented posterior spinal fusion extending from the upper thoracic spine to the pelvis would be performed using pedicle and iliac screws. In this patient, we would use sacroiliac fixation given her likely poor bone quality and the length of the fusion that she will require. The fusion to the pelvis would be performed with bilateral sacral pedicle screws augmented with iliac screws. In our hands these procedures can be performed in a single stage. Cross-links could then be used to supplement the fixation. Iliac crest would be harvested from the patient and combined with local bone and cancellous allograft to promote fusion. The role of postoperative bracing is unclear as its use was not specified in the literature cited in our table and evidence to support this is of poor quality.[79]

Grading the Evidence for this Plan

The best available evidence to support the technical aspects of our treatment selection would be considered low quality as it is derived from retrospective cohort or prospective case series. In accordance with the method of grading recommendations set forth by Schunemann et al.,[80] our proposed treatment would be considered a **weak recommendation**. The grading paradigm utilized is necessary because it not only considers the quality of evidence but also addresses the benefits, harms, and burdens of the proposed interventions. Furthermore, the benefits of posterior fusion outweigh the harms and burdens of such an intervention. The weak recommendation means that the majority of patients and clinicians would choose the intervention, but some would not be based on various patient and clinical factors.

PREDICTING OUTCOMES

Our main goals for the treatment of this patient are pain relief, improved function, and patient satisfaction. Very few data have been reported on the treatment outcomes of AS, particularly in an elderly population. There is some evidence that successful fusion for AS has been shown to reliably result in pain improvement, good functional outcome, and high patient satisfaction.[81,82] However, this patient's age makes her outcome somewhat less predictable. In addition, this patient has several patient specific factors that have been shown to have a negative impact on perioperative outcomes in AS patients, including a history of depression,[17] ischemic heart disease,[18,19] and certain arrhythmias,[18,19] and the patient should be counseled regarding this preoperatively. Despite this, there are several radiographic parameters in this patient that if successfully addressed would favor a successful self-assessed outcome. Pain scores following treatment have been shown to be strongly correlated with the loss of lumbar lordosis and lumbar vertebral obliquity, while functional scores are strongly correlated with global imbalance, apical level of a scoliotic deformity, and intervertebral subluxation.[13,15,26] Hu et al.[80] retrospectively evaluated the outcomes of patients over 40 years of age who underwent major spinal reconstructive surgery and found over 81% patient satisfaction rates with significant improvements in many areas of functional status. Dickson et al.[37] compared the self-reported pain and functional outcomes of 81 adult patients undergoing operative treatment for idiopathic scoliosis with that of 30 patients who declined operative management. After an average of 5-year follow-up, they found that the surgically treated patients reported a significantly greater decrease in pain and fatigue and a greater increase in self-image and function when compared to the nonsurgically treated group. Albert et al.[23] also evaluated the outcomes of a prospective series of adult deformity patients using self-reported assessments of health and functional status and showed statistically significant improvements in functional outcome, pain, and body image in adults following spinal reconstructive surgery. Recently, Kluba et al.[83] compared the outcomes of surgical and conservative treatment for degenerative lumbar scoliosis in 55 patients older than 42 years. They observed that the surgical treatment of decompensated degenerative lumbar scoliosis improved function and quality of life as determined by self-assessment outcome measures. Furthermore, they found a significant improvement in walking distance and a diminished use of analgesics in the operatively treated group.

These results are in keeping with our experience. We studied a series of elderly AS patients to look at radiographic measurements and self-reported outcome measures of patients older than 65 years of age undergoing either operative or nonoperative treatment for scoliosis with a minimum 2-year follow-up. Overall, the results showed that the patients treated operatively reported significantly less pain, had a better health-related quality of life, self-image, and mental health, and were more satisfied with their treatment than patients treated nonoperatively. After a 2-year follow-up, the operative group had significant improvements in their outcome scores (ODI, SF-12, and SRS 22), while in the nonoperative group, no significant differences in outcome scores were noted. Compared with nonoperative treatment at a 2-year follow-up, operative treatment in this series resulted in significantly less pain (pain $p = 0.001$), better health-related quality of life, self-image, mental health, and greater satisfaction as measured with SRS 22 as well as EQ5D instruments. Based on the available data regarding validated patient-derived outcome measures, we anticipate that our patient's overall outcome will be improved following surgical management than she would if she underwent conservative management.

Patient preference is an important component of evidence-based medicine. Preoperative counseling requires a frank discussion of the treatment options and their inherent risks, benefits, potential outcomes, and associated burdens. The information conveyed must contain the best available evidence and expert opinion. Importantly, the delivery must consider the fact that operative intervention for AS carries significant risk. Less invasive surgical techniques and attempts and determining optimal fusion levels are important considerations that require further investigation.

SUMMARY

We are presented with a 68-year-old woman who has progressive symptoms related to her thoracolumbar AS. The most appropriate treatment for this patient's spinal deformity, considering the severity of the deformity as well as the lack of response to conservative treatment, would consist of operative correction and posterior fusion extending from the upper thoracic spine to the pelvis. She will likely experience an improvement in several radiographic parameters with some degree of persistent physical impairment. Her functional outcome will likely be improved with surgical intervention although her medical comorbidities may compromise her result.

REFERENCES

1. Schwab FJ, Smith V, Biserni M, et al. Adult scoliosis: a quantitative radiographic and clinical analysis. *Spine*. 2002;27:387–392.
2. Biot B, Pendrix D. Frequence de la scoliosi lombaire a l'age adulte. *Ann Med Phys*. 1982;25:251–254.
3. Carter OD, Haynes SG. Prevalence rates for scoliosis in US adult: results from the first National Health and Nutritional Examination Survey. *Int J Epidemiol*. 1987;16:537–544.
4. Perennou D, Marcelli C, Herisson C. Adult lumbar scoliosis: epidemiologic aspects in a low-back pain population. *Spine*. 1994;19:123–128.
5. Francis RS. Scoliosis screening of 3,000 college-aged women. The Utah Study-Phase 2. *Phys Ther*. 1988;68:1513–1526.
6. Schwab F, Dubey A, Gamez L, et al. Adult scoliosis: prevalence, SF-36, and nutritional parameters in an elderly volunteer population. *Spine*. 2005;30:1082–1085.
7. Kostuik JP, Israel J, Hall JE. Scoliosis surgery in adults. *Clin Orthop Relat Res*. 1973;93:225–234.
8. Winter RB, Lonstein JE, Denis F. Pain patterns in adult scoliosis. *Orthop Clin North Am*. 1988;20:339–345.
9. Jackson RP, Simmons EH, Strippins D. Incidence and severity of back pain in adult idiopathic scoliosis. *Spine*. 1983;8:749–756.
10. Korovessis P, Piperos G, Sidiropoulos P, et al. Adult idiopathic lumbar scoliosis: a formula for prediction of progression and review of the literature. *Spine*. 1994;19:1926–1932.
11. Kostuik JP. Recent advances in the treatment of painful adult scoliosis. *Clin Orthop*. 1980;147:238–252.
12. Kostuik JP, Bentivoglio J. The incidence of low-back pain in adult scoliosis. *Spine*. 1981;6:268–273.
13. Schwab F, Dubey A, Pagala M, et al. Adult scoliosis: a health assessment analysis by SF-36. *Spine*. 2003;28:602–606.
14. Berven S, Deviren V, Demir-Deviren S, et al. Studies in the modified scoliosis research society outcomes intrument in adults: validation, reliability, and discriminatory capacity. *Spine*. 2003;28:2164–2169.
15. Schwab F, Benchik-el Fegoun A, Gamez L, et al. Lumbar classification of scoliosis in the adult patient: preliminary approach. *Spine*. 2005;30:1670–1673.
16. Birknes JK, White AP, Albert TJ, et al. Adult degenerative scoliosis: a review. *Neurosurgery*. 2008;63:A94–A103.
17. Rosenberger PH, Jokl P, Ickovics J. Psychosocial factors and surgical outcomes: an evidence-based literature review. *J Am Acad Orthop Surg*. 2006;14:397–405.
18. Mangano DT, Layug EL, Wallace A, et al. Effect of atenolol on mortality and cardiovascular morbidity after noncardiac surgery. *N Engl J Med*. 1996;335:1713–1720.
19. Auerbach AD, Goldman L. Beta-blockers and reduction of cardiac events in noncardiac surgery: clinical applications. *JAMA*. 2002;287:1445–1447.
20. Hart RA, Prendergast MA. Spine surgery for lumbar degenerative disease elderly and osteoporotic patients. *Instr Course Lect*. 2007;56:257–272.
21. Waters JM, McClaran JC. The elderly surgical patient. In: Wilmore DW, ed. *American College of Surgeons: Care of the Surgical Patient*. Vol I. New York, NY: Scientific American, 1991.
22. Theiss SM, Boden SD, Hair G, et al. The effect of nicotine on gene expression during spine fusion. *Spine*. 2000;25:2588–2594.
23. Balderston RA, Albert TJ. Adult Scoliosis: evaluation and decision making. In: Wiesel SW, Weinstein JN, Herkowitz H, et al., eds. *The Lumbar Spine*. 2nd ed. Philadelphia, PA: WB Saunders, 1996.

24. Gupta MC. Degenerative scoliosis: options for surgical management. *Orthop Clin North Am*. 2003;34:269–279.

25. Pritchett JW, Bortel DT. Degenerative lumbar scoliosis. *Spine*. 1993;18:700–703.

26. Glassman S, Berven S, Bridwell K, et al. Correlation of radiographic parameters and clinical symptoms in adult scoliosis. *Spine*. 2005;30:682–688.

27. Jackson RP, Simmons EH, Stripinis D. Coronal and sagittal plane spinal deformities correlating with back pain and pulmonary function in adult idiopathic scoliosis. *Spine*. 1989;14:1391–1397.

28. Schwab F, Lafage V, Farcy JP, et al. Surgical rates and operative outcome analysis in thoracolumbar and lumbar major adult scoliosis. *Spine*. 2007;32:2723–2730.

29. Jackson RP, Simmons EH, Strippins D. Incidence and severity of back pain in adult idiopathic scoliosis. *Spine*. 1983;8:749–756.

30. Kim YJ, Bridwell KH, Lenke LG, et al. An analysis of sagittal spinal alignement following long adult lumbar instrumentation and fusion to L5-S1: Can we predict ideal lumbar lordosis? *Spine*. 2006;31:2342–2352.

31. Luk KD, Cheung KM, Lu DS, et al. Assessment of scoliosis correction in relation to felxibilty using the fulcrum bending correction index. *Spine*. 1998;23:2303–2307.

32. Swank S, Lonstein JE, Moe JH, et al. Surgical treatment of adult scoliosis: a review of two-hundred and twenty-two cases. *J Bone Joint Surg Am*. 1981;63:268–287.

33. White AA, Panjabi MM. *Practical Biomechanics of Scoliosis and Kyphosis*. 2nd ed. Philadelphia, PA: J.B. Lippincott Co., 1990.

34. Polly D, Sturm P. Traction versus supine side bending: Which technique best determines curve flexibility. *Spine*. 1998;23:804–808.

35. Delecrin J, Brossard D, Takahashi S, et al. Correction of stiff thoracic idiopathic adult scoliosis. Prediction from the traction radiograph. *Rev Chir Orthop Reparatrice Appar Mot*. 2007;93:783–788.

36. Bridwell KH. Selection of instrumentation and fusion levels for scoliosis: where to start and where to stop. Invited submission from the Joint Section Meeting on Disorders of the Spine and Peripheral Nerves. *J Neurosurg Spine*. 2004;1:1–8.

37. Dickson JH, Mirkovic S, Noble PC, et al. Results of operative treatment of idiopathic scoliosis in adults. *J Bone Joint Surg Am*. 1995;77:513–523.

38. Ponder RC, Dickson JH, Harrington PR, et al. Results of Harrington instrumentation and fusion in the adult idiopathic scoliosis patient. *J Bone Joint Surg Am*. 1975;57:797–801.

39. Byrd AJ, Scoles PV, Winter RB, et al. Adult idiopathic scoliosis treated by anterior and posterior spinal fusion. *J Bone Joint Surg Am*. 1987;69:843–850.

40. Nuber GW, Schafer MF. Surgical management of adult scoliosis. *CORR*. 1986;208:228–237.

41. Sponseller PD, Cohen MS, Nachemson AL, et al. Results of surgical treatment of adults with idiopathic scoliosis. *J Bone Joint Surg Am*. 1987;69:667–675.

42. Everett CR, Patel RK. A systematic literature review of nonsurgical treatment in adult scoliosis. *Spine*. 2007;32:S130–S134.

43. King HA, Moe JH, Bradford DS, et al. The selection of fusion levels in thoracic idiopathic scoliosis. *J Bone Joint Surg Am*. 1983;65:1302–1313.

44. Lenke LG, Betz RR, Harms J, et al. Adolescent idiopathic scoliosis: a new classification to determine extent of spinal arthrodesis. *J Bone Joint Surg Am*. 2001;83-A:1169–1181.

45. Mummaneni PV, Haid RW, Sasso RC. Principles of spinal deformity: Part I. Evaluation of thoracolumbar deformity and nonoperative treatment strategies. *Contemp Neurosurg*. 2002;24:1–9.

46. Wiggins GC, Shaffrey CL, Abel MF, et al. Pediatric spinal deformities. *Neurosurg Focus*. 2003;14:e3:2003.

47. Aebi M. The adult scoliosis. *Eur Spine J*. 2005;14:925–948.

48. Lowe T, Berven SH, Schwab FJ, et al. The SRS classification for adult spinal deformity: Building on the King/Moe and Lenke classification systems. *Spine*. 2006;31:S119–S125.

49. Schwab F, Farcy JP, Bridwell K, et al. A clinical impact classification of scoliosis in the adult. *Spine*. 2006;31:2109–2114.

50. Baron EM, Albert TJ. Medical complications of surgical treatment of adult spinal deformity and how to avoid them. *Spine*. 2006;31:S106–S118.

51. Schwab FJ, Smith V, Farcy JP. Endoscopic thoracoplasty and anterior spinal release in scoliotic deformity. *Bull Hosp Jt Dis*. 2000;59:27–32.

52. Anand N, Baron EM, Thaiyananthan G, et al. Minimally invasive multilevel percutaneous correction and fusion for adult lumbar degenerative scoliosis: a technique and feasibility study. *J Spinal Disord Tech*. 2008;21:459–467.

53. Dick J, Boachie-Adjei O, Wilson M. One-stage versus two-stage anterior and posterior spinal reconstruction in adults: comparison of outcomes including nutritional status, complication rates, hospital costs, and other factors. *Spine*. 1992;17:S310–S316.

54. Bradford DS, Tay BK, Hu SS. Adult scoliosis: surgical indications, operative management, complications, and outcomes. *Spine*. 1999;24:2617–2629.

55. Hamzaoglu A, Ozturk C, Aydogan M, et al. Posterior only pedicle screw instrumentation with intraoperative halo-femoral traction in the surgical treatment of severe scoliosis (>100°). *Spine*. 2008;33:979–983.

56. Deviren V, Patel VV, Metz LN, et al. Anterior arthrodesis with instrumentation for thoracolumbar scoliosis: comparison of efficacy in adults and adolescents. 2008;33:1219–1223.

57. Kim YB, Lenke LG, Kim YJ, et al. Surgical treatment of adult scoliosis: is anterior apical release and fusion necessary for the lumbar curve? *Spine*. 2008;33:1123–1132.

58. Kim YK, Bridwell KH, Lenke LG, et al. Is the T9, T11, or L1 the more reliable proximal level after adult lumbar or lubosacral intrumented fusion to L5-S1? *Spine*. 2007;32:2653–2661.

59. Boachie-Adjei O, Dendrinos GK, Ogilvie JW, et al. Management of adult spinal deformity with combined anterior-posterior arthrodesis and Luque-Galveston instrumentation. *J Spinal Disord*. 1991;4:131–141.

60. Eck KR, Bridwell KH, Ungacta FF, et al. Complications and results of long adult deformity fusions down to L4, L5, and the sacrum. *Spine*. 2001;26:E182–E192.

61. Emani A, Deviren V, Berven S, et al. Outcome and complications of long fusions to the sacrum in adult spine deformity: Luque-Galveston, combined iliac and sacral screws, and sacral fixation. *Spine*. 2002;27:776–786.

62. Grubb SA, Lipscomb HJ, Suh PB. Results of surgical treatment of painful adult scoliosis. *Spine*. 1994;19:1619–1627.

63. Horton WC, Holt RT, Muldowny DS. Controversy: fusion of L5-S1 on adult scoliosis. *Spine*. 1996;21:2520–2522.

64. Kostuik JP, Musha Y. Extension to the sacrum of previous adolescent scoliosis fusions in adult life. *Clin Orthop*. 1999;364:53–60.

65. Edwards CC, Bridwell KH, Patel A, et al. Long adult deformity fusions to L5 and the sacrum a matched cohort analysis. *Spine*. 2004;29:1996–2005.

66. Kuhns CA, Bridwell KH, Lenke LG, et al. Thoracolumbar deformity arthodesis stopping at L5: Fate of the L5-S1 disc, minimum 5-year follow-up. *Spine*. 2007;32:2771–2776.

67. Lebwohl N, Cunningham BW, Dmitriev A, et al. Biomechanical compression of lumbosacral fixation techniques in a calf spine model. *Spine*. 2002;27:2312–2320.

68. Ozgur BM, Aryan HE, Pimenta L, et al. Extreme lateral interbody fusion (XLIF): A novel surgical technique for anterior lumbar interbody fusion. *Spine J*. 2006;6:435–443.

69. Shen FH, Samartzis D, Khanna AJ, et al. Minimally invasive techniques for lumbar fusions. *Orthop Clin North Am*. 2007;38:373–386; abstract vi.

70. Cook SD, Salkeld SL, Stanley T, et al. Biomechanical study of pedicle screw fixation in severely osteoporotic bone. *Spine J*. 2004;4:402–408.

71. Halvorson TL, Kelley LA, Thomas KA, et al. Effects of bone mineral density on pedicle screw fixation. *Spine*. 1994;19:2415–2420.

72. Hilibrand AS, Moore DC, Graziano GP. The role of pediculolaminar fixation in compromised pedicle bone. *Spine*. 1996;21:445–451.

73. Sarzier JS, Evans AJ, Cahill DW. Increased pedicle screw pullout strength with vertebroplasty augmentation in osteoporotic spines. *J Neurosurg*. 2002;96:309–312.

74. Rohmiller MT, Schwalm D, Glattes RC, et al. Evaluation of calcium sulfate paste for augmentation of lumbar pedicle screw pullout strength. *Spine J*. 2006;2:E277–E284.

75. Dick JC, Zdeblick TA, Bartel BD, et al. Mechanical evaluation of cross-link designs in rigid pedicle screw systems. *Spine*. 1997;22:370–375.

76. Luhmann SJ, Bridwell KH, Cheng I, et al. Use of bone morphogenic protein-2 for adult spinal deformity. *Spine*. 2005;30:S110–S117.

77. Pradham BB, Bae HW, Dawson EG, et al. Graft resorption with the use of bone morphogenetic protein: Lessons from anterior lumbar interbody fusion using femoral ring allografts and recombinant human bone morphogenetic protein-2. *Spine*. 2006;31:E277–E284.

78. McKay B, Sandhu HS. Use of recombinant human bone morphogenic protein-2 in spinal fusion applications. *Spine*. 2002;27:S66–S85.

79. Weiss HR, Dallmayer R. Brace treatment of spinal claudication in an adult with lumbar scoliosis—a case report. *Stud Health Technol Inform*. 2006;123:586–589.

80. Schunemann HJ, Jaeschke R, Cook DJ, et al. ATS Documents Development and Implementation Committee. An official ATS statement: grading the quality of evidence and strength of recommendations in ATS guidelines and recommendations in ATS guidelines and recommendations. *Am J Respir Crit Care Med*. 2006;174:605–614.

81. Ali RM, Boachie-Adjei O, Rawlins BA. Functional and radiographic outcomes after surgery for adult scoliosis using third-generation instrumnetation techniques. *Spine*. 2003;28:1163–1169.

82. Simmons ED, Kowalski JM, Simmons EH. The results of surgical treatment for adult scoliosis. *Spine*. 1993;18:718–724.

83. Kluba T, Dikmenli G, Dietz K, et al. Comparison of surgical and conservative treatment for degenerative lumbar scoliosis. *Arch Orthop Trauma Surg*. 2009;129:1–5.

Adult Scoliosis II

STEVEN D. GLASSMAN AND LEAH Y. CARREON

A 55-year-old woman has a complaint of thoracolumbar low back pain that is aggravated with activity and relieved with rest. She has no lower extremity complaints and no report of weakness, numbness, or tingling. Her pain has been present for at least 10 years, recently becoming progressively worse. She also feels that her deformity has become increasingly more pronounced. She has had a long course of nonoperative treatment that has included pain medication and therapy. She is now requiring narcotic agents for pain control. She is otherwise healthy and has no other comorbidities.

Examination demonstrates that she has normal gait. She has about a 1-cm coronal imbalance to the left. Her sagittal balance appears to be normal upon inspection. She has a thoracolumbar flank hump, with smaller rib and lumbar humps. She has minimal tenderness to palpation of the thoracolumbar junction but has moderate tenderness to palpation of the lower lumbar spine. She is neurologically intact.

Plain radiographic and magnetic resonance images are shown in Figure 31.1A–D, 31.2 and 31.3A–C.

INTERPRETATION OF CLINICAL PRESENTATION

This case example is a fairly common presentation of a 55-year-old female with adult scoliosis who reports progressive symptoms and change in body shape over a 5- to 10-year period.[1-6] Prior x-rays are not available; however, her report of increasing deformity suggests some form of curve progression or increased rotational deformity. This may occur as a result of

lumbar degeneration leading to loss of long-standing curve stability,[7-9] or occur simply due to a decrease in mechanical support secondary to deterioration in core muscle strength. While degeneration within or subadjacent to the inferior aspect of a thoracolumbar curve may be associated with stenosis,[10] her lack of neurogenic symptoms makes this etiology unlikely.

Although severe back pain alone may be sufficient to require surgical treatment,[3,8,11,12] patients with thoracolumbar deformity often tolerate moderate or intermittent back pain symptoms.[13] For that reason, it is important to verify that the nonsurgical treatment has been appropriate and sufficient. In particular, aquatic therapy and core strengthening may play an important role. Curve progression may also occur as a result of osteoporotic changes, and bone quality should be assessed in relation to both diagnostic evaluation and as a parameter in treatment planning.[14,15]

Beyond the complaint of severe back pain, patients often elect surgery based on the presence of radiculopathy (not noted in this patient) and based upon change in body shape. Despite the fact that cosmetic issues are not as frequently discussed with regard to adult versus pediatric deformity, patient-based evaluations clearly emphasize the importance of this treatment driver.[16,17]

Review of the plain radiographs reveals a 64-degree left thoracolumbar curve from T6 to L2. The curve is moderately flexible, bending out to 40 degrees on lateral side bending films. There is significant lumbar degeneration and a rigid 35-degree compensatory deformity from L2 to L5, but no spondylolisthesis. MRI demonstrates severe degeneration at L3-4 and L4-5 but age-appropriate disc dehydration at L5-S1. No significant disc herniation or stenosis is detected. This is consistent with the absence of neurogenic complaints. If the patient reported either radiculopathy or neurogenic claudication, then further evaluation by CT myelography would be appropriate to look for weight-bearing accentuated foraminal or central stenosis.

Figure 31.1 ▪

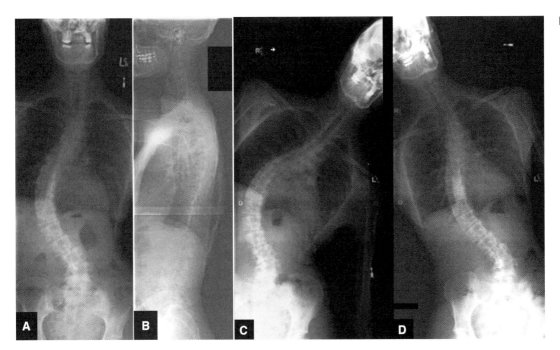

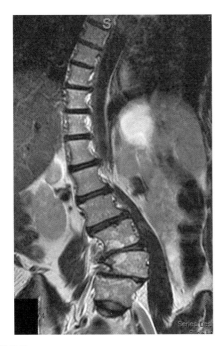

Figure 31.2 ▪

Another critical aspect of the radiographic evaluation is the relatively normal sagittal and coronal balance noted on standing AP and lateral 36 in radiographs. While coronal balance is only moderately associated with clinical symptoms, the positive sagittal balance is the radiographic parameter most highly correlated with adverse health status measures.[18–20] The fact that this patient has a reasonably well-maintained sagittal balance will have a significant impact upon clinical evaluation and any subsequent surgical treatment.

DECLARATION OF SPECIFIC DIAGNOSIS

64-degree adult thoracolumbar scoliosis without neurogenic symptoms or loss of global sagittal balance.

BRAIN STORMING: WHAT ARE THE TREATMENT GOALS AND SURGICAL OPTIONS?

The treatment goals are

1. Control the incapacitating back pain that has been unresponsive to conservative treatment
2. Restore stability of this long-standing adult scoliotic curve, by modification of the therapy regimen if possible or by surgical stabilization if necessary
3. Maintain normal sagittal and coronal balance
4. Preserve lumbar motion segments to as great a degree as possible
5. Improve clinical function and decrease disability as measured by standardized health status measures including SRS-22, ODI, and SF-36

The treatment options are

1. Aquatic therapy and core strengthening if not previously utilized
2. Surgical correction via posterior-only approach with preservation of the L5-S1 level

Figure 31.3 ■

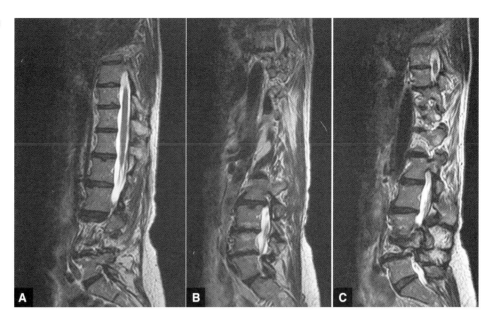

3. Surgical correction of the deformity via an anterior and posterior approach with preservation of the L5-S1 segment

4. Correction of the deformity and extension of the fusion to the pelvis with interbody support via an anterior or posterior approach at L4-5 and L5-S1

EVALUATION OF THE LITERATURE

A computer-aided search that included MEDLINE, EMBASE, HealthSTAR, Cumulative Index to Nursing & Allied Health Literature, Cochrane Database of Systematic Reviews, ACP Journal Club, Database of Abstracts of Reviews of Effects, and Cochrane Central Register of Controlled Trials from the beginning of the databases up to September 2008 was done using the search strategy outlined in Table 31.1. Two hundred sixteen articles were identified. No randomized clinical trials on adult scoliosis were identified. An evidentiary table of all pertinent articles is presented in Table 31.2.

Scoliosis that presents in adulthood may be idiopathic, degenerative, or idiopathic with superimposed degenerative changes in the spine. The reported incidence of scoliosis in adults range from 2% to 68%[3,8,21–25]; this incidence increases with age.[6,8,15,22] Robin and Perennou both reported development of scoliosis in previously straight spines, termed "de novo" scoliosis[15] in an estimated 10% of adults with scoliosis.[6,24] These de novo curves were usually small and accompanied by degenerative changes associated with the aging spine. A study by Schwab reported a 68% incidence of scoliosis (defined as a Cobb angle >10 degrees) in

a group of volunteers aged 60 or older; the majority were asymptomatic.[25]

In the aging spine, disc degeneration with disc collapse and facet joint arthrosis leads to loss of structural integrity of the motion segment. This, in turn, may produce increasing deformity, back pain, and radiculopathy. This is especially pronounced in patients with asymmetric disc collapse, leading to rotatory subluxation and/or lateral listhesis.[7,9]

Symptoms

Our patient presents with progressive low back pain for the past 10 years along with increasing deformity. Low back pain is common among scoliotic adults.[2,5,26] The back pain associated with adult scoliosis is characterized as progressive, increasing in a relatively insidious manner,[11,12,24,27,28] as in this patient. Other symptoms more common in patients with adult scoliosis compared to other degenerative lumbar conditions is the presence of inguinal and anterior thigh pain.[11]

Imaging Studies

Standing 36 in posteroanterior and lateral radiographs are necessary to assess segmental, regional, and global alignment and to determine the degree of spinal curvature, the patient's sagittal balance, the presence of rotatory subluxation or lateral listhesis, the presence of spondylolisthesis, and the status of the L5-S1 disc.

Measurement of the Cobb angle and documentation of end vertebra are necessary to document progression, decompensation, or adding on. Several studies have shown a correlation between patients' symptoms and the severity of the curvature,[8,11,29–32] although other studies have not found this to be true.[17,33] Patients with thoracolumbar and lumbar

TABLE 31.1	Search Strategy.	
1	controlled trial {Including Limited Related Terms}	5196
2	clinical trial {Including Limited Related Terms}	3965
3	1 or 2	9092
4	adult.ti,ab.	419178
5	scoliosis.ti,ab.	11738
6	4 and 3 and 5	0
7	4 and 5	512
8	adolescent.ti,ab.	62137
9	pediatric.ti,ab.	128765
10	congenital.ti,ab.	148731
11	juvenile.ti,ab.	42871
12	neuromuscular.ti,ab.	36470
13	blood loss.ti,ab.	24930
14	analgesia.ti,ab.	47698
15	adolescents.ti,ab.	93680
16	screen$.ti,ab.	349408
17	brac$.ti,ab.	56529
18	neurofibromatosis.ti,ab.	8691
19	infantile.ti,ab.	21412
20	syndrome.ti,ab.	544364
21	dystrophy.ti,ab.	28147
22	familial.ti,ab.	72275
23	child$.ti,ab.	891874
24	11 or 21 or 17 or 22 or 18 or 23 or 16 or 13 or 9 or 12 or 14 or 15 or 20 or 8 or 10 or 19	2178201
25	7 not 24	252
26	limit 25 to English language	231
27	limit 26 to English	231
28	limit 27 to humans	215
29	remove duplicates from 28	166

curves have less favorable clinical outcome scores than thoracic curves. The presence of vertebral rotation[11,19] and rotary subluxation,[11,33] which may be indicative of instability, has been shown to correlate with the severity of the back pain. Our patient has both rotation in the lumbar curve as well as lateral listhesis of L2 over L3. Although scoliosis is generally perceived as a deformity in the coronal plane, a positive sagittal balance[18] and the loss of lumbar lordosis[19] have been found to correlate with the patient's function and disability. In a study by Pritchett of patients with degenerative scoliosis, 55% had additional degenerative spondylolisthesis.[34]

Treatment

Treatment algorithms for patients with adult scoliosis are poorly defined and complex since patients can present with any number of symptoms, signs, and imaging findings. Back pain, postural changes, radiculopathy, neurogenic claudication, and curve progression are all potential factors that have to be addressed during treatment.

Nonoperative Treatment

Surgeons are generally conservative in the treatment of adult deformity because of less predictable outcomes and higher complication rates associated with surgery. However, there are very few well-designed studies evaluating nonoperative treatment options for adult scoliosis.[35] Thus, there is no consensus on the most efficacious conservative clinical treatment for adult scoliosis.[36–38] Conservative management for these patients consists of a regimen similar to that prescribed for patients with common mechanical back pain.[13,35,37] In a study by Glassman comparing two matched cohorts who had surgical and nonsurgical treatments, patients with significant preoperative risk factors and poorer health tended to be treated nonsurgically. Patients with high body mass index also tended to be treated nonsurgically, which may be due to a perceived increased risk with surgery as well as masking of the deformity in heavier patients.

Operative Treatment

The goal of surgery in adult scoliosis is not necessarily curve correction but achieving a stable, well-balanced, and pain-free spine.[10] This must be balanced against the extent of surgery necessary to achieve these goals.[39,40] Most studies report a 60% to 95% reduction in the severity of pain and a 30% to 50% correction of deformity. The presence of osteopenia, disc degeneration, spinal stiffness, rotational deformity, and lateral listhesis, as well as sagittal and coronal imbalance must be considered.[1,41–43] The surgical risks and complications are also substantial.[44–47]

The pseudoarthosis rate in primary fusions for adult scoliosis using current segmental fixation ranges

TABLE 31.2	Evidentiary Table.		
Paper Author (Year)	**Study Design, Description**	**Summary of Results**	**Quality of Evidence**
Everett et al. (2007)	Systematic review of surgical vs. nonsurgical treatment	Nonsurgical treatments may be helpful for patients with adult scoliosis, but evidence is lacking.	Moderate
Glassman et al. (2007)	Case-control matched by propensity scoring of patients with adult scoliosis treated surgically and nonsurgically	Nonsurgical patients had greater preoperative medical risk factors. Surgical patients had larger curves, more frequent leg pain, a higher level of daily back pain, and more frequent moderate-to-severe back pain.	Moderate
Pateder et al. (2006)	Cohort comparing patients undergoing posterior-only vs. anterior-posterior surgery	In patients with curves between 40 and 70 degrees, no significant differences in curve correction, sagittal and coronal balance correction, and major complication rates between posterior-only and combined anterior-posterior groups.	Low
Bridwell et al. (2003)	Review	Authors delineate definite indications for fusion to the sacrum and acknowledge that circumstances in which fusion to L5 or the sacrum is not clear cut.	Very low
Edwards et al. (2003)	Cohort of patients fused to L5 followed up to a minimum of 2 y	Fusion to L5 produces a good functional result in a high percentage of patients. Degeneration of the L5-S1 disc is associated with loss of sagittal balance and an increased incidence of reoperation. Risk factors for degeneration of the L5-S1 disc include preoperative sagittal imbalance and the presence of preoperative disc degeneration.	Low

from 0% to 27%.[48–50] The risk of pseudoarthosis is greater in patients with sagittal plane imbalance[49,51,52] and is most common at the lumbosacral of thoracolumbar junction. After a repair of the pseudoarthrosis 90% go on to eventual fusion.[48] Other complications include residual pain, neurologic deficit, infection, and implant failure.[3]

Lumbosacral Fusion

Surgeons treating adult spinal deformity have to decide whether to stop a long fusion at L5 or the sacrum.[3,42,53–55] Fusion to the L5 is a less complex procedure, preserves motion at the lumbosacral junction with less risk for pseudarthrosis. In a study by Edwards,[54] 61% of patients fused to L5 developed advanced L5-S1 disc degeneration. Risk factors for the development of L5-S1 disc degeneration were preoperative positive sagittal balance, younger age, and the presence of even mild radiographic degeneration before surgery. These patients had a significant loss of sagittal alignment and an increased need for revision surgery.[54]

Fusion of the lumbosacral junction increases risk of pseudoarthrosis and the need for an anterior fusion and adds to the length, complexity, and morbidity to the surgery.[56] However, fusion of the lumbosacral junction is indicated when there is significant L5-S1 disc degeneration, L5 spondylolysis or spondylolisthesis, significant lumbosacral obliquity, previous L5-S1 decompression, or current lumbosacral stenosis requiring decompression.[56–58] In the absence of these indications, for patients with a healthy disc at L5-S1, there is no consensus on the appropriate distal fusion level. In comparing patients fused to L5 or S1, patients fused to the sacrum had better correction of sagittal balance, required more surgical procedures, and had a greater incidence of complications, including nonunion. On the other hand, patients fused to L5 developed disc degeneration at L5-S1 with a trend toward a forward shift in sagittal balance. The SRS-24 outcome scores were similar for both patients. The ultimate influence of these factors on long-term outcomes remains to be seen.

Nonsurgical Versus Surgical Treatment

No definite treatment algorithms exist for determining the proper treatment regimen for patients with adult scoliosis. However, since the patient has had a long course of nonoperative treatment and continues to worsen, surgery becomes a more viable option. Prior to opting for surgery, verification that nonsurgical treatment has been appropriate and sufficient should be undertaken. Delaying surgery, by seeking out other nonsurgical options such as aqua therapy and core strengthening exercises, will give the patient and her medical doctors time to optimize her medical status.

Posterior-Only or Anteroposterior Fusion

The patient has a relatively flexible curve as well as a good sagittal and coronal balance. A posterior-only approach with multiple level Smith-Petersen osteotomies may be adequate.

Distal Extent of the Fusion

In the absence of significant L5-S1 disc degeneration, L5 spondylolysis or spondylolisthesis, significant lumbosacral obliquity, previous L5-S1 decompression, or current lumbosacral stenosis and the presence of a good sagittal balance in this patient, fusion to the sacrum will not be necessary. L3 is the stable vertebra; however, there is significant tilt to L3, and degeneration at the L3-4 and L4-5 motion segments. Fusion has to be carried down to L5.

Outcomes

Since the patient has good sagittal balance and has no risk for pseudoarthrosis, the patient is expected to have substantial improvement in clinical outcomes.[16–19] Long-term outcome depends on the status of the L5-S1 motion segment.[52,56,58]

DEFINITIVE TREATMENT PLAN

Assuming that the patient has, in fact, received an adequate and appropriate trial of therapy, this 64-degree adult thoracolumbar scoliosis would be appropriately treated by surgical correction and stabilization.[1,16,19,39–41] Although findings of neural compression or positive sagittal balance may represent a more definitive target for surgical treatment in adult scoliosis patients,[3,18,29] studies demonstrate a marked improvement in back pain with curve correction and stabilization in severely symptomatic patients.[3,16,39,43] Recent studies also demonstrate a greater improvement in standardized health status measures including SRS-22, ODI, and SF-12 with surgical treatment as compared to continued nonoperative treatment.[16,20,59] Primary surgical goals for this patient are stabilization and safe correction of the deformity with maintenance of acceptable coronal and sagittal balance.

Based on the relative flexibility of the primary curve as well as the acceptable baseline sagittal and coronal balance, a posterior-only approach will most likely afford adequate curve correction in this case.[60] Curve correction via a posterior-only approach is dependent upon adequate bony and soft tissue release, which in this case will probably include multiple level Smith-Petersen osteotomies and transforaminal interbody fusions at L3-4 and L4-5. With a greater magnitude of deformity and in particular with greater sagittal imbalance, more extensive osteotomies such as pedicle subtraction osteotomy or vertebral column resection may be necessary.[61] Although probably not relevant to this particular deformity, it is critical to remember that the success of a posterior-only procedure is contingent upon a release that is equivalent to what would be achieved if an anterior approach were utilized.

The decision regarding distal fusion level depends firstly upon the extent of degeneration in the distal lumbar segments.[56,58] This patient has a reasonable well-maintained L5-S1 motion segment, providing the option to avoid fusion to the pelvis.[53,54,56,58] However, this patient has neither substantial degeneration nor neurogenic complaints. Another important consideration is the magnitude of correction and in particular the need to correct sagittal imbalance. When pedicle subtraction osteotomies are performed or significant sagittal balance correction is undertaken, then extension to the pelvis with iliac fixation becomes critical to maintaining that correction.[3,42,53–55] In this case, the relatively acceptable sagittal balance obviates the need for extension to the pelvis on that basis. The role of interbody fusion would be either to obtain adequate release for correction or to assure bony healing. In this instance, without the need to protect a fusion carried to the pelvis, interbody fusion would only be necessary if the patient had other substantial risk factors for nonunion such as cigarette smoking.

With regard to specific surgical planning, the primary goals are to obtain adequate correction, to maintain coronal and sagittal balance, and to protect neurologic function. While the trend is to utilize an all-pedicle screw construct, there is limited evidence that the added correction obtained versus a hook construct translates into improved clinical outcome. There is some evidence that the use of a pedicle screw construct results in a lower incidence of pseudoarthrosis.[48,49,62] Given this, our preferred surgical technique is to obtain segmental fixation with pedicle screws through the lumbar spine and then to proceed with more proximal pedicle screw fixation to the extent that well-fixed screws can be obtained without risk to neural or vascular structures. In the event that adequate pedicle screw fixation is difficult to obtain, I see limited disadvantage to the use of proximal hook fixation in a hybrid construct. The exception to this would be in the patient with proximal kyphosis where the relative advantage of pedicle screw fixation might justify a more aggressive surgical approach.[62,63]

Selection of fusion levels is critical. While most of the discussion usually revolves around selection of the distal fusion level, proximal fusion level may be equally as important.[39–41] In this case, the appropriate distal fusion level is L5, which falls within a stable zone and saves the L5-S1 motion segment. The use of transforaminal interbody lumbar fusion (TLIF) at L3-4 and L4-5 will improve lumbar lordosis and the likelihood of a successful fusion.[49,60] At times, a compromise is necessary such that a distal fusion level slightly outside the stable zone is chosen in order to leave additional lumbar motion segments. In this instance, the patient's reasonable coronal and sagittal balance obviates that decision-making conflict. The appropriate proximal fusion level is T3. This decision is made primarily based upon sagittal rather than coronal plane constraints. It is important to extend the fusion to the proximal aspect of the thoracic kyphosis if at all possible. Progressive kyphosis at the top of the instrumentation construct is a frequent mode of failure in these adult scoliosis patients, particularly in the setting of associated osteoporosis.[64]

The extent of curve correction, while important, should be balanced with the increased risks associated with forced correction. The use of osteotomies increases the magnitude of the surgical procedure but also improves the safety of correction maneuvers. In this instance, multiple Smith-Petersen osteotomies should be sufficient because of the moderate flexibility and absence of significant sagittal plane imbalance.[52,61] It is critical to remember that more aggressive releases and progressive osteotomies are a much safer and more effective reduction techniques as compared to increased forced application through the instrumentation construct. In this case, much of the correction will be achieved following Smith-Petersen osteotomies, with subsequent cantilever maneuvers and in situ bending affording additional reduction. In considering the extent to which curve reduction is pursued, it is important to remember the poor correlation between curve correction and postoperative health status measures.[17,19,20,60]

Fixation techniques, including screw only, hook only, and hybrid constructs, have been utilized with limited evidence that the specific construct alters ultimate outcome.[65,66] As opposed to adolescent spine deformity, the instrumentation construct for adult scoliosis is relevant both in deformity correction and as an adjunct to fusion. The initial surgical strategy would be to obtain pedicle screw fixation in the lumbar segments and to extend the screw fixation proximally to the extent that screw placement was achieved safely and easily. If pedicle anatomy or curve rotation made upper thoracic screw fixation difficult, conversion to hook fixation would be a completely reasonable option. Also, screw fixation at every level is not necessary. It is, however, important to have adequate fixation particularly at the proximal and distal anchors.

With regard to bone grafting options, adult scoliosis cases represent a very substantial challenge. There is preliminary evidence that bone morphogenetic protein may be a useful adjunct in these cases, but the amount of BMP necessary has not been well delineated and the use of large quantities of BMP may be cost prohibitive.[67] A reasonable consideration at this juncture is the use of multimodality grafting including local bone, iliac crest, bone bank bone, bone morphogenetic protein, and demineralized bone matrix in some combination. A reasonable strategy is to use the highest quality graft material at the distal segments and the thoracolumbar junction that seem to be at greatest risk for nonunion.

PREDICTING OUTCOMES

Predicting outcomes for adult scoliosis patients is difficult because of the complexity of the problem and the array of complaints that bring patients to surgical treatment.[4,16,19,20,38–40] Recent studies indicate reasonable overall patient-based outcomes for patients undergoing adult deformity correction; however, assessment and management of patient expectations are critical. In this patient, in particular, the presence of reasonable coronal and sagittal balance as well as moderate deformity as a baseline means that dramatic changes in alignment are unlikely to be appreciated postoperatively. The patient does have substantial and unremitting back pain and an expectation for significant improvement in that back pain is realistic. An expectation for complete resolution of the patient's back pain is unrealistic. Beyond the treatment of her back pain, surgery is likely to prevent further progression of her deformity. While this seems to be one of the patient's stated concerns preoperatively, avoidance of future problems is something the patient seems less able or willing to appreciate postoperatively.

An important concern is the fate of the L5-S1 disc. Subsequent deterioration and need for extension to the pelvis are legitimate concerns that need to be discussed preoperatively. This risk is balanced against the benefit of a smaller operation and better motion in the short-term.[3,42,53–55]

SUMMARY

In summary, our patient is a 55-year-old with progressive adult deformity and a primary complaint of back pain. She has failed conservative treatment but has no evidence for neurologic compromise or significant global balance deficits. Her distal lumbar motion segments show only age-appropriate degenerative changes.

This case presents some of the easiest and some of the most complicated elements of adult deformity surgery decision making. From a technical standpoint, this curve is not difficult to treat because it is relatively flexible and does not require surgical stabilization extending to the pelvis. Further, the patient's coronal and sagittal balance is good avoiding the need for extensive osteotomies. On the other hand, this patient has a primary complaint of back pain and thus runs the risk that her moderate improvement in back pain postoperatively may not satisfy her preoperative expectations. Only extensive counseling and a clear understanding between the patient and the physician can guide appropriate decision making in this regard.

REFERENCES

1. Aebi M. The adult scoliosis. *Eur Spine J*. 2005;14(10): 925–948. [Epub 2005 Nov 18.]
2. Fowles JV, Drummond DS, L'Ecuyer S, et al. Untreated scoliosis in adult life. *Clin Orthop*. 1978;134:212–217.
3. Grubb SA, Lipscomb HJ, Coonrad RW. Degenerative adult onset scoliosis. *Spine*. 1988;13:241–245.
4. Lonstein JE. Scoliosis: surgical versus nonsurgical treatment. *Clin Orthop*. 2006;443:248–259.
5. Nachemson A. A long term follow-up study of non-treated scoliosis. *Acta Orthop Scand*. 1968;39:466–476.
6. Pérennou D, Marcelli C, Hérisson C, et al. Adult lumbar scoliosis. Epidemiologic aspects in a low-back pain population. *Spine (Phila Pa 1976)*. 1994;19:123–128.
7. Kobayashi T, Atsuta Y, Takemitsu M, et al. A prospective study of de novo scoliosis in a community based cohort. *Spine*. 2006;31:178–182.
8. Kostuik JP, Bentivoglio J. The incidence of low back pain in adult scoliosis. *Spine*. 1981;6:268–273.
9. Murata Y, Takahashi K, Hanaoka E, et al. Changes in scoliotic curvature and lordotic angle during the early phase of degenerative lumbar scoliosis. *Spine*. 2002;27: 2268–2273.
10. Shapiro GS, Taira G, Boachie-Adjei O. Results of surgical treatment of adult idiopathic scoliosis with low back pain and spinal stenosis: a study of long-term clinical radiographic outcomes. *Spine*. 2003;28(4):358–363.
11. Gremeaux V, Casillas JM, Fabbro-Peray P, et al. Analysis of low back pain in adults with scoliosis. *Spine*. 2008;33(4):402–405.
12. Jackson RP, Simmons EH, Stripinis D. Incidence and severity of back pain in adult idiopathic scoliosis. *Spine*. 1983;8:749–755.
13. van Dam BE. Nonoperative treatment of adult scoliosis. *Orthop Clin North Am*. 1988;19:347.
14. Healey JH, Lane JM. Structural scoliosis in osteoporotic women. *Clin Orthop Relat Res*. 1985;195:216–223.
15. Vanderpool DW, James JI. Scoliosis in the elderly. *J Bone Joint Surg Am*. 1969;51:446–455.
16. Glassman SD, Schwab F, Bridwell KH, et al. The selection of operative versus nonoperative treatment in patients with adult scoliosis. *Spine*. 2007;32(1):93–97.

17. Glassman SD, Berven S, Bridwell K, et al. Correlation of radiographic parameters and clinical symptoms in adult scoliosis. *Spine*. 2005;30(6):682–688.
18. Glassman SD, Bridwell K, Dimar JR, et al. The impact of positive sagittal balance in adult spinal deformity. *Spine*. 2005;30:2024–2029.
19. Schwab F, el el-Fegoun AB, Gamez L, et al. A lumbar classification of scoliosis in the adult patient: preliminary approach. *Spine*. 2005;30:1670–1673.
20. Schwab FJ, Smith VA, Biserni M, et al. Adult scoliosis: a quantitative radiographic and clinical analysis. *Spine*. 2002;27(4):387–392.
21. Biot B, Pendrix D. Frequence de la scoliose lombaire an l'age adult. *Ann Med Phys*. 1982;25:251–254.
22. Carter OD, Haynes SG. Prevalence rates for scoliosis in US adults: results from the first National Health and Nutrition Examination Survey. *Int J Epidemiol*. 1987;16:537–544.
23. Francis RS. Scoliosis screening of 3,000 college-aged women. The Utah Study–phase 2. *Phys Ther*. 1988;68: 1513–1516.
24. Robin GC, Span Y, Steinberg R, et al. Scoliosis in the elderly: a follow-up study. *Spine*. 1982;7:355–359.
25. Schwab F, Dubey A, Gamez L, et al. Adult scoliosis: Prevalence, SF-36, and nutritional parameters in an elderly volunteer population. *Spine*. 2005;30(9):1082–1085.
26. Nilsonne U, Lundgren KD. Long-term prognosis in idiopathic scoliosis. *Acta Orthop Scand*. 1968;39:456–465.
27. Ascani E, Bartolozzi P, Logroscino CA, et al. Natural history of untreated idiopathic scoliosis after skeletal maturity. *Spine*. 1986;11:784–789.
28. Trammel TR, Schroeder RD, Reed DB. Rotatory olisthesis in idiopathic scoliosis. *Spine*. 1988;13:1378–1382.
29. Jackson RP, Simmons EH, Stripinis D. Coronal and sagittal plane spinal deformities correlating with back pain and pulmonary function in adult idiopathic scoliosis. *Spine*. 1989;14(12):1391–1397.
30. Weinstein SL, Dolan LA, Spratt KF, et al. Health and function of patients with untreated scoliosis: a 50 year natural history study. *JAMA*. 2003;289:559–567.
31. Weinstein SL, Ponseti IV. Curve progression in idiopathic scoliosis. *J Bone Joint Surg*. 1983;65:447–455.
32. Weinstein SL. The natural history of scoliosis in the skeletally mature patient. In: Dickson JH, ed. *Spinal Deformities*. Vol 1. Philadelphia, PA: Hanley and Belfus, 1987:195–212.
33. Schwab F, Farcy JP, Bridwell K, et al. A clinical impact classification of scoliosis in the adult. *Spine*. 2006;31: 2109–2114.
34. Pritchett JW, Bortel DT. Degenerative symptomatic lumbar scoliosis. *Spine*. 1993;18:700–703.
35. Everett CR, Patel RK. A systematic literature review of nonsurgical treatment in adult scoliosis. *Spine*. 2007;32(19 suppl 1):S130–S134.
36. Fast A. Degenerative adult scoliosis. *Phys Med Rehabil*. 1999;13:525–530.
37. Ogilvie JW. Adult scoliosis: evaluation and nonsurgical treatment. *Instr Course Lect*. 1994;44:251–255.
38. Winter RB. Adult scoliosis. *Instr Course Lect*. 1983;32: 170–191.
39. Kostuik JP. Decision making in adult scoliosis. *Spine*. 1979;4:521–525.

40. Bradford DS, Tay BK, Hu SS. Adult scoliosis: surgical indications, operative management, complications, and outcomes. *Spine.* 1999;24:2617–2629.

41. Kostuik JP, Israel J, Hall JE. Scoliosis surgery in adults. *Clin Orthop Rel Res.* 1973;93:225–234.

42. Ponder RC, Dickson JH, Harrington PR, et al. Results of Harrington instrumentation and fusion in the adult idiopathic scoliosis patient. *J Bone Joint Surg Am.* 1975;57: 797–801.

43. Swank S, Lonstein JE, Moe JH, et al. Surgical treatment of adult scoliosis: a review of two hundred and twenty-two cases. *J Bone Joint Surg Am.* 1981;63:268–287.

44. Winter R. Neurologic safety in spinal deformity surgery. *Spine.* 1997;22:1527–1533.

45. Bridwell K, Lenke L, Baldus C. Major intraoperative neurologic defects in pediatric and adult spinal deformity patients: incidence and etiology at one institution. Presented to the Scoliosis Research Society, Ottawa, Ontario, Canada, 1996.

46. Letts R, Hollenberg C. Delayed paresis following spinal fusion with Harrington instrumentation. *Clin Orthop.* 1977;125:45–48.

47. MacEwen G, Bunnell W, Sriram K. Acute neurologic complications in the treatment of scoliosis: a report of the Scoliosis Research Society. *J Bone Joint Surg Am.* 1975;57:404–408.

48. Kim YJ, Bridwell KH, Lenke LG, et al. Pseudarthrosis in long adult spinal deformity instrumentation and fusion to the sacrum: prevalence and risk factor analysis of 144 cases. *Spine.* 2006;31(20):2329–2336.

49. Kim YJ, Bridwell KH, Lenke LG, et al. Pseudarthrosis in primary fusions for adult idiopathic scoliosis: incidence, risk factors and outcome analysis. *Spine.* 2005;30: 468–474.

50. Weistroffer JK, Perra JH, Lonstein JE, et al. Complications in long fusions to the sacrum for adult scoliosis: minimum five-year analysis of fifty patients. *Spine.* 2008;33(13):1478–1483.

51. Kostuik JP, Maurais GR, Richarson WJ, et al. Combined single stage anterior and posterior osteotomy for correction of iatrogenic lumbar kyphosis. *Spine.* 1988;13: 257–266.

52. Pateder DB, Park YS, Kebaish KM, et al. Spinal fusion after revision surgery for pseudarthrosis in adult scoliosis. *Spine.* 2006;31(11):E314–E319.

53. Eck KR, Bridwell KH, Ungacta FF, et al. Complications and results of long deformity fusions down to L4, L5 and the sacrum. *Spine.* 2001;26:182.

54. Edwards CC II, Bridwell KH, Patel A, et al. Thoracolumbar deformity arthrodesis to L5 in adults: the fate of the L5-S1 disc. *Spine.* 2003;28(18):2122–2131.

55. Kostuik JP. Treatment of scoliosis in the adult thoracolumbar spine with special reference to fusion to the sacrum. *Orthop Clin North Am.* 1988;19:371–381.

56. Bridwell KH, Edwards CC II, Lenke LG. The pros and cons to saving the L5-S1 motion segment in a long scoliosis fusion construct. *Spine.* 2003;28(20):S234–S242, Review.

57. Bridwell KH, Lewis SJ, Lenke LG, et al. Pedicle subtraction osteotomy for the treatment of fixed sagittal imbalance. *J Bone Joint Surg Am.* 2003;85-A(3):454–463.

58. Bridwell KH. Where to stop the fusion distally in adult scoliosis-L4, L5, or the sacrum? In: Pritchard DJ, ed. *Instructional Course Lectures.* Vol 45. Rosemont, IL: American Academy of Orthopaedic Surgeons, 1996:101–107.

59. Albert TJ, Purtill J, Mesa J, et al. Health outcome assessment before and after adult deformity surgery. A prospective study. *Spine.* 1995;20(18):2002–2004.

60. Deviren V, Berven S, Kleinstueck F, et al. Predictors of flexibility and pain patterns in thoracolumbar and lumbar idiopathic scoliosis. *Spine.* 2002;27(21):2346–2349.

61. Berven SH, Deviren V, Smith JA, et al. Management of fixed sagittal plane deformity: outcome of combined anterior and posterior surgery. *Spine.* 2003;28(15):1710–1715; discussion 1716.

62. Marchesi DG, Aebi M. Pedicle fixation devices in the treatment of adult lumbar scoliosis. *Spine.* 1992;17(8 suppl):S304–S309.

63. Lippman CR, Spence CA, Youssef AS, et al. Correction of adult scoliosis via a posterior-only approach. *Neurosurg Focus.* 2003;14(1):e5.

64. Glattes RC, Bridwell KH, Lenke LG, et al. Proximal junctional kyphosis in adult spinal deformity following long instrumented posterior spinal fusion: incidence, outcomes, and risk factor analysis. *Spine.* 2005;30(14): 1643–1649.

65. Kuklo TR, Potter BK, Lenke LG, et al. Surgical revision rates of hooks versus hybrid versus screws versus combined anteroposterior spinal fusion for adolescent idiopathic scoliosis. *Spine.* 2007;32(20):2258–2264.

66. Lehman RA Jr, Lenke LG, Keeler KA, et al. Operative treatment of adolescent idiopathic scoliosis with posterior pedicle screw-only constructs: minimum three-year follow-up of one hundred fourteen cases. *Spine.* 2008;33(14):1598–1604.

67. Mulconrey DS, Bridwell KH, Flynn J, et al. Bone morphogenetic protein (RhBMP-2) as a substitute for iliac crest bone graft in multilevel adult spinal deformity surgery: minimum two-year evaluation of fusion. *Spine.* 2008;33(20):2153–2159.

INDEX

Note: Page numbers in italics refers to figures and page numbers with 't' refers to tables.